Comprehensive
ABSITE Review

Steven M. Fiser MD

The Comprehensive ABSITE Review

Steven M. Fiser MD
Hancock Surgical Consultants, LLC
Richmond, Virginia

This book is not intended for clinical use. Extreme care has been taken to ensure the accuracy of the information contained in this book and to devise the safest and most conservative way of practicing general surgery. However, the authors and publishers are not responsible for errors or omissions in the book itself or from any consequences from application of the information in the book and make no warranty, expressed or implied, with respect to the currency, completeness, or accuracy of the contents of the publication. Application of this information remains the professional responsibility of the practitioner. The specific circumstances surrounding any individual patient requires individual diagnosis and treatment.

Extreme care has been taken to ensure that the drug dosages herein are accurate, however illness such as renal failure and other disease states can affect dose. The reader should check the package insert for any drug being prescribed to see the current recommended indications, warnings, and precautions.

Some drugs and devices in this text have FDA clearance only for certain indications. It is the responsibility of the health care provider to ascertain the FDA status of any drug or device before use.

The American Board of Surgery Inc. does not sponsor nor endorses this book.

The author has never had access to the ABSITE exams used by the American Board of Surgery Inc. other than to take the exam. This book is meant to educate general surgery residents, not reconstruct the ABSITE.

Contents:

<u>Cell membrane</u> (plasma cell membrane)
  Cell membrane structure
    Lipid bilayer with protein channels, enzymes, and receptors
    Cholesterol increases plasma membrane fluidity
    Cells are **negative inside** compared to outside due to membrane enzyme
      Na/K ATPase
    Transports 3 Na^+ out for very 2 K^+ in (cell becomes negative inside)
    Creates a **Na^+ gradient**
    Na^+ gradient - is used to co-transport molecules needed by cells (eg
      Na^+-glucose, Na^+-protein)
    Intra-cellular fluid
      Cations: ↑ K^+ (150 mEq/L, *MC intra-cellular cation*)
                    ↓ Na^+ (12 mEq/L), <u>*extremely low Ca^{++}*</u>
      Anions: protein (impermeable) and ↑ $PO4^-$, ↓ Cl^-
    Extra-cellular fluid
      Cations: ↑ **Na^+** (140 mEq/L, *MC extra-cellular cation*)
                    ↓ K^+ (4 mEq/L)
      Anions: ↑ Cl^- (*MC extra-cellular anion*)
    Osmotic equilibrium – water moves from area of low solute concentration
      to high solute concentration to approach **osmotic equilibrium**
  Special cell membrane structures
    ABO blood group type: glycol-lipids on cell membrane serve as antigens
    HLA blood group type: glycol-proteins on cell membrane serve as antigen
    Desmosomes and **hemidesmosomes** – anchor cells
      (cell–cell and cell–extracellular matrix molecules, respectively)
    Tight junctions – occluding junctions that occur between cells
      Water impermeable barrier (eg epithelium of skin)
    Gap junctions – formed between cells to allow communication
      Composed of **2 connexon** subunits (eg myocytes in heart – signal for
        myocardial contraction is efficiently passed between cells)
    G proteins (type of GTPase) – intra-membrane protein
      Responsible for transducing a signal from a **receptor protein**
        attached to outside surface of the cell membrane (eg beta
        adrenergic receptor) to a **response enzyme** attached to the
        inside of the membrane (eg adenylate cyclase)
    Transmembrane receptor – the receptor and response enzyme form a
      single unit that spans the cell membrane (eg **receptor tyrosine
      kinase** for Insulin-like growth factor)
    Adenylate cyclase – synthesizes **cAMP,** which serves as a second
      messenger to activate various cell enzymes and processes
      depending on cell type
    Guanylate cyclase – similar to above but has second messenger **cGMP**
    Tyrosine kinases (receptor and cytoplasmic types) – phosphorylate
      proteins at tyrosine residues causing activation or deactivation
    Protein hormones that bind cell surface receptor → effect is rapid (eg
      epinephrine binding beta-1 adrenergic receptors in heart)

<u>Nucleus</u>
  Nucleus – bilayer lipid membrane
    Outer membrane continuous w/ rough endoplasmic reticulum
  Nucleolus – found inside nucleus, has <u>no</u> membrane, **ribosomes** made here
  Transcription - DNA strand serves as a template for **RNA polymerase**, which
    synthesizes **messenger RNA** (mRNA) strands
  Transcription factors
    Bind <u>DNA</u> and induce transcription of genes
    Steroid hormones – binds receptor in **cytoplasm**, then enters nucleus
      and acts as transcription factor (**delayed effect**, takes 1-2 hours)
    Thyroid hormone – binds receptor in **nucleus**, then acts as a transcription
      factor (delayed effect, takes 1-2 hours)
    Other transcription factors – NFḰB

Initiation factors
>   Bind <u>RNA polymerase</u> and induce transcription of genes

RNA and DNA building blocks
>   **Purines** – guanine, adenine
>   **Pyrimidines** – cytosine, thymidine (only in DNA), uracil (only in RNA)

Translation
>   After synthesis, mRNA travels out of the nucleus to the **cytoplasm** or
>   **rough endoplasmic reticulum**
>   Is then used as a template by **ribosomes** for synthesis of **proteins**

Ribosomes – have small and large subunits that 1) read mRNA, then 2) bind
>   appropriate **transfer RNAs** (tRNAs) that have attached amino acids, and
>   3) eventually make proteins

DNA polymerase chain reaction – uses oligonucleotides to amplify specific
>   DNA sequences (a tool used in research)

Cell cycle

4 phases:
>   1) **G1**
>   Most variable part, determines <u>cell cycle length</u>
>   *Growth factors affect cell during G1*
>   Cells can also go to G0 (quiescent) from G1
>   2) **S** (synthesis)
>   **Protein** synthesis
>   **DNA replication** (DNA polymerase)
>   Cell is preparing for division
>   3) **G2**
>   **G2 checkpoint** – stops cell from proceeding into mitosis if there is
>   damage to DNA to allow for repairs
>   Helps maintain genomic stability
>   4) **M** (mitosis) - cell divides

Mitosis
>   **Prophase**
>   **Centrosomes** move to opposite sides of cell
>   **Nucleus disappears**
>   **Mitotic apparatus** formed (**microtubules** between centrosomes and
>   centromeres on chromosomes)
>   **Metaphase** – chromosome alignment in middle of cell
>   **Anaphase** – chromosomes are pulled apart
>   **Telophase** – separate nucleus re-forms around each set of chromosomes

Cellular metabolism

Glycolysis
>   Occurs in **cytoplasm**
>   1 glucose molecule generates 2 ATPs and 2 pyruvate molecules

Mitochondria (the major site of **ATP production**)
>   Composed of 2 membranes
>   **Krebs cycle**
>   Occurs in **mitochondrial matrix** (surrounded by inner membrane)
>   The 2 pyruvate molecules (from breakdown of one glucose) create
>   **NADH, NADPH,** and **FADH** → these then enter the **electron
>   transport chain** (within the inner membrane) to create **ATP**
>   Overall, 1 molecule of glucose produces **36 ATP**

Free fatty acids + certain **amino acids** can also enter Krebs cycle

Gluconeogenesis (glucose synthesis)
>   **Liver** is by far the **largest site** of gluconeogenesis
>   Occurs in **cytoplasm**
>   Mechanism by which **lactic acid** (ie Cori cycle) and **amino acids** are
>   converted to **glucose** (is basically glycolysis in reverse)
>   Used in times of starvation or stress
>   ***Free fatty acids and lipids <u>cannot</u> be used for gluconeogenesis***
>   because acetyl CoA (breakdown product of fat metabolism) cannot
>   be converted back to pyruvate

Glycerol – breakdown product from **triacylglycerides** (TAGs)
Can be used for gluconeogenesis
Free fatty acids from TAG breakdown, however, cannot be used

Organelles, enzymes, and structure

Rough endoplasmic reticulum
Synthesizes proteins that are exported (eg pancreatic acinar cells)
Smooth endoplasmic reticulum
1) Lipid + steroid synthesis (eg adrenal cortex); 2) detoxifies drugs (liver)
Golgi apparatus
Modifies proteins w/ **carbohydrates**, then transports them to cell
membrane; proteins are then 1) secreted *or* 2) targeted to lysosomes
Lysosome - contain digestive enzymes that degrade 1) engulfed particles from
phagocytosis and 2) worn out organelles
Phagosome – engulfed large particles; fuse w/ lysosomes for degradation
Endosome – engulfed small particles; fuse w/ lysosomes for degradation
Myosin (**thick** filaments)
Uses ATP to slide along actin to cause muscle contraction (requires Ca^{++}
release from **sarcoplasmic reticulum**)
Actin (**thin** filaments) - interacts w/ myosin to cause muscle contraction
Intermediate filaments:
Keratin (hair and nails)
Desmin (muscle tissue)
Vimentin (fibroblasts)
Microtubules
Form **specialized cell structures** (eg cilia, axons)
Involved in **transport of organelles** within the cell (lattice work)
Involved in **cell division** (mitotic apparatus)
Protein kinase C
An intracellular enzyme activated by $\underline{Ca}^{++}$ and diacylglycerol (**DAG**)
Phosphorylates other enzymes and proteins (signal transduction pathway)
Protein kinase A
An intracellular enzyme activated by c$\underline{A}$MP
Phosphorylates other enzymes and proteins (signal transduction pathway)

Gastric acid secretion as an example of signal transduction:
1) **Acetylcholine** (vagus) activates **phospholipase** and creates PIP
PIP then converted to DAG + IP_3
DAG + IP_3 cause Ca^{++} **release**
Ca^{++} then activates **phosphorylase kinase**
Phosphorylase kinase then ↑s HCl secretion
2) **Histamine** activates **adenylate cyclase** and creates cAMP
cAMP activates **protein kinase A**
Protein kinase A then ↑s HCl secretion
Phosphorylase kinase and **protein kinase A** phosphorylate
H^+/K^+ **ATPase** to ↑ HCl secretion
Omeprazole *blocks* H^+/K^+ *ATPase in parietal cell membrane (final
pathway for H^+ release**)*
Gastrin
Targets parietal cells through enterochromaffin cell intermediary
(these cells release histamine)
Histamine then stimulates parietal cells in a paracrine manner as
above

Normal coagulation

Three initial responses to **vascular injury**:
1) **Vasoconstriction** (TXA_2 release)
2) **Platelet adhesion** (vWF links GpIb to exposed collagen)
3) **Thrombin generation** (occurs on platelets) leading to **platelet plug**

Coagulation Pathway

Contact Activation Pathway
(Intrinsic pathway)
Exposed collagen
+ Prekallikrein
+ HMW kininogen
+ Factor XII
↓
activate XI
Tissue Factor Pathway   ↓
(Extrinsic pathway)   activates IX, *add* VIII
Tissue factor (on injured cell surface)   ↓
+ Factor VII   →   →   →   **activate X,** *add* V
↓
convert **prothrombin** (factor II) to **thrombin**
↓
thrombin then converts **fibrinogen** to **fibrin**
↓
Fibrin + platelets = platelet plug (hemostasis)

Factor X is the **convergence point** and common to both pathways
Prothrombin complex (Xase complex)
    X, V, calcium, platelet factor 3, and **prothrombin**
    Forms on platelets
    Catalyzes formation of <u>thrombin</u>
Tissue factor pathway inhibitor – inhibits Factor X
Factor XIII – crosslinks fibrin
Thrombin
    Key to coagulation cascade
    1) Converts **fibrinogen** to **fibrin** (and fibrinogen degradation products)
    2) Activates **factors V** and **VIII**
    3) Activates **platelets**
    Generated on platelet surface (prothrombin complex above)

Coagulation Factors
Factor VII – shortest half-life
Factors V and **VIII** – labile factors (activity is lost in stored blood)
    Activity <u>not</u> lost in fresh frozen plasma (FFP)
All are synthesized in liver *except* **Factor VIII** (synthesized in endothelium)
    vWF (cofactor for VIII) – also synthesized in endothelium
Vitamin K–dependent factors – II, VII, IX, and X; protein C and protein S
    Coumadin ↓s Vit K dependent co-factors
All are serine proteases *except*:
    Factors V and **VIII** – glycoproteins
    Factor XIII - transglutaminase

Correction of coagulopathy (↑PT or ↑INR; eg **liver disease** or on **coumadin**)
    *FFP** – effect is <u>immediate</u> and lasts 6 hours *(best for emergent / urgent reversal)*
    *Vitamin K** (intravenous) – requires <u>6 hours</u> to take effect

Normal half-life
RBCs	120 days
Platelets	7 days (hold platelet inhibitors for 7 days to reverse)
PMNs	2 days

Normal Anticoagulation

Anti-thrombin III (AT-III)
Key to anticoagulation
1) Binds and inhibits **thrombin**
2) Binds and inhibits **Factors IX, X,** and **XI**
Heparin binds **AT-III** (increases activity 1000 x)
Protein C
Degrades **Factors V** and **VIII**
Degrades **fibrinogen**
Protein S - protein C cofactor
Tissue plasminogen activator (tPA)
Released from **endothelium**
Induces **fibrinolysis** by converting **plasminogen** to **plasmin**
Plasmin
Degrades **Factors V** and **VIII**
Degrades **fibrinogen** and **fibrin**
→ lose platelet plug
→ get fibrin degradation products (FDPs, eg **D-dimer**)
Alpha-2 antiplasmin
Natural inhibitor of plasmin
Released from endothelium
Prostate surgery can release **urokinase**
Induces fibrinolysis (converts plasminogen to plasmin)
Causes bleeding
Tx: aminocaproic acid (inhibits plasmin)

Prostacyclin (PGI_2)
Released from **endothelium**
Inhibits platelet aggregation and causes **vasodilation**
↑s **cAMP** in platelets
ASA irreversibly binds **cyclooxygenase**, but cyclooxygenase is **re-synthesized** in endothelium (have nuclear material unlike platelets)
→ result is **normal PGI_2 production** and platelet inhibition

Thromboxane (TXA_2)
Released from **platelets**
Causes **platelet aggregation** and **vasoconstriction**
↑s **calcium** in platelets → exposes **GpIIb/IIIa** and **GpIb receptors** (induces **platelet binding**)
ASA irreversibly binds **cyclooxygenase**, decreasing TXA production for the life of the platelet (7 days, platelets do not have nuclear material to re-synthesize cyclooxygenase)

Coagulation measurements

PT (prothrombin time)
Evaluates **tissue factor pathway** (extrinsic pathway)
Measures Factors II, V, VII, and X; also fibrinogen
**Best test for liver synthetic function
PTT (partial thromboplastin time)
Evaluates **contact activation pathway** (intrinsic pathway)
Does <u>not</u> measure **Factors VII** and **XIII**
Detects congenital **Factor VIII, IX** and **XI** deficiencies but <u>not</u> Factor VII
Also measures fibrinogen
Want **PTT 60–90** for heparin anticoagulation
ACT (activated clotting time, similar to PTT)
150–200 for routine anticoagulation
> 460 for cardiopulmonary bypass
Bleeding time – measures platelet function
INR > 1.5 – relative contraindication to performing surgical procedures
INR > 1.3 – relative contraindication to central line placement, percutaneous needle biopsies, and eye surgery

THE COMPREHENSIVE ABSITE REVIEW

Hypercoaguable States

MC *congenital* hypercoaguable disorder – resistance to activated protein C
MC *acquired* hypercoaguable disorder – smoking
Key elements in development of venous thromboses (ie Virchow's triad) –
    stasis. endothelial injury, and hypercoaguability
Key element in development of arterial thrombosis – endothelial injury

Congenital Hypercoaguable States

1) **Resistance to activated protein C** (MC; 5% of population)
    Factor V Leiden mutation (mutation is on Factor V)
2) **Hyperhomocyteinemia** (MTHFR mutation *or* folate,B6,B12 deficiency)
3) **Prothrombin Gene Mutation** (G20210A)
4) **Protein C** and **S deficiencies**
5) **Anti-thrombin III deficiency**
    Heparin does not work in these pt
    Have to give **AT-III first** (either recombinant AT-III or FFP)
    FFP has highest concentration of AT-III of all blood products
    Can develop after previous heparin exposure
6) **Plasminogen** and **fibrinolysis disorders** (very rare)
Tx:
    For all (*except* AT III deficiency and hyperhomocysteinemia) →
        Tx: post-op heparin, then coumadin
    For AT III deficiency →
        Tx: give recombinant AT III or FFP, heparinize, then coumadin
    For hyperhomocysteinemia – folate, pyridoxine, cyanocobalamine

Acquired Hypercoaguable States

1) **Smoking** - MC
2) **Anti-Phospholipid Antibody Syndrome** (APAS)
    Causes **thrombosis** (venous or arterial) *and/or* **loss of pregnancy**
    Need **1 clinical** *and* **1 laboratory** criteria:
        Clinical – any **thrombosis** *or* **complication of pregnancy**
            ($\geq$ 3 abortions before 10 weeks, $\geq$ 1 abortions after 10
            weeks, or premature birth before 34 weeks)
        Lab – ↑ed **anticardiolipin** *or* **lupus anticoagulant Ab's**
            ($\geq$ 2 occasions at least 6 weeks apart)
    Anti-cardiolipin Ab – cardiolipin is a mitochondrial phospholipid
    Lupus anticoagulant Ab
        Prolongs phospholipid-dependent coagulation reactions
        Elevated PTT that does not correct w/ FFP
            (but will correct w/ phospholipids or platelets)
        Positive Russell viper venom time
        False-positive RPR test for **syphilis**
    Catastrophic APAS – widespread thrombosis w/ multi-organ
        damage (high mortality)
    Causes – primary or from autoimmune disease (eg SLE)
    Tx: heparin, then coumadin after surgery (lifelong)
3) **Polycythemia vera**
    ↑ed **RBCs**
        Can be: 1) relative – dehydration *or* 2) absolute - more RBCs
    Sx's: Hyperviscosity (HA, dizziness)
        Thrombosis (transient visual problems, Budd Chiari)
        Bleeding (loss of coagulation factors)
        Gout (↑ uric acid from RBC turnover)
    Dx: ↓ed **EPO** (if not, R/O hypoxia or carboxyhemoglobinemia)
        ↑ed **RBC mass** *(best test)*
        Peripheral smear – normal
        Bone marrow Bx – hypercellular, megakaryocyte hyperplasia
    Preop Tx:
        Keep Hct < 48 + platelets < 400 before surgery (phlebotomy)
    Postop Tx:
        Phlebotomy (Hct < 45%)

            Low dose ASA (all pts)

            Hydroxyurea if **high risk** (age $\geq$ 60 or prior thrombosis)

            Allopurinol for gout

            H2 blockers and **antihistamines** for pruritis

4) **Cardiopulmonary bypass** – **Factor XII** (Hageman factor) is activated; results in hypercoaguable state; Tx: heparin to prevent

5) **Others** – CA, inflammatory states (eg inflammatory bowel DZ), infection, OCPs, Tamoxifen, pregnancy, rheumatoid arthritis, surgery, myeloproliferative D/Os, post-splenectomy

Warfarin induced skin necrosis

Skin sloughs off extremities

Occurs when placed on coumadin without being heparinized first

Due to **short half-life of proteins C and S** ($\downarrow$ in levels before procoagulation factors; get **hypercoaguable state $\rightarrow$ thrombosis)**

Pts w/ **protein C deficiency** especially susceptible

Tx: heparin if it occurs; prevent by placing pt on Heparin *before* starting Warfarin

Deep Venous Thrombosis (DVT)

MC DVT location - calf

MC location to result in PE – Ilio-femoral

10% incidence of PE w/ DVT

Sx's - pain, tenderness, and swelling in extremity

    Calf DVT – minimal swelling

    Femoral DVT – ankle and calf swelling

    Iliofemoral DVT – severe leg swelling

    Phlegmasia alba dolens – tender, pallor (white), edema

    Phlegmasia cerulea dolens – tender, cyanosis (blue), massive edema

Left leg 2x MC than right (left iliac vein compressed by right iliac artery in pelvis)

RFs: Virchow's triad $\rightarrow$ venous stasis, hypercoaguability, endothelial wall injury

Dx: Duplex U/S

Tx:

    Heparin, leg elevation, no walking for 5 days, coumadin (INR 2-3)

    Hypercoaguability W/U

    If you suspect HITT (see below) - Tx: stop heparin; start direct thrombin inhibitor (eg Argatroban), send HITT screen; transition to coumadin

    1st DVT or PE (surgery or hospitalization associated)– coumadin **6 months**

    2nd DVT or PE, CA, or non-modifiable RF– coumadin for **1 year**

    3rd DVT or PE, a life-threatening PE, or idiopathic spontaneous DVT/PE (ie pt was at home w/ no illness or predisposition)–coumadin **lifetime**

    Phlegmasia alba dolens (swollen **white** leg) - less severe then below

        Tx: leg elevation, heparin, thrombolytics if heparin fails

    Phlegmasia cerulea dolens (swollen **blue** leg)

        Tx: leg elevation, heparin, thrombolytics

        Emergent **Fogarty balloon thrombectomy** if extremity **threatened** (eg loss of sensation and motor function)

    Coumadin contraindicated in pregnancy $\rightarrow$ Tx: SC enoxaparin

DVT Risk Category	Incidence of DVT *without prophylaxis*
1) **Low**	**1-2%**
Minor surgery, age < 40, anesthesia, < 30 min	
No RFs	
2) **Moderate**	**15%**
Major surgery w/ age < 40, no RFs	
Minor surgery w/ age 40-60 or RFs	
3) High	**30%**
Major surgery w/ age > 60, age 40-60 w/ RFs, or recent MI	
4) **Highest**	**60%**
Major surgery w/ CA, hypercoaguable state or previous DVT	
Major ortho surgery (eg hip surgery or hip fx) stroke, multiple trauma, or spinal cord injury	

Post-op DVT Prevention
1) **Low risk** – early ambulation
2) **Moderate to high risk**
   Early ambulation
   SCDs ($\downarrow$ venous stasis, $\uparrow$ AT-III, tPA, and fibrinolysin)
   LMWH (enoxaparin 0.5 mg/kg BID)
3) **Highest risk**
   Early ambulation
   SCDs
   LMWH (enoxaparin 0.5 mg/kg BID)
   Possible coumadin
   Majority of adult surgery in-patient's should receive LMWH prophylaxis unless contraindicated

IVC filter Indications
1) DVT or PE with **contraindication** to anticoagulation
2) DVT or PE in pt w/ a **complication** while on anticoagulation
3) **Failure of anticoagulation** (recurrent PE or DVT)
4) **Free-floating iliofemoral or caval thrombus**
5) After **pulmonary embolectomy**
6) **Prophylaxis**
   a. Patients w/ DVT undergoing surgery (lower-extremity orthopedic surgery, major abdominal surgery, neurosurgery)
   b. Patients w/ chronic pulmonary hypertension and a marginal cardiopulmonary reserve

Studies have <u>not</u> shown benefit in trauma pts w/ neuro injury or multiple long bone fractures
Ensure there is **not thrombus in femoral or iliac vein** before inserting filter – go through **internal jugular vein** if present
Confirm position of filter by injecting contrast and looking for renal veins – ***want filter below renal veins***
Accidentally gets launched above renal veins – **leave it** (unless it's a removable filter)
Pulmonary embolism w/ filter in place – comes from ovarian veins, IVC superior to filter, or SVC route (upper extremities)

Catheter-induced Venous Thrombosis (central line induced)
Remove if not needed and give heparin to prevent thrombus extension
Can **infuse tPA** down line if running out of access sites (eg dialysis pt)
If infected, the line will need to be removed

<u>HITT</u> (Heparin-induced thrombocytopenia thrombocytosis)
Anti-platelet Ab's [IgG to platelet factor 4 (PF4)] causes **platelet destruction** and at times **thrombosis**
Forms a white clot
Can occur w/ just one low dose of heparin
Type I – direct effect of heparin (no antibody, platelet nadir > 100); **no sequelae**
Type II – IgG to **PF4-heparin complex**; platelet nadir 40, **thrombosis in 40%**
Clinical suspicion of Type II HITT includes:
1) **platelet drop** < 100 or 50% baseline <u>or</u>;
2) **arterial** or **venous thrombosis** (eg cold leg or DVT)
Dx for Type II HITT:
   ELISA for PF4-heparin Ab
   1) If **strongly positive**, the pt has HITT
   2) If **mildly** positive, perform ^{14}**C-serotonin release assay**
      i. if **positive** → pt has HITT
      ii. If **negative** → pt does <u>not</u> have HITT
Tx:
   D/C heparin
   Start **direct thrombin inhibitor** (eg Argatroban, bivalirudin)
   Convert to **Warfarin** (3 months for thrombosis, 1 month for no thrombosis)
   History of HITT Type II and now **PF4 Ab negative** – risk of HITT recurrence low

Pulmonary Embolism (PE) – see Critical Care chp

Coagulopathic States

1) **MC bleeding problem in surgery** – inadequate hemostasis intra-op

2) **von Willebrand's disease** (vWD)
    MC congenital bleeding disorder (AD)
    MC sx – epistaxis (also for Glanzman's and Bernard Soulier below)
    vWF (von Willebrand's Factor) **production** occurs in **endothelium**
    vWF links **GpIb receptor** on **platelets** to **collagen** (main effect)
    Dx:
        PT normal
        PTT normal or slightly prolonged
        Prolonged bleeding time (ristocetin test)
    Tx:
        DDAVP in general is 1st line tx for vWF disease _except_ **Type III**
        Type I (MC type, 70%)
            Reduced quantity of circulating vWF (usually mild sx's)
            Tx: **DDAVP** _(best Tx)_
                   Factor VIII-vWF complex (Humate P)
                   Cryoprecipitate (highest concentration of VIII-vWF)
        Type II
            Have enough vWF but doesn't work well
            Tx: ± DDAVP (may not work, try test dose if possible)
                   Factor VIII-vWF complex (Humate P)
                   Cryoprecipitate
        Type III
            Almost no vWF – can get **severe bleeding**
            Tx: **Factor VIII-vWF complex** (Humate P)
                   Cryoprecipitate
                   (_DDAVP does _not_ work_)
        Conjugated estrogens can also release of VWF and VIII

3) **Glanzmann's thrombocytopenia** (congenital)
    GpIIb/IIIa receptor deficiency on platelets (plts can't bind each other)
    Fibrin normally **cross-links GpIIb/IIIa receptors** together (platelet plug)
    Tx: **platelets**
4) **Bernard-Soulier thrombocytopenia** (congenital)
    GpIb receptor deficiency on platelets (can't bind to collagen)
    vWF normally links **GpIb to collagen**
    Tx: **platelets**
5) **Acquired thrombocytopenia** – can be caused by H2 blockers, heparin
6) **Uremic coagulopathy**
    Occurs w/ BUN > 60-80
    Uremia **inhibits release of vWF**
    Tx:
        DDAVP for **acute reversal** of coagulopathy
            (emergent or urgent procedure, eg mesenteric ischemia)
            Stimulates release of factor VIII and vWF from endothelium
            30 minute time of onset and lasts 4 hours
        Hemodialysis (reverses uremia and coagulopathy)
            Best option for **elective surgery or procedures**
            (ie hemodialysis day before procedure commonly performed)
7) **Disseminated intravascular coagulation** (DIC)
    Often initiated by **tissue factor**
    Dx:
        ↓ed platelets
        prolonged PT, prolonged PTT
        ↓ed fibrinogen, ↑ FDPs (including D-dimer)
    Tx: **treat underlying cause 1st**, FFP, cryoprecipitate, platelets

8) **Hemophilia A**
   Factor VIII deficiency, sex linked recessive
   MC Sx - hemarthrosis; others – muscle, GI tract, or brain hemorrhages
   Factor VIII **crosses placenta** → newborns may not bleed at circumcision
   Dx: **prolonged PTT** and a normal PT
   Tx:
   a.) **Recombinant Factor VIII** (best Tx)
   b.) DDAVP (effective only for <u>mild disease</u>; ie Factor VIII activity >5%)
   c.) **Cryoprecipitate**
   Surgery - want levels **100% pre-op** and **50% post-op** (for 3-5 days)
   Monitor PTT every 8-12 hours
   Hemophiliac joint
   Do <u>NOT</u> aspirate
   Recombinant Factor VIII, ice, and range of motion exercises
   Epistaxis, intracerebral hemorrhage, or **hematuria**
   Recombinant Factor VIII
   Spontaneous bleed – occurs at levels < 1%
   Conjugated estrogens – can release vWF + VIII from endothelium
9) **Hemophilia B**
   Factor IX deficiency, sex linked recessive
   MC Sx - hemarthrosis; others – muscle, GI tract, or brain hemorrhage
   Dx: **prolonged PTT** and normal PT
   Tx:
   a.)   **Recombinant Factor IX**
   b.)   **FFP**
   Surgery - want levels **50% pre-op** and **50% post-op** (for 3-5 days)
10) **Hemophilia C**
   Factor XI deficiency – usually only mild bleeding
   Dx: **prolonged PTT** and normal PT
   Tx: **Recombinant Factor XI** or **FFP**
11) **Factor VII deficiency**
   Dx: *prolonged PT* and normal PTT
   Tx: **Recombinant Factor VII** or **FFP**

Recommendations for Clopidogrel (Plavix) and coronary stents
   High risk of **stent thrombosis** (and myocardial infarction) if Plavix is stopped
   early after stent placement
   Elective Surgery Recommendations:
   Bare metal stents – Plavix for **6 weeks** before elective surgery
   Drug eluding stents – Plavix for **1 year** before elective surgery
   Continue ASA throughout the peri-operative period
   Stop Plavix for 5-7 days before elective surgery
   Restart Plavix ASAP post-op
   Semi-Urgent surgery within window of anti-platelet Tx for coronary stent
   (eg colon CA, breast CA)
   Is the surgical procedure a clear contra-indication to Plavix?
   No → continue Plavix w/ surgery, have platelets available
   Yes → hold Plavix for 5 days, continue ASA, bridge w/ short-acting
   IIb/IIIa inhibitors; re-start Plavix ASAP post-op
   Emergent surgery within window of anti-platelet Tx for coronary stent
   (eg mesenteric ischemia) → operate on Plavix and have platelets available

Mechanical valve on coumadin now w/ GIB or need for emergency surgery
   Completely reverse w/ FFP and limited amount of vitamin K
   Tx underlying problem (eg GI bleeding or acute abdomen)
   Start heparin after 48 hrs, then coumadin (thrombosis risk <u>low</u> w/ this method)

Anticoagulation agents
Platelet inhibitors
Cyclooxygenase inhibitor - ASA (irreversible)
ADP receptor inhibitors (↓ GpIIb/IIIa activation) - Clopidogrel (Plavix)
Adenosine re-uptake inhibitor - Dipyridamole (Persantine)
cAMP phosphodiesterase inhibitors (↑ cAMP) - Pentoxifylline (Trental)
Glycoprotein IIb/IIIa Inhibitors - Eptifibatide (Integrilin)
PCN/cephalosporins – bind platelets, can ↑ **bleeding time**
Direct thrombin Inhibitors
1) **Argatroban**
Reversible, **liver metabolism,** 1/2 life 50 min
Want PTT 60–90 (same as heparin)
MC use - HITT
*Falsely elevates **PT and INR*** (when transitioning to coumadin, **follow Factor X activity** levels)
2) **Bivalirudin** (Angiomax)
Reversible, **proteinase enzyme metabolism** (blood); 1/2 life 30 min
Want PTT 60–90 (same as heparin)
MC use - percutaneous transluminal coronary angioplasty (PTCA)
Thrombolytics
1) **Tissue plasminogen activator** (tPA, Alteplase)
2) **Urokinase**
3) **Streptokinase**
Indications - acute MI, stroke, PE, or limb ischemia
Streptokinase has ↑**antigenicity** (*contraindicated* if previous streptokinase exposure)
Tx:
For thrombolytics to work, a **guidewire** must get past the obstruction, and an **infusion catheter placed inside thrombus**
Given w/ **heparin**
Usually for **8-24 hours**
Follow **fibrinogen levels** → <100 associated w/ ↑ bleeding risk
Thrombolytic overdose Tx – aminocaproic acid
Contraindications
Absolute
Active **internal bleeding**
Recent CVA (< 2 months)
Cranial pathology (eg brain tumor)
Relative
Recent (<10 days) surgery, organ biopsy, obstetric delivery, or major trauma
Left heart thrombus (left ventricle or left atrium)
Recent serious GI bleed (< 90 days)
Uncontrolled hypertension
Minor - minor surgery, recent CPR, bacterial endocarditis, hemostatic problems (eg renal or liver DZ), diabetic hemorrhagic retinopathy, pregnancy
Heparin - activates **antithrombin III**
Want PTT 60-90
1/2 life 60–90 minutes
Cleared by **reticuloendothelial system** (mostly macrophages in spleen)
Long-term heparin S/Es – osteoporosis, alopecia
Does <u>not</u> cross placental barrier (Warfarin does)
Pts on Heparin - hold heparin 6 hours before surgery; may not be possible in emergency; re-start 48 hrs post-op if pt not bleeding
Protamine – binds and reverses heparin (1.25 mg protamine/100 U heparin)
Cross-reacts w/ **NPH insulin** (eg diabetic) or **previous protamine exposure** → can cause **protamine reaction**
Protamine reaction (1%, anaphylactic reaction; MC S/E) → hypotension, bradycardia, and ↓ed heart function
Tx: Volume, epinephrine, and inotropes
Can **re-heparinize** and go back on bypass if during cardiac surgery

Low molecular weight heparin (eg enoxaparin, dalteparin, fondiparinux)

    Fondaparinux (Lovenox) is a selective **Xa inhibitor**

    Smaller risk of HITT

    Do not need to monitor PTT

    Not reversed w/ Protamine

Warfarin (coumadin)

    Prevents **vitamin K–dependent decarboxylation of glutamic residues**
        on vitamin K–dependent factors (II, VII, IX, and X; protein C and
        protein S)

Sequential compression devices (SCDs) – improve venous return but also
    induce fibrinolysis with compression (release of tPA)

Procoagulant agents

    Aminocaproic acid (Amicar) - **plasmin inhibitor** (inhibits thrombolysis)

        Indications:

            DIC

            Persistent bleeding following cardiopulmonary bypass

            Thrombolytic overdose

    DDAVP – stimulates factor VIII and vWF release from endothelium

Other coagulation issues

    ASA

        Stop 7 days before surgery

        Prolongs bleeding time

        Inhibits cyclooxygenase in platelets which **decreases TXA$_2$**

    Coumadin

        Stop 7 days before surgery

        Consider starting heparin while coumadin wears off

    Platelets

        keep > 50,000 before surgery

        keep > 20,000 after surgery

        1/3 of all platelets stored in spleen

        GpIb – vWF connects GpIb on platelets to exposed collagen

        GpIIb/IIIa – fibrin cross-links GpIIb/IIIa receptors on platelets (platelet plug)

        Other platelet receptors – ADP, epinephrine

    H and P – best way to predict bleeding risk

    Normal circumcision

        Does not R/O bleeding disorders

        Can still have clotting factors from mother (eg Hemophilia A, Factor VIII
            crosses the placenta)

    Abnormal bleeding w/ tooth extraction or tonsillectomy

        Picks up 99% pts with bleeding disorder

    Menorrhagia – heavy bleeding w/ menses; common with bleeding disorders

    Joint and muscle hemorrhage – common w/ hemophilias (eg hemophilia A, B,
        and C)

    Epistaxis – common w/ vWF deficiency and other platelet disorders

BLOOD PRODUCTS

Packed red blood cells (PRBCs)

Medical State	*Appropriate Hgb*
Critical illness	hgb 7-9 adequate
Coronary ischemia	hgb 10-12 adequate
Ongoing blood loss	hgb 10-12 (target; room for loss)

1 unit pRBCs raises hgb by 1 gm/dl

PRBCs stored in **citrate** (CDPA) for preservation – citrate **binds Ca^{++}**

Can get ↓ Ca^{++} level w/ **massive transfusions** (≥ 10 units PRBCs)

Stored PRBCs last **3 weeks**

Storage - ↓ 2.3 DPG, ↓ pH, ↑ K^{+} and ↑ lactic acid

Massive transfusion – can ↓ Ca^{++}, ↓ **coagulation factors** and ↓ **body temp**

Max blood product temp prior to infusion – 49.0 C (protein denaturation occurs at temp's higher than this)

Platelets

Platelet transfusion indications:

1) **< 10,000** - high risk **spontaneous bleeding**

2) **< 20,000** w/ **infection or bleeding risk** (eg post-op pts)

3) **< 50,000** w/ **active bleeding or pre-procedure**

Contraindications – TTP, HUS, HELLP, HITT (may need to give platelets to control severe bleeding w/ these syndromes)

6 units (6 pack) – ↑s platelets by **50,000**

< 5000 increase suggests allo-immunization, try **ABO matched platelets**

If still < 5000, check panel reactive antibody for **HLA antibodies** (may need **HLA matched platelets**)

Fresh frozen plasma (FFP)

Contains **all of the coagulation factors** (includes protein C, protein S, and AT-III)

Good for **deficiencies of all coagulation factors** (dilutional coagulopathy from massive transfusion, DIC, liver disease, Warfarin, PT > 17 pre-procedure)

Cryoprecipitate

Has highest levels of vWF, Factor VIII, fibrinogen, and **Factor XIII**

Good for bleeding with low fibrinogen (< 100) or bleeding in vWD

Special products and procedures

Irradiated blood products

Kills T cells in blood product

Used in pts at risk for transfusion related **graft versus host disease** (hematopoietic stem cell TXP, hematologic malignancies, congenital immunodeficiency)

CMV negative (from CMV negative donors)

Used for CMV sero-negative pregnancy, organ and bone marrow TXP candidates/recipients, AIDS, low birth weight infants

Leukoreduced

WBCs can cause **HLA allo-immunization, fever** (cytokine release) and **carry CMV**

Used for chronically transfused pts, potential TXP recipients, previous **febrile non-hemolytic transfusion reaction**, or when CMV products are desirable but unavailable

Immunoglobulin (intravenous, IV-Ig)

Used for post-exposure prophylaxis (eg Hep A), some autoimmune D/Os (eg ITP, myasthenia gravis)

Plasmapheresis - removes **immunoglobulins** (eg TTP)

Transfusion reactions

Febrile non-hemolytic transfusion reaction   1:100
    MC transfusion reaction
    Sx's - Fever and rigors 0-6 hrs after transfusion
    Preformed recipient Ab's against **donor WBCs**
    Causes **cytokine release**
    Tx:
        Stop transfusion
        Acetaminophen (R/O infection and hemolysis)
        WBC filters for subsequent transfusions
Allergic reaction   1:150
    MC Sx - urticaria (rash)
    Rare anaphylaxis (sx's - bronchospasm and hypotension)
    Reaction to plasma proteins in blood product
    MCC - IgA deficient pt (w/ **preformed Ab's** to IgA) receiving **IgA blood**
    Tx:
        Urticaria – diphenhydramine (Benadryl), H2 blockers
        Anaphylaxis – epinephrine, fluids, possible steroids
Delayed hemolytic transfusion reaction   1:2500
    Sx's- usually **minimal** (often goes unnoticed)
        Possibly **unexplained fever, jaundice**, or **drop in hct**
        Usually get sx's **5-10 days** after transfusion
    Preformed **recipient Ab's** against donor minor RBC antigens (HLA)
    Urinalysis shows urobilinogenuria
    W/U includes LFTs, clotting and red cell antibody screens
    Tx: nonspecific
    Dx impt for future transfusion (HLA match next time)
Transfusion related acute lung injury (TRALI)   1: 15.000
    Sx's – hypoxia, diffuse alveolar infiltrates, fever
    Non-cardiogenic pulmonary edema **< 6 hours** after transfusion
    Donor Ab's bind <u>recipient</u> **WBCs** and lodge in lung
        Release mediators causing ↑ **capillary permeability**
    Tx: may require intubation; Tx same as ARDS
Acute hemolytic transfusion reaction   1: 250,000
    Sx's - fever, hypotension, tachycardia, flank pain, hematuria
        Can lead to renal failure, shock and DIC
        Anesthetized pts can present as **diffuse bleeding**
    Cause - ABO incompatibility
        Preformed recipient Ab's against **donor RBCs**
        Results in acute hemolysis
    Dx:
        Haptoglobin < 50 (binds Hgb, then gets degraded)
        Free hemoglobin > 5
        ↑ed **unconjugated bilirubin**
    Tx:
        Stop transfusion
        Fluid resuscitation for **BP** and to maintain **good UOP**
        Diuretics (lasix and mannitol)
        HCO3- (prevent Hgb precipitation in kidney and ATN)
        Pressors for refractory hypotension
Fatal hemolytic transfusion reaction   1: 500,000

MCC death from transfusion reaction – Clerical error resulting in ABO
    incompatibility
Non-immune hemolysis – from squeezing the blood bag
Severity of transfusion reactions are inversely proportional to frequency

Infectious Complications of Transfusion

Bacterial (in platelets)	**1: 50,000**
Bacterial (in pRBCs)	**1: 500,000**
Hep B	**1: 200,000**
Hep C	**1: 2,000,000**
HIV	**1: 2,000,000**

Blood is also tested for syphilis, HTLV, and West Nile virus
MC blood product w/ bacterial contamination – platelets (not refrigerated)
    Platelets are stored at **room temp** – good medium for bacterial growth
    Platelets last for **5 days** at room temp
    Not cold-stored because **half-life** would be decreased
MC bacterial contaminant – GNRs (MC **E. coli**)

Other transfusion problems
Cold body temp
    Poor clotting can be caused by cold products or cold body temp
    Pts need to be warm to clot correctly
    Due to **slowing of enzymatic reactions**
Dilutional thrombocytopenia
    Occurs w/ 10 units pRBCs
    Tx: platelets
Hypocalcemia
    Occurs w/ massive transfusion
    Ca^{++} required for clotting cascade
    Tx: calcium
Antiplatelet antibodies – develop in 20% after 10-20 plt transfusions
Hetastarch (eg Hespan) – volume expander
    Can use up to 1 L w/o risk of bleeding Cx's
Chagas disease – can be transmitted with blood transfusion
All blood products carry risk of **HIV** and **hepatitis** _except_ → **albumin** and
    immunoglobulins (these are heat treated)

Trying to raise hemoglobin without giving blood
(eg Jehovah's Witness w/ low Hct before surgery)
Epoetin
Fe supplementation
Should raise hemoglobin 1-2 pts/week

Iron deficient anemia (microcytic anemia) in **post-menopausal female or male** –
    screen for colon CA or another GI source

INNATE IMMUNE SYSTEM
(Inflammation and Complement)

Inflammation Response (part of **innate immune system**)
Tissue Injury (eg trauma or infection) →
1) Exposes **collagen**
2) **PAF** release (from endothelium) – recruits platelets, leukocytes
3) **Tissue factor** release (from endothelium) – starts clotting cascade
4) **Vasoconstriction** (early) – from **platelet** and **endothelial TXA$_2$**

Platelets bind collagen (vWF mediated) →
1) Platelets release **growth factors** (eg PDGF) → PMN and macrophage recruitment
2) **Coagulation cascade** (prothrombinase complex forms on platelets)
   Fibrin crosslinks platelets → **platelet plug**
3) **Vasodilation** (late) – from platelets releasing **histamine**
   Increased **porosity** (edema) facilitates **leukocyte migration**

PMN's
Arrive within **1 hour** → phagocytosis and remove debris

Macrophages
*Have the **dominant role** in inflammation and wound healing*
Release important **growth factors** (PDGF) and **cytokines** (IL-1 and TNF-alpha) to attract other inflammatory cells and fibroblasts
Phagocytosis + remove debris (monocytes→ macrophages after activation)

Order of cell arrival in wound
1) **Platelets**
2) **PMNs**
3) **Macrophages**
4) **Fibroblasts**
5) **Lymphocytes**

Predominant cell type by day
Days 0–2	PMNs
Days 3–4	Macrophages
Days 5 and on	Fibroblasts

Inflammation is 1st step in normal wound healing

Wound Healing:
1) **Inflammation** (PDGF, PAF)
2) **Proliferation** (PDGF, FGF, EGF)
3) **Remodeling**

Growth factors
PDGF (platelet-derived growth factor) – *__key growth factor__ in wound healing*
Chemotactic and activates **inflammatory cells**
Chemotactic and activates **fibroblasts**
Angiogenesis
Epithelialization
Chemotactic for **smooth muscle cells**
Accelerates **wound healing**

PAF (platelet-activating factor)
Activates **platelets**
Chemotactic and activates **inflammatory cells**
↑s **adhesion molecule** expression
Not stored, generated by **phospholipase** in endothelium and other cells
(PAF is a **phospholipid**)

FGF (fibroblastic growth factor)
Chemotactic and activates **fibroblasts**
Angiogenesis
Epithelialization

EGF (epidermal growth factor)
Chemotactic and activates **fibroblasts**
Angiogenesis
Epithelialization

TGF-beta (transforming growth factor-beta)
Primarily **immunosuppressive** - inhibits lymphocytes and leukocytes

Chemotactic factors
>For inflammatory cells – PDGF, PAF, IL-8, LTB-4, C5a and C3a
>For fibroblasts – PDGF, FGF, EGF

Angiogenesis factors – PDGF, FGF, EGF, IL-8, hypoxia
>Produced by **macrophages** and **platelets** in response to **hypoxia**

Epithelialization factors – PDGF, FGF, EGF

Macrophages – main producers of **growth factors**

PMNs – last 2 days in tissue (last 7 days in blood)

Platelets – last 7 days

Innate Immune System Cytokines

Main cytokines released w/ inflammation - TNF-alpha (#1) and IL-1
>Vast majority of cytokines are produced by **macrophages**

TNF-alpha (tumor necrosis factor-alpha)
>**Main source** - macrophages
>↑ **cell adhesion molecules** (eg ICAM, selectins)
>**Procoagulant**
>Activates **PMNs** and other **macrophages**
>>→ leads to **growth factor** production → **cell recruitment**
>↑ HR, ↑ cardiac output, ↓ SVRI
>>→ high concentration can cause **myocardial depression**, circulatory collapse and multi-system organ failure
>Causes **cachexia** in pts w/ CA

IL-1
>**Main source** - macrophages
>Effects similar to TNF and synergizes TNF
>Induces **fever** (**PGE_2 mediated** in hypothalamus)
>>Raises thermal set point, causing fever
>>**NSAIDs** – ↓ fever by reducing PGE_2 synthesis.
>>**Alveolar macrophages** – cause fever w/ **atelectasis** by releasing **IL-1**

IL-6
>Primary function is ↑**hepatic acute phase proteins** (see below)

IL-8
>Primary function is **chemotaxis of PMNs** (+ other inflammatory cells)
>**Angiogenesis**

IL-10
>Primary function is **down regulation inflammatory response**
>(↓ TNF-alpha, IL-2, IL3, and interferons; down-regulates APCs)

IL-15
>Primary function is **activation of natural killer cells** in response to **viral infection**

IL-18
>Primary function is to ↑ **interferon release** from **natural killers cells** and **T cells**

Interferons
>Released by **lymphocytes** and **natural killer cells** primarily in response to **viral infection** (IL-18 mediated)
>1) Activate **macrophages, natural killer cells,** and **cytotoxic T cells** (cell mediated immunity)
>2) **Inhibit viral replication** (esp RNA viruses)
>3) Upregulate **MHC expression**

Hepatic acute phase proteins
IL-6 – most potent stimulus

Increased – <u>C-reactive protein</u> (an opsonin, activates complement), amyloid A and P, fibrinogen, haptoglobin, ceruloplasmin, alpha-1 antitrypsin, alpha-1 antichymotrypsin and C3 (complement)

**Decreased – albumin, prealbumin, and transferrin

Innate Immune System Cells
Macrophages
1) ***Dominant cell type*** *in inflammation and wound healing* mainly through the release of **growth factors** and **cytokines**
2) **Phagocytose** pathogens or cells infected w/ pathogen followed by **respiratory burst**; also remove debris
   Respiratory burst releases reactive oxygen species (free radicals, H_2O_2) into pathogen or cell infected w/ pathogen, killing it
3) Involved in **antibody-dependent cell mediated cytotoxicity**
   Macrophages help clear cells with **intracellular** viral and bacterial pathogens (eg mycobacterium)
   Requires **adaptive immune system** for **Ab production 1st**

PMNs
Main function is **phagocytosis** (pathogens, cells infected w/ pathogens, debris)

Dendritic Cells – main function is to **bridge the innate** and **adaptive immune** systems by serving as APCs (antigen presenting cells)

Natural Killer T Cells
Attack **host cells** that have been infected by microbes
Do <u>not</u> directly attack microbe
Do <u>not</u> need MHC-antigen complexes
Attack cells w/ **low expression of MHC** (missing self)
   Occurs w/ cell infection (esp. viral infection)

Mast cells – main cell type involved in Type I hypersensitivity reactions
Basophils – Type I Hypersensitivity reactions
Eosinophils – parasitic infections and Type I hypersensitivity reactions (late)

Cell mediated immunity
Involves both the **innate** and **adaptive immune systems**
Cells involved – macrophages, PMNs, eosinophils, natural killer cells, cytotoxic T cells
Intradermal skin test (eg PPD for TB) – used to test cell-mediated immunity
Infections associated w/ defects in cell mediated immunity – *intra-cellular pathogens (eg TB, other mycobacterium, viruses)*

Antibody dependent cell-mediated cytotoxicity (ADCC)
Involves both the **innate** and **adaptive immune systems**
Cells involved - Macrophages, PMNs, eosinophils, and natural killer cells
These cells have **Fc receptor** (for constant region of antibody)
Requires **antibody production** from **adaptive immune system** to bind to antigen 1st

Innate immune system response to pathogens

***Extra*-cellular Bacterial Infection**
   **Macrophages
   **PMNs
   Complement

***Intra*-cellular Bacterial Infection** (eg mycobacterium, legionella)
   **Natural Killer Cells (primary cell)^
   Macrophages (only w/ ADCC and adaptive immunity)

***Intra*-cellular Viral Infection**
   **Natural Killer cells (primary cell)^
   Macrophages (only w/ ADCC and adaptive immunity)

^**Note** – natural killer cells are involved in ADCC as well but can also attack cells infected w/ intra-cellular pathogens without antibody binding; macrophages cannot perform this later function

Cell adhesion molecules

Selectins – involved in **rolling adhesion** (1st step in transmigration process)
> **L-selectins** (on leukocytes) bind to **E-selectin** (endothelial) and **P-selectin** (platelets)

Beta-2 integrins (CD 11/18 molecules)
> Found on **leukocytes** and **platelets**
> Involved in **anchoring adhesion** and **transendothelial migration**
> Bind ICAM, VCAM, etc

ICAM, VCAM, PECAM, and ELAM
> Found on **endothelial cells**
> Involved in **anchoring adhesion** and **transendothelial migration**
> Bind **beta-2 integrin molecules** (above)

Complement

Part of **innate immune system**

1) **Classic pathway**
> **Activation Mechanisms**
> > a) Antigen–antibody complex (IgG or IgM *only*) *or;*
> > b) Direct binding of pathogen to C1
> **Initial step** is formation of **C1 complex** (2 C1 molecules)
> **Factors C1, C2,** and **C4** – found *only* in the classic pathway

2) **Alternative pathway**
> **Activation mechanisms** - Endotoxin, bacteria, other stimuli activate
> **Initial step** is **C3 activation**
> **Factors B, D,** and **P** (properdin) – found *only* in alternate pathway

C3 activation – common to and convergence point for both pathways
Mg^{++} required for both pathways
Complement proteins synthesized in **liver**
Products:

1) **Anaphylatoxins** – C3a, C4a and C5a
> ↑ vascular permeability
> Bronchoconstriction
> Activate mast cells and basophils
2) **Membrane attack complex** – C5b–C9b (C5bC6bC7bC8bC9b)
> Inserted into **pathogen cell membrane** → makes hole → cell lysis
> Can also **attack normal cells infected w/ bacteria**
3) **Opsonization** – C3b and C4b
> Enhances **phagocytosis of antigen**
4) **Inflammatory cell chemotaxis** (PMNs, macrophage) – C3a and C5a

Oxidants generated in inflammation (oxidants and producers)

Superoxide anion radical (O_2^-)	NADPH oxidase
Hydrogen peroxide (H_2O_2)	Xanthine oxidase, NADPH oxidase
Hydroxyl radical (-OH)	Fe mediated (very destructive)
Hypochlorous acid ($HOCl^-$)	Myeloperoxidase

Cellular defenses against Oxidative Species

Superoxide anion radical	**Superoxide dismutase** (need Cu + Zn)
	Converts to hydrogen peroxide
Hydrogen peroxide	**Glutathione peroxidases**
	Catalase, Peroxiredoxins
Hydroxyl Radical	*Cannot* be eliminated
	(although ½ life is short, 10^{-10} s)
Hypochlorous acid	**Taurine scavenger**

**Primary injuring mechanism of oxygen radicals – DNA damage
Also cause lipid (eg cell membrane) and protein oxidation
Respiratory burst (from macrophages and PMNs) – releases superoxide anion and hydrogen peroxide
Red blood cells – have antioxidant properties (superoxide dismutase and catalase)
Chronic granulomatous disease
> NADPH-oxidase system enzyme defect in PMNs and macrophages
> Results in ↓ superoxide radical (O_2^-) formation

Lipid mediators

Mainly involved in **inflammation regulation**
Initial substrate is **phospholipid essential fatty acids** (from cell membrane)
    Phospholipids → (*phospholipase*) → **Arachadonic acid**
    *Glucocorticoids inhibit phospholipase and production of everything below
Arachadonic acid (an eicosanoid, along w/ everything below)
    Enters either: 1) **cyclooxygenase pathway** *or* 2) **lipoxygenase pathway**
1) **Cyclooxygenase (COX) pathway** (produces prostaglandins)
    a) **PGI_2** (prostacyclin) and **PGE_2**
        Systemic and pulmonary **vasodilation** ($\downarrow$ SVR, $\downarrow$ PVR)
        $\downarrow$ platelet aggregation
        Bronchodilation
    b) **PGG_2, PGH_2**, and **TXA_2** (thromboxane)
        Systemic and pulmonary **vasoconstriction** ($\uparrow$ SVR, $\uparrow$ PVR)
        $\uparrow$ platelet aggregation
    c) **PGF_2** – primarily uterine contraction (**Dinoprost**, induces labor)
    d) **PGD_2** – primarily a brain neurotransmitter
2) **Lipoxygenase pathway** (produces leukotrienes and lipoxins)
    Are **leukocyte derived** molecules
    a) **Leukotrienes**
        LTC_4, LTD_4, LTE_4 – Slow-reacting substances of anaphylaxis
        Bronchoconstriction
        Vasoconstriction followed by $\uparrow$permeability (**wheal and flare**)
        LTB_4 – chemotaxis for PMNs and eosinophils
    b) **Lipoxins** - anti-inflammatory ($\downarrow$ chemotaxis, $\downarrow$ transmigration)

NSAIDs (COX inhibitors, reversible) – inhibit prostaglandin synthesis
    COX-1 – constitutively expressed in essentially all mammalian cells
    COX-2 – inducible variant produced at sites of inflammation
    Non selective COX inhibitor (both COX-1 and COX-2 enzymes inhibited)
        $\uparrow$ ulcer risk due to $\downarrow$ed prostaglandins in stomach ($\downarrow$ mucus barrier)
    Selective COX-2 inhibitor – more specific for inflammatory tissue
        $\downarrow$ed incidence of ulcers, some $\uparrow$ in **cardiovascular S/Es**
ASA (non-selective COX inhibitor, irreversible) – inhibits prostaglandin synthesis
    $\downarrow$s platelet adhesion by $\downarrow$ TXA_2 from platelets
Glucocorticoids – inhibits **phospholipase** and prostaglandin synthesis
    → inhibits inflammation
(see Pharmacology chp for selective / non-selective COX inhibitors)

Platelet granules

Alpha granules
    Aggregation Factors– platelet factor 4, vWF, fibrinogen, fibronectin
    Beta-thromboglobulin – binds thrombin
    PDGF and TGF-beta
    Factors V and XIII
Dense granules (ASC)
    Adenosine (as ATP or ADP)
    Serotonin
    Calcium
Other factors in platelets – PAF, beta-lysin (antimicrobial)

Other Inflammation

Catecholamines (neural response to injury) - peak 24–48 hours after injury
    Norepinephrine released from **sympathetic chain neurons** (post-
        ganglion) and **adrenal medulla**
    Epinephrine released *only* from **adrenal medulla** *(only site of production)*
Neuroendocrine response to injury
    Afferent nerves from site of injury stimulate ACTH, ADH, growth hormone,
        epinephrine, and norepinephrine release
Thyroid hormone – does not play a major role in injury
Chemokines (CXC) – primary role is chemotaxis (eg IL-8)
    C = cysteine; X = another amino acid

WOUND HEALING

Wound healing phases

1) **Inflammation** (1-10 d, see previous Chp for details)
   Main growth factors – PDGF and **PAF**
   Platelet aggregation, coagulation cascade, cell recruitment, phagocytosis

2) **Proliferation** (5 days to 3 weeks)
   Main Growth Factors – PDGF, FGF, and **EGF**
   a) **Granulation tissue** (= vascularized ECM)
      Provisional extracellular matrix (ECM) - platelets, fibrin, fibronectin
         and **hyaluronic acid** (ground substance, glycosaminoglycan)
      Fibroblasts very early (5-7d) produce **fibronectin** and **hyaluronic
         acid** to build provisional ECM
      Fibroblast, inflammatory cells + myofibroblasts migrate over ECM
         Fibroblasts attracted by PDGF, FGF, EGF and fibronectin
      Neovascularization
         Endothelial cells attracted to area (PDGF. FGF, EGF, hypoxia
            , lactic acid) form **pseudopodia** that infiltrate ECM
            MMPs (matrix metalloproteinases; need Zn^{++}) + **collagenase**, +
               plasmin digest ECM to allow **endothelial proliferation**
   b) **Epithelialization** (1–2 mm/day, requires **granulation tissue**)
      Keratinocytes (epithelial cells) from **hair follicles** *(#1 source)* +
         wound edges + sweat glands **migrate** across granulation tissue
      Cell division occurs *only* at wound edges, sweat glands, and hair
         follicles until entire wound is covered
      Migration stimulated by - lack of inhibition, NO, PDGF, FGF, EGF
      Quicker migration results in **less scarring**
      Epithelial cells phagocytose **debris and scab** in their way; secrete
         MMPs and **tPA** (plasmin activation) **which** dissolve scab
      Migration facilitated by **moist environment**
      After migration, epithelial cells form a **new basement membrane**
   c) **Wound contraction** - peaks at **10** (±5) **days**
      Myofibroblasts (differentiated fibroblasts, have actin) contract wound
   d) **Collagen Deposition** – maximum (peak) at **3 weeks**
      Produced by **fibroblasts**; provides **wound strength**
      Initially, synthesis of Type III collagen predominates (2d), then Type I
         *Although **Type I is *always*** the predominant collagen in wound
         Pre-existing Type I at wound site far greater than Type III
      Breakdown of provisional ECM and ↑ed chondroitin sulfate →
         Signals fibroblasts to stop migrating and proliferating (entering
            maturation and remodeling phase)

3) **Maturation and Remodeling** (3 weeks to 1 year)
   Decreased cellular presence (mostly just collagen)
      Apoptosis of blood vessels, fibroblasts, and myofibroblasts
   Maximum collagen synthesis occurs at **3 weeks →** net amount then
      does not change although production + degradation occurs
   Type III collagen replaced w/ **Type I**
   Collagen cross-linking occurs along **tension lines**
   ↓ed vascularity
   At 8-12 weeks wound strength is 80% normal (most it ever gets)

Macrophages – most essential cell in wound healing (growth factors, cytokines)
Fibronectin – chemotactic for macrophages and fibroblasts
Thrombin and fibrin – act as growth factors for endothelial cells, fibroblasts
Accelerated wound healing – reopening a wound results in quicker healing the
   2nd time (healing cells there already)
Myofibroblasts
   Fibroblast w/ smooth muscle cell components
   Communicate by **gap junctions**
   Involved in **wound contraction** and **healing by secondary intention**
   Perineum (more redundant tissue) has better wound contraction than leg
When wound healing cells are no longer needed, they undergo **apoptosis**
Peripheral nerves – regeneration at **1 mm/day**

Order of cell arrival in wound
1) **Platelets**
2) **PMNs**
3) **Macrophages**
4) **Fibroblasts**
5) **Lymphocytes**

Predominant cell type by day

Days 0–2	PMNs
Days 3–4	macrophages
Days 5 and on	fibroblasts

Zinc and **Copper** – impt in many enzyme systems of wound healing
Phosphate – important for leukocyte **chemotaxis** and **phagocytosis**
(↓ed phosphate results in ↓ed ATP)

Epithelial integrity

Most impt factor in healing **open wounds** (*secondary intention*)
Epithelial cell **migration** occurs from wound edges, sweat glands, and **hair
   follicles** (#1 source)
Dependent on **granulation tissue**
Unepithelialized wounds leak serum and protein → **promote bacteria growth**

Tensile strength

Most impt factor in healing **closed incisions** (*primary intention*)
Depends on **collagen deposition** and **cross-linking**
Submucosa – strength layer of bowel
Weakest time point for small bowel anastomosis – 3-5 days
Tensile strength after wound healing never equal to prewound (80%)
At 6 weeks – wound 60% original strength
At 8-12 weeks – wound **maximum tensile strength** (80% original strength)
Suture removal
Face or cosmetic area – 1 week
Other areas – 2 weeks

Delayed primary closure

- wound left open for a couple of days to make sure it is not
infected, then close it primarily. There is a risk of abscess and wound infection
with this method

Collagen

I	**MC type in body**
	Skin, bone, tendons, **cornea** (not lens)
	Primary collagen in **healing wound**
II	**Hyaline Cartilage** → MC collagen in **cartilage**
III	**Granulation tissue**; blood vessels, fetal skin
IV	**Basement membrane, eye lens**, glomeruli
V	most interstitial tissue (associated w/ Type I)

Many other types

Collagen has **proline** every 3rd amino acid; also has abundant **lysine**
Proline residues must undergo **hydroxylation** *(prolyl hydroxylase)* and
   subsequent **cross-linking** which requires:
Alpha-ketoglutarate
Vitamin C
Oxygen
Iron
Hydroxylysine also undergoes cross-linking
Scurvy – vitamin C deficiency
d-Penicillamine – inhibits collagen cross-linking

Essentials for clinical wound healing

1) **Moist environment** (avoid desiccation)
2) **Oxygen delivery**
   Optimal fluids, no smoking, pain control, arterial revascularization if needed, supplemental oxygen
   Want transcutaneous oxygen measurement (TCOM) **> 25 mmHg**
3) **Avoid edema** – leg elevation, light compression
4) **Remove necrotic tissue**

Impediments to wound healing

1) **Bacteria >10^5/ cm^2** (wound infection) - ↓s oxygen content, ↑s collagen lysis, prolongs inflammation, inhibits epithelial cell migration, causes edema
2) **Devitalized tissue and foreign bodies** – retards granulation tissue formation, impedes epithelial cell migration
3) **Cytotoxic drugs** (eg cyclosporine, FK-506, 5-FU, methotrexate)
   Chemotherapy – has no effect on wound healing after 14 days
4) **Diabetes**
   Glycosylation of **inflammatory cells** slows chemotaxis and inflammation
   Glycosylation of **RBCs** impairs oxygen delivery
   Small artery disease impairs oxygen delivery
   Neuropathy – pts don't realize the wound (delayed Dx)
5) **Albumin < 3.0** = poor nutrition = poor wound healing
6) **Steroids**
   Inhibit macrophages, PMNs, and fibroblasts
   Also ↓ **wound tensile strength** from ↓ed **collagen deposition**
   **Vitamin A (25,000 IU qd) – counteracts steroid effects on wound healing
7) **Wound Ischemia**
   Fibrosis (chronic scarring)
   Pressure (sacral or calcaneus decubitus ulcers)
   Poor arterial inflow or venous outflow
   Smoking
   Previous XRT
   Edema

Diseases w/ abnormal wound healing

Osteogenesis imperfecta   **Type I collagen defect**
Ehlers-Danlos syndrome (10+ types)   **Collagen defects** (many)
Epidermolysis bullosa   **Excessive fibroblasts**
     Tx: phenytoin
Scurvy   **Vit C deficiency**
Pyoderma gangrenosum   **Immune dysfunction**
Marfan's syndrome (*minimal effect* on healing)   **Fibrillin defect**

Other wound healing

Scars – proteoglycans, hyaluronic acid, and water (may take a while for this to get replaced w/ Type I collagen)
   Scar revision – wait for 1 year for maturation; may improve w/ age
Infants can heal with little or no scarring
Cartilage – no blood vessels (get nutrients and oxygen by diffusion)
Denervation – no effect on wound healing
Malnutrition – MC immune deficiency
Diabetic foot ulcers – **Charcot's joint** (2nd MTP joint) and **heel** MC sites
   Neuropathy leads to pressure ischemia + necrosis (see Vascular chp)
Leg ulcers – 90% due to **venous insufficiency** (see Vascular chp)
Pressure sores – see Skin and Soft Tissue chp

Wound dehiscence

RFs – deep wound infection (*largest RF*), poor nutrition, COPD, cougher, DM, PNA, stroke, emergency surgery, long operative time, prolonged ventilation

If fascial sutures have pulled through→ back to OR, place retention sutures

Tx:

> **Examine fascia** for signs of infection
>> Examine anastomoses (if present) for leak
>> Run the small bowel looking for leaks
>> Send cultures of fluid and fascia
>
> Figure of 8 stitches (0-PDS sutures, 1cm intervals and 1 cm back on fascia)
> Retention sutures (0 nylon 3 cm back at 3 cm intervals – full thickness
>> missing the peritoneum, rubber booties to protect the skin)
>
> Leave the skin open to heal by secondary intention
> WTD dressings TID

Wound drainage post-op

DDx: Dehiscence (or evisceration), necrotizing fascitis, wound infection, seroma, urine leak, bowel or anastomotic leak (< 7 days), fistula (≥ 7 days)

For all post-op drainage:

> 1) Drape pt out and evaluate wound every time
> 2) Pull out a few staples or look into opening to **assess fascia:**
>> **Sutures pulled through** fascia **→ dehiscence →** laparotomy
>> **Fascia infected → possible necrotizing fascitis →** laparotomy
>
> 3) Assess and send **Fluid drainage**:
>> a) **Clear pink** or **salmon** colored **→** possible **dehiscence or just a seroma →** assess fascia
>> b) **Yellow + thick →** likely a **wound infection →** assess fascia
>> c) **Gray + foul smelling →** reop for **necrotizing fascitis**
>>> (see Infection chp)
>> d) **Green →** injury or leak from **small bowel** or **bile duct**
>>> **< 7 days** (this is a leak) **→** re-operate and fix problem
>>> **≥ 7 days** (this is a fistula) **→** conservative Tx if fascia is intact and no signs of 1) fascitis, 2) peritonitis (peritoneal signs) or 3) sepsis (see Small Bowel or Biliary System chp)
>> e) **Brown** (stool) **→** injury or leak from **large bowel**
>>> **< 7 days** (this is a leak) **→** re-operate and washout
>>>> After **LAR w/o ileostomy →** takedown LAR, place colostomy + HP or MF; leave drains – redo LAR when infection clears (*safest answer*)
>>>> After **right hemicolectomy →** takedown anastomosis and place ostomy + HP or MF
>>> **≥ 7 days** (this is a fistula) **→** conservative Tx if fascia is intact and no signs of 1) fascitis, 2) peritonitis (peritoneal signs) or 3) sepsis
>> f) **Clear yellow tinged →** likely **urine** (send fluid for **Creatinine**)
>>> (eg after APR, large pelvic tumor resection)
>>> **< 7 days →** re-operate and repair (see Trauma chp)
>>> **≥ 7 days →** place drain (or ostomy) and repair in 6-8 weeks
>> g) **Clear fluid after pancreatic surgery →** likely pancreatic fistula
>>> *Regardless* if early or late, **want conservative Tx** (pancreatic tissue too fragile and edematous post-op – would do more harm then good w/ re-op; see Pancreas chp)
>>> If 1) fascitis, 2) peritonitis (peritoneal signs) or 3) sepsis present **→** reoperate (washout, place drains)

If you re-operate – assess anastomoses, run bowel to look for enterotomies, assess fascia, find problem, send off cultures of fluid and fascia

If not re-operating– local wound care; abx's for 7 days

> If fistula - other specific measures depending on fistula type

> 7 days is a bad time to re-operate due to friable tissue and dense adhesions

> (↑ **iatrogenic injury**) **→** better to **reoperate at 6-8 weeks** (thin adhesions)

ADAPTIVE IMMUNE SYSTEM

Innate Immune system

Includes **inflammation + complement** systems

Cells - phagocytes (eg PMNs, macrophages), natural killer cells, mast cells,
eosinophils, and basophils

Defend host in a **non-specific manner**

Does not confer long lasting protection or immunity

Newborns – innate immunity has **poor phagocyte chemotaxis (PMNs +
macrophages); susceptible to **cutaneous infections** → **wash hands**

Adaptive Immune System

T cells – are presented non-self antigens by **APCs** (in lymph nodes, spleen)

B cells – recognize circulating non-self antigens

Generation of responses **tailored** to pathogen or pathogen infected cells:

    1) Involved in **cell mediated immunity** (along w/ innate immune system;
eg macrophage, cytotoxic T and natural killer cells)

    2) Responsible for **antibody mediated immunity** (B cells, humeral)

    3) Development of **immunologic memory**

Primary response – **slower** than innate immune system (takes days)

Secondary response (after memory established) – much faster

Newborns – have **IgG (from mother through placenta; *the only Ig that crosses
placenta*) and **IgA** (from breast milk); provide humeral immunity while
newborn immune system develops

T cells [maturation in Thymus, all have **T cell receptors** (CD3]

    1) **Helper T cells** (CD4)

        Functions:

            a) **IL-2** release - activates **cytotoxic T** and **natural killer cells**

            b) **INF-gamma** release (from T_H1 cells) - ↑s bactericidal activity of
macrophages (and other phagocytes)

            c) **IL-4** release (from T_H2 cells) - ↑s **Ab production** (B-cell divides,
forms many plasma cells) and **class switching** (IgM → IgG)

        T Helper cells (T_H) differentiate into:

            Effector T_H cells – secrete cytokines that interact w/ other leukocytes

            Memory T_H cells – can act later as effector T cells w/ **second
immune response** (immunologic memory)

        Effector T_H cell subtypes:

            T_H1 cells

Major cytokine produced	**INF-gamma**	
Main target cell	**Macrophages**	
Immune response	Cell mediated immunity	

            T_H2 cells

Major cytokine produced	**IL-4**	
Main target cell	**B cells**	
Immune response	Ab mediated immunity	

    2) **Regulatory T cells** (ie suppressor T cells, can be CD4+,CD8+ or both)

        Suppress immune response and helps prevent autoimmunity

        Regulate CD4 and CD8 cells

    3) **Cytotoxic T cells** (CD8+, activated by **IL-2**, cell-mediated immunity)

        Attack cells that are infected, damaged, or dysfunctional

        Have **T cell receptor** that recognizes and attacks specific non-self antigens
attached to **MHC class I** receptors (eg viral gene protein)

            CD8 protein on cytotoxic T cell stabilizes interaction

        Release **perforin + granulysin** (creates pores in target cell membrane →
cell lysis) and **granzymes** (activates caspase cascade → apoptosis)

        Cytotoxic T cells cause *nearly all* of the liver injury from w/ HepB infection

    4) **Natural killer T cells** (activated by **IL-2**, cell-mediated immunity)

        Not involved in T cell receptor and antigen-MHC class recognition

        a) **Attack cells** w/ **low expression of MHC** (missing self)

            Occurs w/ cell infection (esp. viral infection)

        b) **Attack cells** w/ **bound Ab** (have Fc receptor)

B cells (maturation in **B**one)
    Antibody-mediated (humoral) **immunity**
    Have a **B cell receptor** (immobilized Ab molecule that binds antigens)
    Recognizes antigens in their **native form** (<u>not</u> in processed form, such as with
        APC and T cell interaction)
    Once it encounters antigen (and is activated by T_H2 **cell**), it differentiates and
        divides into many **plasma cells** (live 2-3 d), which secrete **Ab's** to antigen
    10% of plasma cells become memory B cells
        Can be re-activated if pathogen re-infects host
        IgG secreted (as opposed to IgM) with re-infection (class switching)

MHC classes (major histocompatibility complex or HLA classes)
    MHC class I (A, B, and C)
        Interacts w/ **CD8 cells** (mostly cytotoxic T cells)
        Class I MHC found on **all nucleated cells** (not RBCs)
        Presents *endogenous* antigen from cytosolic protein breakdown or
            endogenous antigen pathway (ie viral proteins produced inside cell)
        Cytotoxic T cells → recognize and attack non–self-antigens attached to
            MHC class I receptors
        Single chain with 5 domains
    MHC class II (DR, DP, and DQ)
        Interacts w/ **CD4 cells** (*exclusively* T helper cells)
        Class II MHC found on **antigen presenting cells** (APCs)
            APCs include dendritic cells, macrophages, and B cells
            Dendritic cells are the most impt **APC** (present antigen to T cells)
        Present *exogenous* antigen (exogenous antigen pathway, eg
            phagocytosis of extra-cellular bacterial proteins)
        T helper cells (T_H cells) are **activated** by MHC class II-antigen complex
        2 chains with 4 domains each

Viral infection**
    Endogenous viral proteins produced inside cell
    Are bound to **MHC class I**
    MHC class I – antigen complex goes to cell surface, is recognized by CD8
        cytotoxic T cells
    Cytotoxic T cell then **attacks the cell expressing the complex**

Bacterial infection (extracellular)***
    Dendritic cells (APCs) engulf exogenous pathogens (eg bacteria, toxins)
        Migrate to T cell enriched lymph nodes
        Display non-self antigen coupled to **MHC class II** molecule
        This is recognized by **T Helper cells** passing through lymph node
    T Helper cells then become **Effector T_H cells** (see above):
        Effector T_H-1 cells – Secrete **interferon gamma** and activate
            macrophages which have already bound the antigen
        Effector T_H-2 cells – secrete **IL-4** and activate **B cells** which have already
            bound the antigen

**These pathways are the general mechanisms by which viral and bacterial infections
    are handled. There are examples of crossover between MHC class I and class II
    immunity, meaning viruses get presented through MHC II pathway and bacteria
    through MHC I pathway.

Intradermal skin test (eg PPD for TB) – used to test cell-mediated immunity
***Infections associated w/ defects in cell mediated immunity** – intracellular
    pathogens (eg TB, viruses)*

Antibodies (immunoglobulins)

IgM

MC Ab in **spleen**
Responsible for **primary immune response** (initial exposure to antigen)
Largest antibody - 5 domains and 10 binding sites (pentamer)
Activates **complement**
Opsonization for phagocytosis
Does not cross placenta
    If elevated in neonate – indicates **intra-uterine infection**
Primary Ab against **A** and **B antigens on RBCs** (ABO blood type)
    Causes **clumping** of RBCs and **thrombosis** w/ ABO incompatibility
Lack of IgM after splenectomy results in **overwhelming post-splenectomy infection** (OPSI, see spleen chp)

IgG

MC Ab overall (75% of all immunoglobulins)
Responsible for **secondary immune response**
Activates **complement** (takes 2 IgGs)
Opsonization for phagocytosis
Crosses placenta and provides protection in newborn period
    The only immunoglobulin able to do this
Impt in **antibody dependent cell mediated cytotoxicity** (ADCC eg natural killer cells, macrophages, and eosinophils – all have **Fc receptor**)
Associated w/ **Type II and III hypersensitivity reactions**

IgA

Critical role in **mucosal immunity** (MC immunoglobulin in mucosal linings)
Found in majority of **secretions**, Peyer's patches in gut, respiratory lining, saliva, intestinal juice, breast milk
Plasma cells release IgA, which is taken up by **epithelial cells** and released on mucosal **luminal surface** (eg gut, respiratory epithelium)
IgA **binds pathogens** to prevent adherence and invasion
    Coats bacteria so that it cannot bind to mucosal epithelium

IgD

Membrane-bound receptor found on B cells
IgD is expressed when **young B cells in the spleen are ready to be activated** and take part in the immune system

IgE

Involved in **Type I Hypersensitivity** and **parasite infections**
Type I hypersensitivity reactions (see section below)
    IgE molecule bound to surface of mast cells and basophils through **Fc receptor**
    Antigen binds to IgE, activating mast cell or basophil

IgM and IgG are **opsonins**
IgM and IgG activate (fix) **complement** (requires 2 IgGs or 1 IgM)
Variable region – antigen recognition
Constant region (Fc portion) – recognized by macrophages, PMNs, natural killer cells and eosinophils; Fc fragment does not carry variable region
All immunoglobulins have **2 binding sites** except IgM (has 10 binding sites)
Polyclonal antibodies
    Have multiple binding sites to the antigen at multiple epitopes
Monoclonal antibodies
    Have only one binding site to only one epitope

Hypersensitivity reactions

Type I – immediate hypersensitivity reaction
- **Ex**: **allergies** (pollen), **asthma, allergic reactions** (eg bee stings, peanuts, lymphazurin blue dye for SLNBx) and **anaphylaxis**
- Provoked by **re-exposure**
- **Mediator** – IgE
  - Antigen interacts w/ IgE bound to **mast cells** and **basophils**
- **Response** – Degranulation of mast cells and basophils
  1) **Histamine** <u>(main response)</u> → vasodilation + bronchoconstriction
  2) **TNF-alpha** → vasodilation + inflammation
  3) **Leukotrienes** (LTC_4, LTD_4, LTE_4, slow reacting substance of anaphylaxis → bronchoconstriction + inflammation
  4) **Bradykinin** → pain, pulmonary arteriole constriction
- **Effects:**
  - **Local effects** (eg allergies and asthma)
    1) **Bronchoconstriction**
    2) **Rhinorrhea**
  - **Systemic Effects** (eg allergic reactions, anaphylaxis)
    1) **Flushing**
    2) **Hypotension**
    3) **Respiratory compromise** (severe bronchoconstriction)
    4) **Angioedema** (swelling of face, neck and throat)
- **Tx:**
  - **Acute airway management** if necessary (eg angioedema)
  - **Epinephrine, anti-histamines** (diphenhydramine), **corticosteroids**

Type II – antibody dependent cytotoxicity
- **Ex: acute hemolytic transfusion reaction, hyperacute rejection, ITP**
- **Mediator** – IgG or IgM
  - IgG or **IgM** binds to **cell bound antigen** (or foreign cells w/ TXP hyperacute rejection or ABO transfusion reaction)
- **Response:**
  1) **Cell mediated immune response** to bound **IgG or IgM** via Fc receptor on macrophage, PMNs, natural killer cells, eosinophils
  2) Bound IgM or IgG **activates complement**
- **Effects and Tx:** (see specific disease process for above examples)
- Note - Grave's disease and myasthenia gravis are considered Type II but don't result in cytotoxicity

Type III – immune complex deposition
- **Ex: serum sickness** (eg anti-venom), **SLE**
- Large Antigen-Ab immune complexes deposited in vessel walls and induce inflammatory response
- Ab's are <u>not</u> bound to cell surfaces like Type II
- **Mediator** – IgG
- **Response** - rashes, arthralgia, fever, lymphadenopathy, splenomegaly
- **Tx: corticosteroids, antihistamines**, possible **plasmapheresis**

Type IV – delayed type hypersensitivity reaction
- **Ex: chronic rejection** (TXP tissue sensed as foreign), **PPD** (TB skin test), **graft versus host disease** (T cells in graft sense host as foreign), **contact dermatitis** (eg poison ivy)
- **Mediator** - T cell mediated immune response (*antibody independent*)
  - Takes **2-3 days** to develop (or years w/ TXP)
- **Response** (T cell mediated) - APCs present **MHC class II**-antigen complex to **T helper cells** → create effector T_H1 **cells** → activate **macrophages** which destroy antigen

Adaptive Immunity for Cancer Therapy

1) **IL-2** helps convert harvested **lymphocytes** into **lymphokine-activated killer** (LAK) cells after exposure *in vitro* to tumor antigens
2) **IL-2** helps convert harvested **lymphocytes** into **tumor-infiltrating lymphocytes** (TILs) after exposure *in vitro* to tumor antigens
3) **IL-2** therapy enhances endogenous T cell immune response to tumor
4) **Tumor vaccines** (ie CA antigens) are injected into the pt in an effort to stimulate **adaptive immunity against the tumor** (antigen engulfed by APCs, presented, etc)

Some success w/ melanoma for above

Other Immunology

Primary lymphoid organs – liver, bone, thymus
Secondary lymphoid organs – spleen and lymph nodes
Immunologic chimera – 2 different cell lines in one individual (eg allogenic bone marrow TXP)
Malnutrition – most common immune deficiency
Mast cells - main source of <u>histamine</u> in **tissues** other than stomach
Basophils - main source of <u>histamine</u> in **blood**
   Basophils are generally <u>not</u> found in tissue
Angiotensin-converting enzyme (ACE) – inactivates bradykinin

TRANSPLANTATION

Transplant immunology

Major transplant antigens – ABO blood type and MHC

MHC (Major Histocompatibility Complex)
> Thought to be the major factor leading to acute and chronic rejection
> **HLA** (Human Leukocyte Antigen) is the MHC form in humans
>> **HLA class I antigens:** HLA -A, –B, and -C
>> **HLA class II antigens:** HLA -DP, -DQ, and -DR
> **A, B,** and **DR** are used for kidney allocation
>> *HLA-DR* – *most impt antigen in donor/recipient matching*
> **Time on list + HLA matching** - criteria used for cadaveric kidney allocation in US
> Can place non-US citizens on TXP waiting lists and give them same priority as non-US citizens

ABO blood compatibility
> Generally need **ABO compatibility for TXP***
> Would cause **hyperacute rejection**
> **Recipient AB blood type** (ie has no A or B Ab's) – can receive Type A, Type B, Type AB, or Type O organs
> **Recipient O blood type** (ie has Ab's to A and B antigens) – need Type O organ
> *Non-ABO compatible organs have been transplanted w/: 1) pre-op plasmapheresis and IV-IG *or* 2) in recipients aged < 1 year

Crossmatch (lymphocyte crossmatch)
> Detects **recipient preformed Ab's** by mixing recipient serum w/ donor lymphocytes → would result in **hyperacute rejection** (termed *positive crossmatch*)
> **Indications:**
>> 1) **All kidney TXPs** and **pancreas TXPs** require pre-op crossmatch
>>> Every 3 months pt must send serum for potential crossmatching
>> 2) **Heart** and **Lung**
>>> If **PRA > 10%** *or* if specific HLA abs (-A, -B, or -DR) are identified pre-op, need pre-op crossmatch (see below)
>> 3) **Liver TXPs** do not require a pre-op crossmatch
>>> *(Liver TXPs almost never get hyperacute rejection)*

Panel reactive antibody (PRA) – used for either heart or lung TXPs
> Techniques identical to crossmatch; detects preformed recipient Ab's using a panel of typing cells
> Get a percentage of cells that the serum reacts with (0-100%)
> **RFs for high PRA** – previous transfusions, pregnancy, previous TXP, and autoimmune diseases can all ↑ PRA
> High PRA indicates recipient has Ab's against many pre-formed antigens and is less likely to find a compatible donor
> Can try to **reduce PRA %** (ie reduce circulating Ab's) w/ **plasmapheresis, IV-IG,** or **Rituximab**
> **If pre-transplant PRA > 10%** → need crossmatch before heart or lung TXP
> **If pre-transplant HLA -A, -B,** or **-DR Ab's** detected → need cross-match before heart or lung TXP

Rejection

1) **Hyperacute rejection** (minutes to hours after TXP)
    Preformed recipient Ab's to donor antigens
    This should have been identified w/ the **crossmatch**
    MC problem – ABO blood type incompatibility
    Results in:
        1) **Type II Hypersensitivity Reaction**
        2) **Complement** activation (from Ab binding) + **vessel thrombosis**
            (graft thrombosis usually occurs before Type II reaction)
    Sx's – organ turns blue and mottled, hemorrhages, edema, rupture
    Tx: remove organ and **emergency re-transplantation** (if kidney, just
        remove organ)

2) **Accelerated rejection** (within 1st week)
    Pre-sensitized recipient <u>T cells</u> (cytotoxic and T helper) to donor antigens
    T cell sensitization from previous transfusion, childbirth, previous TXP or
        autoimmune DZ
    Causes a **secondary immune response**
    Tx: ↑**immunosuppression** (eg pulse steroids, thymoglobulin, ↑
        maintenance drugs)

3) **Acute rejection** (1 week to 6 months)
    Recipient <u>T cells</u> against donor antigens (cytotoxic and helper T cells)
    T cells need **1 week** for APC recognition, to differentiate and to mount a
        response (reason for delay after transplantation)
    Tx: ↑ **immunosuppression** (eg pulse steroids, thymoglobulin, ↑
        maintenance drugs)

4) **Chronic rejection** (months to years)
    Specifically a chronic immune response to transplanted tissue
    Etiologies - MHC (Minor Histocompatibility Complex), others
    Effects:
        1) **<u>T cells</u>** (Type IV hypersensitivity; APCs → helper T cells →
            macrophages)
        2) **<u>Ab production</u>** (B cells)
    Different from chronic allograft vasculopathy
    Tx: ↑ **immunosuppression** (eg pulse steroids, thymoglobulin, ↑
        maintenance drugs) → <u>not</u> effective long term
    Re-transplantation is the only definitive tx

Chronic Allograft Vasculopathy
    Fibrosis or accelerated atherosclerosis of **internal blood vessels** of
        transplanted tissue
    Likely due to **chronic rejection of blood vessels**
    Impt problem (main mechanism of chronic rejection after Heart TXP)
    Tx: ↑ **immunosuppression** (eg pulse steroids, thymoglobulin, ↑
        maintenance drugs) → <u>not</u> effective long term
    Re-transplantation is the only definitive tx

Antibody mediated rejection
    Can occur at any time point
    Usually Ab's against HLA antigens
    Dx: serum **HLA Ab levels** and **C4d tissue staining** on biopsy
        (complement degradation product)
    Tx options: ↑ immunosuppression, IVIG, plasmapheresis, Rituximab
        (anti-CD 20, B cells), splenectomy

Immunosuppressive Drug Classes

1) **Calcineurin Inhibitors**

Cyclosporin (Neoral, CSA)

Binds **cyclophilin protein** and inhibits genes for cytokine synthesis (**IL-2**, IL-4, INF-gamma) blocks activation of **T- and B-cells**

S/Es: nephrotoxicity, hepatotoxicity, HUS, tremors, seizures

Undergoes **hepatic metabolism** and **biliary excretion**

Undergoes **enterohepatic re-circulation (reabsorbed in the gut)

Biliary drain will decrease levels and cause rejection

Trough level 200–300

Tacrolimus (Prograf, FK-506)

Binds **FK binding protein**; similar action as CSA (ie inhibits **IL-2**, IL-4, INF-gamma), 50 x more potent

S/Es: same as CSA

Hepatic metabolism (highly metabolized) - enterohepatic recycling much less of an issue

Trough level 10–15

****Generally, fewer acute rejection episodes than cyclosporin**

2) **mTOR inhibitors**

Sirolimus (Rapamycin)

Binds **FK-binding protein** similar to tacrolimus

However inhibits **mammalian target of rapamycin** (mTOR) pathway

Inhibits **response to IL-2** (instead of blocking production like tacrolimus) and blocks activation of T- and B-cells

****Is _not_ nephrotoxic** (chief advantage over CSA and tacrolimus)

3) **Anti-proliferative agents**

Azathioprine (Imuran)

Inhibits de novo **purine synthesis**, which **inhibits T cells**

6-mercaptopurine is active metabolite (formed in liver)

S/Es: myelosuppression, GI intolerance

Keep WBCs > 3

Mycophenolate (MMF, Cellcept) – same profile as azathioprine

4) **Steroids**

Inhibit **macrophages** and genes for **cytokine synthesis** (IL-1, IL-6)

S/Es – Cushing's syndrome

5) **Antibodies**

Daclizumab (Zenapax) and **Basiliximab** (Simulect)

Monoclonal anti -IL-2 receptor Ab's *(is not cytolytic)*

Used w/ **induction**

↓s acute rejection *without* ↑ *in infection*

S/Es - should not be combined w/ other cytolytic Ab's (eg ALG and ATG) → ↑ infection and ↑ mortality

Anti-thymocyte globulin (thymoglobulin, ATG, Rabbit Ab's)

Polyclonal Ab's directed against antigens on T cells (CD2, CD3, CD4, and CD8)

Used for **induction** or **refractory acute rejection**

Complement dependent opsonization of T cells (cytolytic)

Keep **WBCs > 3**

S/Es:

PTLD (see below)

Myelosuppression

Cytokine release syndrome –Ab's bind T cell receptor causing release of cytokines, results in SIRS reaction w/ hypotension, fever, rigors, and pulmonary edema

Pre-tx pt w/ steroids and **antihistamines** → ↓ed severity and ↓ incidence of cytokine release

↓ use since anti-IL-2R receptor Ab's

Anti-lymphocyte globulin (ATGAM, ALG, Rabbit Ab's)

Polyclonal Ab's - similar profile as ATG (cytolytic)

↓ use since anti-IL-2R receptor Ab's

OKT3 (monoclonal Ab to CD3) - Rare use now due to high incidence of cytokine release syndrome and PTLD

Malignancy related to TXP Immunosuppression

MC malignancy following TXP - skin cancer (MC squamous cell CA)

Post-transplant lymphoproliferative disease (PTLD)
2nd MC malignancy following TXP
Highest risk - **children** and **heart TXPs**
Epstein-Barr virus (EBV) mediated **B cell proliferation**
Mechanism - calcineurin inhibitors, anti-T cell Ab's, and anti-proliferative
agents ↓ **suppressor T cell population** so **B cell proliferation** after
EBV infection goes unchecked → can progress to Non-Hodgkins
Lymphoma
Tx: **Significant lowering or withdrawal of immunosuppression**
CHOP-R (± XRT) for NHL (see Spleen chp)

Infections following transplantation

1st month
*   *****Bacterial** (MC, 80%) - related to surgery (eg UTI,
PNA, line infection)
CMV (15%)
Non CMV viral* and fungal** (5%)

2-6 months
*   *****CMV** (MC, 60%)
Bacterial (30%) -
Community acquired PNA + UTI's
Non CMV viral* and fungal** (10%)

> 6 months
*   *****CMV** (45%)
*****Bacterial** (45%) - community acquired PNA, UTI's
Non CMV viral* and fungal** (10%)

*EBV, varicella (Zoster) HSV, adenovirus
**PCP (bactrim Px), aspergillus, nocardia, toxoplasmosis, cryptococcus, candida
Highest risk period for any infection – 1st month
Lowest risk period for any infection - > 6 months

Cytomegalovirus infection (CMV)
Transmitted via **leukocytes** (use leukoreduced or CMV negative blood)
MC infectious agent in TXP recipients
Causes PNA, gastritis, colitis, ophthalmitis, and mononucleosis
MC manifestation - febrile mononucleosis (sore throat, adenopathy)
Most deadly form - CMV pneumonitis
Bx - characteristic **cellular inclusion bodies**
Tx:
Gangciclovir
Usually given prophylactically in TXP pts
S/Es – CNS toxicity, bone marrow suppression
CMV-IVIG (CMV immunoglobulin)
Given for severe infections
Also given after TXP for CMV negative recipient and CMV
positive donor
S/Es – N/V, flushing
Varicella (Zoster) – dissemination can be life-threatening
Tx: acyclovir, IVIG, ↓ immunosuppression
HSV – Tx: acyclovir

Kidney transplantation

MC etiology for ESRD leading to kidney TXP – Diabetes

Contraindications

Severe cardiac, pulmonary or hepatic insufficiency

Recent CA, active substance abuse, poor compliance

Not a contraindication - HIV infection

Donor Kidney (cadaveric or living donor)

Can store **48 hours**

UTI in donor – can still use kidney

Acute ↑ in creatinine (1.0–3.0) – can still use kidney

Attach to **iliac vessels** w/ **ureteral-bladder anastomosis**

Cx's

MCC Postop Oliguria	ATN (**path** → dilation and loss of tubules)
MCC Postop Diuresis	High urea and glucose pre-TXP
MCC new Proteinuria	Renal vein thrombosis (Dx – U/S)
MCC Postop Diabetes	S/E of CSA or FK, steroids

Urine leaks (MC complication)

Sx's: ↓ed UOP <u>early</u> (1st week), ↑Cr

Dx: Duplex U/S – hypoechoic mass early, aspirate fluid (shows ↑Cr)

Tx: percutaneous drainage + stent *(best Tx);* reop if that fails

Renal artery stenosis (or thrombosis)

Sx's: ↓ed UOP, ↑Cr

Dx: Duplex U/S – shows flow acceleration, narrowing at anastomosis

Tx: PTA + stent [also the Tx for **renal vein stenosis** (less common)]

Lymphocele – MCC of **external compression** (MC 3 weeks after TXP)

Sx's: ↓ed UOP <u>late</u> (**compression of ureters**); ± pain

Dx: Duplex U/S - hypoechoic mass, hydronephrosis from ureter
compression, good graft perfusion, fluid has normal Cr

Tx: **1st** – percutaneous drainage

2nd – If that fails need **intraperitoneal marsupialization** (95%
successful) → drain through window in peritoneum

Viral infections

CMV Sx's: PNA, gastritis, colitis

Dx (path); <u>inclusion bodies</u> (in **leukocytes**)

Tx: Gangciclovir

HSV – Tx: Acyclovir

Acute rejection

MC 1 week to 6 months

Dx: Duplex U/S and renal Bx

Path – tubulitis (vasculitis w/ severe form)

Tx: pulse steroids, other immunosuppressive agents (eg Daclizumab)

Repeat Bx after tx to make sure rejection is cleared

Chronic rejection – usually don't see until after 1 year; no good Tx

MCC mortality after kidney TXP – myocardial infarction

5-year graft survival – 75% (cadaveric 70%, living donors 80%)

Median survival – 15-20 years (Kidney TXP **extends survival 15 years**)

S/P kidney TXP, now w/ **↑Cr** or **↓UOP** post-op →

DDx – acute rejection, vascular problem, urine leak w/ compression,
lymphocele (late)

Initial Tx - Try **fluid challenge, lasix trial, or both;** check bladder catheter

Dx and Tx:

Duplex U/S w/ **biopsy** *(best test)*

Check for vascular problem, urine leak, acute rejection

Empiric ↓ in **CSA or FK** (these can be nephrotoxic)

Pulse steroids (often empirically given); further Tx based on cause

Living kidney donors

MC Cx – wound infection (1%); **MCC of death** – fatal PE

The remaining kidney hypertrophies

Contraindications to living kidney donation – cardiovascular DZ (eg
uncontrollable HTN), DM, HIV, current cocaine usage, Hep B and C,
concurrent CA, current infection

Dual collecting systems is <u>not</u> a contraindication to TXP

Liver transplantation

MC indication for liver TXP – chronic hepatitis from **Hep C**
   Children – biliary atresia

Contraindications to liver TXP
- **Current ETOH** (< 6 mos) or **other substance abuse**
- **Acute ulcerative colitis**
- Severe **cardiac or pulmonary insufficiency**
- **Poor compliance**
- Active **septic infections**
- **CA** (*except* hepatocellular CA, *see below*)

Some Hepatocellular CA can undergo TXP:
1) Single tumor <5 cm *or;*
2) $\leq$ 3 tumors, each <3 cm *or;*
3) Favorable histology (eg fibrolamellar)

Cannot have mets or vascular invasion; *No* cholangiocarcinoma
Not contraindications – HIV, portal vein thrombosis, recipient age

Donor Liver (cadaveric or living related)
- Can store **24 hours**
- **Macrosteatosis** (cadaveric)
  - Extracellular fat globules in liver allograft
  - Best overall predictor of **primary non-function**
  - If 50% of cross section is macrosteatic in potential donor, there is a 50% chance of primary non-function
- **Living related**
  - **MC for adult donation** - right portion of liver
  - **MC for pediatric donation** – left lateral (segments 2 and 3)
  - Donor liver regenerates to 100% in **6-8 weeks**

Liver TXP criteria for **acute fulminant hepatic failure:**
Acetaminophen Toxicity
1) **pH < 7.3** (regardless of other values) *or;*
2) PT > 100, Cr > 3.4, and stage III or IV coma
All other causes
1) **PT > 50** (regardless of other values) *or;*
2) Any 3 of the following:
    Age < 10 or > 40
    Halothane, drug, or idiopathic hepatitis
    Jaundice > 7 days before encephalopathy
    PT > 25
    Bilirubin > 17.5

Liver TXP criteria for cirrhosis: (see liver chapter for MELD score)
- **MELD score $\geq$ 15** more likely to get benefit from liver TXP
- **MELD score < 15** more likely to die from liver TXP itself than their underlying liver disease

Procedure
- **IVC sewn 1ˢᵗ**
- **Bile duct last** (after restoration of blood flow)
  - Duct-to-duct anastomosis, hepaticojejunostomy in kids
- Right subhepatic, right and left subdiaphragmatic drains
- **Biliary system** (eg ducts) depend on **hepatic artery** blood supply.
- **MC arterial anomaly** – aberrant right hepatic artery coming off SMA
- Considered **orthotopic TXP** (liver is replaced)
- Partial caval bypass needed if IVC removed (**piggy-back** technique does not remove IVC)
- **Tx of pre-op portal vein thrombosis** – thrombectomy or vein graft bypass to SMV or other portion of portal venous system at time of liver TXP

Cx's
- **Biliary Leak** (MC complication)
  - Tx: percutaneous drainage and ERCP w/ sphincterotomy and stent (across leak if possible)
- **Biliary stenosis** – ERCP w/ dilatation and stent

Primary non-function
   1st 24 hour
      Total bilirubin >10
      Bile output < 20 cc/12 hr
      PT and PTT 1.5x normal
   After 96 hours
      Hyperkalemia
      Mental status changes (lethargy)
      ↑ LFTs
      Renal failure
      Respiratory failure
   Dx: Duplex U/S and Bx to help figure out problem
   Tx: re-transplantation
Vascular Cx's
   Early Hepatic artery thrombosis
      MC early vascular Cx
      Sx's: ↑ LFT's, ↓ed bile output, fulminant hepatic failure
      Tx: Can try angio w/ PTA ± stent or reop
              MC will need **emergent re-transplantation** for ensuing
                 fulminant hepatic failure
   Late Hepatic artery thrombosis results in biliary strictures and
      abscesses (not fulminant hepatic failure)
   IVC thrombosis / stenosis (rare)
      Sx's: edema, ascites, renal insufficiency
      Tx: angio w/ thrombolysis, PTA and stent
   Hepatic vein thrombosis (rare)
      Sx's: ↑ LFT's
      Tx: PTA and stent
   Portal vein thrombosis (rare)
      Sx's: Early- abd pain; Late- UGI bleed, ascites, asymptomatic
      Tx: reop thrombectomy + revise anastomosis; possible re-TXP
   MCC Hepatic Abscess after liver TXP – hepatic artery thrombosis
Cholangitis – see **PMNs** around portal triad, not mixed infiltrate (DDx vs.
   acute rejection)
Hyperacute rejection – rare w/ Liver TXP; can be done w/ **ABO-
   incompatibility** (large reticuloendothelial system of liver absorbs Ab)
Acute rejection
   T cell mediated against **blood vessels**, MC in 1st 2 months after TXP
   Sx's: fever, jaundice, ↓ bile output
   Dx: ↑ WBCs, ↑ LFTs, and ↑ PT; get **liver Bx** (duplex U/S + Bx)
   Path:
      Portal venous lymphocytosis
      Endothelitis (mixed infiltrate, not just PMNs)
      Bile duct injury
   Tx: pulse steroids; other immunosuppressive agents
Chronic rejection
   **very low chronic rejection compared to other TXPs (only 5%)
   Path
      Disappearing bile ducts (abs + cellular attack on bile ducts)
      ↑ **alk phos**, portal fibrosis
   RFs for chronic rejection - ↑ acute rejection episodes (biggest RF)
   S/P liver TXP, now w/ ↑ed LFTs or ↓ed bile output early post-op →
      Dx: Duplex U/S w/ Liver Bx (best test; will Dx vascular problem,
      acute rejection, primary non-function, bile leak)]
5-year survival – 70%
   Median Survival – 15-20 years
   APACHE score – best predictor of 1-year survival
   ETOH – 20% will start drinking again (recidivism)
   Retransplantation rate – 20%
Living Liver Donor – 10% complication rate (MC bile leak), Mortality < 1%
Recurrence of primary biliary cirrhosis – 20%
Recurrence primary sclerosing cholangitis – 20%

Hepatitis B Recipient

Tx: **HBIG** (hepatitis B immunoglobulin) and **lamivudine** (protease inhibitor) post-op to prevent reinfection → reduces reinfection rate to 20%

Hepatitis C Recipient

Disease most likely to recur in the new liver allograft

Reinfects *essentially all* grafts (no immunoglobulin exists); usually indolent

Heart transplantation

Indications - life expectancy <1 year

Can store heart for **6 hours**

Persistent pulmonary hypertension after heart TXP (↑s mortality)

Tx: prostacyclin (inhaled or intravenous), inhaled NO, ECMO if severe

MCC early mortality (< 1 year) – infection

MCC late mortality (> 5 years) – chronic allograft vasculopathy (**accelerated atherosclerosis** of **small coronary vessels** – can't bypass w/ CABG)

MCC mortality overall – chronic allograft vasculopathy

Acute rejection – **perivascular infiltrate** w/ increasing grades of **myocyte inflammation and necrosis**

High risk of **silent MI** due to **vagal denervation** after heart TXP

Median Survival – 10 years

Lung transplantation

Indications - life expectancy <1 year

Can store lung for **6 hours**

**Absolute indication for double-lung TXP – cystic fibrosis

Exclusion criteria for using donor lungs – aspiration, moderate to large contusion, infiltrate, purulent sputum, $PO_2 < 350$ on 100% FiO_2

MCC early mortality (< 1 year) – reperfusion injury (primary graft failure)

MCC late mortality (> 1 year) – bronchiolitis obliterans

MCC mortality overall – bronchiolitis obliterans

Acute rejection – perivascular lymphocytosis

Chronic rejection – bronchiolitis obliterans

Median survival – 5 years

Pancreas transplantation

MC indication – type I diabetes and ESRD

90% of pancreas TXPs are combined **Kidney-Pancreas TXPs**

Need both **donor celiac artery** and **SMA** for arterial supply

Need **donor portal vein** (for venous drainage

Attach to **iliac vessels**

Most use **enteric drainage** for pancreatic duct

Take 2nd portion of duodenum from donor along w/ ampulla of Vater and pancreas

Perform anastomosis of donor duodenum to recipient bowel

Successful pancreas/kidney TXP results in:

Stabilization of retinopathy

↓ **neuropathy** w/ ↑ nerve conduction velocity

↓ **autonomic dysfunction** (gastroparesis)

↓ **orthostatic hypotension**

<u>No</u> reversal of vascular disease

Cx's

Vessel thrombosis (MC Cx) – very hard to treat

Rejection

Hard to Dx if pt lacks kidney transplant

Dx - ↑ glucose, amylase, or trypsinogen; fever, ↑ WBCs

Small bowel transplantation

Need high immunosuppression

↑ed incidence of **PTLD**

Rare graft vs. host disease (even though small bowel filled w/ WBCs)

Acute rejection – can present as diarrhea; Tx: ↑ immunosuppression

Bacterial Pathogens in Surgery

Gram positive Cocci (GPCs)
    Staphylococcus
        1) **Staph Aureus** (coagulase <u>positive</u>)
            MC organism in **SSI** (surgical site infection)
            MC organism in **VAP** (ventilator associated pneumonia)
                and **nosocomial PNA**
            Commonly involved in **nosocomial infections**
            Other infections – endocarditis, line infection
                Prosthetic hardware
                Toxic Shock Syndrome - exotoxin
                Staph scalded skin syndrome
            Have **exoslime biofilm** - adhere to prosthetic material
            Resistance to PCN – beta-lactamase
                Tx: anti-staph PCN (eg oxacillin)
            MRSA (methicillin resistant staph aureus) – have altered
                penicillin binding protein
                Tx: vancomycin
            20% of population are **carriers** (nares)
        2) **Staph Epidermidis** (coagulase <u>negative</u>)
            MC organism in **line infections** and **CRBSI** (catheter-related
                blood stream infection)
            Other infections – endocarditis, prosthetic hardware
            Have **exoslime biofilm** - adhere to prosthetic material
            Common skin organism - usually non-pathogenic
                Most frequent skin contaminant in blood cultures
        3) Other staph species exist – commensal skin organisms, potentially
            cause infection in immunocompromised
    Streptococcus
        1) **Strep pneumoniae**
            Infections – PNA, bacteremia, septic arthritis, endocarditis,
                cellulitis
        2) **Strep pyogenes** (Group A Beta-hemolytic strep)
            Infections – cellulitis, **necrotizing fascitis** (exotoxin)
            Can also cause **Toxic Shock Syndrome** (exotoxin)
        3) **Strep -viridans, -bovis, -sanguinous, -mitis** (endocarditis)
            MC organism involved in **endocarditis** - Strep sanguinous
    Enterococcus
        1) **Enterococcus faecalis**
            Resistant to <u>all</u> cephalosporins
            Common organism of gut (95% of population)
            Infections – UTI, bacteremia, endocarditis, diverticulitis
            Vancomycin resistant enterococcus (VRE)
                Mutation in **cell wall binding protein**
                Tx: Synercid or Linezolid

Gram Positive Rods (GPRs)
    Clostridium (anaerobic)
        1) **Clostridium difficile**
            Pseudomembranous colitis
            Normal colon organism (5% of population)
        2) **Clostridium perfringens**
            Gas gangrene (can cause early serious wound infection)
            Emphysematous cholecystitis
        3) **Clostridium tetani**
            Tetanus
    Corynebacterium (diptheroids) – can cause endocarditis
        Other infections – indwelling catheters, cellulitis

Gram Negative Rods (GNRs, can have **endotoxin**)

1) **H pylori** – ulcer disease
2) **Bacteroides fragilis** (anaerobic)
- **MC organism** in gut (colon)
- **MC anaerobe** in gut
- **MC organism** in **anaerobic peritoneal infections** (eg abscess)
- Infections – peritoneal infections, diverticulitis
- Can be resistant to variety of abx's
3) **E coli**
- **MC GNR in gut** (colon)
- **MC organism** in **UTI** (90%)
- **MC organism** in **biliary tract infections** (cholangitis)
- **MC organism** in **pyogenic liver abscess**
- Other Infections – peritonitis, bacteremia, PNA
- O157:H7 type – food poisoning, HUS
4) **Enterobacter aerogenes, -cloacae**
- Infections – UTI, PNA, VAP, CRBSI, SSI (15% MDR)
- Normal organism of colon (facultative anaerobe)
5) **Proteus mirabilis**
- **MC organism** in **struvite kidney stones**
- **Urease** production
- Infections – UTI, SSI, bacteremia, PNA
6) **Klebsiella pneumonia**
- Infections – PNA, aspiration PNA, VAP, UTI, SSI
- Common **nosocomial infection**
7) **Serratia marcescens**
- Infections – UTI, bacteremia, SSI, PNA, VAP
- Common *nosocomial infection*
- *Resistant to several abx's*
8) **Pseudomonas aeruginosa**
- **MC lung infection w/ cystic fibrosis**
- **MC organism** in **burn wound infections**
- **MC colonizer** of **indwelling catheters**
- Form **alginate mucoid layer** (biofilm) – can colonize tubes
- Infections – VAP, PNA, UTI, burns, wounds, bacteremia
- Common **nosocomial infection**
- ***Difficult to Tx:***
  - **Low antibiotic susceptibility** overall
  - Can undergo ***acquired resistance*** during antibiotic therapy
9) **Acinetobacter baumannii**
- Infections - PNA, VAP (esp. late onset), UTI, bacteremia, SSI
- Can be **very difficult to tx** and cause **life threatening infections**
- ***Naturally resistant to many abx's*** (PCNs, aminoglycosides, often to fluoroquinolones)
- **Best Tx:** carbapenems (eg Imipenem)
10) **Stenotrophomonas maltophilia**
- Infections – UTI, line infections, VAP, bacteremia
- **Frequently colonize tubes** (eg ETT, tracheostomy, central lines)
  - → best tx is to remove tube if possible
- Can be **very difficult to tx** and cause **life threatening infections**
- ***Naturally resistant to many broad spectrum abx's*** (including carbapenems)
11) **Burkholderia cepacia**
- Important resistant organism in pts w/ **cystic fibrosis**
- **Colonization is *contraindication* to lung TXP in some centers**

Gram Negative Cocci (GNCs)

1) **Neisseria gonorrhea** – STD, septic arthritis
2) **Neisseria meningitides** – meningitis
3) **Moraxella catarrhalis** – PNA in COPD pts

Gut Flora

Stomach	Almost sterile few GPCs, some yeast
Proximal small bowel	10^5 bacteria mostly GPCs
Distal small bowel	10^7 bacteria GPCs, GPRs, GNRs
Colon	10^{11} bacteria 99% anaerobes few GNRs and GPCs

Anaerobes (eg Bacteriodies and Clostridium)
>**MC organisms in GI tract**
>**MC organism overall in GI tract** – Bacteroides fragilis
>**MC anaerobe in colon** – Bacteroides fragilis (30%)
>**Anaerobes outnumber aerobic bacteria** in colon (1000:1)
>**Need low oxygen content** – lack superoxide dismutase and catalase
>>(vulnerable to reactive oxygen species)

MC aerobic bacteria in the colon – E. Coli
Gram negative sepsis (GNR sepsis) – much of the pathogenesis is related to
>lipopolysaccharide (LPS, **lipid A**, *endotoxin*) layer in the cell wall
>****Lipid A** is the *most potent* stimulant for **TNF-alpha** release (→ SIRS)

Fever Source

Fever Source	MC Time Frame (post-op day)
Atelectasis	POD 1-2
UTI	POD 3-5
DVT	POD 4-6
Wound infection, medications	POD 5-7
Abscess	POD 7-10
MC fever source within **48 hours**	Atelectasis
MC fever source 48 hours – 5 days	Urinary tract infection
MC fever source after **5 days**	Wound infection

Post-op Fever W/U (after 48 hours)
>Look at wound
>Send blood, sputum, and urine cx's
>Change or remove central lines
>CXR – look for infiltrate
>Check WBC
>Consider Abd CT if post-op to look for abscess
>Consider duplex U/S to look for DVT
>**If under 48 hours** – likely atelectasis but make sure there is not a fast forming
>>wound infection (eg clostridium perfringens or group A beta hemolytic
>>strep)

Nosocomial Infections
>Infections acquired in hospital (> 48 hours after admission or up to 30 d after
>>discharge)
>****Hand washing before each pt contact most effective way of preventing**
>>**transmission**
>>**Judicious use of abx's** also impt
>**35% of all nosocomial infections can be prevented**
>**Nosocomial Infections:**
>>1) **Surgical Site infections** (SSI)
>>2) **Ventilator Associated Pneumonia** (VAP)
>>3) **Catheter Related Blood Stream Infection** (CRBSI)
>>4) **Urinary tract infection** (UTI, MC nosocomial infection, 80% E coli)
>**Highest risk pt group for nosocomial infections overall** – burn patients
>>Also highest specifically for **UTI, VAP,** and **CRBSI**

<u>Surgical Site Infections</u> (SSI, wound infections)

Comorbidity RFs for SSI - advanced age, COPD, renal failure, liver failure, DM, malnutrition, immunosuppression, obesity

Methods to decrease SSI

    1) **Pt factors**

        Do <u>not</u> operate on pts w/ **active infections**

        Stop tobacco (poor healing)

        Clippers to remove hair at surgical site (<u>not</u> shaving)

        Shower night before w/ abx soap

        Abx's 30 minutes to 2 hours prior to incision *and* for **24 hours afterward** (maintain **levels** during procedure)

            1st and 2nd generation cephalosporins usual

            ↓ infection risk 5 x

        Use appropriate **skin prep**

        Maintain blood glucose < 120-150 in diabetic pts

        Keep **PaO$_2$ high** during operation (use 100% FiO2)

        Keep **pt warm** (*best method* → warm air conduction, eg Bair Hugger)

    2) **OR staff factors**

        Exclude infected staff

        Staff scrub hands and keep nails short

        Wear a mask and cover all hair

        Use sterile gloves, gowns and drapes that resist fluid penetration

        Use CDC guidelines for definition and surveillance

    3) **OR**

        Keep OR doors closed

        Sterile instruments and avoid flash sterilization

        Avoid hypothermia (higher risk than previously thought)

            Keep OR temp 70 degrees

        Ensure appropriate operating room ventilation

    4) Procedure

        Avoid unnecessary tissue trauma

        Closed suction drains when appropriate

        Delayed primary closure for heavily contaminated wounds

        Sterile dressing for **24-48 hours**

        Minimize duration of operation (if possible)

        Ensure appropriate **hemostasis**

        Obliterate dead space to prevent seroma formation

    Notably, early foley removal does <u>not</u> matter for SSI but will ↓ UTI's

SSI Incidence

Clean (eg umbilical hernia)	2%
Clean contaminated (elective bowel rsxn w/ prepped bowel):	4%
Contaminated (stab wound to colon w/ repair)	8%
Gross contamination (perforated appendix):	30%

MC organism in SSI – staph aureus; others – staph epidermidis, E. coli

MC GNR in SSI – E. coli

MC anaerobe in SSI – bacteriodies fragilis

Dx of SSI – need ≥ 10^5 bacteria (less if foreign body present)

SSI within 24-48 hours of procedure →

    1) **Large bowel leak**

    2) **Virulent organism**

        a) **Gas gangrene** (clostridial myonecrosis)

        b) **Necrotizing fascitis** (MC - strep pyogenes, others - staph aureus)

        Takes as little as **6-8 hours for both**; both produce **exotoxins**

MC infection in surgical pt – UTI (MC - E. coli)

    Early removal of bladder catheters will ↓ UTI's

    Best tx of UTI - removal of bladder catheter (usually also give abx's)

MC infectious death in surgical pt – nosocomial pneumonia

Prevention of Hypothermia

    Warm **air conduction** (eg Bair Hugger),max temp 43.3 C, *best method*

    Warm **IV fluids** – max temp 65.0 C

    Warm room and **Blankets** around pt

    Effects of hypothermia - ↑ infection, poor coagulation, ↓ C.O.

Ventilator Associated Pneumonia (VAP)

MCC infectious death in surgical pts (25% mortality)

Criteria – hospital acquired PNA in pts on ventilator $\geq$ 48 hours (20% incidence)

MC nosocomial infection in ICU sub-population

UTI MC nosocomial infection overall

RFs – prolonged intubation, advanced age, pre-existing lung DZ, immunosuppression, malnutrition

From **aspiration** of exogenous or endogenous microbes in **oropharynx**

Sx's: fever or low temp, purulent sputum, and hypoxia

Dx: ↑ WBCs

CXR – new infiltrate

Tracheal aspiration or **broncho-alveolar lavage** – send for cultures

BAL or aspirate **> 10,000** (10^4) CFUs/ml = **pneumonia**

Reduction in VAP

Minimize duration of intubation (1% risk VAP / day)

Barrier techniques by staff attending to patient and wash hands

Elevate head of bed 30 degrees

Ventilator circuit change if contaminated (not routine)

Adequate drainage of oral and sub-glottic secretions

Oral hygiene w/ antiseptic

Avoid nasal intubation (sinusitis → PNA)

Daily sedation withdrawal – wake pt up

Avoid unnecessary abx's and transfusions

Stress ulcer prophylaxis w PPI

Tracheostomy when ventilation is needed > 7 days

Blood sugar control (80-120)

Not associated w/ reduction in VAP

Gut decontamination

Routine ventilator circuit changes (only change if contaminated)

VAP pathogens

Staph Aureus - MC organism overall in VAP

Pseudomonas - MC MDR organism in VAP

GNRs (MC class of organism in VAP) – klebsiella, serratia, enterobacter, acinetobacter

Tx:

Vancomycin + (3^{rd}gen. cephalosporin, fluoroquinolone, or antipseudomonal PCN); change abx's w/ susceptibilities

Bronchoscopy if critically ill, not-responding, or immunocompromised

Chest CT if failing to respond to Tx

Can cause **ARDS** (see Critical Care chp)

Hospital acquired PNA (or **aspiration PNA while in hospital**)

Pathogens – same as VAP pathogens; **Tx** – same as VAP

Community aspiration pneumonia

MC site - superior segment of RLL; other – posterior segment of RUL

Gastric fluid w/ **pH < 2.5** and **volume > 0.4 cc/kg** ↑s lung damage

Mendelson's Syndrome – chemical pneumonitis from aspiration of gastric secretions (RFs – ETOH, intubation, pregnancy) → gives ARDS picture

Dx: CXR - may <u>NOT</u> produce CXR findings immediately

Pathogens

MC organism – strep pneumonia

Others – staph aureus, anaerobes (Bacteriodies), oral flora

Tx: (3rd gen cephalosporin *or* fluoroquinolones) ± (clindamycin *or* flagyl)

Lung abscess can form

MC location – superior segment of RLL (see Thoracic chp)

CXR should resolve after **6 weeks** → if not worry about **lung CA** (Dx: chest CT)

Line infections

Sx's of line infection: ↑WBCs, fever, chills, erythema around site
- Can lead to CRBSI (see below)

MC organism – staph epidermidis
- others – staph *aureus* (#2), enterococcus (#3) yeast (#4), GNRs

Central line w/ lowest risk of infection – subclavian
- **Internal jugular lines** higher risk than subclavian
- **Femoral lines** higher risk compared to subclavian and jugular
- ***Contraindications to subclavian line*** – coagulopathy or ↓ platelets (incompressible area), pts in whom a PTX would likely cause death

↑ed length of time catheter is present → ↑ infection

Prevention:
- Wash hands
- **Chlorhexidine** for skin preparation
- Full barrier precautions when inserting (mask, shield, gown)
- Subclavian preferred site
- Remove when unnecessary

Tx:
- **Pt very ill** → change sites
- **Site looks bad** (eg erythema) → change sites
- **If not ill and site OK** → change over wire, send tip (5 cm) + blood cultures
  - **→ central line cultures > 15 colonies** → change sites
  - **→ positive blood cultures** → change sites
- **Does pt need the line?** → maybe get rid of it altogether
- **Infected peripheral IV site** – Tx: remove IV, elevation, warm compresses
  - **Suppurative thrombophlebitis** can occur (see Vascular chp)

Blood stream infection (BSI, bacteremia)

Primary BSI (MC) – direct inoculation of blood (ie intravenous catheter, CRBSI)
Secondary BSI – another site (eg urine, lung, GI) spreading to blood
Sx's: fever and rigors

These pts *do not* necessarily have sepsis
- Represents spectrum of DZ
- **Line infection → CRBSI → Sepsis** (see Critical Care chp for Tx)
- ****Sepsis = SIRS + infection**

CRBSI pathogens
- **MCC CRBSI** – staph epidermidis (coagulase negative staph)
- **Others** – staph aureus, enterococci, yeast, GNR (MC - E coli), strep

Dx:
- **Bacteremia** occurs **1 hour before fever**
  - **Fever** often occurs at same time each day
  - ***Get cultures 1 hour before fever time***
- Sometimes hard to Dx due to skin contamination
- **Higher risk of true bacteremia →**
  - 1) **Culture organism** – staph aureus, group A strep, enterococci, GNRs, strep pneumonia
  - 2) Growth **< 24 hours** after culture
  - 3) **≥ 2 positive blood cultures** for same organism
- **Lower risk for true bacteremia →**
  - 1) **Culture organism** - diptheroid or propionibacterium (<1% bacteremia)
  - 2) Growth **> 72 hours** after culture

Tx:
- **D/C line** if present
- **Empiric abx's** – 2 weeks; include vancomycin (MRSA) until cultures back
- **Staph bacteremia** – ECHO to R/O endocarditis as a complication
- **Attempting to tx through line infection** (eg dialysis catheter)
  - Abx's for 2 weeks
  - **50% line salvage rate overall**
    - 80% successful w/ **staph epidermidis**
    - 20% successful w/ **staph aureus**
  - **Less successful** - tunnel infection or associated clot

Necrotizing fascitis

Rapidly spreading infection involving **superficial** and/or **deep fascia** leading to **soft tissue + muscle necrosis**

RFs – DM, immunocompromised (HIV, CA), peripheral vascular disease, cirrhosis, ETOH, poor hygiene, malnutrition

Can present **within 6-8 hours** after **trauma or surgery** (_**rapid**_ wound infection)

Can also be **community acquired** w/ minor injuries involving fascia (eg stepping on glass); marine vibrio rare type (eg stepping on coral)

Fournier's gangrene describes involvement of perineum (see below)

Sx's:

> **Systemic toxicity** - 1) **N/V,** 2) **fever,** 3) **mental status changes** (lethargy)
> > **Hypotension** related to sepsis

> **Wound**
> > Edema, bullae, crepitus, rapid spread, drainage
> > Erythema that can progress to **purple**
> > If **deep infection:**
> > > → _overlying skin can initially look **normal**_
> > > → _get pain out of proportion to apparent cellulitis_

Path

> **Type I - Poly-microbial** (GPCs GNRs + anaerobes)
> > Often related to surgery; usually more delayed than below
> **Type II - Mono-microbial** (2 types)
> > 1) **Streptococcus pyogenes** (beta hemolytic Group A)
> > > 'Flesh eating strep'
> > > MC monomicrobial cause of necrotizing fascitis
> > > **Release exotoxins** (A + C → SIRS syndrome)
> > > > Major of source of **morbidity** and **mortality**
> > > **Infection → Fever → SIRS → MSOF → death**
> > 2) **MRSA** – also have **exotoxins**
> **Wound Bx for Type II** – _GPCs w/ **paucity** of PMNs_

Dx:

> ****_Clinical Dx_ enough to initiate surgical exploration**

> Following studies if pt not ill and trying to figure out problem:
> > 1) Percutaneous aspiration of necrotic center (gm stain, cultures)
> > 2) Blood cultures
> > 3) CT scan or MRI (tissue destruction, gas)

Tx:

> _**Take to OR for debridement immediately**_
> **Fluid resuscitation + broad spectrum abx's** until organisms isolated
> > **Isolated strep pyogenes** – high dose PCN G + clindamycin
> **Debride all soft tissue and fascia that looks bad**
> > Check bowel anastomoses (if previous surgery)
> > Run bowel to look for leaks (if previous surgery)
> > Send cultures of fascia and fluid
> > May require multiple debridements
> > May need amputation if extremity
> **Closure of previous incision →**
> > **Retention sutures** (0 nylon 3 cm back, 3 cm intervals, full thickness missing the peritoneum); rubber booties to protect skin
> > **Figure of 8's** for fascia if enough left (0-PDS 1cm intervals, 1 cm back on fascia)
> > **If you can't close primarily** (too much fascia taken)
> > > **Detach omentum** from colon and drape over bowel
> > > **Vicryl mesh** over omentum sewn to skin edges (this will absorb w/ time)
> > > **WTD dressing changes TID**; this will granulate over time
> > > > When granulation tissue present and pt stable, **STSG** (meshed) using dermatome; place over omentum
> **Massive skin and soft tissue debridement of extremity →**
> > WTD dressings changes (1/4 strength Dakin's solution)
> > When infection healed, place **STSG** (meshed)

Fournier's Gangrene

A type of **necrotizing fascitis** that affects the perineal region
Results in severe infection → 50% mortality
RFs – **DM** (*classic*), immunocompromised, poor hygiene, malnutrition, ETOH
Path – polymicrobial (GPCs, GNRs, anaerobes)
Sx's:
> Pain and redness in scrotum, penis, labia, perineum
> Crepitance
> Foul smelling gray discharge

Tx:
> **Immediate radical surgical debridement of fascia and soft tissue**
>> (try to preserve testicles; may need diversion of GI tract)
> **Fluid resuscitation + broad spectrum Abx's ASAP** (cover aerobes + anaerobes)

Clostridial Myonecrosis

From **muscle trauma** and **wound contamination** w/ clostridial spores
Need **necrotic tissue** w/ **low oxygen-redux potential** for growth of clostridium
> Clostridial infection implies *dead tissue* in area of infection

MC organism – clostridium perfringens
RFs – **farming** accidents, **CA, delay** in Tx
Incubation time – **6 hours** to 2-3 days
> Can cause **rapid, early wound infection** (can occur after surgery)

Sx's:
> **Systemic toxicity**
>> 1) **acute onset of pain**
>> 2) **fever**
>> 3) **mental status changes** (lethargy)
> **Wound**
>> 1) **Bullae**
>> 2) **Crepitus** (deep in muscle), skin discoloration (bronze)
>> 3) **Gray dish-water fluid** from wound
>> ***Pain may be <u>out of proportion</u> to cellulitis**
>>> Can be **deep infection**

Path
> ***<u>Large GPRs</u>** (long bacilli) and <u>**very few PMNs**</u>
> **Alpha toxin** – inserts into cell membrane, creating gap and cell lysis
>> Major of source of **morbidity** and **mortality**

Dx:
> *<u>Clinical Dx</u> enough to initiate surgical exploration**
> **X-ray** – gas dissecting into muscle

Tx:
> *Take to OR for debridement immediately*
> **Fluid resuscitation + abx's** (high dose **PCN G + Clindamycin**)
> **Debride all muscle and fascia that looks bad**
>> Fasciotomies if necessary, amputation if necessary
>> Check bowel anastomoses (if previous surgery)
>> Run bowel to look for leaks or necrosis (if previous surgery)
>> Send cultures of fascia and fluid
> Important concept here is that **clostridium only grows in necrotic tissue**
>> **(obligate anaerobe)** – something is dead (eg muscle, bowel,) and you need to identify it and resect it
> **Wound closure options** (see necrotizing fasciitis above)

Abscess
90% of **abdominal** abscesses contain **anaerobes**
> **MC anaerobe infection** – bacteriodies fragilis

80% of **abdominal** abscesses contain both **anaerobes** and **aerobes**
MC time frame: 7–10 d after operation
Tx:
> **Drainage** (usually percutaneously for intra-abdominal)
> **Abx's indicated for:**
>> Diabetics
>> Cellulitis
>> Clinical signs of sepsis - fever, elevated WBCs
>> Bioprosthetic hardware (eg mechanical valves, hip replacements)

> **Broad spectrum coverage** (include **Flagyl** for anaerobes)

Special abscesses
> **Lung Abscess** – 95% are treated w/ **abx's alone** (rarely need drainage)
>> MC related to aspiration (see Thoracic chp)

> **Pancreatic abscess** – need open drainage *(safest answer)*
>> Percutaneous drainage generally does not work for these

> **Splenic abscess** – Tx: splenectomy *(safest answer)*
>> Mortality rate 30%
>> **MC source** – endocarditis or IVDA

> **Peri-rectal or peri-anal abscess** – open drainage
> **Epidural abscess** – open drainage usual (esp w/ cord compromise)
> **Retropharyngeal abscess** – *airway emergency*, open drainage
>> Can lead to **mediastinitis**

> **Parapharyngeal abscess** – watch airway, open drainage
>> Can lead to **mediastinitis**

> **Liver abscess** – variety of causes (see Liver chp)
> **Suppurative Flexor Tenosynovitis** (flexor tendon sheath in finger)
>> Tx: Initially just abx's (see Orthopaedic chp)
>> Need **axial longitudinal drainage** if does not respond quickly

Pseudomembranous Colitis (Clostridium difficile Colitis)
Normal colonic flora altered by **abx's**, allowing overgrowth of C. difficile
Incidence – 1:10,000 pts receiving abx's (up to 3 weeks after abx's)
Sx's:
> **Pain** and **cramping**
> **Diarrhea** – watery, green, mucoid, foul (±.blood)
> **Fulminant colitis** or **toxic megacolon** (1%; colon $\geq$ 6 cm on KUB)
> Increased in post-op, elderly, and ICU pts
> Carrier state not eradicated → **15% recurrence**
> Can have **nosocomial spread** (eg nursing homes, hospitals)
> **Toxins A + B** cause **diarrhea** (both kill mucosal cells, A more damaging)

Dx:
> 1) **Stool ELISA** for **toxin A** (enterotoxin, *best*) or **toxin B** (cytotoxin)
>> Takes 2-6 hours; **repeat tests** if initially negative and suspicion high

> 2) **Stool cytotoxin assay** (<u>gold standard</u>; but takes 24-48 hours)
> Fecal leukocytes - not specific; Stool cultures - takes long time

Colonoscopy Key findings:
> 1) **PMN inflammation** of mucosa and submucosa
> 2) **Pseudomembranes** (**yellow** plaques; ring-like lesions)
> 3) MC in **distal colon**

Tx:
> **Fluid resuscitation**, <u>avoid</u> anti-motility agents
> **Abx's:**
>> **IV** – Flagyl
>> **Oral** – Flagyl or vancomycin (very expensive).
>> **Pregnancy** – **PO vancomycin** (<u>no</u> systemic absorption)

> **Lactobacillus**
> **D/C or change other abx's** (can Tx **empirically** if waiting for Dx results)
> Can get **toxic colitis** requiring hemi-colectomy (place colostomy and MF or
>> HP)

Fungal infection

MC organism in fungemia (fungus BSI) – Candida
> Other fungi can cause fungemia but <u>rare</u> (usually immunocompromised)

RFs:
> Use of **broad spectrum abx's**
> Fungal **colonization** (eg Candidiasis)
> **Immunosuppression** – chemo, bone marrow TXP, steroids, TXP drugs
> **Immunocompromised** – neutropenia, HIV, CA
> **Central lines**
> Others – dialysis, DM, severe illness, burns

Path (for fungemia or invasive DZ):
> | | |
> |---|---|
> | Candida albicans | 80% |
> | Candida glabrata | 20% |
> | Aspergillus | < 1% |

Fungal Tx Indications:
> 1) Positive **blood culture** (even just 1)
> 2) ≥ **2 sites** (eg urine and sputum)
> 3) ≥ **1 site w/ severe sx's**
> 4) **Endophthalmitis** (check eyes in any pt w/ suspected fungal infection – fundoscopic exam)
> 5) Pts on **prolonged bacterial abx's w/ failure to improve**
> 6) **Febrile neutropenia**

Empiric Tx: Anidulafungin (Eraxis, *best Tx*) or liposomal amphotercin

Candidemia
> **Tx:** Anidulafungin (Eraxis, *best Tx*) or liposomal amphotercin
>> Much lower toxicity than amphotercin w/ equal efficacy
>
> **Candiduria –** typically from colonization of catheter Tx: remove catheter, likely <u>do not</u> need to Tx w/ anti-fungals

Aspergillosis
> **RFs** – immunocompromised (neutropenia, TXP, steroids, AIDS)
> **Sx's:**
>> **Febrile neutropenic pt w/ new lung nodules** *(classic)*
>> **PNA** w/ **chest pain** and **hemoptysis**
>> CT shows nodules, halo, air crescent sign
>
> **Tx:** Voriconazole *(best Tx)* or amphotercin

Unusual fungal infections
> Rarely cause sx's (usually immunocompromised pts)
> **Tx for severe infections** → amphotercin usual
> **Types**
>> **Histoplasmosis** – pulmonary Sx's: Mississippi, Ohio River valleys
>> **Coccidiomycosis** – pulmonary Sx's: Southwest
>> **Blastomycosis** – pulmonary sx's + **skin lesions**
>> **Cryptococcus** – CNS sx's MC (meningitis, AIDS)
>
> **Actinomyces** (<u>not</u> a true fungus)
>> Pulmonary sx's MC
>> Can cause **tortuous abscesses** in neck, chest, and abdomen
>> Can be **confused w/ CA** (eg tortuous abscess in cecum)
>> **Path** – yellow sulfur granules
>> **Tx:** drainage + PCN-G
>
> **Nocardia** (<u>not</u> a true fungus)
>> Pulmonary and CNS sx's
>> **Tx:** drainage + bactrim (sulfonamides)

Surgical indications for fungal infection:
> 1) **Inability to R/O lung CA** (MC surgical indication; ie granulomas)
>> MC organism – Histoplasmosis, Dx: lung Bx or wedge resection
> 2) **Broncholith –** calcified granuloma (MC source – Histoplasmosis)
>> Sx's – hemoptysis; Tx: thoracotomy for resection
> 3) **Aspergilloma w/ persistent hemoptysis** (anti-fungals ineffective)
>> **Tx:** surgery (if pt can tolerate resection) or embolization
> 4) **Mucormycosis** (diabetic in **DKA** + **neutropenia** + coughing up **black pus** + lung **infiltrate**) - Tx ampho; resection if refractory and localized

Spontaneous bacterial peritonitis (SBP)

Occurs in pts w/ **cirrhosis** and **ascites**

Mortality rate – 30%

RFs – ascites fluid total protein < 1, previous SBP, current GI bleed

Sx's:

Fever and **abd pain** (peritonitis) ± N/V

Hepatic encephalopathy may be the only sx

→ Pts w/ **encephalopathy** need **paracentesis to R/O SBP**

Dx:

Fluid

1) **WBCs > 500** *or:*
2) **PMNs > 250** *or:*
3) **positive cultures**

Gram stain (less sensitive, more helpful for free perforation)

Fluid cultures negative in some cases

Path

Secondary to ↓**ed host defenses** (intrahepatic shunting + impaired bactericidal activity in ascites); *not due to transmucosal migration*

MC organism – E. coli (50%), others - pneumococci, klebsiella

**Should be mono-microbial → if not, worry about bowel perforation or abscess (need exploratory laparotomy)

Tx:

3rd gen. cephalosporin

Usually respond in 48 hrs

If not getting better - confirm your dx by repeating paracentesis or laparotomy if suspected bowel perforation or abscess

IV albumin – ↑s survival w/ SBP (1.5 gm/kg at Dx + 1 gm/kg on HD #3)

Liver TXP **not** an option w/ active SBP

Weekly prophylactic abx's after episode of SBP indicated (eg norfloxacin)

Pts w/ **bleeding esophageal varices** should also receive **prophylactic abx's for SBP** (high risk)

Polymicrobial infection (likely abscess or perforation) → laparotomy usual

Secondary bacterial peritonitis

Intra-abdominal source (eg perforated viscus, abscess)

Polymicrobial – *Bacteroides fragilis, E. coli, Enterococcus*

Tx: laparotomy to find source (usual)

Peritoneal dialysis catheter infections

Sx's: cloudy fluid, abd pain, fever

MC organism – staph aureus (70% GPC's)

Tx:

Intravenous – **vancomycin + gentamicin**

Peritoneal – **vancomycin + gentamicin**

↑**ed dwell time** and **intraperitoneal heparin** may help

Removal of catheter for peritonitis that lasts for 4–5 days

70% catheter preservation rate

Fecal peritonitis requires **laparotomy** to find perforation

Usually need to **remove catheter** w/ certain organisms (eg **fungus, pseudomonas, TB**)

Osteomyelitis
Path:
1) **Hematogenous osteomyelitis** – staph aureus
2) **Contiguous focus** →
    a) **Open fx or ortho surgery** – staph aureus, staph epidermidis
    b) **Diabetic foot** – polymicrobial

Sx's: fever, night sweats, bone pain (eg back pain)

Dx osteomyelitis
Needle Bone Bx *(best Dx test)* – not swabs of fistula or openings
Blood cultures – *only* 10% positive; more often w/ acute
Plain X-rays – shows changes after 2-6 weeks
CT scan – periosteal reaction; cortical and medullary destruction
MRI – can detect early changes
False positives w/ MRI *or* **CT scan**
    1) **Contiguous infection** w/ periosteal reaction
    2) **Charcot changes** (eg bony destruction, resorption, deformity)
Tagged WBC scan
    Usually for Dx of chronic osteomyelitis
    Highest sensitivity but not specific (false positive w/ soft tissue
        inflammation)

Tx:
Abx's for 4-6 weeks (wound Bx to figure out organism)
Surgery indicated for:
    1) **Diabetic foot ulcer** w/ osteomyelitis (debridement; see Vascular
        chp)
    2) **Open wound** w/ osteomyelitis
    3) **Acute or chronic hematogenous osteomyelitis** that fails to
        respond to medical tx
    4) **Cx's of pyogenic vertebral osteomyelitis** (cord compression,
        spinal instability, epidural abscess)
    5) **Infected bioprosthesis**

Tetanus Prophylaxis

Previous Vaccines	Clean, minor wounds	Contaminated wounds*
Unknown or < 3	Td only, <u>No</u> TIG	Td and TIG
3 or more^	<u>No</u> Td**, <u>No</u> TIG	<u>No</u> Td^^, <u>No</u> TIG

*   Contamination w/ dirt, feces, soil, or saliva; also puncture wounds,
     avulsions, GSW, crush, burns, frostbite, or > 6 hours old
^   Give fourth dose if only 3 give so far
**   Yes, if > 10 years since last dose
^^   Yes if > 5 years since last dose

Td (tetanus toxoid)
TIG (tetanus immune globulin) – give only to pts w/ contaminated wounds who
    lack appropriate immunizations (inject near wound)

Tetanus infection (Lockjaw)
Initial sx – facial spasm
    Followed by dysphagia, respiratory distress, apnea
    Can have fever and profuse sweating; muscle spasms
Mechanism
    Tetanospasmin toxin travels retrograde in nerve roots to CNS
    Blocks release of inhibitory neurotransmitter GABA → muscle spasm
Tx:
    Intubation, sedation and paralysis if needed
        → **tracheostomy** for lock jaw
    Flagyl (replaced PCN which can ↑ spasms) + **TIG**
    Debride wound
    Mg^{++} (can help w/ spasms)
    Diazepam

Viral hepatitis

All hepatitis viruses (A, B, C, D+B, and E) can cause:
  1) **Acute hepatitis** *and:*
  2) **Fulminant hepatic failure** (although <u>rare</u> for HepC)
  HepE causes acute hepatitis in **pregnancy**
  HepB, HepC and **HepD** can also cause **chronic hepatitis** and **hepatoma**

1) **HepA** (RNA)
   Serious consequences uncommon (**fecal-oral** transmission)
   Prevention w/ **HepA vaccine**
2) **HepB** (DNA)
   Blood or **bodily fluid** transmission (10% chronic infection)
   The only **DNA** hepatitis virus (**s** = surface, **e** = envelope, **c** = core)
   Infection
      Anti-HBc IgM is highest in first 6 mos, then **IgG** takes over
   HepB Vaccination
      Have increased **anti-HBs Ab's** <u>only</u>
   Example:
      Pt w/ ↑ed **anti-HBc, anti-HBe** and **anti-HBs** Ab's and <u>no</u> HBs
         antigens → pt had infection w/ recovery + subsequent immunity
   Tx:
      Interferon alpha + reverse transcriptase inhibitor (Entecavir) for:
         1) Proven HepB + continued ↑ed LFTs <u>*or*</u>:
         2) Acute fulminant hepatitis B
      HBIG (HepB immunoglobulin) **+ HepB vaccine** can ↓ mother to
         infant transmission 95% if given **immediately after birth**
   Prevention w/ **HepB vaccine**
3) **HepC** (RNA)
   MC viral hepatitis leading to liver TXP
   Blood transmission
   Can have long incubation period
   <u>No vaccine available</u>
   Path

Fulminant hepatic failure	rare
Chronic infection	60%
Cirrhosis	15%
Hepatocellular CA	5%

   Tx:
      Interferon alpha + anti-viral metabolite (Ribavirin) for either:
         1) proven HepC + continued ↑ed LFTs <u>*or*</u>:
         2) acute fulminant hepatitis C
4) **HepD** (RNA)
   Cofactor for HepB (needs HepB to cause infection)
   ****In combination w/ HepB, has the highest overall mortality rate of all
      the hepatitis infections** (20%; from ↑ed cirrhosis and ↑ed CA)
5) **HepE** (RNA)
   Usually self-limiting (< 1% mortality)
   Disease much worse w/ pregnancy
      Can cause **fulminant hepatic failure in pregnancy**
      MC in **3rd trimester**
      Up to <u>20% mortality</u> if associated w/ pregnancy
   Animals are thought to be a carrier

No surgery in setting of **acute hepatitis** (viral or ETOH) unless emergency (high
   mortality rate)

Human Immunodeficiency Virus (HIV)

Loss of **cell mediated immunity** due to low **T helper cell** (CD4+) counts
Then susceptible to **opportunistic infections**
RNA virus that has a **reverse transcriptase** to make DNA that gets
incorporated into host genome
Exposure risk

HIV blood transfusion	90%
Infant from positive mother	30%*
Needle stick from positive patient	0.3%
Mucous membrane exposure	0.3%

*HAART in mother and **c-section decrease** this to 1%
Testing – ELISA (looks for Ab) followed by Western Blot (detects HIV protein)
Tx:

HAART (Highly Active Anti-Retroviral Therapy)
Need ≥ **3 drugs** in ≥ **2 classes** of the following:
1) **Nucleoside** analogue **reverse transcriptase inhibitor**
(NARTI, eg didanosine)
2) **Non-Nucleoside** analogue **reverse transcriptase inhibitor**
(N-NARTI, eg efavirenz)
3) **Protease inhibitor**
Average life expectancy is 32 years from time of infection w/ HAART (vs.
9 years w/o HAART)
Noncompliance is reason most pts fail
S/Es – pancreatitis in many of these drugs
Post-exposure prophylaxis (eg needle stick from HIV pt)
1) **Begin HAART Tx <u>immediately</u> after exposure**
Within 1 hour (go to occupational health)
2) Usually 4 weeks of tx
3) ELISA at time of exposure and at 4 weeks
Opportunistic infections
MC indication for laparotomy in HIV pts
MC infection requiring laparotomy - CMV colitis
CMV colitis – MC intestinal manifestation of AIDS
Sx's: bleeding or perforation from **ulcers**
Tx: ganciclovir; surgery for perforation or refractory bleeding
Ulcers - need Bx to figure it out
HSV – **MC rectal ulcer w/ HIV**; can cause **proctitis**
HIV – can cause idiopathic mucosal ulcers (esophagus, rectum)
Lymphogranuloma venereum (rectal ulcers w/ adenopathy,
chlamydia); Tx: tetracycline
Non-Hodgkin lymphoma – can look like rectal ulcer or abscess
Toxoplasmosis – MC focal brain lesion in HIV pt (Tx – bactrim)
Neoplastic disease
2nd MC reason for laparotomy in HIV pts
MC malignancy requiring laparotomy – lymphoma (bleeding, perforation)
Lymphoma w/ HIV (usually NHL, 70% B cell)
**MC get solid organ lymphoma w/ HIV – <u>stomach</u> (#2 – rectum)
Tx: CHOP-R (± XRT) – see Spleen chp
Anal CA (squamous cell CA) - ↑ed in HIV due to HPV
May not tolerate Nigro protocol (immunosuppression) – possible
upfront resection
Condyloma accuminata – can grow very rapidly w/ HIV (felt to be low
grade verrucous CA w/ HIV) – Tx: resection
Kaposi's sarcoma– see purple nodule w/ ulceration (Skin,Soft Tissue chp)
MC CA in pts w/ AIDS
Rarely need surgery (want to palliate these)
Rarely a cause of death w/ AIDS; _exception_→intestinal hemorrhage
Tx:
HAART Tx usually shrinks AIDS related Kaposi's Sarcoma
Local Tx – XRT, intra-lesional vinblastine, cryosurgery
Systemic Tx (for disseminated DZ) – interferon, paclitaxel

GI bleeds w/ HIV:
>   **Lower GI bleeds** > upper GI bleeds
>   **Upper GI bleeds** – **Kaposi's sarcoma** (MC), lymphoma
>   **Lower GI bleeds** – **CMV** (MC), bacterial, HSV

CD4 counts
>   800–1200 normal
>   300–400 symptomatic disease
>   < 200 opportunistic infections

Bactrim or Pentamidine used for prophylaxis against PCP

Other infections
Brown recluse spider bites (necrosis from vasculitis)
>   Tx: oral **dapsone** *(avoid surgery early)* WTD dressings TID
>   **Late** – possible resection and STSG for large ulcers

Acute septic arthritis
>   **Etiology** – gonorrhea, staph, strep (check cultures)
>   Tx: **open drainage** and **3rd gen. cephalosporin + vancomycin**

Diabetic foot infections – GPCs, GNRs, anaerobes
>   Tx: broad-spectrum abx's (eg Unasyn, Zosyn)

Human bites – polymicrobial
>   **MCC** – **closed fist injury** (hitting someone in teeth)
>   **MC organism** – strep pyogenes (other strep species)
>   **Staph aureus** causes some of the most serious bite wound infections
>   ****Eikenella** – only found in human bites; risk for permanent joint injury
>   Tx: broad-spectrum abx's (eg Augmentin), tetanus

Cat and dog bites – polymicrobial
>   **Pasteurella multocida** – MC isolated organism
>   >   Only found in cat and dog bites
>   Tx: broad-spectrum abx's (eg amoxicillin-clavulanic acid), tetanus

Impetigo, erysipelas, cellulitis, folliculitis, furuncle, carbuncle
>   **MC organism** – staph; others - strep
>   **Folliculitis** – infection of hair follicle
>   **Furuncle** – boil (abscess of hair follicle); Tx: drainage ± antibiotics
>   **Carbuncle** – a multi-loculated furuncle (often have sinuses); ↑ed in **DM**

Sinusitis
>   **RFs** – NG tubes, nasal intubation, severe facial fractures
>   MC polymicrobial
>   Dx: CT head shows air-fluid levels in sinus
>   Tx: Broad-spectrum abx's
>   >   Rare to have to tap sinus percutaneously for systemic illness
>   >   Remove NGT if possible

Increased infection risk in diabetics due to →
>   1) **PMN dysfunction** (glycosylation ↓s chemotaxis)
>   2) **↓ed blood flow** – arteriopathy (narrowing of blood vessels)

Most commons
MC organism in gram negative sepsis – E Coli
MC organism in surgical wound infections – staph aureus
MC anaerobe in surgical wound infections – bacteriodies fragilis
MC fungal infection – Candida
MC infection in surgical pts – urinary tract infection
MCC of infectious death after surgery – nosocomial pneumonia
MC organism for nosocomial pneumonia – staph aureus
MC class of organism for nosocomial pneumonia – GNR's
MC organism in spontaneous bacterial peritonitis (SBP) – E. Coli
MC organism in line infection – staph epidermidis

ANTIBIOTICS

Mechanism of action

Inhibition of cell wall synthesis
Penicillins
Cephalosporins
Carbapenems (ertapenem, imipenem, meropenem)
Monobactams (aztreonam)
Vancomycin

Inhibition of small subunit ribosome (30S; inhibits protein synthesis)
Tetracyclines (doxycycline, tigecycline)
Aminoglycosides (**irreversible** inhibition of 30s; tobramycin, gentamicin, amikacin)
Linezolid (**irreversible**)

Inhibition of large subunit ribosome (50s; inhibits protein synthesis)
Macrolides (telithromycin, azithromycin, erythromycin)
Clindamycin
Chloramphenicol
Synercid (**irreversible**)

Inhibitor of DNA helicase (DNA gyrase)
Quinolones (ciprofloxacin, levofloxacin, moxifloxacin)

Inhibitor of RNA polymerase
Rifampin

Produces oxygen radicals that breakup DNA
Metronidazole (Flagyl)

Membrane depolarizer (leads to ↓ed DNA, RNA, and protein synthesis)
Daptomycin

Sulfonamides – has a PABA analogue which inhibits purine synthesis

Trimethoprim – inhibits dihydrofolate reductase which inhibits purine synthesis

***Bacteriostatic* antibiotics**
Chloramphenicol
Tetracycline
Clindamycin
Macrolides (telithromycin, azithromycin, erythromycin)
(all above have reversible ribosomal binding)
Bactrim

Other antibiotics considered ***bacteriocidal***

Aminoglycosides – have irreversible binding to ribosome and are considered **bactericidal**

Plasmids

Transfer of plasmids – MC method of antibiotic resistance

MDR (multi-drug resistance)

Examples of Beta lactamase type Plasmids:

1) **Penicillinase**
Resistant to PCNs

2) **Inducible AmpC Beta-lactamase** (**C**ephalosporinase)
Resistant to PCNs, cephalosporins, and monobactams
This enzyme is often **inducible** and resistance can occur during the course of treatment (eg serratia, enterobacter)

3) **Inhibitor resistant beta-lactamase** (extended spectrum beta-lactamase)
Resistant to PCNs w/ inhibitors clavulanic acid or sulbactam

4) **Carbapenemase** (ie **Zinc** metallo-beta lactamase); resistant to →
PCNs
Beta-lactamase PCNs (eg Unasyn, Augmentin)
Extended spectrum PCNs (eg Zosyn, Timentin)
Cephalosporins
Carbapenems
Can be very hard to tx
Tx: aztreonam

Most Commons
MC resistance mechanism for most **PCNs, cephalosporins, monobactams and carbapenems** – beta lactamase type plasmids

Exception– MRSA (see below)

MC mechanism for **gentamicin resistance**

Modifying enzymes leading to **decreased active transport** into cell

MC mechanism for **fluoroquinolone resistance**

Modified **DNA gyrase** (spontaneous mutations) – can't bind

MC mechanism for **macrolide resistance** (eg azithromycin, clarithromycin)

Modified **ribosomal subunit** (spontaneous mutations) – can't bind

MC mechanism for **metronidazole resistance**

Plasmid or gene for **nitroreductase** which catalyzes drug uptake and reduction w/o formation of damage inducing nitro-radicals

Methicillin-resistant *Staph aureus* (MRSA)

Resistance develops from **mutation in cell wall binding protein**

Vancomycin-resistant *Enterococcus* (VRE)

Resistance develops from **mutation in cell wall binding protein**

MDR *Pseudomonas*

Acquired mutations in **efflux pumps** which remove abx's from cell

MDR *Klebsiella*

Beta-lactamase type plasmids

MDR *Serratia*

Beta-lactamase type plasmids including **Inducible AmpC beta-lactamase**

Resistance can be acquired <u>during</u> the course of therapy

MDR Enterobacter

Beta-lactamase type plasmids including **Inducible AmpC beta-lactamase**

Resistance can be acquired <u>during</u> the course of therapy

Carbapenemase – can be very hard to Tx

Penicillins
Natural Penicillins (eg PCN G, PCN V)

GPCs – *Strep* species including Group A beta-hemolytic strep, *Syphilis*, *N. meningitides* (GNC), *C. perfringens* (GPR), *Anthrax*

<u>Not</u> effective for *Staph* or *Enterococcus*

Anti-staph penicillins (eg oxacillin, nafcillin, methicillin) - *Staph only*

Beta-lactamase resistant

A̲mino-penicillins (eg a̲mpicillin and a̲moxicillin)

Same as natural penicillins but also picks up *Enterococci*

Amino-penicillins w/ beta-lactamase inhibitors

[a̲mpicillin + sulbactam (Unasyn), a̲moxicillin + clavulanic acid (Augmentin)]

Broad spectrum

GPCs (*Staph, Strep,* and *Enterococci*)

GNRs

± anaerobic coverage

<u>Not</u> effective for *Pseudomonas, Acinetobacter*, or *Serratia*

Extended Spectrum Penicillins (eg ticarcillin, piperacillin)

GNRs

Enteric bacteria (eg *E coli, Enterobacter*)

Pseudomonas

Acinetobacter

Serratia

S/Es: platelet inhibition; high salt load

Extended Spectrum Penicillins w/ beta-lactamase inhibitors

Ticarcillin + clavulanic acid (Timentin); piperacillin + sulbactam (Zosyn)

Broad spectrum

GPCs (*Staph, Strep* and *Enterococci*)

GNRs (see above)

± anaerobic coverage

S/Es: platelet inhibition, high salt load

Beta-lactamase inhibitors – prevent drug breakdown

Carbapenems (eg meropenem, imipenem, ertapenem)
- **Widest spectrum** of all PCNs and cephalosporins
- **Resistant to beta-lactamase type enzymes**
- **Broad spectrum**
  - **GPCs** (*except* Enterococcus)
  - **GNRs**
  - **Anaerobes**
- Not effective for **MEPP**:
  - **MRSA**
  - *Enterococcus*
  - *Proteus*
  - *Pseudomonas* (which can develop resistance)
- **Cilastatin** – prevents renal hydrolysis of the drug and increases half-life
- **S/Es**: seizures

Cephalosporins
- *Cephalosporins are not effective for Enterococcus*
- 10% w/ PCN allergy have cephalosporin allergy
- **First-generation** (eg cefazolin, cephalexin)
  - **GPCs** (*Staph* and *Strep*)
    - Not effective for *Enterococcus*
    - Does not penetrate CNS
  - Cefazolin has longest half-life → best for prophylaxis
  - **S/Es:** can produce positive Coombs test
- **Second-generation** (eg cefoxitin, cefotetan, cefuroxime)
  - **GPCs**
    - Not effective for *Enterococcus*
    - Lose some *Staph* activity
  - **GNRs**
    - Effective only for community-acquired GNRs
    - Not effective for *Pseudomonas, Acinetobacter,* or *Serratia*
  - **± anaerobic coverage**
  - Cefotetan has longest half-life → best for prophylaxis
  - **S/Es:** prolonged PT
- **Third-generation** (eg ceftriaxone, ceftazidime, cefepime)
  - Not effective for *Enterococcus*
  - **GNRs**
    - Effective for *Pseudomonas, Acinetobacter*, and *Serratia*
  - **± anaerobic coverage**
  - **S/Es**: cholestatic jaundice, sludging in gallbladder (ceftriaxone)

Vancomycin (glycopeptides)
- **GPCs** – includes *Enterococcus,* MRSA, *C. difficile* (w/ PO intake)
- Binds cell wall proteins
- Resistance develops from change in **cell wall binding sites**
- **S/Es**: HTN, Redman syndrome (histamine release), nephrotoxicity, ototoxicity

Synercid (streptogramin, quinupristin-dalfopristin)
- **GPCs** – includes MRSA, VRE

Linezolid (oxazolidinones)
- **GPCs** – includes MRSA, VRE
- **S/Es**: low platelets, rare mitochondrial inhibition leading to lactic acidosis

Daptomycin
- **GPCs** – includes MRSA, VRE, *Corynebacterium*
- ****Not used for pneumonia** (*inactivated* by **pulmonary surfactants)**
- Mostly just for bacteremia and right sided endocarditis

Monobactam (eg aztreonam)
> **GNRs**
>> Effective for *Pseudomonas, Acinetobacter*, and *Serratia*
>> <u>Not</u> effective for *Enterococcus*
>
> Resistant to some beta-lactamases
> **S/Es** – toxic epidermal necrolysis (rare), hemolytic anemia (rare)

Bactrim
> **GNRs** ± GPCs
>> <u>Not</u> effective for *Enterococcus*
>> <u>Not</u> effective *Pseudomonas, Acinetobacter*, and *Serratia*
>
> **S/Es** (numerous): teratogenic, allergic reactions, renal damage, Stevens-Johnson syndrome (erythema multiforme), hemolysis in G6PD-deficiency

Quinolones (eg ciprofloxacin, levofloxacin, trovafloxacin)
> **GPCs** - 50% of MRSA is sensitive
> **GNRs**
>> Effective for *Pseudomonas, Acinetobacter*, and *Serratia*
>> <u>Not</u> effective for *Enterococcus*
>
> Good for intra-cellular pathogens (eg *Mycoplasma*) – enters cell easily
> Same efficacy PO and IV
> **S/Es:** tendon ruptures (esp w/ concomitant steroid use), peripheral neuropathy

Aminoglycosides (eg gentamicin, tobramycin, amikacin)
> **GNRs**
>> Effective for *Pseudomonas, Acinetobacter*, and *Serratia*
>> Synergistic w/ **ampicillin** for *Enterococcus*
>> **Beta-lactams** (ampicillin/amoxicillin) facilitate aminoglycoside penetration
>
> <u>Not</u> effective for anaerobes (needs O_2 to work)
> Resistance due to modifying enzymes leading to **decreased active transport**
> **S/Es:** reversible nephrotoxicity, irreversible ototoxicity

Macrolides (eg erythromycin, azithromycin, clarithromycin)
> **GPCs** and **GNRs** (best for community-acquired PNA and atypical PNA)
> **Erythromycin** also binds motilin receptor and is prokinetic for bowel
> **S/Es:**
>> Nausea (PO) and Cholestasis (IV)
>> **QT prolongation**
>> **Macrolides** and **statins** should be avoided (peripheral neuropathy)

Tetracyclines
> **GPCs** and **GNRs**
> <u>Not</u> used for serious infections due to high rate of resistance
>> (membrane pump that effluxes the antibiotic and altered ribosomes)
>
> Avoid in children < 8
> **S/Es**: tooth discoloration and growth problems in children
>> Faconi syndrome (acute tubular dysfunction)

Clindamycin
> **Anaerobes**, some GPCs
> Good for **aspiration pneumonia**
> Can be used to treat *Clostridium perfringens*
> **S/Es: pseudomembranous colitis**

Metronidazole
> **Anaerobes**
> Active metabolite – **ferredoxin** (creates oxygen radicals that disrupt DNA)
> **S/Es:** disulfiram-like reaction, **peripheral neuropathy** (chronic use)

Chloramphenicol
> **Anaerobes**
> **S/Es:** gray baby syndrome, bone marrow suppression, aplastic anemia

<u>**Effective for *Enterococcus***</u>
Ampicillin / amoxicillin
Gentamicin with ampicillin
Timentin / Zosyn
Vancomycin

<u>**Effective for *Pseudomonas, Acinetobacter, and Serratia***</u>
Ticarcillin / piperacillin, Timentin / Zosyn
3rd generation cephalosporins
Aminoglycosides (gentamicin and tobramycin)
Carbapenems (resistance can develop in *Pseudomonas*)
Fluoroquinolones
Double cover *Pseudomonas*

<u>**Appropriate drug levels**</u>
Vancomycin – peak 20–40 ug/ml; trough 5–10 ug/ml
Gentamicin – peak 6–10 ug/ml; trough <1 ug/ml
Peak too high → decrease amount of each dose
Trough too high → decrease frequency of doses (increase time interval
between doses)

Broad-spectrum antibiotics can lead to **superinfection**
MRSA Tx: vancomycin
VRE Tx: Synercid or Linezolid
Special Dosing:
levofloxacin – 500 mg PO QD
ciprofloxacin – 500 mg PO BID
piperacillin – 3.375 IV Q 6
Oral fluoroquinolones have the same bioavailability as intravenous

<u>**Anti-fungals**</u>
1) **Amphotercin** (polyene)
Creates **channels** w/ ergosterol in cell wall (causes cell lysis)
S/Es: renal toxicity (nephrogenic diabetes insipidus), hypotension, fever, ↑
LFTs, anemia, ↓ K+
S/Es less w/ **liposomal variant** (liposomal amphotercin B)
Used less since introduction of less toxic drugs w/ equal efficacy
2) **Anidulafungin** (echinocandin, Eraxis)
Inhibits synthesis of **cell wall glucan**
***1st line therapy for suspected Candidemia**
Used for serious ***Candida*** infections or **refractory *Aspergillus***
S/Es → Very few S/Es and equally effective as amphotercin
Spontaneous degradation, safe w/ renal or hepatic disease
Alternate – Caspofungin, **S/Es -** ↑ LFTs, less renal failure than ampho
3) **Voriconazole** (triazole, Vfend)
Inhibition of **fungal P-450** oxidase dependent synthesis of **ergosterol**
***Standard of care for invasive Aspergillosis**
Also used for **serious *Candida*** and other **fungal infections**
S/Es: visual disturbances, ↑ LFTs
Less renal toxicity than liposomal ampho (better tolerated overall)
4) **Itraconazole** (triazole, mechanism as above)
Broader spectrum than fluconazole
<u>Not</u> used for *Aspergillosis*
Can be used for *Candida, Blastomycosis, Histoplasmosis, and
Cryptococcus*
<u>No</u> CNS penetration
S/Es: ↑ LFTs
5) **Nystatin** – for oral thrush

Anti-tuberculosis drugs

1) **Isoniazid** – inhibits **mycolic acids** (cell wall)
   S/Es: hepatotoxic, peripheral neuropathy prevented w/ pyridoxine **(Vit B$_6$)**
2) **Rifampin** – inhibits **RNA polymerase**
   S/Es: hepatotoxic; GI symptoms; high rate of resistance
3) **Pyrazinamide** – inhibits **arabinogalactan synthesis** (cell wall)
   S/E: hepatotoxic
4) **Ethambutol** – inhibits **fatty acid synthesis**
   S/E: retrobulbar neuritis
5) **Streptomycin** – inhibits **small ribosomal subunit** (30S)
   S/E – ototoxicity, nephrotoxicity

Positive TB skin test (PPD, mantoux) → get CXR and sputum culture
Usually use 4 or 5 drugs initially for TB (**positive AFB sputum** or **high suspicion**) until sensitivities back
Total length of Tx – 9-12 months (need to make sure sputum converts to negative)

Antiviral drugs

HSV infection – Acyclovir (inhibits DNA polymerase)
CMV infection – Ganciclovir (inhibits DNA polymerase)
   S/Es: bone marrow suppression, CNS toxicity

Perioperative antibiotics

Prevents incisional wound infections
Need to be given between 30 minutes and 2 hours before incision

Antiseptic – antimicrobial that kills and inhibits organisms on body (skin)
   (eg chlorhexidine, betadine)
Disinfectant – antimicrobial that kills and inhibits organisms on inanimate objects
Sterilization – all organisms killed (eg autoclave)

Common antiseptics in surgery

Iodophors (eg Betadine) – GPCs, GNRs, poor fungi
Chlorhexidine gluconate (eg Hibiclens) – GPCs, GNRs, and fungi
   Better coverage overall compared to betadine type drugs

PHARMACOLOGY

Pharmacokinetics
Absorption
Sublingual and rectal medications – do not pass through liver first so do not undergo first pass metabolism

Skin – ↑ed **lipid solubility** increases absorption through epidermis

CSF– usually restricted to non-ionized, lipid-soluble drugs

Kinetics
0 order kinetics – constant amount of drug eliminated regardless of dose (increasing dose will not increase amount eliminated)
Enzyme and elimination systems saturated

1st order kinetics – amount of drug eliminated is proportional to dose (increasing does will increase amount eliminated)
Enzyme and elimination systems are likely not saturated

Need 5 half-lives for drug to reach steady-state

1) **Volume of distribution** = amount of drug in body divided by amount of drug in plasma (blood)
Drugs w/ a high volume of distribution have higher concentrations in the **extravascular compartment** (eg fat) compared to intravascular compartment

2) **Bioavailability**
Fraction of unchanged drug reaching systemic circulation
100% for IV drugs, less for other routes (eg oral)

ED_{50} – drug level at which **desired effect** occurs in 50% of pts

LD_{50} – drug level at which **death** occurs in 50% of pts

Drug Effects
Hyperactive – effect at an unusually low dose

Tachyphylaxis – tolerance after only a few doses

Potency – dose required for effect

Efficacy – ability to achieve result without untoward effect

Drug metabolism
Converts **lipophilic** (more lipid soluble) chemical compounds into more readily excreted **hydrophilic** polar products (more water soluble)
99% of the time this is associated w/ **detoxification** of drug

1) **Primary system** – hepatocyte **smooth endoplasmic reticulum** *and* **cytochrome P-450** mono-oxygenase system

Phase I (non-synthetic reactions)
Involves demethylation, oxidation, reduction, hydrolysis cyclization, and decyclization
Mixed function oxidases, requires **NADPH** and **oxygen**

Phase II (conjugation reactions)
Glucuronic acid (MC) and **sulfates** attached to drug
Form **water-soluble metabolite** (usually inactive) → excretion
Drugs excreted in bile may become **deconjugated** in intestines w/ **reabsorption**, some in active form (eg cyclosporin) → process is termed **entero-hepatic recirculation**
Pt w/ **biliary drainage tube** that bypass intestines will not have this reabsorption [eg kidney TXP pt requiring bile duct T-tube has acute rejection episode (↑ Cr, ↓ UOP) due to low cyclosporin levels]

Inhibitors of P-450 – isoniazid, ketoconazole, erythromycin, fluoroquinolones, metronidazole, allopurinol, verapamil, amiodarone, MAOIs, disulfiram

Inducers of P-450 – cruciform vegetables, ETOH, cigarette smoke, phenobarbital (barbiturates), phenytoin, theophylline, Warfarin

P-450 system can transform aromatic hydrocarbons to **carcinogens**

2) **Hoffman elimination** (does not rely on organ metabolism)
These drugs can be used in pts w/ liver or kidney failure without worry about toxic buildup of metabolites (eg cisatricurium)
Drug is metabolized in blood

Drug Elimination
- **Kidney** – most impt organ for eliminating most drugs (glomerular filtration and tubular secretion)
- **Biliary system** – may be subject to entero-hepatic recirculation (see above)
- **Polar drugs** (ionized) – more **water soluble** and more likely to be eliminated in unaltered form
- **Non-polar drugs** (non-ionized) – more **lipid soluble** and more likely to be metabolized before excretion

Important drug interactions
- **Albumin** – largely responsible for binding drugs (PCNs and Warfarin 90% bound)
- **Sulfonamides** (eg bactrim) – displace unconjugated bilirubin in newborns Cause kernicterus
- **Tetracycline** and **heavy metals** – stored in bone, avoid in children

Gout Therapy
- Due to **uric acid** buildup (end product of purine metabolism)
- **Colchicine** – anti-inflammatory; binds tubulin and inhibits migration
- **Indomethacin** – non-selective COX inhibitor
- **Allopurinol** – xanthine oxidase inhibitor, blocks uric acid formation from xanthine (nucleic acid breakdown); used in chronic setting for **overproduction**
- **Probenecid** – inhibits renal reabsorption of uric acid

Lipid lowering agents
- **Bile acid sequestrants** (in gut, **cholestyramine**, ↓fat absorption and ↓LDL)
  - **S/Es:** can bind Vit K leading to bleeding tendency
- **Cholesterol absorption inhibitors** [in gut, **ezetimibe** (Zetia) - ↓LDL]
  - **S/Es:** ↑ LFTs and myalgias
- **HMG-CoA reductase inhibitor** (**statins**, simvastatin, ↓cholesterol syn., ↓LDL)
  - **S/Es:** ↑ LFTs and rhabdomyolysis
- **Niacin** (blocks fat breakdown → ↓free fatty acids, ↓LDL, some ↑HDL)
  - **S/Es:** flushing; Tx: ASA
- **Fibrates** (eg **gemfibrozil** - ↑lipoprotein lipase → ↓TAGs, some ↓ LDL, ↑ HDL)
  - **S/Es:** myopathy and rhabdomyolysis increased when combined w/ statins

GI Drugs
Antiemetics
- **Promethazine** (Phenergan) – **dopamine receptor blocker**
  - **S/Es:** tardive dyskinesia, Tx: diphenhydramine (Benadryl)
- **Droperidol** – **dopamine receptor blocker**
  - **S/Es:** rare QT prolongation
- **Ondansetron** (Zofran) – central brain **serotonin (5-HT) receptor blocker**

Prokinetics
- **Metoclopramide** (Reglan, prokinetic) – **dopamine receptor blocker**
  - ↑ gastric motility and gut motility in general
- **Erythromycin** – can act on **motilin receptor** (pro-kinetic)
  - Motilin receptor is found primarily in **stomach** (MC – antrum), **duodenum,** and **colon**
- **Alvimopan** (Entreg) – **μ-opioid antagonist**
  - For post-op ileus (restores bowel function about 1 day earlier)
- **Methyl-naltrexone** (Relistor) – **μ-opioid antagonist**
  - Used for opioid induced ileus
- **Loperamide** (Imodium) – slows down gut by **stimulating μ-opioid receptors** in myenteric plexus; <u>no</u> systemic absorption
- **Omeprazole** – proton pump inhibitor; blocks H/K ATPase in stomach
- **Ranitidine** and **famotidine** – histamine H_2 receptor blockers; ↓ acid in stomach

Glucagon
- Tx of **hypoglycemia**
- Tx of **beta-blocker overdose**

Megestrol (Megace) – increases appetite in pts w/ advanced CA

Octreotide – somatostatin analog that is longer acting; **uses →**
1) Potent **splanchnic vasoconstrictor** (useful for GI bleeding, eg esophageal varices, gastric ulcers)
2) **↓s biliary, pancreatic** and **gastric secretions** (good for **fistulas**)
3) Carcinoid syndrome
4) Short gut syndrome
5) Chylothorax
6) Most metastatic islet cell tumors
7) Acromegaly

Vasopressin (DDAVP, Desmopressin) – used for:
1) Potent **splanchnic vasoconstrictor** (useful for GI bleeding, eg esophageal varices, gastric ulcers) – give NTG during Tx
2) **Refractory shock** (esp septic shock)
3) ACLS code drug
4) Release of vWF and factor VIII in von Willebrand's DZ and Factor VIII deficiency
5) Tx of diabetes insipidus (same mechanism as ADH)

Cardiac Drugs (also see ICU chp)

Digoxin

Inhibits **Na/K ATPase** and **↑s myocardial calcium**
↑ atrial contraction rate but **slows AV conduction**
Also acts as an **inotrope**
S/Es

> **↓ blood flow to intestines** – implicated in **mesenteric ischemia**
> Hypokalemia ↑s the sensitivity of heart to digitalis which can precipitate **arrhythmias** or AV block
> <u>Not</u> cleared w/ dialysis
> Other - visual changes (yellow hue), fatigue

Anti-arrhythmics for ACLS

1) **Amiodarone**
   First line drug for tx of atrial fibrillation, ventricular tachycardia, and ventricular fibrillation
   Cautious use in pts w/ pre-existing pulmonary dysfunction
   S/Es:
   > **Inhibits p-450**
   > **Pulmonary fibrosis** – w/ short or long term use (↓s DLCO)**
   > **Hypothyroidism or hyperthyroidism**
   > **↑ LFTs**

2) **Lidocaine** (see Anesthesia chp)
   Used for ventricular tachycardia or ventricular fibrillation
   S/Es
   > CNS (eg seizures) and cardiovascular collapse
   > CNS sx's occur at much lower levels then cardiovascular sx's

3) **Magnesium** – used to treat torsades de pointes (ventricular tachycardia)

Adenosine

Causes transient interruption of AV node
Good for **supraventricular tachycardia** (SVT)
<u>Not</u> used w/ Wolff Parkinson White (AV nodal re-entry; get heart block)

Atropine – acetylcholine antagonist; increases heart rate

ACE inhibitors (angiotensin-converting enzyme inhibitors, eg captopril)

Best single agent to ↓ mortality in CHF
Best single agent to ↓ mortality after MI
> Can prevent CHF post-MI
Can prevent progression of **renal dysfunction** w/ HTN and DM
S/Es
> Cough, angioedema (due to ↑ed Bradykinin), hyperkalemia
> Can exacerbate renal impairment in pts w/ **renal artery stenosis**

Angiotensin II receptor blockers (ARB)

Similar results as ACE inhibitors (although not quite as good)
Usually used when there is a contraindication to ACEI (eg cough)
(see Critical Care chp for ACE inhibitor and ARB mechanism)

Beta-blockers
  ↓ mortality w/ CHF _and_ ↓ mortality after **MI**
  ↓ risk of **atrial fibrillation** after cardiac surgery
Endothelin receptor antagonist (bosentan, ambrisentan)
  Oral pulmonary vasodilators used in pts w/ pulmonary HTN
Diuretics
  1) **Loop diuretics** [eg furosemide (Lasix), bumetanide (Bumex)]
      Inhibit Na-K-2Cl transporter
      Over-diuresis results in **metabolic alkalosis** and hypokalemia
  2) **Thiazide** [eg hydrochlorothiazide (HCTZ)]
      Inhibits Na/Cl symporter
      Over-diuresis results in **metabolic alkalosis**

  3) **Carbonic anhydrase inhibitor** [eg acetazolamide (Diamox)]
      Inhibits bicarbonate formation and reabsorption → leads to ↑ed Na
          and K excretion w/ concomitant water excretion
      Over-diuresis results in **metabolic acidosis** and **hypokalemia**
      Good diuretic choice in pts previously tx'd w/ lasix who developed
          metabolic alkalosis
  4) **Potassium sparing diuretics** (eg spironolactone)
      Inhibits Na/K exchanger (and Na/H exchanger)
      Over-diuresis results in **metabolic acidosis** and **hyperkalemia**

Diabetic Drugs
  NPH insulin – exposure to protamine after receiving NPH increases risk of
      protamine reactions upon exposure
  Metformin (Glucophage) – **1st line drug for type II DM**
      ↓s hepatic glucose production
      S/Es: should be held **at least 48 hours** before getting **IV contrast** (risk of
          lactic acidosis w/ temporary renal dysfunction associated w/
          contrast dye→ potentially life threatening)
  Sulfonylurea (Glipizide) – ↑s insulin release from pancreatic beta insulin cells
      S/Es: teratogenic
  Rosiglitazone (Avandia) – ↓s insulin resistance through up-regulation of
      peroxisome proliferator-activated receptors (PPAR)
      S/Es: ↑ risk of fractures

Chronic Kidney Disease (stage 5; chronic renal failure; end-stage renal DZ)
  Control underlying etiology (eg DM, HTN)
  Erythropoietin (epoetin) – ↑s RBC production (low epo production w/ ESRD)
  Phosphate binder - calcium acetate(Phoslo), sevelamer hydrochloride(Renagel)
  Vit D and **calcium**
  ACE inhibitors and **ARBs** can slow progression
  Avoid Mg^{++} containing compounds (eg laxatives) and K^{+}

COPD and Asthma drugs
  Inhaled corticosteroids (↓inflammation)
      Beclomethasone (Beconase), Fluticasone (Flovent)
      Combination fluticasone/salmeterol (Advair Discus)
  Inhaled Beta-2 adrenergic receptor agonist (bronchodilators)
      Salbutamol (Albuterol, short acting); S/E - ↑ HR
      Salmeterol (Serevent, long acting, maintenance)
  Inhaled Anti-cholinergics (bronchodilator)
      Ipratropium (Atrovent, short acting)
      Piotropium (Spiriva, long-acting)
  Leukotriene Receptor Antagonists (↓ inflammation, ↓ bronchoconstriction)
      Montelukast (Singulair, maintenance)
      Block LTC$_4$, LTD$_4$, LTE$_4$ (Slow-reacting substances of anaphylaxis)
      Not used for acute exacerbations
      Not used for COPD
  Oral steroids – for acute exacerbations
  Home oxygen – _only agent to improve survival in pts w/ severe COPD_

Anti-Inflammatory Drugs (NSAIDs)

Non-selective COX inhibitors
Inhibit both **constitutive** (COX-1) and **inducible** (COX-2) **cyclooxygenase** and **prostaglandin** synthesis (all reversible *except* ASA)

S/Es (dose-dependent):
1) **GI bleeding** (gastric ulcers and gastritis)
   Inhibition of prostaglandin synthesis leads to:
   - ↓ mucus and HCO_3^- secretion (↓ed protection)
   - ↑ acid production

   PPIs and **misoprostol** can be given for protection
2) **Renal insufficiency**
   Inhibition of prostaglandin synthesis leads to **vasoconstriction of renal afferent arterioles**
   PGEs usually keep the arterioles vasodilated
   Refrain from use in pts w/ ↑ed creatinine

Types - **naproxen** (Naprosyn), **ketorolac** (Toradol), **ibuprofen** (Motrin)
Indomethacin
1) Prevents pre-term labor
2) Helps close patent ductus arteriosus (PDA)
3) Treatment for gout and other inflammatory conditions

ASA (*irreversible* non-selective COX inhibitor)
S/Es (ie poisoning) – HA's, N/V
1st – respiratory alkalosis
2nd – metabolic acidosis

Selective COX-2 inhibitors (celecoxib)
Inhibit inducible form of cyclooxygenase (COX-2)
Expressed at sites of inflamed tissue
S/Es

Less ulcers and renal failure
↑ **risk of cardiovascular events** (2-3 x, eg MI, stroke)
↓s number of **polyps** in FAP

Colchicine – inhibits microtubule formation by **binding tubulin** (↓ inflammatory cell chemotaxis)
Misoprostol – PGE_1 derivative
A **protective prostaglandin** used to prevent peptic ulcer disease
Consider in pts on **chronic NSAIDs** (or just use COX-2 inhibitor)

Neuro Drugs
Haldol – **inhibits dopamine receptors**; good for **ICU psychosis**
S/Es

Extrapyramidal manifestations (Tx: diphenhydramine)
Prolonged QT syndrome (risk of ventricular tachycardia or fibrillation)
Clonidine
CNS acting alpha-2 adrenergic receptor agonist used for **HTN**
↓s cardiac output and SVR to <u>lower</u> blood pressure
Also used to help control ETOH withdrawal sx's
Zolpidem (Ambien) – **GABA receptor agonist** for **insomnia**
Tramadol (Ultram) – **CNS acting opioid**; used for **pain control**
S/Es – seizures (esp when combined w/ SSRIs); possible dependency
Gabapentin (Neurontin) – **CNS calcium channel blocker**
↓ glutamate and ↓ substance P
Used to tx diabetic **peripheral neuropathy**
Duloxetine (Cymbalta) - **serotonin-norepinephrine reuptake inhibitor** (SNRI)
Used for diabetic **peripheral neuropathy**

Metyrapone and aminoglutethimide– inhibit adrenal steroid and metabolite synthesis
Used in pts with adrenocortical CA

Infliximab (Remicade)

    Ab's to **TNF-alpha** (others adalimumab, certolizumab)

    Used for **inflammatory bowel DZ** (Crohn's Disease, Ulcerative Colitis)

    Contraindications – allergy to rodents, active infection, CHF

    S/Es:

        1) **Infection Risk** (MC serious complication)

            MC serious infection → tuberculosis

                ↑ed re-activation and ↑ed incidence of acquiring TB

                PPD placed before starting drug

                When treating pts w/ Infliximab who have a positive PPD,

                    isoniazid should be started as well

            Other infections – fungal infections, PCP, legionella, listeria

        2) **Abscess** can form when fistulas heal over with the drug (Tx: drainage)

        3) **Serum sickness** can occur after being on the drug for some time

        4) **Allergic Reactions** (10%; rash, chest tightness, dyspnea)

        5) **Progressive multifocal leukoencephalopathy** (PML) opportunistic

            viral brain infection; ↑mortality (↑ed risk w/ **interferon** co-therapy)

        6) **Lymphoma** – 6x risk compared to general population

Gadolinium (Gd) – used in MRI as a contrast agent

    Should <u>not</u> be used in pts w/ **renal insufficiency** (GFR < 60), buildup of **Gd^{+++}**

    S/Es: 1) **Acute renal dysfunction**

            2) **Nephrogenic systemic fibrosis** (fibrosis of skin, joints, eyes, organs)

               From Gd^{+++} deposition

Antidotes

Tylenol overdose	N-acetylcysteine
Digoxin overdose	Digibind
Benzodiazepine overdose	Flumazenil
Wilson's Disease (copper)	Penicillamine
Hemochromatosis (iron)	Deferasirox
(also chronic blood transfusion and	
thalassemia major)	
Lead poisoning	Dimercaptosuccinic acid

GCSF (granulocyte colony stimulating factor)

    ↑s granulocytes and stem cells

    Used to ↑ PMNs in neutropenic states

    (eg neutropenic -typhlitis, -mucormycosis infection, -aspergillus infection)

Xigris (Drotrecogin alfa activated)

    Activated protein C – thrombolytic used to prevent microthrombi in pts w/ sepsis

    S/Es: bleeding

    Indications (*many* requirements):

        1)   In **ICU** w/ **ICU attending**

        2)   **APACHE score > 25**

        3)   Evidence of an **infection**

        4)   **≥ 3 signs of SIRS** (see critical care chp)

        5)   **≥ 1 organ w/ dysfunction**

        6)   **therapy started ≤ 48 hours** after meeting inclusion criteria

        7)   <u>*Not*</u> used in children

        8)   **± heparin**

        9)   *Absolute contraindications* – active internal bleeding, recent

              hemorrhagic stroke (< 3 mos), recent intracranial or spine surgery or

              head trauma (< 2 mos), epidural catheter, intracranial neoplasms or

              mass, hypersensitivity to protein C

       10) *Relative contraindications* – many (all deal w/ ↑ risk of bleeding)

Induction

Can use either **inhalational agent** (MC sevoflurane) or **IV agent** (MC propofol)

Inhalational agents (volatile anesthetics)
- **MAC** (minimum alveolar concentration)
  - = smallest concentration of inhalational agent at which 50% of pts will not move w/ incision
  - **Small MAC** = more lipid soluble = more potent
  - **High MAC** = less lipid soluble = less potent
  - **Speed** of induction is inversely proportional to lipid solubility
    - Nitrous is fastest but has high MAC (and low potency)
- **Effects of inhalational anesthetics** (mechanism unknown)
  1) **Anesthesia** (unconsciousness)
  2) **Amnesia**
  3) ± **Analgesia** ($\downarrow$ pain)
  - Blunt **hypoxic respiratory drive**
  - Most have some **myocardial depression**, $\uparrow$ **cerebral blood flow**, and $\downarrow$ **renal blood flow**
  - **Short acting** (5-10 min) – redistributes into body fat and muscle
- **Types**
  - **Sevoflurane** (MC used inhalational anesthetic) – high cost
    - Fast onset, less myocardial depression, less laryngospasm
  - **Desflurane** – very pungent odor, irritates airways, not used to induce
  - **Isoflurane** – very pungent odor, irritates airways, not used to induce
  - **Enflurane** – S/Es: seizures (not used in pts w/ epilepsy)
  - **Halothane** – slow
    - Highest myocardial depression + arrhythmias
    - Least pungent (good for children)
    - **Halothane hepatitis** – fever, eosinophilia, jaundice, $\uparrow$ LFTs
  - **Nitrous oxide** (NO_2) – fast, minimal myocardial depression
    - Usually used as a carrier gas for sevoflurane or desflurane

IV agents
- **Etomidate** – few hemodynamic effects; fast acting (unknown mechanism)
  - Often used for **rapid sequence intubation**
  - Good anesthetic and amnesic properties, **no analgesic properties**
  - **S/Es:** continuous infusion leads to **adrenal suppression**
- **Sodium thiopental** (barbiturate, GABA receptor agonist) – fast acting
  - Good anesthetic and amnesic properties, **no analgesic properties**
  - **S/Es: hypotension**, $\downarrow$ cerebral blood flow
- **Propofol** – very rapid distribution and **on/off** (unknown mechanism)
  - Good anesthetic and amnesic properties, **no analgesic properties**
  - Metabolized in **liver** and by **plasma cholinesterases**
  - **S/Es: hypotension**, respiratory depression
  - Do not use in pts w/ **egg** or **soybean allergy**
  - ****Avoid in children** - prolonged use has been associated with **metabolic acidosis** and **death**
- **Ketamine** – dissociation of thalamic and limbic systems
  - Places pt in cataleptic state (**amnesia**, **analgesia**)
  - **No respiratory depression**
  - Good for **children**
  - **S/Es: hallucinations**, catecholamine release ($\uparrow$ CO2, tachycardia), $\uparrow$ airway secretions, $\uparrow$ cerebral blood flow
  - *Contraindicated* in pts w/ **head injury**

Rapid sequence intubation - used in pts w/ $\uparrow$ed risk of **aspiration**
- **RFs for aspiration** - recent oral intake, GERD, delayed gastric emptying (gastroparesis), pregnancy, bowel obstruction
- **Sequence:**
  1) **Pre-oxygenation** (tight fitting mask)
  2) **IV induction agent** (eg Etomidate, thiopental, Propofol)
  3) **IV paralytic** (eg succinylcholine or rocuronium)

<u>**Best indicator of successful tracheal intubation**</u> – ET-CO2 (end tidal CO2)
   ET-CO2 specifically reflects exchange of CO2 from blood to alveolus
   1) **Sudden ↑ ET-CO2** → MCC - alveolar hypoventilation (atelectasis)
      Tx: ↑TV (expands lungs, ↓s atelectasis) or ↑RR
   2) **Sudden ↓ ET-CO2** → MCC - became disconnected from the vent
      Others (associated w/ hypotension) – PE, CO2 embolus
   Endotracheal tube – should be placed 2 cm above the carina
   MC PACU complication – nausea and vomiting

<u>**Maintenance Anesthesia**</u>
   Usually combination 1) **nitrous oxide**, 2) **oxygen**, and 3) **volatile anesthetic** w/
      supplemental IV opioids and benzodiazepines
   Propofol can be used alone for maintenance
   Fentanyl + versed drips can be used for maintenance
   Dexmedetomidine (Precedex)
      Provides anesthesia and analgesia _without_ decreasing respiratory drive
      Good for **early extubation protocols** (eg cardiac surgery)
      Mechanism – CNS alpha-2 receptor agonist

<u>**Narcotics**</u> (opioids)
   Types - morphine, fentanyl, meperidine (Demerol), codeine, hydromorphone
      (Dilaudid), oxycodone (Percocet), hydrocodone (Vicodin), oxycontin,
      oxymorphone, dextropropoxyphene (Darvocet)
   All act on **µ-opioid receptor** in **CNS**
   ***All are reversed w/ Narcan** (naloxone)*
   Effects:
      1) **Profound analgesia** (euphoria)
      2) **Respiratory depression** (↓ CO_2 drive)
      3) Blunt sympathetic response
   Liver metabolism and **kidney excretion**

   1) **Morphine**
         S/Es: miosis, ↓cough, ↑constipation, **histamine release** (mild ↓BP)
         Active metabolites can build up in pts w/ renal failure
   2) **Demerol**
         S/Es: miosis, tremors, fasciculations, seizures; **No histamine release**
         Avoid **high doses**
         Avoid in pts w/ **renal failure**
            → can get buildup of **normeperidine analogue** (→ seizures)
         Avoid in pts on **MAOIs** (monoamine oxidase inhibitors)
            → leads to **serotonin syndrome** (↑↑ serotonin release in CNS)
               Sx's – agitation, tremor, severe fever, tachycardia, HTN,
                  severe muscle rigidity, seizures, shock, coma
               Tx:
                  D/C offending meds
                  Benzodiazepines for myoclonus
                  Control fever, cardiac and respiratory support
                  Serotonin antagonists (cyproheptadine)
                  intubate, sedate and **paralyze if severe**
   3) **Fentanyl** – 80x strength of morphine
         Does <u>not</u> cross react w/ morphine allergy
         No histamine release
   4) **Sufentanil, alfentanil,** and **remifentanil** – very fast-acting w/ short half-lives

   Careful w/ opioid and benzodiazepine combinations (have **synergistic effect**)
   Methadone – binds **CNS µ-opioid receptor**, less euphoria

   Note – resident work hour restrictions in large part resulted from the Libby Zion
      case, in which the combination of an MAOI and Demerol led to Serotonin
      Syndrome

Muscle relaxants (paralytics)

    Diaphragm – last muscle to go down and 1st muscle to recover from paralytics

    Neck muscles and face – 1st to go down and last to recover from paralytics

Depolarizing agent (only agent is **succinylcholine**)

    Succinylcholine – fast, short-acting; fasciculations at first, _**many**_ **S/Es**

        1) **Malignant hyperthermia**

            Defect in calcium metabolism

            Calcium released from sarcoplasmic reticulum causes **muscle excitation–contraction syndrome**.

            Sx's:

                ****1st sign** is ↑ **end-tidal** CO_2

                Then **fever**, tachycardia, **rigidity**, acidosis, hyperkalemia, hypoxia

                Rhabdomyolysis can lead to **myoglobin release**

            Tx:

                Dantrolene – inhibits Ca release and decouples excitation complex

                Cooling blankets, HCO_3, glucose, supportive care

            Can also be caused by volatile anesthetics

            Mechanism - **ryanodine receptor defect** on sarcoplasmic reticulum

        2) **Hyperkalemia**

            Depolarization releases **potassium**

            Don't use in pts w/ **severe burns, neurologic injury, neuromuscular disorders, spinal cord injury** (all have up-regulation **of ACh receptors** in muscle which dramatically ↑s potassium release)

            Don't use in **massive trauma pts** (↑ potassium from muscle injury)

            Don't use w/ **acute renal failure**

        3) **Open-angle glaucoma** can become closed-angle glaucoma.

        4) **Atypical pseudocholinesterases** – prolonged paralysis (Asians)

        5) ↑ed **intracranial pressure** (ICP)

    Metabolism - degradation by **plasma cholinesterases**

Non-depolarizing agents

    Inhibit neuromuscular junction by competing w/ ACh at the ACh receptor (competitive antagonist)

    Not as fast as depolarizing agent

    Types

        1) **Rocuronium**– very fast acting, intermediate duration(good for **RSI**)

            Metabolism – hepatic

        2) **Pancuronium** – slower acting, long duration (good in **ICU**)

            <u>No </u>hypotension

            Metabolism – renal

            ****MC S/E:** <u>tachycardia</u>

        3) **Cis-atracurium** – slower acting, intermediate duration

            Good in pts w/ **liver** or **renal failure**

            Metabolism – Hoffman elimination

            S/Es: Histamine release (hypotension)

        4) **Vecuronium** – fast acting, short duration, few S/Es

            Metabolism – Hepatic-biliary excretion (MC in unaltered form)

    Reversing drugs for non-depolarizing agents

        Neostigmine – blocks **acetylcholinesterase**, ↑s acetylcholine

        Edrophonium – blocks **acetylcholinesterase**, ↑s acetylcholine

        Atropine or glycopyrrolate (ACh antagonists) given w/ <u>neostigmine or edrophonium</u> to counteract effects of generalized acetylcholine overdose (salivation, diarrhea)

Critical illness polyneuropathy – widespread motor weakness and neurologic dysfunction; RFs – SIRS, steroids, paralytics, ↑ glucose

Benzodiazepines
Effects: anxiolytic, anticonvulsant, amnesic, respiratory depression
Not analgesic
Metabolism – hepatic
Mechanism – bind GABA receptor (most prevalent inhibitory receptor in brain)
1) **Versed** (midazolam) – short acting
   Contraindicated w/ pregnancy, crosses placenta
2) **Ativan** (lorazepam) – long acting
3) **Valium** (diazepam) – long acting

Overdose Tx: flumazenil
   Competitive inhibitor; may cause seizures and arrhythmias;
   Contraindicated in pts w/ elevated ICP or status epilepticus

Local anesthetics
Mechanism – increase action potential threshold, preventing Na influx
Infected tissues – hard to anesthetize secondary to **acidosis**
Length of action: bupivacaine > lidocaine > procaine
Epinephrine allows higher doses to be used, stays local
   No epinephrine with arrhythmias, unstable angina, uncontrolled
      hypertension, poor collaterals (penis and ear), uteroplacental
      insufficiency
Neuro blockade: sensory > motor
Allergic reactions
   Amides (all have an "i" in first part of name) – lidocaine, bupivacaine,
      mepivacaine; *rare* **allergic reactions**
   Esters – tetracaine, procaine, cocaine
      ↑ **allergic reactions** secondary to PABA analogue
Max Dosage:
   Lidocaine max dosage – 5 mg/kg (w/ epi 7 mg/kg)
      Can use 0.5 cc/kg of 1% lidocaine
   Bupivicaine max dosage – 2 mg/kg (w/ epi 3 mg/kg)
Lidocaine toxicity progression:
   1st sx → Peri-oral paresthesias (tingling, numbness)
   2nd sx → Visual and auditory hallucinations
   Sedation
   Unconsciousness
   Seizures
   Respiratory depression
   Cardiac arrhythmias
   Cardiovascular collapse
   ***Neuro S/Es** occur at lower doses than cardiovascular S/Es*

Epidural anesthesia

Epidural (outside dura)

Causes **sympathetic denervation** and **sensory blockade**

Pain receptors affected much more than motor receptors

Motor affected only w/ large dosages

Does <u>not</u> provide good paralysis

Good for control of **post-op pain**

Finding epidural space – loss of resistance w/ injection

Bloody tap – insert at new level

Block height is 3-4 levels above site of insertion

T-5 epidural – affects cardiac accelerator nerves

Contraindications to epidural and spinal:

Hypertrophic cardiomyopathy (↓ afterload causes LV outflow tract collapse)

Cyanotic heart disease (↓ afterload shunts blood away from lungs)

Aortic stenosis (↓ afterload impairs coronary blood supply)

Liver DZ (bleeding risk → epidural hematoma)

Infection (worry about epidural abscess)

Coagulopathy (INR > 1.5, low plts, uremia, heparin → bleed risk)

Anatomic abnormalities (spina bifida, meningomyelocele)

Elevated ICP

Cx's:

Morphine component – respiratory depression (esp high spinal)

Tx: Turn off epidural, airway management

Avoid respiratory depression by using **Dilaudid**

Lidocaine component - ↓ heart rate and ↓ blood pressure

Tx for hypotension and bradycardia:

1) Turn epidural down

2) Fluids, phenylephrine, atropine

3) Make sure hypotension not due to another source (eg bleeding)

Urinary retention (all need bladder catheter)

Spinal headaches – HA gets worse <u>sitting up</u>

Tx: rest, increased fluids, caffeine, analgesics

Blood patch to site if persists >24 hours

Falls

Abscess (risk greatest if left in > 72 hours)

Sx's: back pain, fevers, sensory or motor deficits

Dx: MRI

Tx: usually requires drainage w/ laminectomy

Epidural Hematoma

Classic clinical course of epidural hematoma:

1) **sudden localized back pain** or discomfort at epidural site ± paresthesias

2) **within 1-2 hours → motor + sensation loss** ± loss of bladder and bowel function

Dx: emergent MRI

Tx: decompressive laminectomy

Decreased motor in legs

Often unilateral

MC from medication overdose (majority, leg should feel <u>warm</u>)

Consider epidural hematoma (see above)

Tx: Turn down epidural and monitor, if no recovery, emergent MRI to R/O epidural hematoma

Benefits – ↓ respiratory cx's (eg PNA), ↓ myocardial infarction, ↑ return of bowel function, no survival difference

Spinal anesthesia – sensory *and* motor blockade

Sensory blockade is above motor blockade

Can perform any surgery below umbilicus w/ spinal anesthesia <u>alone</u>

(eg C-sections, hernia, LE orthopedic, hysterectomy, appendectomy)

Caudal block – through sacrum, good for pediatric hernias and perianal surgery

ASA class (American Society of Anesthesiologists)
Class I – healthy patient
Class II – mild disease without limitation (HTN, DM, obesity, smokers)
Class III – severe disease (stable angina, previous MI, moderate COPD)
Class IV – disease is a severe constant threat to life (unstable angina, renal or liver failure, severe COPD)
Class V – moribund patient (eg ruptured AAA, saddle pulmonary embolus)
Class VI – organ donor

Revised Cardiac Risk Index (modified; Circulation 1999; 100:1043-1049)
Each risk factor is assigned one point (6 points max):
1. **High-risk surgical procedures**
    Intra-peritoneal
    Intra-thoracic
    Major vascular (eg AAA repair, lower extremity bypass)
2. History of **ischemic heart disease**
    History of MI
    Positive stress test
    Current angina
    Nitrate use
    ECG w/ Q waves
3. History of **congestive heart failure** (CHF)
    Pulmonary edema
    Paroxysmal nocturnal dyspnea
    Bilateral rales or S3 gallop
    CXR w/ pulmonary congestion
4. History of **cerebrovascular disease**
    History of transient ischemic attack or stroke
5. Preop Tx w/ **insulin** (ie diabetic)
6. Preop **creatinine > 2.0**

RISK OF MAJOR CARDIAC EVENT

# of points	Class	Risk of Major Cardiac Event
0	I	0.5%
1	II	1%
2	III	7%
3 or more	IV	11%

Major cardiac event – MI, pulmonary edema, ventricular fibrillation, cardiac arrest, and complete heart block

Tx:
    Class III and IV – get non-invasive cardiac testing
    Class II – if poor or indeterminant functional status → get noninvasive cardiac testing (lean towards testing)
    Class I – do not need testing
Class III and **IV** – benefit from beta-blocker which reduces mortality
Class I – do not benefit from beta-blocker (may be harmful)

CABG within last 5 years and no return of sx's – no testing
PTCA within last 2 years w/ good result and no return of sx's – no testing

Wait 6-8 weeks after MI for elective surgery
    10% mortality if < 6-8 weeks
Aortic and **lower extremity procedures** are generally considered **high risk**

Largest risk factor for cardiac complication – *uncompensated CHF* (as evidence by JVD, ↑ed CVP or S3 gallop; *11 points* on Goldman criteria)
    Recent MI (#2) – *10 points*

<u>General criteria for non-invasive cardiac testing prior to non-cardiac surgery:</u>
Angina (any) or **shortness of breath** ($\leq$ 2 blocks)
PTCA > 2 years ago or **CABG > 5 years ago**
Peripheral vascular disease (eg claudication, previous stroke)
Age > 70
Previous MI and <u>not</u> revascularized
> 20 pack year smoking (or FEV-1 < 70% predicted)
Diabetes
EKG - Q waves, ST changes, T wave changes, LBBB, heart block (second or
third degree), rhythm other than sinus, multiple PVC's (> 5/min)
CHF
Left ventricular hypertrophy
Uncontrolled HTN (DBP > 110 mmHg)
Pt undergoing **major vascular surgery**
Low functional capacity (**< 4 METS**)
Creatinine $\geq$ 2
Aortic stenosis

Non-invasive cardiac testing
[eg dobutamine-thallium, stress-thallium (walking), adenosine-thallium scans]
Looking for areas of ischemia (ie decreased thallium uptake) w/:
1) the heart under **stress** (eg Dobutamine or walking) or
2) **coronary vasodilatation** (eg adenosine or dipyridamole)
Positive stress test = chest pain, ST changes, hypotension, or areas of
reversible ischemia $\rightarrow$ all indications for **coronary angiogram**

Coronary Angiogram Indications:
1) **Positive non-invasive cardiac testing**
2) **Acute ST elevation MI** (STEMI) – standard is 90 minutes ER door to PTCA
time (termed door to balloon time)
3) **Non-ST elevation MI** – most get cath before discharge
Ongoing chest pain or ischemia despite medical therapy $\rightarrow$ cath
Unstable angina $\rightarrow$ cath
Possible PTCA w/ stent or CABG depending on findings

Perioperative Complications
CHF and **renal failure** – highest RFs for post-op hospital mortality
Post-op MI – may have no pain or EKG changes; can have hypotension,
arrhythmias, $\uparrow$ filling pressures, oliguria, bradycardia

Emergency non-cardiac surgery in patients w/ cardiac disease
1) Place a **swan, a-line, and foley**
2) Try to maximize **wedge pressure** (15-20) w/ fluid
3) **Beta-blocker** (want HR of 60 if pressure tolerates)
4) **Nitropaste** (1/2 - 2 inches as pressure tolerates)
5) Optimize **Hct $\geq$ 30**
6) **FiO2 100%**
7) Add low dose **inotrope** (dopamine, dobutamine, milrinone) if $\downarrow$ed C.O.

Pre-op issues
Check **b-HCG** w/ elective surgery in women < 50
Laparoscopy $\rightarrow$ place **NGT** and **Foley**
Do not perform a whipple, APR, or total gastrectomy unless you have **tumor**
or a very good reason for a benign situation (this is rare)

Myasthenia Gravis

Sx's: ocular muscles MC involved; generalized skeletal involvement (90%)

Dx *(confirmatory testing essential):*

    1) **EMG** *(best test,* Jolly test) – shows **jitter** (non-uniform NMJ destruction)

    2) **Anti-cholinesterase test** (Edrophonium) – sx's get better in 30 sec's

    3) **Chest CT** to look for thymoma (10%)

Path

    Ab's to ACh receptors at the NMJ → ACh receptors get destroyed

    Myeloid cells in thymus may serve as Ag source

Tx:

    Cholinesterase inhibitors (pyridostigmine)

        S/Es – salivation, diarrhea, bradycardia

        Cholinergic crisis – too much ACh (see below)

    Steroids

    Plasmapheresis – short term improvement

    Azathioprine

    IVIG

Thymectomy

    Indications – thymomas or severe MG

    Want sx's under control before you operate

    Anesthesia

        Avoid NMJ blocking agents – prolonged effect w/ incomplete reversal

            by neostigmine

        Give succinylcholine (less potent)

    Thymus receives branches from **inferior thyroid artery** and **internal**

        mammary artery

    Careful narcotic administration → potential for respiratory depression

    Cholinesterase inhibitors re-started post-op and gradually weaned

    Results of Thymectomy – 80% get improvement

Myasthenia Crisis (too little ACh)

    Respiratory Failure - caused by infection, stress, sepsis

    NO surgery – *no role for emergency thymectomy for myasthenia gravis*

    Tx: pyridostigmine, plasmapheresis, steroids; may need to intubate

Cholinergic Crisis (too much ACh)

    Overdose of cholinesterase inhibitor

    Causes too much ACh at NMJ – results in **depolarization blockade**

    Effects – paralysis, respiratory failure, salivation, sweating

    May need intubation

Advanced oral directives

Take precedence when determining a pts treatment in cases where the pt is

    otherwise not able to make informed choices about their care.

The next order of precedence is **living will**

Followed by **durable power of attorney** (eg wife or husband)

Hierarchy for life support decisions / organ donation (if no advanced oral

    directives or living will):

        1)   wife or husband

        2)   adult son or daughter

        3)   parent

        4)   adult brother or sister

        5)   guardian

National Surgical Quality Improvement Program (NSQIP) - seeks to collect

outcome data to measure and improve surgical quality in the U.S.

Iodine Allergy

MC reaction to iodine – **nausea** (others include urticaria, itching, heat)

MC reaction requiring medical tx – **dyspnea** (others include hypotension,

    LOC, cardiac arrest)

FLUIDS and ELECTROLYTES

Total body water

2/3 of total body weight is water (<u>infants</u> little more body water, <u>women</u> little less)

    2/3 of water is intracellular (mostly muscle).

    1/3 of water is extracellular

Protein – main determinant of intravascular and interstitial compartment **_oncotic pressure_**

Na^+ – main determinant of intracellular and extracellular **_osmotic_** pressure

Volume overload: MCC → **iatrogenic**; 1st sign is **weight gain**

    3rd space fluid (edema) is in the **interstitial space**

Cellular catabolism – can release a significant amount of H_2O

Normal saline (NS, 0.9%) - Na 154 and Cl 154

    3% saline - Na 513, Cl 513; **0.45% saline** - Na 77, Cl 77

Lactated Ringer's (LR; ionic composition of plasma)

Na^+	130
K^+	4
Ca^{++}	2.7
Cl^-	109
lactate	28

Plasma osmolarity = (2 x Na) + (glucose/18) + (BUN/2.8) → **Normal: 290 ± 10**

Normal K^+ requirement: 0.5 - 1.0 mEq/kg/day

Normal Na^+ requirement: 1 - 2 mEq/kg/day

Hemodialysis (HD) can remove **K, Ca, Mg, and PO4**; also removes **urea + Cr**

Volume replacement

Maintenance IVFs:

    4 cc/kg/hr for 1st 10 kg

    2 cc/kg/hr for 2nd 10 kg

    1 cc/kg/hr for each kg after that

Best indicator of adequate volume replacement → **urine output**

Open abdominal operations - fluid loss is **0.5–1.0 L/hr** unless there is a measurable blood loss

Usually do <u>not</u> replace blood lost unless it's **> 500 cc**

Insensible fluid losses – 10 cc/kg/day (75% sweat, 25% respiratory, hypotonic)

IV replacement after major adult GI surgery

    During operation and **1st 24 hours** → use lactated ringers

    After 24 hours → switch to D5 ½ NS with 20 mEq K^+.

        5% dextrose stimulates **insulin release** (↑glucose and amino acid uptake, protein synthesis, prevents protein catabolism)

        D5 ½ NS @ 125/hr provides 150 gm glucose per day (525 kcal/day)

	Fluid Secretion (cc/d)	Electrolyte Loss	*Maintenance IVFs
Sweat	300 - 500	**Water**, some NaCl	**1/2 NS** (if excessive loss)
Saliva	Normally negligible	**K** (highest K concentration in body)	**1/2 NS w/ 20 mEq K** (if excessive loss)
Stomach	1000-2000	H+ and Cl-	**D5 1/2 NS w/ 20 mEq K**
Pancreas	500-1000	HCO3-	**LR****
Biliary System	500-1000	HCO3-	**LR****
Small Intestine	*Fluid absorption unless fistula*	HCO3-, ± K+	**LR**** (eg fistula)
Large Intestine	*Fluid absorption unless diarrhea*	K+	**LR**** (eg diarrhea)

*Above are **maintenance**, <u>not</u> resuscitation IVFs for dehydration (see below)

May need additional **HCO3- replacement

***May need additional **K** replacement

Moderate to Severe Dehydration (related fluid loss / replacement)
    1) **Sweat** (eg marathon runner)   **NS bolus**
    2) **Gastric** (eg gastric outlet obstruction w/ profuse N/V)   **NS bolus**
    3) **Pancreatic. biliary, or small bowel** (eg high output fistula)   **LR bolus**
    4) **Large intestine** (eg C. diff colitis w/ severe diarrhea)   **LR bolus**
    **Never bolus normal saline w/ K added (cardiac arrest)
GI losses – should generally be replaced **cc/cc**
Urine output – keep at least 0.5 cc/kg/hr; <u>not</u> replaced, sign of normal post-op diuresis

<u>Sodium</u> (nl 135 - 145)
    Hypernatremia
           Synonymous w/ **dehydration** 99% of the time
           MCC – poor fluid intake (95%); others – *over-diuresis, diabetes insipidus*
           Sx's: irritability, restless, ataxia, weakness, seizures
           Tx: D5 water
           Correct slowly to avoid **brain swelling** ($\leq$ 0.7 meg/L/hr)

           Free water deficit = 0.6 x pts weight (kg) x $[(Na^+/140) - 1]$

    Hyponatremia
           Synonymous w/ **fluid overload** 99% of the time
           MCC – iatrogenic (1st sign – **weight gain**), others - *SIADH*
           Sx's: N/V, headaches, delirium, seizures, stupor, coma
           Tx:
                1) **Water restriction** (1st line), *if that fails;*
                2) **Diuresis,** *if that fails;*
                3) **Hypertonic saline****
           Correct Na slowly to avoid **central pontine myelinosis** ($\leq$ 0.5 mEq/L/hr)
           ****If symptomatic** (eg N/V, mental status changes, coma) $\rightarrow$ go right to
                hypertonic saline
           1 L of 3% hypertonic saline contains 513 mEq/L each of Na^+ and Cl^-
                Will change Na^+ in 70 kg man apx **10 mEq/L** (eg Na^+ 130$\rightarrow$140)
           Pseudohyponatremia – from **hyperglycemia** (eg DKA) or
                hyperlipidemia (eg acute pancreatitis);Tx: nothing, <u>underlying illness</u>

<u>Potassium</u> (nl 3.5 - 5.0)
    Kidneys regulate serum K^+
    Hyperkalemia
           MCC – renal disease (80%), others – *meds* (eg spironolactone, ACE
                inhibitors, ARBs), *diabetic nephropathy, aldosterone deficiency,*
                adrenal insufficiency, calcineurin inhibitors
           EKG – initial peaked T waves deteriorates to ventricular fibrillation
           Tx:
                1) **1 amp calcium gluconate** (heart membrane stabilizer)
                   $\rightarrow$ *1st drug to give*
                2) **1 amp sodium bicarbonate**
                   Alkalosis causes K to enter cell in exchange for H
                3) **10 U insulin** and **1 ampule of 50% dextrose**
                   K driven into cells w/ glucose
                4) **Kaexylate**
                5) **Lasix 40 mg IV**
                6) **Albuterol Nebs**
                7) **Dialysis** if refractory
           Addison's disease (ie adrenal insufficiency) – $\downarrow$ aldosterone
                $\uparrow$K, $\downarrow$Na, $\downarrow$ glucose; fever, hypotension, abd pain (see Adrenal chp)
           Type IV renal tubular acidosis (hyperkalemia type RTA)
                Cardinal feature is **hyperkalemia**
                MC etiology – diabetic nephropathy (resistance to aldosterone)
                Others – meds (spironolactone, ACEI, ARBs, NSAIDs)
           Pseudohyperkalemia – hemolysis of blood sample

Hypokalemia

MCC – diuretics
> others – *poor intake* (eg TPN), *GI losses* (eg N/V, NG tube, diarrhea)

EKG – T waves disappear

Tx: potassium chloride (10 mEq ↑s serum K by 0.1 mEq/L)

May need to **correct magnesium before you can correct potassium

Calcium

Normal total   8.5 - 10.5 mg/dl (2.0 - 2.5 mmol/L)

Normal ionized   4.5 - 5.5 mg/dl (1.0 - 1.5 mmol/L)

Ca absorbed in GI tract (**calcium binding protein**) + reabsorbed in kidney (**PTH**)

Ca also *excreted* into GI tract

Hypercalcemia

Hyperparathyroidism + malignancy account for 90% of all cases
> (see Parathyroid chp)

MCC hypercalcemia – hyperparathyroidism (MC- parathyroid adenoma)

MC malignant cause of hypercalcemia – lung CA and breast CA (tied for #1)

MCC hypercalcemic crisis – previous primary hyperparathyroidism undergoing another procedure

Sx's: lethargy, weakness, N/V, hypotension, arrhythmias, shortened QT
> kidney stones, stomach ulcers, ↓ DTRs (deep tendon reflexes)
>
> **Ca > 13 mg/dl** (ionized >6) → symptoms
>
> **Ca > 15 mg/dl** (ionized > 7) → risk for cardiac arrest

Tx Hypercalcemic Crisis (Ca 13-15):
> 1) **Rapid volume infusion** – Normal Saline at 200-300 cc/hr
>   *No lactated ringers* (contains Ca)
> 2) **Lasix** (do *not* use thiazide diuretics which cause Ca resorption)
> 3) **Dialysis** if refractory to above
> 4) **If malignancy** →
>   **Bisphosphonates** [*best therapy*, eg alendronate (Fosamax)]
>   Inhibits osteoclast bone resorption
>   **Calcitonin** – inhibits osteoclast bone resorption
>   **S/Es**: quick onset of tachyphylaxis
>   **Glucocorticoids**
>   **Mithramycin** – inhibits osteoclast bone resorption
>   **S/Es**: liver, renal, hematologic
> 5) **If hyperparathyroidism** → parathyroidectomy after recovery

Just to re-state:
> *No lactated ringers (contains Ca)*
> *No thiazide diuretics (these retain Ca)*

Hypocalcemia

MCC – previous thyroid surgery (iatrogenic injury→ hypoparathyroidism)
> others – *rapid blood transfusion* (citrate), *renal failure, pancreatitis*

Ca < 8 (ionized <4) → symptoms

Sx's:
> **1st sx - Perioral tingling**
> Chvostek's sign (tapping facial nerve causes face twitching)
> Trousseau's sign (carpopedal spasm after occluding arm blood flow)
> Laryngospasm
> Hyper-reflexia
> Prolonged QT on EKG → can get ventricular arrhythmias

Tx: calcium gluconate (calcium chloride if coding), Vit D

May need to correct **magnesium** before being able to correct calcium

Hypoproteinemia (↓ed albumin) causes **artificially low Ca**
> For every 1 g decrease in protein, add 0.8 to Ca level

Can occur after surgery for **hyperparathyroidism**
> Caused by **bone hunger** (bone repleting lost supply) or **failure of parathyroid remnant or graft**
> Remember to give Ca post-op

Magnesium (nl 2.0 - 2.5 mg/dl)

Hypermagnesemia
MCC – renal failure *combined* w/ Mg intake (eg laxatives, antacids)
  others - burns, trauma
Sx's: lethargy, weakness, N/V, hypotension, arrhythmias, ↓ DTRs
  > 10 → complete heart block
  > 13 → risk for cardiac arrest
Tx: calcium (*best Tx*, competitive antagonist to Mg), **diuretics**, **dialysis**

Hypomagnesemia
MCC
  Symptomatic – diuretics (massive diuresis); others - *ETOH abuse,*
    malnutrition (TPN)
  Asymptomatic - 70% of all ICU pts have low Mg^{++}
Sx's start when **Mg < 1**
Sx's: (similar to hypocalcemia) irritability, tremors, confusion, hyper-
  reflexia, tetany, seizures, prolonged QT, ventricular arrhythmias
  (torsades de pointes, others)
Tx: magnesium

Phosphate (nl 2.5 - 4.5 mg/dl)

Hyperphosphatemia
MCC – renal failure (80%; often have co-existent **hypocalcemia)**
  others – *hypo-parathyroidism* (MC related to previous thyroid surgery),
    tumor lysis syndrome
Sx's:
  Majority asymptomatic
  May have sx's associated w/ hypocalcemia (see above)
  Ectopic calcification, renal osteodystrophy (see Parathyroid chp)
Tx: sevelamer chloride (Renagel, phosphate binder in gut), low
  phosphate diet (eg avoid dairy products), **dialysis** (removes PO4)

Hypophosphatemia
Usually due to **PO4 shift from extra-cellular to intracellular**
Usually in setting of **ETOH abuse**
MCC– re-feeding syndrome (phosphorylation of glucose in cell)
  Others – *respiratory alkalosis* (PO4 moves into cells), *TPN,*
    hyper-parathyroidism, DKA Tx (intracellular glycolysis uses
    PO4)
Sx's:
  **Failure to wean from the ventilator (↓ ATP production)
  Muscle weakness (lack of PO4 for ATP production)
  ↑ **infection risk** (impaired leukocyte chemotaxis due to ↓ ATP)
  Mental status changes (including coma)
Tx: potassium phosphate

Electrolyte abnormalities w/ renal failure
Volume overload
↓ **Na$^+$ and Ca^{++}**
↑ **K$^+$, PO4$^-$, and Mg^{++}**
Avoid Mg containing antacids and laxatives

Indications for dialysis
Fluid overload
↑ed K$^+$, Mg^{++}, PO4$^-$, or BUN
Metabolic acidosis
Uremic encephalopathy
Uremic coagulopathy
Poisoning

Acid-Base

		pH	pCO$_2$	HCO$_3$
	Respiratory acidosis	↓	↑ (1° problem)	↑
	Respiratory alkalosis	↑	↓ (1° problem)	↓
	Metabolic acidosis	↓	↓	↓ (1° problem)
	Metabolic alkalosis	↑	↑	↑ (1° problem)

Normal values

pH 7.35-7.45 (**7.4**)

CO2 35-45 (**40**)

HCO3⁻ 22-26 (**24**)

$$H+ + HCO_3^- = H_2CO_3 = H_2O + CO_2$$
(bicarb)   (carbonic acid)

Lung controls pH through **pCO2 regulation** (*rapid process*)
Kidney controls pH primarily through **HCO3- regulation** (proximal tubule
NaHCO3 reabsorption, carbonic anhydrase mediated, *slow → days*)
Secondary regulation through NH4+ (as urea) and H+ excretion
Henderson-Hesselbach equation: pH = pK + log [HCO$_3^-$] / [0.03 x CO$_2$]
Ratio of base to acid (HCO$_3^-$ to CO$_2$) of 20:1 = pH of 7.4

<u>**Reparatory Alkalosis**</u> - from hyperventilation (eg PE causes hypoxia and hypocarbia)
Chronic cases associated w/ hypokalemia
<u>**Respiratory Acidosis**</u> - from hypoventilation (eg COPD exacerbation → ↑ pCO2)

Metabolic alkalosis

Mechanism – Loss of H+ or **gain of HCO3** (GI tract or kidneys)
Associated w/ **hypokalemia** (K+ moves intracellular in exchange for H+)
Etiologies
1) **Gastric fluid loss** (gastric outlet obstruction, NG tube, severe vomiting)
Loss of gastric fluid results in **hypochloremic, hypokalemic,
metabolic alkalosis**, and **paradoxical aciduria** (see below)**
2) **Over-diuresis** (furosemide or hydrochlorothiazide) or **dehydration**
Results in **contraction alkalosis** (fluid loss causes relative ↑ in
HCO3- mass in body)
w/ lasix or HCTZ over-diuresis, **hypokalemia** stimulates renal **K+/H+
exchanger** (excretes H+ in exchange for K+) → ↑ed alkalosis
3) **Hypertensive Types** (mineralocorticoid excess; saline resistant)
Primary hyperaldosteronism (Conn's Syndrome)
Aldosterone activates Na/K ATPase (reabsorbs Na, excretes K)
Also Na/H exchanger (reabsorb Na, excrete H) - alkalosis
Hypokalemia stimulates **K+/H+ exchanger** (excretes H+ in
exchange for K+) → ↑ed alkalosis
Secondary hyperaldosteronism (renin secreting tumor or renal
artery stenosis) – similar mechanism as above
Cushing's Syndrome – high levels of corticosteroids have
mineralocorticoid effects (same mechanism as above)
Tx for **gastric loss** type → **NS bolus** for resuscitation (corrects volume +
chloride) followed by D5 NS w/ 20 mEq K maintenance (switch to 1/2 NS
when chloride corrected; adults)
Tx for **Lasix** or **HCTZ over-diuresis** type → **NS bolus**
If pt still **fluid overloaded** → **acetazolamide** diuresis; <u>No NS bolus</u>
If pt **fluid overloaded + renal insufficiency** →**HCL drip**, possible **dialysis**
Tx for **hypertensive** types (ie Na⁺ + water reabsorption causing fluid overload) →
spironolactone (aldosterone inhibitor) initially, correct underlying D/O

****Mechanism of hypochloremic, hypokalemic, metabolic alkalosis w/
paradoxical aciduria** (gastric fluid loss)
Loss of Cl⁻ and H ion from stomach (**hypochloremic alkalosis**)
Water loss causes kidney to reabsorb Na (+ water) in exchange for K⁺
(Na/K ATPase) resulting in **hypokalemia**
K⁺/H⁻ exchanger activated (reabsorbs K, excrete H)→ **paradoxic aciduria**

Metabolic acidosis
Gain of acid or **loss of HCO3-**
2 types (anion gap and non-anion gap)
    Anion Gap = Na^+ – ($HCO3^-$ + Cl^-)
        {normal < 10-15}
Etiologies
    1) **Anion gap metabolic acidosis**
        All are gaining acid <u>and</u> unmeasured anions
        Diabetic Ketoacidosis (DKA; ↑ed ketones)
        Ingestions (eg methanol, ethylene glycol, ASA)
        Renal failure [uremia (BUN), ammonia, sulfates, phosphates]
        Lactate Acid (eg shock, ↑ed lactic acid)

    2) **Non-anion gap metabolic acidosis**
        All gaining HCL or losing NaHCO3
        GI losses of HCO3- (eg ileostomy, small bowel fistula)
        Over-diuresis w/ spironolactone (aldosterone inhibitor – gain H+)
            or **acetazolamide** (carbonic anhydrase inhibitor – lose HCO3-)
        Dilutional (rapid infusion of HCO3- deficient fluids)
        Lactulose (for liver failure; metabolized to short chain fatty acids,
            which acidifies colon, leading to increased H+ absorption)
        Hyperparathyroidism (gain HCL)
        Renal tubular acidosis (RTA, 4 types)
            Either failure to 1) reabsorb $HCO3^-$ <u>or</u> 2) excrete H^+
        Hypoaldosteronism (ie Type IV RTA)
            Etiologies
                Diabetic nephropathy (resistance to aldosterone)
                     MC Type IV RTA
                Addison's Disease (↓ aldosterone production)
                   ↓ed aldosterone leads to **hyperkalemia** →
                   K+/H+ exchanger then excretes K^+ + reabsorbs H^+

Tx: treat underlying pathology (keep **pH >7.25 w/ HCO3** to avoid myocardial
    depression)

Diabetic Ketoacidosis (DKA)
Precipitants (I's)
    Insulin deficiency
    Infection / inflammation (PNA, UTI, appendicitis, cholecystitis, pancreatitis)
    Intoxication (ETOH, drugs)
    Ischemia or Infarction (MI, stroke, mesenteric ischemia)
    Iatrogenic (steroids, thiazide diuretics)
Occurs almost <u>exclusively</u> in type I DM
Glucose cannot be taken up by cells due to lack of insulin (↑ glucose, ↑ ketones
    from fatty acid oxidation in the liver)
Sx's: polydipsia, polyuria, dehydration, N/V, abd pain, Kussmaul's respirations,
    acetone breath, mental status changes (**somnolence**)
Dx: anion gap metabolic acidosis; ketones in urine, ↑ glucose (> 500 usual)
    ↓ed Na^+ (pseudohyponatremia)
    Possible ↑ed BUN and Cr from dehydration
    K^+ usually elevated initially (but total body K^+ usually low)
Tx:
    1) **R/O precipitants** – infection, inflammation, MI (see above precipitants)
    2) **Hydration – NS 10 cc/kg/hr** (adjust to BP and UOP)
    3) **Insulin** (10 U IV push; 0.1 u/kg/hr drip) – continue until anion gap normal
        (if glucose < 250 and anion gap still high – add glucose to the insulin
        drip and continue to metabolize ketones)
    4) **Potassium** – will initially be high but will be driven back into cells w/
        glucose; add potassium to drip if K < 4.5 (careful if renal failure)
    5) **HCO3-** → add if pH < 7.25 or cardiac instability
    6) **PO4-** → replete if < 1

NUTRITION

Calories

Fat	9 kcal/g
Protein	4 kcal/g
Oral carbohydrates	4 kcal/g
Dextrose	3.4 kcal/g

Caloric need
Need 25 kcal/kg/day (resting energy expenditure) *plus* stress factor
- **20% protein** (1-1.5 g protein/kg/d), 20% essential amino acids
- **30% fat** (impt for essential fatty acids)
- **50% carbohydrates**

Typical 70 kg adult male needs 1500-1750 calories/d
If overweight, use →
- Weight = [(actual weight – ideal body weight) x 0.25] + IBW

Majority of surgery pts can go NPO for **7 days** safely

Stress Factor

Trauma, surgery, or sepsis	↑ kcal requirement **20%–60%**
Pregnancy	↑ kcal requirement **300** kcal/d
Lactation	↑ kcal requirement **500** kcal/d

Protein requirement also ↑s w/ above

Burns (start nutrition early in burn pts)

Calories	25 kcal/kg/day + (30 kcal/day x % burn)
Protein	1–1.5 g/kg/day + (3 g x % burn)

Energy expenditure
Much of the energy expenditure is used for **heat production**

Basal metabolic rate (BMR, resting energy expenditure) ↑s **10%** for each degree above 38.0°C.

Harris-Benedict equation calculates BMR from **weight, height, age,** and **gender**

Fat and cholesterol digestion
Triacylglycerides (TAGs), **cholesterol** and **lipids** are digested

Broken down by pancreatic **lipase, cholesterol esterase, phospholipase,** and **bile salts** → form **micelles** and **free fatty acids** (FFAs) in the intestinal lumen

**Micelles

Aggregates of **bile salts, long-chain FFAs, monoacylglycerides,** and **cholesterol**

Fat-soluble vitamins (A, D, E, K) – also absorbed in micelles
Enter enterocyte by **fusing w/ membrane**
Bile salts – help form **micelles** (↑s absorption area for fats)

Medium- and short-chain FFAs – enter enterocyte by simple diffusion (<u>not</u> in micelles)

Micelles and **medium- + short- chain FFAs** enter **enterocytes**

TAGs are re-synthesized in intestinal cells → placed in **chylomicrons**

**Chylomicrons then enter <u>lymphatics</u> (terminal lacteals → thoracic duct)
Chylomicrons contain - **90% TAGs**, + 10% phospholipids, proteins, and cholesterol

Long-chain FFAs – enter <u>lymphatics</u> along w/ chylomicrons

Medium- and short-chain FFAs – enter <u>portal system</u> (same as amino acids and carbohydrates).

Lipoprotein lipase – located on <u>endothelium</u>

Clears **chylomicron content** from blood → breaks down **TAGs** to **FFAs** and **glycerol**, then taken up by cells through fatty acid binding protein

Fatty acid–binding protein – located on <u>cell membranes</u>

Transfers fatty acids from extra-cellular to intra-cellular

Saturated fatty acids (and ketone derivatives – acetoacetate, beta-hydroxybutyrate) used as **energy** by **liver** and **heart**

Unsaturated fatty acids – used as structural components for cells

Fatty acid synthesis can occur in **cytoplasm**

Lipoproteins
- Transport lipids around the body
- **Chylomicrons** – carry TAGs (fat) from intestines to liver, skeletal muscle, and adipose cells
- **Very low density lipoproteins** (VLDL) – carry newly synthesized TAGs and cholesterol from liver to adipose tissue.
- **Low density lipoproteins** (LDL) – formed from VLDL after removal of TAGs by lipoprotein lipase; carry cholesterol from liver to other cells; "bad cholesterol" lipoprotein
- **High density lipoproteins** (HDL) – collects cholesterol from cells in body and brings it back to the liver; "good cholesterol" lipoprotein

- **LDL receptor** on cells at **clathrin coated pits** – binds LDL, followed by endocytosis
- The majority of **total body cholesterol** is *synthesized in tissues* (liver #1; others - adrenal cortex, sex organs), rather than dietary uptake
- 95% of the cholesterol released into bile is **reabsorbed** (termed entero-hepatic recirculation)

Hormone-sensitive lipase
- Located in **adipose cells**
- Breaks down stored **TAGs** (storage form of fats) **to FFAs** and **glycerol**
- These are released into blood
- Sensitive to growth hormone, catecholamines, glucocorticoids, glucagon

Essential <u>fatty acids</u> – linolenic and linoleic
- Needed for prostaglandin synthesis (long-chain fatty acids)
- Important for immune cells
- 1) **Omega-3 fatty acids** - considered essential fatty acids
  - Includes **linolenic acid**, the simplest fatty acid in the category, the others can be synthesized from this
  - These fatty acids are thought to have **anti-oxidant properties** important for heart disease, CA, and inflammation
- 2) **Omega-6 fatty acids** – considered essential fatty acids
  - Includes **linoleic acid,** the simplest fatty acid in the category, the others can be synthesized from this

<u>Carbohydrate digestion</u>
- **Carbohydrates** are the body's key source of **energy**
  - Glucose is prime energy source for **brain**
  - **Obligate glucose users**-peripheral nerves, adrenal medulla, RBCs, WBCs
  - **Glucose** either 1) enters **glycolysis pathway** to produce **energy** (ATP) *or:* 2) is stored as **glycogen**
- Digestion begins w/ **<u>salivary amylase</u>**, then **pancreatic amylase** and **intestinal brush border disaccharidases** (eg maltase, sucrase, lactase)
- **Disaccharides**
  - **Sucrose** = fructose + glucose
  - **Lactose** = galactose + glucose
  - **Maltose** = glucose + glucose
- **Transport**
  - **Glucose** and **galactose** – absorbed by secondary active transport (Na^+ gradient); released into **<u>portal vein</u>**
  - **Fructose** – facilitated diffusion; released into **<u>portal vein</u>**
- **Glucose** ingestion causes **insulin release** from **beta cells in pancreas,** which results in cellular uptake of circulating glucose
- **Primary storage areas for glucose** (as **glycogen**) – <u>skeletal muscle</u> (#1), <u>liver</u>
- **Glucagon**
  - Has opposite effect of insulin, causes breakdown of glycogen to glucose
  - Glucose from glycogen breakdown in **liver** is released into **circulation**
    - Released in times of **stress** or **fasting**
    - Body glycogen stores are **depleted** after **18-24 hours of fasting**
  - Glucose from glycogen breakdown in **muscle *stays in muscle***
    - (muscle lacks **glucose-6 phosphatase**, *glucose-6 <u>can't</u> be released*)
- **<u>Cellulose</u>** (fiber) – non-digestible carbohydrate chains

Protein digestion

Digestion begins w/ **stomach pepsin**, then **pancreatic proteases** (eg trypsinogen, chymotrypsinogen, and pro-carboxypeptidase)

Pepsin <u>not</u> required; **pancreas enzymes** are required for absorption

Trypsinogen is released from pancreas and activated by **enterokinase** released from duodenum

Other pancreatic proteases then activated by trypsin

Trypsin can also autoactivate other trypsinogen molecules

Protein broken down to amino acids, di-peptides, and tri-peptides

Absorbed by **secondary active transport** (Na^+ gradient) into enterocytes (primarily **jejunum**) and released as free amino acids into **portal vein**

Then taken up by various cells under the influence of **insulin**

During **starvation**, protein shunted to **liver** for **gluconeogenesis**

Liver is prime regulator of **amino acid** (AA) **production** and **breakdown**

Nonessential AAs – those that begin with **A, G or C**, plus **serine, proline, tyrosine,** and **histidine**

Essential AAs – leucine, isoleucine, valine, lysine, methionine, phenylalanine, threonine, tryptophan

Branched-chain AAs (all essential) – leucine, isoleucine, valine ("LIV")

Can be metabolized in **muscle** (only AAs metabolized <u>outside</u> liver)

Impt source of **protein calories** (energy source) in pts w/ **liver failure**

Are **essential AAs**

Glutamine

MC AA in **bloodstream** and **tissue**

Can be used as an **energy source** (TCA cycle, see below)

Can be used for **gluconeogenesis** (see below)

Also used in **urea cycle** (see below)

Limit protein intake in pts w/ **liver failure** to avoid **ammonia buildup** and worsening **encephalopathy**

Limit protein intake for pts w/ **end stage kidney DZ** (to limit urea buildup)

Nitrogen balance (N balance)

6.25 g of protein contains 1 g of nitrogen

N balance = (N in – N out) = ([protein/6.25] – [24 hr urine N + 4 g])

Positive N balance (anabolism) – more nitrogen ingested (in form of protein) than excreted (in form of urea)

Negative N balance (catabolism) – more nitrogen excreted than taken in

Total protein synthesis for a healthy, normal 70-kg male is **250 g/day**

Liver

Responsible for **AA production** and **breakdown**

Site of **urea cycle** (gets rid of NH_3^+ from AA breakdown, see below)

Majority of protein breakdown from skeletal muscle is in the form of **glutamine** and **alanine**

Normal Major Fuel Source (non-stress, non-starvation)

Stomach - glutamine

Small bowel enterocytes - glutamine

Pancreas - glutamine

Spleen - glutamine

Liver - ketones (acetoacetate + beta hydroxybutyric acid; from FFA breakdown)

Large bowel colonocytes - <u>short</u> chain fatty acids [eg butyric acid (butyrate)]

Heart - <u>short</u> chain fatty acids

Skeletal muscle - glucose

Brain - glucose

Kidney - glucose

Peripheral nerves, adrenal medulla, RBCs, PMNs - <u>obligate</u> glucose users

WBCs;

Lymphocytes and **macrophages** - glutamine

PMNs - glucose

MC primary fuel for <u>neoplastic cells</u> - glutamine (glucose #2)

Glutamine, ketones, and **short chain fatty acids** - enter TCA cycle for NADP, NADPH and FADH production → eventual ATP production (see below)

Respiratory quotient (RQ)

Ratio of CO_2 produced to O_2 consumed (CO_2 / O_2)

Measures **energy expenditure** (metabolic cart, indirect calorimetry)

RQ > 1 = lipogenesis (<u>overfeeding</u>; sx's - ↑ RR, ↑pCO2)

↑ed **metabolic rate**

High carbohydrate intake leads to **CO_2 buildup** (eg **failure to wean from ventilator**; lungs working hard to get rid of CO2)

CO2 produced when **excess carbohydrates** are converted to **fat**

Tx: ↓ carbohydrates and caloric intake

RQ < 0.7 = fat oxidation and **ketosis** (<u>starvation</u>)

↓ed **metabolic rate**

Fat breakdown does <u>not</u> ↑CO2 and O2 consumption ↑s w/ starvation

Tx: ↑ carbohydrates and caloric intake

Pure **fat** metabolism	RQ = 0.7
Pure **protein** metabolism	RQ = 0.8
Pure **carbohydrate** metabolism	RQ = 1.0
Balanced Feeding	RQ = 0.825

Cori cycle

Glucose is utilized and converted to **lactate** in muscle

Lactate then goes to liver and is converted back to **pyruvate** and eventually **glucose** via <u>gluconeogenesis</u>

Glucose is then transported back to muscle

Urea cycle (90% of all nitrogen loss)

Glutamine is principal NH_3^+ donor to remove **excess** NH_3^+ from body in form of **urea**; reactions occur and urea is formed in **liver; urea** removed by **kidney**

Preoperative nutritional assessment

Approximate half-lives

Albumin	20 days
Transferrin	8 days
Prealbumin	2 days

Normal albumin level: 3.5 - 5.5; **Normal pre-albumin level**: 15 - 35

Acute indicators of nutritional status – pre-albumin, transferrin, retinal binding protein, total lymphocyte count

Ideal body weight (IBW)

Men = 106 lb + 6 lb for each inch over 5 feet

Women = 100 lb + 5 lb for each inch over 5 feet

Preoperative signs of poor nutritional status

Acute weight loss > 10% in 6 months

Weight < 85% of IBW

Albumin < 3.0 – strong RF for cx's and mortality after surgery

Normal Postoperative phases

Catabolic phase	postop days 0–3 (negative nitrogen balance)
Anabolic phase	postop days 3–6 (positive nitrogen balance)
Diuresis phase	postop days 2–5

Enteral Tube Feeds (TFs)

Standard TFs (Jevity, 1-1.5 kcal/cc)

Diarrhea Tx: slow rate, add **fiber** (bulk) to slow transit time, use **less concentrated** feeds (prevent osmotic diarrhea)

High gastric residuals (stomach feeds) **Tx:** Reglan or erythromycin

Renal formulation (Nepro) – low in K and PO4; low protein

Try to feed gut (rather than use TPN) to avoid **bacterial translocation** (bacterial overgrowth and increased permeability due to starved enterocytes)

Early enteral feeding ↑s survival w/ **sepsis and pancreatitis**

<u>TPN composition</u> (total parenteral nutrition)

> **Apx 20% calories** as **protein** (1-1.5 g protein/kg/day, 20% essential AAs)
>> Usually a 5-10% amino acid solution ($\downarrow$ protein w/ liver or renal failure)
> **Apx 30% calories** as **fat** (lipids, 500 cc of 10% lipid solution - contains 550 kcal)
>> 10% lipid solution has 1.1 kcal/cc, 20% lipid solution has 2 kcal/cc
> **Apx 50% calories** as **dextrose** (consists of a 15-25% dextrose solution)
> **Additives:**
>> **Electrolytes**
>>> Na^+ (2 mg/kg/day), K^+ (1 mg/kg/day), Ca^{++}, Mg^{++}, $PO4^-$, Cl^-
>>> **Acetate** – buffer to $\uparrow$ pH of solution (prevents met. acidosis)
>> **Trace minerals** – Zn, Cu, Mn, Cr, Se (see below for deficiencies)
>> **Vitamins**
>>> ***Need to add <u>Vit K separately</u>*** – <u>Not</u> normally added to TPN
>>> Vit A, Vit D, Vit E, ($\rightarrow$ fat soluble, rest water soluble), Vit C, thiamine,
>>>> folate, riboflavin, niacin, pantothenic acid, pyridoxine (B6),
>>>> biotin, cyanocobalamine (B12) – see below for deficiencies
>> **Special additives**
>>> **ETOH abuse** – $\uparrow$ thiamine and folate
>>> **Promote wound healing** – $\uparrow$ Zinc and Vitamin C
>>> **Diabetics** – insulin can be added (want blood glucose 100-140)
> **Total volume** = 2-3 liters / day usual (apx. rate $\rightarrow$ 100-150 cc/hr)
> **Indications for TPN** – short gut, high output fistulas, other situations where
> enteral feeding can't be used
> **Central line TPN** – glucose based; maximum glucose administration – **3 g/kg/hr**
> **Peripheral line parenteral nutrition** (PPN) – <u>fat</u> based (high glucose
> concentration damages peripheral veins)
> **Elemental formula** – all protein given in form of amino acids (given IV, costly)
> **Stopping TPN –** cut rate in 1/2 for 1-2 hours 1st (avoids hypoglycemia)
> **Short term TPN** – complicated by issues associated w/ **indwelling catheters**
> (line sepsis, pneumothorax, etc.)
> **Long term TPN** – can eventually lead to **cirrhosis**

<u>Post-op Nutrition</u>

> Most pts can tolerate a **15% weight loss** w/o major cx's
> Pts can tolerate about **7 days** w/o eating; if longer than that, place a **feeding
> tube** or start **TPN**; enteral feeding is preferred
> **PEG** – consider when regular feeding not possible (eg CVA) or predicted to not
> occur for > 4 weeks

<u>Response to Starvation and Major Stress</u> (eg abdominal surgery, trauma, sepsis)

> **Glycogen stores**
>> **Depleted after 24 hours of starvation or major stress**
>>> 2/3 stored in skeletal muscle, 1/3 stored in liver (liver is the source of
>>> systemic glucose in times of stress)
>>> Skeletal muscle lacks **glucose-6-phosphatase** (found only in **liver**)
>>> Glucose-6-phosphate stays in muscle after breakdown from glycogen
>>> and is utilized there (<u>cannot</u> be released into circulation)
>> Body **switches to fat** after glycogen stores run out (fat is largest potential
>> energy source)
> **Adipose stores**
>> **Fat** is main energy source w/ **starvation** and **major stress**
>> **Hormone sensitive lipase** is activated, TAGs broken down, FFAs
>> released into circulation along w/ glycerol
>> **FFA oxidation** and the **TCA cycle** (Kreb's cycle) occur in the
>> **mitochondrial matrix** (inner mitochondrial space)
>>> **FFAs** are **oxidized** and enter Krebs cycle as either **acetyl-CoA** or
>>> **succinyl-CoA**
>>> **Krebs cycle** produces **NADPH, NADH,** and **FADH** from **FFAs**,
>>>> lactate (pyruvate), and **AAs** (AAs, pyruvate $\rightarrow$ acetyl-CoA 1st)
>> **Electron transport chain** – **NADPH, NADH,** and **FADH** are used to
>> produce **ATP**; occurs on **inner mitochondrial membrane**

Gluconeogenesis
Precursors – #1 alanine, others - lactate, pyruvate, glycerol, amino acids
Alanine
Primary substrate **for gluconeogenesis**
Simplest amino acid precursor for gluconeogenesis
Alanine and phenyl-alanine – only amino acids to ↑w/ stress
Gluconeogenesis primarily occurs in **liver**; in late starvation also occurs in
kidney (glutamine precursor)
Occurs to much greater degree w/ **major stress** than w/ starvation
*****Fatty acids are not used in gluconeogenesis because Acetyl-CoA
cannot be converted back to pyruvate***
Protein
Protein-conservation occurs w/ **starvation**
Protein-conservation *does not occur* after **major trauma** or **surgery**
secondary to **catecholamine** and **cortisol** release
Simple Starvation
↓**ed metabolic rate** (↓ insulin, ↑ glucagon)
Fat is major energy source, ↑↑ **ketone production**
Protein conserved → significant gluconeogenesis does not occur until late
Major stress
↑ **catecholamines, cortisol** and **cytokines** → all ↑metabolic rate
↓ insulin and ↑ glucagon
Fat is main energy source, however significant **protein breakdown** and
gluconeogenesis also occur (catecholamine + cortisol effect)
Hepatic urea formation and **negative nitrogen balance** also occur w/
protein breakdown
Progressive starvation primary fuel changes (when glucose levels low)
Skeletal Muscle and **Kidney** – switch to fatty acids (eg butyric acid)
Brain – switches to ketones (from fatty acid breakdown in liver)
Peripheral nerves, adrenal medulla, RBCs, PMNs – all obligate glucose
users

Systemic Effects of Major Stress
(fight or flight response; trauma, major surgery, sepsis)
Pancreas - ↓ insulin and ↑ glucagon
Cardiovascular - ↑ HR, ↑ SVR
Adrenal - ↑ cortisol, ↑ epinephrine + norepinephrine
Adrenal medulla is the *exclusive producer* of epinephrine in the body
Other tissues lack **PNMT enzyme** (converts norepinephrine→ epinephrine)
Protein breakdown in skeletal muscle
Renal - ↑ renin → ↑ aldosterone
Cytokines - ↑ TNF-alpha and IL-1
CNS - ↑ ACTH, ↑ ADH, ↑GH
Sympathetic nervous system - ↑ norepinephrine (no epinephrine directly);
blood loss acutely ↑s NE release (baro-receptors release NE)
Blood - activation of complement, coagulation, inflammatory cascades

Refeeding syndrome
Occurs w/ feeding after prolonged starvation or malnutrition (eg ETOH abuse)
MC on **Day 4** of refeeding
Sudden shift from fat metabolism to carbohydrate metabolism results in
↓K^+, ↓Mg^{++}, and ↓PO_4^- (all move intracellular along w/ glucose)
Effects →
Encephalopathy (↓ PO_4^-)
Cardiac arrhythmias (↓K^+, ↓ Mg^{++})
Profound weakness (↓PO_4^- – lack of ATP)
CHF (↓PO_4^- – lack of ATP)
Failure to wean from vent or **respiratory difficulty** (↓PO_4^- – lack of ATP)
Prevent this by starting feeds at a **low rate** (10–15 kcal/kg/day) and monitoring
electrolytes w/ replacement

Specific Deficiencies
Cachexia – anorexia, weight loss, wasting
Thought to be mediated by **TNF-alpha**
Glycogen breakdown, lipolysis, protein catabolism
Kwashiorkor – protein deficiency
Marasmus – starvation

TPN calorie calculation
A pt receives a 1000 cc bag of TPN which contains 20% dextrose and 7% protein. In addition, this pt receives 250 cc of a 20% fat emulsion solution
A 1000 cc bag of 20% dextrose is equal to 200 gm of dextrose (0.20 x 1000 = 200 gm), which is 640 calories (200 gm x 3.4 calories/gm)
A 1000 cc bag of 7% protein is equal to 70 gm of protein (0.07 x 1000 = 70 gm), which is 280 calories (70 gm x 4 calories/gm)
A 250 cc bag of 20% fat emulsion has 2 kcal/cc = 500 kcal (fat has 9 kcal/gm, the clinical lipids emulsions have 1.1 kcal/cc for 10% fat emulsion and 2.0 kcal/cc for 20% emulsion)
Then just add them up 680 + 280 + 500 = 1460 calories

Deficiency	Causes	Sx's
Chromium (Cr)	TPN *without* trace minerals	**Hyperglycemia**, confusion, peripheral neuropathy
Selenium (Se)	TPN *without* trace minerals	**Cardiomyopathy** (myocardial necrosis) hypothyroidism, neuro changes
Copper (Cu)	TPN *without* trace minerals gastric bypass	**Pancytopenia** neuropathy w/ ataxia
***Zinc** (Zn)	TPN *without* trace minerals gastric bypass, Crohn's chronic liver or renal DZ	**Rash w/ blisters** (peri-orbital) **chronic non-healing wounds**, wasting
Trace minerals in general	TPN *without* trace minerals	**Poor wound healing** (esp copper, zinc); often 1st manifestation
***Phosphate**	See fluid and electrolytes chapter	**Weakness** (failure to wean off ventilator), **encephalopathy** ↓ WBC chemotaxis, phagocytosis
***Thiamine** (B₁)	ETOH abuse, white rice diet	**Wernicke's encephalopathy** (ataxia) **lateral gaze palsy** (abducens nerve) **cardiomyopathy** (beri-beri), ± CHF peripheral neuropathy
Pyridoxine (B₆)	Very rare, usually children	**Seizures**, cheilitis (lip inflammation) peripheral neuropathy
Cobalamin (B₁₂)	Gastric bypass, malabsorption intrinsic factor deficiency	**Megaloblastic anemia**, beefy tongue **peripheral neuropathy**
Folate	Inflammatory bowel DZ, malabsorption, sulfasalazine	**Megaloblastic anemia**, beefy tongue
Niacin	ETOH abuse, psych pts lack of protein (esp tryptophan)	**Pellagra** (diarrhea, dermatitis, dementia)
Essential fatty acids	Steatorrhea, pancreatic insufficiency	**Thrombocytopenia**, dermatitis, hair loss, **poor wound healing**
Vitamin A	Diet deficiency - major problem in African nations; steatorrhea	**Night blindness**
Vitamin D	Poor fat absorption (eg steatorrhea) coupled w/ lack of sunlight	**Rickets, osteomalacia**
Vitamin E	Poor fat absorption (eg steatorrhea) almost never from diet deficiency	**Neuropathy**, spinocerebellar ataxia
****Vitamin K**	Inflammatory bowel disease, steatorrhea, abx's that clear gut	**Coagulopathy** (↑pre-thrombin time, PT)

TPN main cause of trace mineral deficiency
****Most Vit K produced by **bacteria** in the intestines
Steatorrhea can cause deficiency of fat soluble vitamins
Transferrin – transporter of iron; **Ferritin** – storage form of iron

ONCOLOGY

Most commons (MC)

Cancer #2 cause of death in US (MC – heart disease)
MC CA in women – breast CA
MCC of CA death in women – lung CA
MC CA in men – prostate CA
MCC of CA death in men – lung CA

Oncogenesis (cancer transformation)

Cancer - heritable alteration in genome leading to **loss of growth regulation**
Neoplasms can arise from:
Carcinogens (eg smoking, XRT)
Viruses (eg EBV, HPV, HepB, HepC, HepD)
Immunodeficiency (eg AIDS, TXP pts)
Spontaneous gene mutation (eg 25% MEN syndromes)
Latency period – time between exposure and formation of detectable tumor
Tumor doubling time: 20-100 d
Proto-oncogenes – normal human genes that regulate cell growth; mutations or over-expression can transform proto-oncogenes into oncogenes
Oncogenes – genes that can participate in the onset and development of CA
Retroviruses can contain **oncogenes**
Epstein-Barr – Burkitt's lymphoma (8:14 translocation, B cell, mandible)
Nasopharyngeal CA (c-myc)
Post-transplantation lymphoproliferative DZ (PTLD)
HPV – cervical CA
HepB, -C, -D - hepatocellular CA
Tumor Suppressors – have 1 or both of the following functions
1) **Inhibit cell cycle**
2) **Induce apoptosis** (programmed cell death)
Generally need multiple oncogenic gene transformations and mutations in tumor suppressors to get cancer

Proto-oncogenes

Growth factors (eg c-*sis* – PDGF)
Receptor Tyrosine Kinases [eg HER/neu (EGFR), PDGFR, VEGFR]
Cytoplasmic Tyrosine Kinases (eg *src* family)
GTPase (G proteins; eg *ras* family) – usually transmembrane
k-ras oncogene - ras protein is a GTPase involved in transmembrane signal transduction and cell cycle regulation
Transcription factors (eg *myc* family)
DCC gene (deleted in colorectal cancer) ? mechanism

Tumor suppressor genes

APC (chr 5; adenomatous polyposis coli) - protein binds glycogensynthasekinase (GSK) and is involved **in cell cycle regulation** and **cell movement**
p53 (chr 17) - protein is a **transcription factor** involved in **cell cycle regulation** and **apoptosis** (normal gene induces cell cycle arrest and apoptosis; abnormal gene allows unrestrained cell growth)
BRCA 1 and **2** (chr 17 and chr 13) - proteins involved in **DNA damage repair** and are also **transcription factor** in **cell cycle regulation**
Bcl-2 - governs mitochondrial outer membrane permeabilization
Involved in **apoptosis**
Retinoblastoma (Rb1, chr 13) - involved in **cell cycle regulation**

Carcinogens

Coal tar – larynx, skin, bronchial CA
Beta-naphthylamine – urinary tract CA (bladder CA)
Benzene – leukemia
Asbestos – mesothelioma
Tobacco – lung CA
UV radiation – skin CA

Cancer Immunology

Innate and **adaptive immune systems** involved in CA immunosurveillance

Natural killer cells can independently attack tumor cells (attack cells w/ ↓ed MHC expression)

Cytotoxic T cells need MHC complex to attack tumor

Tumor antigens are random unless viral-induced tumor

Immunodeficiency or immunosuppression can lead to ↓ CA surveillance

HIV-related malignancies – Kaposi's sarcoma (MC), NHL

Transplant related malignancies – skin CA (MC), PTLD

Cancer spread

Resection of a normal organ to prevent cancer

Breast – BRCA I or II with strong family history

Thyroid – RET proto-oncogene w/ family history of MEN or thyroid CA

Also (although organ not totally normal)

Undescended testicle in adults (testicular CA)

Colon (FAP, long standing ulcerative colitis)

Gallbladder [polyps (esp w/ sclerosing cholangitis) or porcelain gallbladder] → gallbladder CA

En bloc multi-organ resection can be attempted for some tumors (colon into bladder, adrenal into kidney, gastric into liver or spleen)

**Local invasiveness is different from metastatic disease

Palliative surgery may be indicated – tumors of hollow viscus causing obstruction or bleeding (colon CA, gastric CA), pancreatic CA w/ biliary obstruction, breast CA w/ skin or chest wall involvement

MC CA in suspicious axillary lymph node (or any other site) – lymphoma

Other supraclavicular – neck, breast, lung, stomach, pancreatic CA's

Other axillary – breast CA, melanoma

Other peri-umbilical – pancreatic CA (Sister Mary Joseph's node)

Lymph nodes have poor barrier function

→ better to view them as signs of **probable systemic mets**

Sentinel lymph node biopsy – *no role for clinically palpable nodes*; you need formal lymphadenectomy

Discovery of a metastasis

Metastasis Site	MC Primary Source
Bone	breast CA, prostate (males)
Skin	breast CA, melanoma (males)
Lung	breast CA (contra-lateral lung males)
Breast	melanoma
Small bowel	melanoma (causes intussusception)**
Liver	colorectal CA
Spleen (rare)	colorectal CA
Ovary	colorectal CA
Brain	lung CA
Heart	lung CA
Adrenal	lung CA

Krukenberg tumor – gastric CA mets to ovary (also colorectal CA)

Most successfully cured isolated mets w/ surgery (5-year survival)

Germ cell (eg seminoma) to lung	**75% *(best)***
Colon CA to liver (≤ 3 mets)	35%
Sarcoma (eg osteogenic CA) to lung	35%
Renal cell CA to lung	35%
Melanoma to lung or liver	25%
Lung CA to brain	20%

Breast CA rarely presents w/ isolated mets

Multiple mets isolated to a single organ can be resected if you leave enough of the organ behind for function or if organ is non-essential

Chemotherapy agents

Cell cycle–nonspecific agents ($\rightarrow$ all DNA cross-linking and binding agents)
Act at all phases of the cell cycle
Linear response to cell killing ($\uparrow$ dose $\rightarrow$ $\uparrow$ killing)
Alkylating agents – add **alkyl groups** to DNA, forms **covalent bond**
    Cisplatin (platinum) – nephrotoxic, neurotoxic, ototoxic
    Carboplatin (platinum) – **bone** (myelo-) suppression
    Oxaliplatin (platinum) – nephrotoxic, neuropathy, ototoxic (all less
        than cisplatnin), cold sensitivity; used for **colon CA**
    Cyclophosphamide – **acrolein** is active metabolite
        S/Es: gonadal dysfunction, SIADH, hemorrhagic cystitis
        Mesna can help w/ hemorrhagic cystitis.
    Busulfan: S/Es – pulmonary fibrosis
    Streptozocin (nitrosurea) – use for **pancreatic islet cell tumors**
        'Glucose mimic' to islet cells only $\rightarrow$ kills islet cells
    Dacarbazine – used for **metastatic melanoma**; often as single agent
Streptomyces Agents
    Bleomycin – crosslinks and interferes w/ DNA
        S/Es – pulmonary fibrosis
    Actinomycin – binds DNA, blocks RNA polymerase and DNA
        polymerase (less)

Cell cycle–specific agents
Act at specific stages of cell cycle **(S or M)**; only cells <u>at that stage</u> affected
Exhibit **plateau** in cell-killing ability (at certain point, $\uparrow$ dose$\rightarrow$ killing same)

1) S Phase
    Anti-metabolites – interfere w/ metabolites used to form DNA
        Methotrexate – inhibits <u>dihydrofolate reductase</u> (DHFR), which
            inhibits purine and DNA synthesis
            S/Es: renal toxicity, radiation recall
            Leucovorin rescue (tetrahydrofolic acid) - reverses
                effects of methotrexate
        5-Fluorouracil (5FU) – inhibits <u>thymidylate synthase</u> (TS),
            which inhibits purine and DNA synthesis
            Leucovorin – $\uparrow$ toxicity of 5FU
        Pemetrexed – inhibits <u>DHFR</u> and <u>TS</u> above plus <u>GARFT</u>
            (glycinamide ribonucleotide formyltransferase)
            Use – advanced squamous type non-small cell lung CA
                (pemetrexed + cisplatin), malignant mesothelioma
            Need to give **folate** and **B-12** (avoids deficiencies) w/ Tx
                in addition to **steroids** (avoid skin rash)
        Gemcitabine – <u>nucleoside analogue</u> gets inserted into DNA
            and arrests replication
            Use – pancreatic CA, bladder CA
    Topoisomerase Inhibitors (etoposide, topotecan) – interfere w/
        DNA transcription and replication by <u>inhibiting topoisomerase</u>
        S/Es – bone marrow suppression
        Topoisomerase normally unwinds DNA for DNA duplication
    Anti-tumor antibiotics
        Doxorubicin (Adriamycin) – <u>DNA intercalator</u>
            S/Es: cardiomyopathy (CHF) secondary to O_2 **radicals** at
                >500 mg/m^2

2) M phase (<u>m</u>icrotubule <u>m</u>odulators – arrest <u>m</u>itosis)
    Alkaloids
        Vincristine (microtubule inhibitor) – peripheral neuropathy,
            neurotoxic
        Vinblastine (microtubule inhibitor) – **bone** (myelo) suppression
    Taxanes (docetaxel, paclitaxel) – promotes microtubule **formation**
        and stabilization that cannot be broken down; S/E- neuropathy

Hormonal Therapy
Selective Estrogen Receptor Modulators (SERMs)
Tamoxifen – Tx and prevention of <u>breast CA</u> (see Breast chp)
> Preferred for **pre-menopausal: 1) prevention** and 2) **receptor positive breast CA** (or unknown receptor status)

Raloxifene - prevention of <u>breast CA</u> (see Breast chp), also ↓s fx's
> Preferred for **post-menopausal prevention**

S/Es: blood clots (1%), endometrial CA (0.1%) – less w/ Raloxifene

Aromatase Inhibitors (anastrozole, letrozole - ATAC trial)
Block conversion of androgens to estrogen

Preferred for **post-menopausal receptor positive breast CA** (or unknown receptor status)

S/Es: fractures (2x more common than SERMs)

GnRH analogues (leuprolide, goserelin): ↓ FSH + ↓LH → ↓ testosterone
Used for hormone sensitive <u>prostate CA</u>

Anti-androgens (flutamide, bicalutamide) – inhibit androgen receptors (testosterone + DHT receptors); used in <u>prostate CA</u>

Monoclonal Antibody Therapy
Trastuzumab (Herceptin) – binds **HER/neu receptor**, used for <u>breast CA</u>
HER/neu-Human Epidermal Growth Factor Receptor tyrosine kinase

Bevacizumab (Avastin) – binds **VEGF** and acts as angiogenesis inhibitor
Use in metastatic: 1) <u>colorectal CA</u>, 2) <u>non-small cell lung CA</u>

Rituximab (Rituxan) - binds B cell **CD20**, for <u>Non-Hodgkins lymphoma</u>

Receptor Tyrosine Kinase Inhibitors (multi-RTKI)
Imatinib (Gleevac)
> Binds **c-kit** (stem cell growth factor receptor)
> Used for <u>malignant GIST tumors</u> (very effective)
> **S/Es**: CHF (uncommon)

Immunotherapy
Interferon-alpha (2b) – metastatic <u>melanoma</u> or <u>renal cell CA</u>
Chronic Hep C and Hep B

IL-2 – metastatic <u>melanoma</u> or <u>renal cell CA</u> (can be used as single Tx)

Vaccines to prevent CA – HepB vaccine, HPV vaccine (Gardasil)

Adaptive immunity (see Adaptive Immune System chp)
> 1) **IL-2** can be used to enhance immunity to tumor
> 2) **Tumor antigen** given to pt, induces tumor immune response

Other
Mitotane (DDD) – cytolytic for adrenal cortex
> **Use** - unresectable or metastatic <u>adrenocortical CA</u>

Alitretinoin – topical retinoid used for isolated <u>Kaposi's Sarcoma</u>

Octreotide – used for <u>pancreatic islet cell tumors</u> (including gastrinoma) and <u>carcinoid syndrome</u>

Levamisole – **anti-helminthic drug** that ↑s immune system against CA

Important S/Es
Bleomycin and **busulfan** – can cause pulmonary fibrosis

Least myelosuppression – bleomycin, vincristine, busulfan, cisplatin hormonal Tx, monoclonal antibody Tx

GCSF (granulocyte colony-stimulating factor) – ↑s PMN recovery after chemo
> **S/Es: Sweet's syndrome** (acute febrile neutropenic dermatosis) → tender erythematous plaques filled w/ PMNs→ Tx: **steroids** *(best Tx)*

Radiation therapy (XRT, ionizing radiation)

    M phase – most vulnerable stage of cell cycle for XRT

    Most damage done by formation of **oxygen radicals**

        → maximal effect w/ **high oxygen levels**

    Main target is DNA – oxygen radicals damage DNA and other molecules

        W/ damaged DNA, the cell is **no longer able to divide** successfully

    Higher-energy radiation has skin-preserving effect (maximal ionizing

        potential not reached until deeper structures).

    Fractionate doses

        Allows **repair** of normal cells

        Allows **reoxygenation** of tumor

        Allows **redistribution** of tumor cells in cell cycle to **M phase**

    Very radiosensitive tumors – seminomas, lymphomas

        The more frequently the cells divide, the more sensitive to XRT

        Kidneys, lungs, liver, and lymphocytes have ↑ed sensitivity to XRT.

    Very radioresistant tumors – epithelial, sarcomas

        Large tumors – less responsive to XRT due to **lack of oxygen in tumor**

    Brachytherapy – source of radiation in or next to tumor (Au-198, I-128); delivers

        high, concentrated doses of radiation

    Gamma knife – high intensity cobalt XRT directed at brain tumors

    XRT sensitizers – oxygen, chemo, hyperthermia

    XRT can be used for **painful bony mets**

Tumor markers

    ABC-B5 – melanoma

    CEA – colon CA, others

    AFP-L3 – L3 form specific for hepatocellular CA

    DCP (des gamma carboxyprothrombin) – high specificity for hepatocellular CA

        (not present in other diseases)

    CA 19-9 – pancreatic CA

    CA 125 – ovarian CA, endometrial CA

    Beta-HCG – testicular CA, choriocarcinoma

    PSA – prostate CA (thought to be the tumor marker w/ **highest sensitivity,** low

        specificity)

    NSE – small cell lung CA, neuroblastoma

    BRCA I and II – breast CA

    Half-lives – CEA: 18 days; PSA: 18 days; AFP: 5 days

Tumor lysis syndrome

    Rapid tumor lysis following chemo can lead to **acute metabolic disarray**

        Destroyed cell releases of **purines** and **pyrimidines** (→ uric acid)

        K^+ and PO_4^- also leaked from cell

    Leads to:

        1) **acute renal failure** (uric acid nephropathy)

        2) **arrhythmias** (↑K^+)

        3) **seizures** (↓Ca^{++}; low levels from precipitation w/ PO4⁻)

    RFs – lymphomas, leukemias

    Path

        ↑ uric acid, ↑PO_4^-, ↑K^+, ↓Ca^{++}

        ↑ **BUN** and **creatinine** (from renal failure)

    Tx

        Aggressive hydration

        Allopurinol (↓ uric acid production)

        Rasburicase (converts **uric acid** to inert metabolite **allantoin**)

        PO_4^- **binding antacids** before chemo

        Loop diuretic

        HCO3⁻ (alkalinize urine, prevent uric acid precipitation)

        Calcium

        HD if previous fail

<u>PET</u> (positron emission tomography)

18-FDG (fluorodeoxyglucose) metabolized to **FDG-6-phosphate** by **hexokinase**
PET detects **FDG-6-phosphate**

SUV (standardized uptake value, ratio)
- **SUV** = ratio of activity in area of interest/cc^3 compared to activity in injected dose/patient weight
- **< 2.5** considered benign
- 5-10% false positive rate (**inflammatory DZ** – histoplasmosis, TB)
- 5-10% false negative rate (**slow metabolizing tumors** – carcinoid, bronchoalveolar lung CA)
- Accuracy for **brain** low because of **increased glucose uptake in brain**
- Test may not work in **diabetics** or **hyper-insulinemia**
    - (hyperglycemia competes w/ 18-FDG uptake; insulin promotes 18-FDG uptake into normal cells)

PET good for detecting recurrent CA – need to wait 6 months for inflammation to go down

Best tumors for pre-op staging w/ PET scan (initial tumor W/U, not recurrence)
1) **Lung CA**
2) **Esophageal CA**
3) **Melanoma** (stage III or IV)

<u>SLNBx</u> (sentinel lymph node biopsy)

Sentinel lymph node – hypothetical first lymph node(s) reached by cancer cells from a tumor

Lymphazurin blue dye and **technetium labeled sulfur colloid radiotracer**
- Are injected around primary tumor area
- Need 1-4 hours for uptake → dye + radiotracer travel to sentinel node(s)
- **Type I hypersensitivity reactions (1%)** have been reported w/ lymphazurin blue dye

Usually find 1-3 nodes; send for permanent

All blue nodes and **nodes within 10%** of highest gamma count node should be taken

Can't find dye or gamma counts in OR → **formal lymph node dissection**
Tumor found in LN's along path → **formal lymph node dissection**

For a high gamma count in a lymph node basin you were not expecting (eg you are doing a sentinel lymph node biopsy in a pt for breast cancer and the supra-clavicular region lights up), you should sample lymph nodes in the area that has the high count if it is at least 10% of the highest count node

MC uses – breast CA and melanoma

<u>Bone Marrow TXP</u> (BMT)

Treatment mortality – 10%

Sequence: Peripheral blood stem cells harvested, then chemo ± XRT given to get rid of the primary disease process, stem cells given back

Cx's

Graft versus host disease
- **Most serious Cx w/ allogenic BMT**
    - <u>Not</u> seen w/ **autologous** (peripheral blood stem cells used)
- MC in **1st 3 months**
- **Tx: steroids**

Opportunistic Infections

Hepatic veno-occlusive disease (SOS, sinusoidal obstructive syndrome)
- Hepatic venules become **occluded** causing liver injury
- Can result in **mortality**
- **Ursodiol** can help prevent

BMT allows higher doses of chemo to be given

Occasionally indicated for:
- Stage IV Neuroblastoma
- Stage IV Non-Hodgkins Lymphoma
- other advanced CA's

Most impt prognostic factor of breast CA devoid of systemic mets – nodal status
Most impt prognostic factor of sarcoma – tumor grade

Ovarian CA – one of the few tumors for which **surgical debulking** improves
    chemotherapy (not seen in other tumors, see Gynecology chp)
Colon CA
    Genes involved in development include **APC, p53, DCC, and K-ras**.
    APC – thought to be the initial mutation in the development of colon CA
    Colon CA does not usually go to bone
Curable solid tumors w/ chemo only – Hodgkin's lymphoma and NHL
    Most lymphomas are **B cell**
T-cell lymphomas – HTLV-1 (skin lesions), mycosis fungoides (Sezary cells)

Types of Tx
    Induction – sole treatment; often used for advanced disease (eg metastatic lung
        CA) or when no other better treatment exists (eg lymphoma)
    Primary (neoadjuvant) – chemo given <u>1st</u>, followed by another (secondary)
        therapy (XRT, surgery, or both)
        Common indications
            Esophageal CA (> stage I)
            Stage III lung CA (some)
            Stage III breast CA (some)
            Sarcomas for limb preservation
    Adjuvant – chemo given <u>after</u> another therapy is used (XRT, surgery, or both)
    Salvage – for tumors that fail to respond to initial chemotherapy

Definitions
    Hyperplasia – increased number of cells
    Metaplasia – replacement of one tissue with another (GERD w/ squamous
        epithelium in esophagus changed to columnar epithelium → Barrett's
        esophagus)
    Dysplasia – altered size, shape, and organization (Barrett's Dysplasia)

Clinical trials
    Phase I – is it safe and at what dose?
    Phase II – is it effective?
    Phase III – is it better than existing therapy?
    Phase IV – implementation and marketing

Core needle biopsy (CNBx) – gives architecture
Fine needle aspiration (FNA) – gives cytology (just cells)

TRAUMA

Trauma Sequence for Blunt Trauma
(stay in order, go back to the top for clinical change)

A - Airway – awake and alert, assess for hoarseness or stridor
> **Intubation**
>> **In-line traction**
>> Avoid succinylcholine w/:
>>> **Severe head injury** (↑'s ICP)
>>> **Hyperkalemia** – burns, compartment syndrome
>> 7.5 tube for adult (in child use child's little finger to size)
>>> Adult ET tube 22-24 cm at lip
>> **Cricoid pressure** to prevent aspiration
> **Cricothyroidotomy** in a crunch (facial trauma)
> **Tracheostomy** (local, awake) or **fiberoptic intubation** if injury is below
> cricothyroid (laryngeal trauma)
> **Needle cricothyroidotomy** in a child as opposed to open

B - Breathing – assess bilateral breath sounds, look for subcutaneous air
> Bowel sounds in chest → *no chest tube* (diaphragm rupture)

C- Circulation – **BP** and **HR**; look for **JVD** (tension PTX or cardiac tamponade), **muffled heart sounds**
> **Place 2 large bore IV's**
>> 16 gauge in antecubital fossa
>> **Saphenous vein** at ankle – best site for cut-down for access (if you can't get central line)
>> **Intra-osseous** (tibia) for children
> **Fluid bolus 2 L lactated ringers**
>> Then switch to **O negative blood;** then switch to **type specific blood**
>> **Children** – 20 cc/kg bolus of LR x 2; then switch to blood 10cc/kg boluses
> **T and C** for 6 units of PRBCs
>> **If bleeding** have available FFP (6), platelets (6), and cryoprecipitate (6)
>> **Trauma labs** - T and C, PT/PTT, CBC, LFTs. amylase, lipase, chemistries, lactic acid, UA
> Order **Lateral C spine, PA CXR,** and **Inlet PXR** while finishing primary survey
> **Feel abdomen** (distension?) and **pelvis** (stable to rock?)

D - Deformity – assess pulses, moves everything; anything broken or bleeding; pupils
E - Exposure – clothes off; c-spine collar, backboard

Head to toe assessment after above
Foley if no blood at the urethral meatus
NGT if no facial fx's
XR of anything that's possibly broken
Head, chest (as screen for aortic injury if mechanism suggests), abdominal, and pelvic CT scans
C/T/L spine x-rays if appropriate
Unit or floor depending on injuries
Follow serial exams or Hct's if worried about something and not going to OR
Obvious fx's (eg femur fx) – splint, finish W/U, repair later depending on pt stability

Blunt trauma
> Stable → w/u as above
> **Unstable** → (SBP ≤ 90 despite 2 L of LR) → **FAST scan** (or DPL)
>> **If positive** (bleeding from **abdominal source**) → OR (for laparotomy)
>> **If negative** → find source of bleeding:
>>> **Pelvic fx** (exam, PXR)
>>> **Chest** – hemorrhage, tension PTX, cardiac tamponade (exam, CXR)
>>> **Extremity bleeding** – lacerations or femur fractures
>>> Neurogenic shock (lateral c-spine) – R/O above, then consider this

Penetrating trauma

ABCs, IV x 2, LR fluid bolus x 2 if hypotensive

T and C for 6 units of blood (same as blunt to this point)

Find exit and **entrance sites** ("box" injuries defined in chest section)

Not sure if it penetrates abdominal fascia – consider diagnostic laparoscopy

Superficial stab wounds:

- **Stable pt** → local exploration
  - If not penetrating fascia → observe
  - If penetrating fascia → follow GSW and deep stab wounds below
- **Unstable pt** → follow GSW or deep stab wounds below

GSW or **deep stab wounds:**

1) **If chest wound** and **stable**

    (injuries at level of nipples or below – will also need **laparotomy**):

    Chest in "box " → get CXR

    - Chest tube on side of injury (you are going to OR) + chest tube on contra-lateral side if PTX or hemothorax on that side
    - To OR for pericardial window, EGD and bronch; gastrograffin/barium swallow (later)

    Chest outside "box" → get CXR

    - Chest tube for PTX, hemothorax, or if going to OR for something else

2) **If chest wound** and **unstable**

    (DDx: hemorrhage, tension PTX, cardiac tamponade)

    Place chest tube(s) right away (diagnoses tension PTX and hemorrhage; consider bilateral chest tubes right away):

    - → If not much blood, go to OR for **pericardial window** and **laparotomy**
    - → If chest tube has **high output** (> 1000-1500) →
      - OR for **anterior thoracotomy** on **bleeding side**
        - (**clamshell incision** if you need to see whole heart)
      - Keep pt **supine** for thoracotomy (anterior thoracotomy)
      - Clamp hilum if **severe lung injury** (then repair)
      - Clamp aorta if **aortic injury** (then repair)
      - Put finger in hole for **heart injury** (then repair)

    Complete the W/U after you repair injury → pericardial window, bronch and EGD; gastrograffin/barium swallow (later)

3) **If abdominal** (stable or unstable) → laparotomy

    4 quadrant packs

    Compress aorta at diaphragm if unstable

    Let anesthesia catch up

    Look for injuries starting w/ quadrants least likely to have an injury 1st

Need Abd CT following blunt trauma for: abd pain, need for general anesthesia, closed head injury, intoxicants, paraplegia, distracting injury, hematuria, pts w/ a negative DPL

CT scan misses (false negatives) – hollow viscous injury, diaphragm injury

If pt taking coumadin → repeat CT scans in 8 hours (looking for delayed bleed)

Laparotomy Indications: peritonitis (suggests hollow viscous perforation), evisceration, positive DPL or FAST, clinical deterioration, free air, diaphragm injury, intraperitoneal bladder injury, positive contrast studies, specific renal, pancreas, biliary tract injuries

Coding in ED
→ possible ED thoracotomy (loss of pulse or SBP < 60)

Blunt trauma – use only if pressure or pulse lost **while in ER**

    Consider immediate reversible cause before thoracotomy (eg tension PTX)

Penetrating trauma – use only if pressure or pulse lost **on way to ER** or **in ER**

ED left anterior-lateral thoracotomy:

    Open pericardium longitudinally and anterior to phrenic nerve
        (decompress possible cardiac tamponade)

    Cross-clamp aorta (open mediastinal pleura, watch for esophagus
        posteriorly)

    Let anesthesia catch up w/ volume resuscitation

    1) **If blunt Injury** → perform FAST (or DPL)

        Positive → OR for laparotomy

        Negative → find source and Tx (pelvic fx, chest, or extremity
            bleeding; neurogenic shock)

    2) **If penetrating injury** → **go to OR and explore area** (laparotomy,
        thoracotomy or both)

    Penetrating right chest injury and pt codes – still do <u>left</u> thoracotomy

        Can extend incision across sternum to right side if needed for
            exposure (clamshell incision)

OR protocol
Rapid infuser blood warmer

Cell saver (not if bowel perforation)

Warming lights and **warm room**

Prep chin to ankles in supine position all the way to both sides

Do not induce until after you have prepped (can drop blood pressure)

Abdominal Injury:

    4 quadrant pack

    Compress aorta at diaphragm if **hypotensive** (go through gastro-hepatic
        ligament if you want to clamp) → **let anesthesia catch up on**
        volume

    Check areas remote from injury 1st, then area of suspected injury

    Address bleeding before any other injury

    At any point during trauma lap, you can **press down on aorta** for
        hypotension or to help **control arterial bleeding**

    Mattox maneuver – left colon, spleen, and pancreas brought up
        Good for retroperitoneal exposure of aorta, left iliac, and left renal

    Cattel maneuver – right colon and duodenum brought up
        Good for retroperitoneal exposure of IVC, right iliac, and right renal

    W/ associated pelvic fx → don't make midline incision below umbilicus to
        avoid releasing retroperitoneal hematoma

Diagnostic peritoneal lavage (DPL)
Used in **hypotensive pts** (SBP ≤ 90) with blunt trauma

Positive DPL (blunt trauma) – >10 cc blood, >100,000 RBCs/cc, food particles,
    bile, bacteria, >500 WBC/cc

Need **emergency laparotomy** if positive

Perform supra-umbilical DPL if pelvic fracture present

DPL misses (false negatives) – retroperitoneal bleed, contained hematomas

FAST scan (focused abdominal sonography for trauma)
U/S used to inspect heart and abdominal compartment (looks for blood in
    peri-hepatic fossa, peri-splenic fossa, pelvis, and **pericardium**)

Morbid obesity can limit viewing

May miss free fluid < 50–80 ml (eg hollow viscous injury)

Need emergency laparotomy if FAST is positive

FAST scan misses (false negatives) – retroperitoneal bleed, hollow viscous
    injury

<u>Head injury</u>
Neuro status – can be due to **head injury** or **carotid injury**

Specific Head Injuries
Subdural hematoma
Greater incidence than epidural
MCC – venous injury; usually from tearing of **bridging veins**
between dura matter and arachnoid plexus
Head CT – crescent-shaped deformity adjacent the skull
Tx: Operate for significant **neuro degeneration** and **mass effect**
(shift **> 10 mm** for subdural)
Chronic subdural hematomas
MC - elderly after minor fall
Operation indications as above
Epidural hematoma
MCC – arterial injury; usually **middle meningeal artery**
Head CT – lenticular (lens-shaped) deformity adjacent the skull
Typical pattern – loss of consciousness (LOC) → then lucid interval
→ then sudden deterioration (N/V, irritability, restless, LOC)
Tx: Operate for significant **neuro degeneration** and **mass effect**
(shift **> 5 mm** for epidural).
Cerebral hematoma and **contusions** – MC in frontal lobe
Coup or contra-coup (typically don't require operation)
Intraventricular hemorrhage – if hydrocephalus → place ventriculostomy
Diffuse axonal injury
Dx: usually CT scan, MRI most sensitive
Tx: supportive care; ventriculostomy and drainage; ± craniotomy
Extremely poor prognosis
Fosphenytoin or **Levetiracetam** (eg Keppra) – prophylactic to prevent
seizures in pts w/ head injury
Do not need to check drug levels w/ these

Dilated pupil (blown pupil)
Possible ipsilateral temporal lobe pressure on **cranial nerve III**
(**oculomotor**, can progress to **temporal uncal herniation**)
If you need to go to OR emergently for something else (and you can't get
head CT) →
1) **Burr hole** on that side and on other side if that's negative
5 cm anterior and superior to external auditory canal
2) Can also just do **craniotomy**
3) Another option is to place **ICP bolt** to see if pressure elevated
(if elevated, perform burr hole)
If in ER w/ blown pupil and **pt stable** →
Go to **Head CT** (could be baseline anisocoria; Don't want Burr hole if
pt had baseline pupil difference)

Cerebral perfusion pressure (CPP)
CPP = Mean arterial pressure (MAP) *minus* intracranial pressure (ICP)
Elevated ICP findings on CT scan
1) **Decrease in size of ventricles**
2) **Loss of sulci** (flattening)
3) **Loss of cisterns**
ICP monitors for:
1) **GCS ≤ 8**
2) **Suspected elevated ICP** based on CT scan
3) **Not able to follow neuro exam** w/ moderate to severe head injury
(eg in OR; paralyzed or sedated)
Peak ICP after head trauma → **48–72 hours** after injury

Supportive treatment for elevated ICP

Normal ICP is 10

ICP > 20 usually requires treatment

Overall, want **goal cerebral perfusion pressure** (CPP) > 60

Sedate and paralyze

Raise head of bed

Relative hyperventilation

Want some cerebral vasoconstriction (keep **pCO$_2$ 30–35**)

Limits brain edema and lowers ICP

Avoid too much hyperventilation (causes cerebral ischemia from vasoconstriction)

Keep sodium 140–150

Serum Osmolarity should be **300 $\pm$ 10**

Normal saline used for volume (draws edema from brain and lowers ICP); also raises MAP

Volume + Pressors to keep **MAP high** (normal saline + phenylephrine)

Mannitol

Loading dose 1 g/kg x 1

Maintenance dose 0.25 mg/kg q4h

(Draws edema from brain and lowers ICP)

Keppra or Fosphenytoin – prophylactic for seizure prevention

Barbiturate coma – if refractory to above

Ventriculostomy

MC placed in **posterior parietal region** (5 cm posterior and superior to external auditory canal)

Removes CSF fluid which can help lower ICP

Craniotomy – if refractory to all of the above (decompresses ICP)

Brain swelling

Maximum brain swelling occurs **48–72 hours after trauma**

Symptoms of ↑ ICP – stupor, headache, N/V, stiff neck

Signs of ↑ ICP – HTN, HR lability (high or low), slow respirations

Intermittent bradycardia is a sign of severely elevated ICP and impending herniation

Cushing's triad – HTN, bradycardia, and slow respiratory rate

Impending herniation

Herniation – shift of brain across structures in skull; usually fatal

Skull Fractures – most do not require surgery

Basal skull fx's

Raccoon eyes (anterior fossa), Battle's sign (mastoid; middle fossa, risk facial nerve injury), hemotympanum, CSF rhinorrhea / otorrhea

Temporal skull fx's

Risk injury to CN VII (facial) and VIII (vestibulocochlear)

MC facial nerve injury site (motor to the face) – geniculate ganglion in temporal bone

MC vestibulocochlear injury site (hearing and head movement) – temporal bone

Operate on skull fx's if either:

1) **Significantly depressed** ($\geq$ 1 cm, needs elevation) *or:*

2) **Contaminated** (dura penetration) *or:*

3) **Refractory CSF leak**

Close dura w/ operation

CSF leaks – treat expectantly w/ epidural drain (↓s pressure to allow closure); may need to close if refractory (wait 4-6 weeks)

If fixing facial fx – close at that time

Usually associated w/ **nasoethmoid fx's**

CSF has **tau protein + beta-transferrin**

Diabetes Insipidus (↓ed ADH)
    Sx's: copious dilute urine output
        ↑ serum Na; ↓ urine Na; ↓ urine spec gravity (dilute; nl 1.002-1.028)
    Tx:
        1) Replace free water deficit w/ **D5 water**
            Correct Na < 0.7 mEq/L/h → avoid **brain swelling**
        2) **DDAVP**

SIADH (syndrome of inappropriate anti-diuretic hormone; anti-diuresis)
    Sx's: low urine output and <u>**no**</u> **edema** despite fluid overload
        ADH acts on distal tubules to reabsorb water (**cAMP** mediated)
        ↓ serum Na; ↑ urine Na, ↑ urine spec gravity (concentrated)
    Tx:
        1) **Fluid restriction + diuresis** (*mainstay*, + treat underlying cause)
        2) ****If symptomatic**, above **Tx fails**, or pt is in a **coma** (eg severe
            head trauma pts) → **3% hypertonic saline**
            Correct Na < 0.5 mEq/L/h → avoid **central pontine myelinosis**

(see Fluids and Electrolytes chp for other sx's of diabetes insipidus
    hypernatremia and SIADH hyponatremia)

Glasgow Coma Scale (GCS)
    Motor Function
        6 follows commands
        5 localizes to the pain site
        4 withdrawals from pain
        3 flexion with painful stimuli (decorticate)
        2 extension with painful stimuli (decerebrate)
        1 no response to painful stimuli
    Verbal Response
        5 oriented x 3
        4 confused but responds
        3 inappropriate words with speech
        2 incomprehensible sounds (grunting)
        1 no response verbally
    Eye opening
        4 spontaneous eye opening
        3 opens eyes to command
        2 opens eyes to pain
        1 no response to eye opening

    Most impt prognostic indicator of the GCS is the **motor score**
    Penetrating head injury has poorest survival of any head injuries given
        equal GCS scores
    GCS score:
        ≤ **14** need head CT
        ≤ **10** need intubation
        ≤ **8** need ICP monitor

Spine Injury

All trauma pts need to be in a **C-collar** and on a **backboard**
Steroid indications (usually for spine injury w/ **neuro deficit**)

Best indication is **worsening neuro deficit**

Methylprednisone – bolus 30 mg/kg, then 5 mg/kg/hr IV for 23 hrs
Neurologic deficits without bony injury → MRI to check for ligamentous injury
**Cervical spine X-ray w/ pre-vertebral soft tissue swelling and no bony
injury** → MRI to check for ligamentous or occult injury
Going to OR for laparotomy in pt w/ cervical spine injury – place sand bags
around head
Facet subluxations – MC in **cervical spine** (90%)
Cervical Facet subluxation (dislocation, jumped facets)

Unilateral – usually no cord injury

Bilateral – 90% have cord injury

Spinal cord injury from displacement

MCC – hyperextension and rotation w/ ligamentous disruption

Tx: open reduction w/ spinal fusion usual for all

Cervical Spine

C1 burst (Jefferson Fx)

Mechanism - impact or blow to back of head (diving in shallow water)

Tx: rigid collar

C2 Hangman's Fx

Mechanism - hyperextension of head

Tx: halo cervical brace (3 mos)

C2 Dens

Mechanism - hyperflexion w/ loading (MC w/ MVA)

Type I (base stable, through tip of Dens)

Tx: rigid collar

Type II (base unstable, through dens base)

Tx: halo cervical brace (3 mos) or internal fixation

Type III (base unstable, through vertebral body)

Tx: halo cervical brace (3 mos) or internal fixation

Dens = odontoid process
MC location for spine injury – cervical spine
MC cervical spine fx – dens fx
RFs – blunt injury above clavicles, MVAs, unconsciousness
The higher the cervical spine fx, the higher the morbidity and mortality

Thoracolumbar Spine

Thoracolumbar spine contains 3 columns (anterior, middle, and posterior)
If ≥ 2 columns are disrupted, spine considered **unstable:**

Wedge Fx's usually anterior column only and considered **stable**

Burst Fx's considered unstable (2 columns – anterior and middle)

Tx: **spinal fusion**
Upright fall – calcaneus, lumbar, and wrist/forearm fractures

Indications for emergent surgical spinal cord decompression:

1) **Significantly displaced fx or dislocation that is non-reducible** w/
distraction
2) **Open** Fx
3) **Spinal cord compression**
4) **Progressive neuro dysfunction**
5) **Anterior Cord Syndrome**

Maxillofacial trauma

Facial trauma at high risk for **cervical spine trauma**

Facial lacerations – preserve skin, avoid trimming edges

Facial Fx's (Le Fort Fx's)

> **Type I** (- across maxilla);
>> **Tx: Maxillo-mandibular fixation** (MMF) ± miniplates (if unstable)
>
> **Type II** (/ \, lateral to nasal bone, underneath eyes, down towards maxilla)
>> **Tx: MMF** ± miniplates (if unstable)
>
> **Type III** (- -, lateral to the orbital wall)
>> **Tx: MMF and miniplates**

Facial nerve injury

> **Penetrating injury** – repair (see below for timing)
>
> **Blunt injury** (no fx) – leave alone, will recover
>
> **Temporal skull fx** – assess amount of nerve injury
>> **Severe** – repair (see below for timing)
>>
>> **Not severe** – leave alone
>
> **Need repair <u>within 3 days</u>** (for knife wound or skull fx)
>> Allows use of a **nerve stimulator** (hard to find nerve after trauma) before **degeneration** sets in (after 3 days); also avoids having to dissect through scar
>>
>> **Contaminated wound** (eg for GSW) – early exploration, washout, tag nerve ends w/ long prolene sutures so you can find them later; **delayed repair** (*within* <u>30 days</u>)
>>
>> **Nerve injuries** repaired w/ **10-0 prolene** (bites just through epineurium)
>
> **MCC facial nerve injury** – temporal bone fracture
>
> **Iatrogenic injury** – repair immediately

Mandibular fx

> **Malocclusion** best indicator of injury
>
> Dx: thin slice CT w/ facial reconstruction
>
> Tx: external or internal fixation

Nasoethmoid fx

> CSF leak in 70%
>> Conservative therapy initially
>>
>> Place epidural catheter to decrease CSF pressure
>>
>> Close dura if that fails (4-6 weeks of conservative therapy)
>>
>> If undergoing facial reconstruction, repair at that time

Nosebleeds

> **Anterior** – vaseline gauze packing
>
> **Posterior** – vaseline gauze deep packing; balloon tamponade if that fails (can use foley catheter)
>> May require **angio-embolization** of internal maxillary artery or ethmoidal artery

Orbital fx (blowout fractures)

> Impaired gaze or diplopia need repair
>
> Tx: restore orbital floor (bone fragments or graft)

Tripod Fx (zygomatic bone) – internal fixation (just for cosmesis; not a functional problem)

Neck trauma

May need emergent airway

Blunt neck injury: **asymptomatic** – neck CT scan, **symptomatic** - explore

**Zone I Neck (penetrating) – explore if symptomatic or significant finding
  Location – *clavicle to cricoid cartilage*
  W/U – angio, bronchoscopy, EGD and swallow (late), $\pm$ pericardial window
  Approach – median sternotomy (or upper sternal split) to reach these
    lesions (especially vascular injuries for proximal control)
Zone II Neck (penetrating) – **explore all (if penetrating platysma muscle)
  Location – *cricoid cartilage to angle of mandible*
  Approach – **lateral neck incision** (trachea, esophagus, blood vessels)
**Zone III Neck (penetrating) – explore if symptomatic or significant finding
  Location – *angle of mandible to the skull base*
  W/U – angio and laryngoscopy
  Approach – jaw subluxation, digastric and sternocleidomastoid muscle
    release, ± mastoid sinus resection to reach vascular (ie carotid) injury

Sx's requiring neck exploration – shock, bleeding, expanding hematoma,
  losing or lost airway (cricothyroidotomy or tracheostomy, then exploration),
  subcutaneous air, stridor, dysphagia, hemoptysis, neuro deficit
Shotgun injury to neck – neck CT-angio, EGD, bronch, and swallow
Esophageal injury (see below for thoracic esophageal injuries)
  Hardest neck injury to Dx
  Best combined Dx modality → esophagoscopy + barium swallow
  No leak - Tx: conservative therapy
  Leak - Tx: **primary 2 layer closure for most,** cover w/ **strap muscle**
    Massive neck injury (can't repair) –cervical esophagostomy (safest)
Laryngeal and Tracheal Injuries (fractures)
  Airway emergencies
  Sx's: crepitus, stridor, respiratory distress, hoarseness
  Secure airway emergently in ER →
    Awake fiberoptic intubation if pt is still breathing
    Awake cricothyroidotomy or tracheostomy if can't get fiberoptic
      Use **local anesthetics** so pt can maintain his airway
  Tx: Primary repair of injury w/ strap muscle covering repair
    Tracheostomy to allow **edema** to subside and to check for **stricture**
    If cricothyroidotomy, convert to tracheostomy (late) to avoid voice
      problems
Carotid artery
  Hemorrhage, pseudoaneurysm, or **AV fistula** (hear a continual bruit)
    Tx: open **primary repair** or interposition graft
  Dissection (needs to be just carotid; not aortic dissection)
    Asymptomatic Tx: anticoagulate (prevent thrombus formation)
    Symptomatic Tx: carotid stenting *(best);* open repair if that fails
  Thrombosis
    If antegrade flow is still present →
      Tx: open **primary repair** or interposition graft
    No antegrade flow → Tx: **anticoagulate** to prevent thrombus
      extension and propagation
  Carotid ligation – stroke in 20%
Vertebral artery
  Hemorrhage, pseudoaneurysm, or **AV fistula** (hear a continual bruit)
    Tx: angio for **embolization** (make sure contra-lateral vertebral artery
      is open; rare subsequent neuro deficit)
      If open ligation necessary→ incision at C1-C2 vertebral space
  Dissection (needs to be just vertebral; not aortic dissection)
    Tx: **anticoagulation** (heparin, coumadin), prevent thrombus forming
  Thrombosis
    Tx: **anticoagulation** (heparin, coumadin) → ↓ thrombus extension
Thyroid gland injury – stop bleeding and place a drain
Recurrent laryngeal nerve injury – repair or reimplant in <u>cricoarytenoid muscle</u>

Chest trauma

Penetrating chest injury (stable)
    Define **entrance and exit** wounds
    1) **Penetrating "box" injuries** - borders are clavicles, xyphoid process, nipples:
        a.) **Pericardial window**
            If there is blood → median sternotomy to fix injury
            Place pericardial drain at the end
        b.) **Bronch**
        c.) **Esophagoscopy**
        d.) **Esophagogram** (gastrograffin followed by thin barium)
            Obtain before commencing regular diet (esophageal injuries notoriously hard to find with EGD alone; combined EGD and swallow studies improve accuracy)
        Esophageal injuries** are the **hardest to Dx
    2) **Penetrating chest wound outside "box"**
        Need chest tube if pt requires intubation or has PTX / hemothorax
        No PTX or hemothorax and No intubation → just follow serial CXRs
    3) **Penetrating injury below nipples** – also need **laparotomy**

Chest tube
    For **hemothorax or PTX**
        May pick these up before CXR w/ **breathing portion of ABC's**
        Do not place chest tube w/ **ruptured diaphragm**
    Indications for OR thoracotomy after chest tube placement:
        1) **> 1000-1500 cc** after initial insertion
        2) **> 250 cc/hr** for 3 hours
        3) **Unstable pt** w/ significant bleeding
    OR Thoracotomy for bleeding
        Keep pt supine in case you need abdominal or contralateral access
        Check intercostal vessels; IMA; lungs and hilum; great vessels; heart
        Perform **clamshell incision** if trouble w/ exposure
    Need to drain all blood from chest w/ chest tubes
        Prevents fibrothorax, pulmonary entrapment, infected hemothorax, and to **stop bleeding**
        Lung inflation compresses area (↓s bleeding)
    Unresolved hemothorax after two well-placed chest tubes
        VATS drainage (wait until pt stable from trauma)
    Persistent large PTX after chest tube
        Check and make sure the **1st chest tube** has **good placement** and **system is working**
        Place 2nd chest tube **anteriorly**
        Still doesn't resolve → **bronch** to look for **tracheo-bronchial injury** or mucus plug

Sucking open chest wound
    Hole needs to be at least 2/3 the size of trachea to cause resp compromise (air will then preferentially be sucked in through hole and not trachea)
    Tx:
        Wound dressing w/ tape on three sides (creates 1 way valve)
            Prevents developing a **tension PTX** while allowing lung to expand w/ inspiration
        Chest tube
        Eventually need closure of defect

Flail chest
    ≥ 2 consecutive ribs broken at ≥ 2 sites → causes paradoxical motion of the chest wall
    ****Underlying *pulmonary contusion* biggest impairment to respiratory status (not the flail chest itself)*
    Tx: may need **intubation** for underlying pulmonary impairment

Multiple rib fx's – thoracic **paravertebral block** best at relieving pain and allowing pt to take deep breaths w/o pain (prevents hypoxemia)

Tracheobronchial Injury
> **Sx's:**
>> **Worsening oxygenation** after chest tube placement (pt takes a deep breath in and goes out chest tube)
>> Large **continuous air leak** after chest tube placement
>> Large **pneumomediastinum** or **severe subcutaneous emphysema**
>> **Persistent PTX** after chest tube placement
>> MC after **blunt trauma**
>
> **Dx:**
>> **Bronchoscopy**
>>> **90% of injuries** within **1 cm of carina**
>>> **MC side** – right (not as flexible as left side)
>
> **Tx:**
>> **Immediate tx** - one of extremely few indications for **clamping a chest tube** (prevents the chest tube from sucking air out the injury and away from the lungs)
>> **Indications for repair:**
>>> 1) Respiratory compromise
>>> 2) Persistent air-leak (1-2 weeks)
>>> 3) Can't get lung up
>>> 4) Injuries > 1/3 the lumen
>>
>> **Surgery**
>>> **Mainstem intubate** unaffected side w/ **long single lumen** tube (double lumen tube likely too large and can **worsen tear**)
>>> **Right thoracotomy** – for *right mainstem, trachea, and proximal left mainstem* injuries (avoiding the aorta here)
>>> **Left thoracotomy** - for *distal left mainstem injuries* (aorta is in the way for more proximal injuries)
>>> Usually close the bronchus (4-0 vicryls) and cover injury w/ intercostal muscle flap or pericardial fat pad

Lung injury bleeding
> **Perform tractotomy w/ GIA 45 stapler** - Place stapler in tract and fire to stop bleeding, resecting lung as you go (<u>no</u> formal lobectomy)
> **Clamp hilum** if having trouble getting control

Esophageal injury (thoracic)
> **Dx:** EGD and **esophagogram** (gastrograffin followed by thin barium)
> **Tx:**
>> 1) **Primary repair usual** (4-0 vicryls mucosa; 4-0 silks muscle; buttress w/ intercostal muscle, drains, feeding J tube)
>>> Absorbable suture for mucosa to avoid stricture
>> 2) **If not able to primarily repair** (ie esophagus too disrupted)
>>> Cervical **esophagostomy** (left neck); staple esophagus in neck and at GEJ <u>(diversion and exclusion)</u>
>>> **Chest tube** drainage
>>> **G-tube** for decompression
>>> **J-tube** for feeding
>>> Esophagectomy later - consider esophagectomy at same time if stable

Diaphragm Injury
> MC on **left side** (liver protects the right side)
> MC after **blunt trauma**
> **Dx:**
>> **CXR** or **CT scan** (can be hard to Dx)
>>> **Air-fluid level** in chest from **stomach herniation through hole**
>>> **NGT in chest**
>
> **Tx:**
>> **Trans-abdominal approach** if < 1 week (look for associated injuries)
>> **Chest approach** if > 1 week (adhesions in chest prevent safe trans-abdominal approach)
>> **Reduce stomach + assess viability** (can infarct, resect if necrotic)
>> **2-0 Tevdeks** (non-absorbable) for repair of diaphragm
>> May need PTFE **mesh** for hole

Aortic transection

MC from rapid deceleration injury (MVAs)

90% of these pts die at scene

Address other life-threatening injuries 1st (eg severe solid organ laceration, pelvic fx w/ hemorrhage) → ***repair aorta when pt stable***

Mediastinal widening is from laceration of bridging veins and arteries (not leaking from aorta itself)

Signs (on CXR):

Widened mediastinum (> 8 cm)

1st and 2nd rib fractures

Apical capping

Loss of aorto-pulmonary window

Loss of aortic knob contour

Left hemothorax

Trachea deviation to right

Displacement of NGT to right

Depression of left mainstem bronchus

MC location for tear - ligamentum arteriosum (slightly distal to left subclavian artery)

Other locations – near base of innominate, near aortic root, at diaphragm

Need aortic evaluation w/ significant mechanism (eg head on car crash >45 mph, fall >15 feet)

Dx: spiral chest CT (to screen; **aortogram** is the *gold standard*)

CXR normal in 5%

Tx:

Control blood pressure w/ **esmolol** (continuous IV beta-blocker)

↓ed HR also ↓s shear stress

Repair options:

1) Left thoracotomy (posterolateral) w/ partial left heart bypass, place interposition graft (*safest answer*)

2) Many being treated w/ stent grafts (off label indication)

**Important that you treat other life-threatening injuries 1st →

Pt w/ positive FAST scan or other life-threatening hemorrhage or injury should have that addressed before aortic transection

Vascular injuries (thoracic)

In general want to get proximal and distal control before repairing these or be on cardiopulmonary bypass through the groin

Median sternotomy for injuries to:

Ascending aorta

Innominate artery

Proximal right subclavian artery

Innominate vein

Proximal left or right common carotid artery

Proximal left subclavian artery (can perform **trap door incision** w/ median sternotomy)

Left thoracotomy for injuries to

Distal left subclavian artery

Descending thoracic aorta

Right mid-clavicular incision ± resection of medial clavicle

Distal right subclavian artery

Cardiac contusion

MCC death after heart contusion – ventricular fibrillation

(highest risk in **1st 24 hours**)

MC arrhythmia after myocardial contusion – SVT

RFs – sternal Fx's, sternal contusion, no seatbelt

Dx: EKG (*best test*) - **conduction abnormalities** most significant finding

Anything other than NSR considered significant

Tx: need telemonitoring for 24 hours

Traumatic causes of cardiogenic shock and arrest
    1) **Tension pneumothorax**
        Sx's:
                Hypotension, ↓ breath sounds, bulging neck veins, tracheal
                    shift away from injury, high airway pressures (if on
                    ventilator)
                ****Hypotension may worsen after being intubated**
                Can see **bulging diaphragm** during laparotomy
                Cardiac compromise due to **decreased venous return**
        Tx: chest tube
    2) **Cardiac tamponade**
        Sx's: hypotension, distended neck veins and muffled heart sounds
           (Beck's Triad)
        Dx: FAST scan
            If FAST scan shows fluid – pericardiocentesis
            FAST scan not available or can't tell – pericardial window in
                OR
        Pt coding → left anterior-lateral thoracotomy in ER; open
           pericardium
        Pericardial window or pericardiocentesis shows blood → need
           median sternotomy

    Cardiac injury near coronary – place mattress stitch under coronary artery w/
        pledgets
    ED thoracotomy and find a hole in the heart → Tx – digital control (finger in
        hole), go to OR to repair

Pelvic Fractures

    Can be a major source of blood loss
    Pt unstable w/ pelvic fx and **negative FAST** (and not bleeding in chest based
        on CXR or from extremity)
        1) **Stabilize pelvis** (cross pelvis w/ sheet or external fixator if ortho there)
        2) **Go to angio** for **embolization** (do <u>not</u> wait for ortho) – they can meet
           you in angio
        Anterior pelvic fractures / dislocations – MC venous bleeding
        Posterior pelvic fractures / dislocations – MC arterial bleeding
    Pt stable w/ pelvic fx – continue w/u
    All pts w/ significant pelvic fx need:
        1) **Proctoscopy** ± sigmoidoscopy
        2) **RUG** (retrograde urethrogram) + **cystogram**
        High risk for **genitourinary** and **rectal injuries**
    Consider **colostomy** for severe rectal or perineal tears
    Operative findings:
        Penetrating injury pelvic hematomas →
           Open (may need Mattox or Cattel for exposure)
           Get proximal control of pelvic vessels 1st
           Dissect directly into hematoma to find problem, pressure, control,
             repair (5-0 prolene) or ligate depending on injury
           At times, may not be able to fix these → **pack and go to angio for**
             embolization
        Blunt injury pelvic hematomas →
           Leave
           If expanding or pt unstable - **stabilize pelvis** (as above), **pack** pelvis,
             go to **angio** for embolization (remove packs when pt stable)
    External fixator – can be left for 5-7 days
    Usually repair pelvic fx 3-7 d after initial trauma if stable

Duodenal trauma
Path
MCC – blunt trauma (crush or tears from deceleration injury)
MC location for tears – 2nd portion of duodenum (near ampulla of vater)
   Can also get tears near ligament of Treitz
MC location for hematoma – 3rd portion (overlying spine)
25% mortality w/ **blunt duodenal injuries** due to associated **shock**
Fistulas – major source of morbidity w/ duodenal injuries

Debridement and either: 1) **primary repair** or 2) **primary anastomosis** treats
85% of all duodenal injuries requiring operation
Used when there is a **leak** or **loss of integrity** of bowel wall
If circumference of wall is reduced by > 50%, can't use primary repair
Segmental resection w/ **primary anastomosis** is possible w/ all portions of
   duodenum *except* **2nd portion** (can do **primary repair** to most 2nd
   portion injuries)
Consider intra-op cholangiogram (IOC) for injuries to 2nd portion of
   duodenum

Dx of suspected duodenal injury
CT scan findings - bowel wall **thickening**, **hematoma**, **air**, contrast **leak**,
   retroperitoneal **fluid/air**
UGI *(best test for Dx of duodenal injury)*
Leak → OR, No leak → conservative tx
If CT scan worrisome for injury but non-diagnostic → **repeat CT** in 8 hours
   or get an **UGI study** (if stable)

Paraduodenal hematomas on CT scan
MC location – 3rd portion of the duodenum overlying the spine
Sx's: high small bowel obstruction 12–72 hours after injury (eg N/V)
Dx:
   UGI study (*best test,* → 'stacked coins' or 'coiled spring' appearance)
      Need to R/O leak w/ this study as well

Tx:
   Conservative Tx 1st
   TPN + NGT resolves 95% of these within **3 weeks (hematoma gets
      reabsorbed)
      Clamp NGT for 4 hours every 3-4 days
         Check residual to see if moving gastric fluid through
            If **< 250 cc** left over 4 hours, **start clears**
   Weekly UGI until resolution and before starting oral feeding
   OR if not resolved within 3 weeks → follow **paraduodenal
      hematoma** below

Paraduodenal hematomas in OR – need to explore these
MC location – 3rd portion of duodenum overlying spine
Kocher maneuver and open **lesser sac through omentum**
   Kocher – peritoneum to right of duodenum incised; duodenum and
      pancreas reflected towards midline (inspects 2nd and 3rd
      portions of duodenum and pancreatic head)
   Assess duodenal wall, pancreas, portal triad, and surrounding areas
   Can give methylene blue down NGT to look for leak in duodenum
1) **No leak →** repair serosa; **overlay omentum**; leave **drains** (19 Fr JP)
2) **Leak or questionable wall integrity →** primary repair or primary
   anastomosis usual (see below)
Consider intra-op cholangiogram (IOC) for injuries to 2nd portion of
   duodenum (also for fat necrosis, bile staining, or any leakage not
   from duodenum)

Kocher maneuver indicated for:
1) **Bile staining** (biliary system or duodenal injury)
2) **Succus drainage** (duodenal injury)
3) **Fat necrosis** (pancreatic injury – pancreatic enzyme release)
4) **Paraduodenal hematomas**

Operative Tx of duodenal injuries

Primary repair or **primary anastomosis** treats 85%

Duodenal Diversion Protocol

Used for the following:

Severe primary repairs

Primary anastomosis

Jejunal serosal patch

Permanent duodenal exclusion

Duodenal-jejunal anastomosis

Swelling and **edema** can eventually cause problem w/ duodenal injuries (duodenal blow-out) – often need to divert

Technique

a) **Pyloric exclusion** (TA 45 stapler – will exclude pylorus but not cut it; this staple line will eventually open up with time)

b) **Gastrojejunostomy** (usually Roux-en-Y)

c) **Distal feeding J-tube**

d) **Consider lateral duodenostomy tube** *or* **retrograde draining J-tube** (esp if duodenal closure looks tenuous) to prevent duodenal stump blow-out

e) Place lots of **Drains**

1) Jejunal serosal patch

Used when:

a) Not enough duodenum is present for primary repair or primary re-anastomosis *or*

b) In 2nd portion of duodenum and too large for primary repair

Jejunal serosal patch sutured to cover hole (just bring up a loop of jejunum)

*Follow **Duodenal Diversion Protocol** above

2) Permanent Duodenal Exclusion

Used when hole too big for primary closure, primary anastomosis or jejunal patch and is **proximal to Ampulla of Vater**

Staple and divide pylorus (GIA 45 - do not want this to ever open up)

Staple off distal end of duodenal injury (needs to be proximal to Ampulla of Vater); can **tack anterior duodenum to posterior duodenum** if not enough room to get stapler

Careful not to occlude the ampulla of Vater

*Follow **Duodenal Diversion Protocol** above (except use GIA 45 instead of TA 45)

3) Duodenal-jejunal anastomosis

Used when hole too big for primary closure, primary anastomosis or jejunal patch and is **distal** to Ampulla of Vater

Bring up **segment of jejunum** (Roux-en-Y; divide jejunum close to ligament of Treitz) and connect to duodenum (this should be able to drain the biliary system)

Will need another Roux limb for the diverting gastro-jejunostomy

Just resect the residual 3rd and 4th portions of the duodenum

4) Trauma Whipple

Rarely if ever indicated acutely (most recommend just placing drains)

Really only if ampulla and its connection to duodenum are blown out (functional Whipple) would you consider this

If just the ampulla is blown out and the duodenum is OK → drains initially, delayed whipple

Drains – remove when patient tolerating diet without an increase in drainage

Duodenal Fistulas – can close with time (duodenal worst at closing)

Tx:

NPO, NGT (decompression), **TPN, octreotide, H2 blockers**

UGI w/ SBFT to R/O distal obstruction

Abd CT to r/o abscess

Conservative management for 6 weeks

Failure to close → repeat UGI w/ SBFT to R/O distal obstruction and abd CT scan to R/O abscess → **OR** after that for repair

<u>Small bowel trauma</u>
MCC – penetrating injury
Can be hard to Dx w/ blunt trauma
Occult small bowel injuries
1) **Abd CT scan** characteristics of occult small bowel injury:
Intra-abdominal **fluid** <u>not</u> associated with a solid organ injury
Bowel wall **thickening**
Mesenteric hematoma
2) **Repeat Abd CT** w/ **delayed PO contrast to R/O leak**
Leak – OR for laparotomy
No Leak – Close observation
Repeat abd CT after 8-12 hours to make sure finding not
getting worse (fluid building up in abdomen), worse → OR
Develops peritoneal signs → OR
Make sure pts w/ non-conclusive findings can tolerate a diet
before discharge
Majority repaired primarily
Repair lacerations **transversely to avoid stricture**
Resection and re-anastomosis for:
1) **Large lacerations** (>50% circumference)
2) If wall circumference is **reduced > 50%** w/ primary repair
3) Significant **tissue destruction**
4) **Multiple close** lacerations
5) **Compromised vascular supply**
Mesenteric hematomas – open (>2 cm or expanding)

<u>Colon trauma</u>
MCC – penetrating injury
Blunt colon trauma w/ significant tissue injury → will need resection
Penetrating colon trauma:
1) **Right** and **transverse colon**
Primary repair or **primary anastomosis** usual (<u>no</u> ostomy)
Knife wounds – can perform primary repair
GSW – can perform primary anastomosis
Need ostomy w/ MF (Mucus Fistula) or **HP** (Hartmann's Pouch) for
right sided or transverse lesions w/ any of the following:
a. Pt in **shock** (will compromise blood supply to anastomosis)
b. **Significant fecal spillage** (tissue too damaged for
anastomosis)
c. **Elapsed time > 6 hours** (tissue too damaged for
anastomosis)
2) **Left colon**
Repair w/ **colostomy** and **HP or MF**(*safest answer*, although some
stab wounds could be primarily repaired)
Para-colonic hematomas – open to look for injury (both blunt and penetrating)
Abscess rate after colon injury – 10%
Fistula rate after colon injury – 2%
Both fistula and abscess <u>higher</u> w/ primary repair

<u>Rectal trauma</u>
MCC – penetrating injury
Can be associated w/ pelvic fx – stabilize pelvic fx, fix rectal injury + colostomy,
colostomy takedown later
1) *Extra*-**peritoneal rectal trauma**
a. **Low rectal** (< 5 cm)
Pelvic stabilization if associated w/ pelvic fx
Primary trans-anal repair
Consider diversion w/ colostomy and MF or HP
Pre-sacral drains
Late colostomy takedown
If no pelvic fx or other injury, may not need to divert

b. **High rectal** (> 5 cm)

Pelvic stabilization if associated w/ pelvic fx

Fecal diversion w/ colostomy

Repair rectal injury if accessible (generally <u>not</u> repaired because of inaccessibility)

Pre-sacral drains

Late colostomy takedown

2) *Intra*-**peritoneal rectal trauma**

Pelvic stabilization if associated w/ pelvic fx

Repair defect

Divert w/ colostomy and MF or HP

Pre-sacral drains

Liver trauma

MCC – blunt trauma

Glisson's capsule covers liver

Lobectomy almost <u>never</u> necessary

Common hepatic artery – can be ligated proximal to the GDA (collaterals through GDA fill the proper hepatic artery)

Hepatic lobar artery – single artery may be ligated as long as pt in NOT hypotensive (would lead to liver ischemia)

Subcapsular hepatic hematomas – leave alone

Portal triad hematomas – open (both blunt and penetrating)

Leave drains w/ liver injuries

Intra-op Hepatic bleeding (both penetrating and blunt)

1) **4 quadrant packs**

Compress aorta and let anesthesia catch up if necessary

2) **Liver fractures**

Look for **bile leaks** and **bleeders** → ligate them

Can use Argon beam, thrombin, chromic suture ligation

Omentum –sutured into liver laceration to help w/ **minor bleeding** and **seal bile leaks**

Leave **drains**

3) **Pringle maneuver**

For severe hepatic bleeding

Consists of intermittent clamping of **portal triad** (leave clamp for 20 minute intervals while you perform repair, 5 min of reperfusion)

Does not stop bleeding from **hepatic veins or IVC**

Effective for liver injuries w/ portal venous or hepatic artery bleeding

Free hepatoduodenal ligament medially (window), finger through foramen of Winslow, soft clamp

4) **Damage Control Peri-hepatic packing**

For severe hepatic bleeding

Can pack severe liver injuries if pt becomes unstable (or severely coagulopathic) in OR and you are not able to easily fix problem

Pack behind, below, lateral, and over top of liver; **lots of packs**

Go to ICU and get pt **warmed, stabilized, correct coags,** transfuse **blood**

Bring back to OR next day

Consider closing abdomen w/ sterile IV bag to prevent compartment syndrome if hard to get abdominal contents back in abdomen (occurs w/ massive resuscitation)

5) **Retro-hepatic venous bleeding** (bleeding from **hepatic veins** or **IVC**)

Pack (*best option*, very hard to fix these injuries; damage control peri-hepatic packing above) and see if its **controlled:**

a. **If bleeding controlled** →go to ICU and follow damage control peri-hepatic packing pathway above

b. If bleeding not controlled → need **Atrio-caval shunt** (32 Fr chest tube) and **repair**

Allows blood diversion while performing repair

Median sternotomy, open pericardium, split diaphragm down to IVC

Vessel loop around IVC in chest

Vessel loop around IVC in abdomen (**above renal veins**)

Divide right triangular ligament and roll liver to left

Place 32 Fr chest tube in IVC for atrio-caval shunt (insert through incision in IVC or injury)

Repair injury

Common bile duct injury

<50% of circumference – primary **repair over stent** (pediatric feeding tube)

>50% of circumference or complex injury – **choledochojejunostomy** (place 14 Fr T-tube across anastomosis to prevent stricture)

Kocher maneuver and dissect out the portal triad to find these injuries

Consider **IOC** to define injury (pediatric feeding tube through purse-string in gallbladder)

10% of duct anastomoses leak so leave drains

Late cx's – biliary stricture at site of repair

Portal vein injury or SMV injury

Need to repair (ligation has 50% mortality)

May need to transect **neck of pancreas** to get to injury

Need to perform **distal pancreatectomy** with that move

Place **side-biting clamp** (allows blood flow while you repair) and perform **lateral venorraphy**

Hemobilia

Sx's: abd pain, jaundice and **hematemesis** (± melena) late after trauma (*classic*; mean **4 weeks**; can also follow hepatic surgery)

MCC - hepatic artery to biliary duct fistula

Follow UGI bleed protocol (see Stomach section)

Will see blood coming out of the ampulla of vater

Tx: **angio embolization;** surgical ligation of fistula if that is unsuccessful

Conservative management of blunt liver injuries (ie found on CT scan)

1) **Active blush** (ie free bleeding) or **pseudoaneurysm** on abd CT → **Go to OR** (no conservative management)

2) **Conservative management:**
   a. **Bedrest for 5 days** (ICU for the 1st day if severe)
   b. **Serial exams**
   c. **Serial Hct checks**

3) **Conservative management has failed if pt** (*apx*):
   a. **Becomes unstable** (HR ≥120 or SBP ≤90) despite aggressive resuscitation including 2-4 units of PRBCs
   b. **Has Hct < 21** despite 2-4 units of PRBCs
   Tx: OR for exploration

4) **Repeat CT scan for grade IV and V injuries** after 5 days (lower extremity duplex to R/O DVT before getting them out of bed, then walk pt around):

   Looking for **bile leak** (fluid collection **bigger** than original CT) or active **extravasation** after getting pt out of bed

   a. **Fluid collection bigger** than original CT and seems like **bile leak**
      → **Percutaneous drain** (if seems like bile on CT)
      → **ERCP** if bile to look for duct injury
         If leak → sphincterotomy + temporary stent
      → If failure of above (give it 6-8 weeks), OR for repair

   b. **Fluid collection bigger** then original CT and seems like **hematoma;** will see sediment area)
      → **bedrest** for another 3 days and re-CT to make sure hematoma not getting worse

   c. **Active extravasation of contrast** → OR

Spleen trauma

MCC – blunt injury (MC organ injured w/ blunt trauma)

Fully heals in 6 weeks

Threshold for splenectomy in **children** is high – unusual for children to have to undergo splenectomy

Subcapsular splenic hematomas – leave

Conservative management of blunt splenic injuries (ie found on CT scan)
1) **Active blush** or **pseudoaneurysm** on abdominal CT →
   Go to OR (no conservative management)
2) **Conservative management:**
   a. **Bedrest for 5 days** (ICU for the 1st day if severe)
   b. **Serial exams**
   c. **Serial Hct checks**
3) **Conservative management has failed if patient** (*apx*):
   a. **Becomes unstable** (HR $\geq$120 or SBP $\leq$90) despite aggressive resuscitation including 2 units of PRBCs
   b. **Has Hct < 21** despite 2 units of PRBCs
   Go to OR
4) **Repeat CT scan for grade IV and V injuries** after 5 days (lower extremity duplex to R/O DVT before getting them out of bed, then walk pt around):
   Looking for **pancreatic leak** (fluid collection <u>bigger</u> than original CT) or **active extravasation**
   a. **Fluid collection <u>bigger</u>** than original CT, and seems like **pancreatic fluid** (injury usually in tail of pancreas)
      → **percutaneous drain** (send fluid for amylase)
         Conservative Tx w/ drain will cure 95%
      → If failure of conservative Tx (give it 6-8 weeks), get ERCP to look for pancreatic duct leak:
         If leak → sphincterotomy + temporary stent
         If that does not work, go to OR (likely distal pancreatectomy or possible whipple if in head of pancreas)
   b. **Fluid collection <u>bigger</u>** than original CT and seems like **hematoma** (will see <u>sediment area</u> on CT scan)
      → bedrest for another 3 days and re-CT to make sure hematoma not getting worse
   c. **Active extravasation of contrast** → OR

Intra-operative splenic salvage

Compress spleen w/ chromic sutures or vicryl mesh (good for large capsular tears); partial splenectomy an option also

Contraindications **to splenic salvage** – unstable, DIC, grade IV (hilar injury) or higher, other serious injuries (ie head injury, liver injury → don't want spleen to be a confounding issue here), penetrating injury to spleen

Transfusion rate increased w/ splenic salvage

Pancreatic leak after splenectomy

Can injure the **tail of pancreas** w/ splenectomy

Tx: *percutaneous drain only (cures 95%)*
   If it persists after 6-8 week, get ERCP to R/O main pancreatic duct injury (see above)

Post-splenectomy issues:

Immunizations after trauma splenectomy (Pneumococcus, Meningococcus, H. influenza)

ASA for platelet count > 1-1.5 x 10^6

Prophylactic Augmentin for 6 months in children < 10 (give every day)

If child, explain to parents need to bring child to ER w/ any fever

Early broad spectrum Abx's in these pts w/ any signs of infection

(see Spleen chp)

THE COMPREHENSIVE ABSITE REVIEW

Pancreatic trauma

MCC – penetrating trauma (80%)

Blunt trauma can cause perpendicular **pancreatic duct fractures**

Intra-op pancreatic hematoma – open (both penetrating and blunt)

Persistent or rising amylase – worry about duct injury

Suspicious fluid around pancreas on CT scan :

    ERCP (or MRCP) to look for duct leak (if pt stable); If ERCP not available
        repeat CT scan in 8 hours to see if the finding is getting worse

    Follow clinical exam over that time period

    CT scan poor at picking up pancreatic injuries acutely (better w/ late
        findings; delayed signs - fluid, necrosis, edema)

    Indications for OR:

        1) **Duct leak** on ERCP (or MRCP)

        2) **Significantly worsening clinical exam**

        3) **Significantly worsening finding on repeat abd CT**

Intra-op Assessment of Pancreas

    Kocher maneuver and open **lesser sac through omentum** to evaluate
        pancreas

    Need to evaluate **duodenum** w/ pancreatic injuries

    80% of pancreatic injuries discovered in the OR are treated w/ just
        drains (ie pancreatic duct not involved)

OR findings suspicious of pancreatic injury:

    1) **Edema**

    2) **Hematoma** (need to open these up for both penetrating and blunt)

    3) **Fluid**

    4) **Fat necrosis**

    Primary concern is to figure out if **duct is injured**

        If pancreatic duct not involved (eg contusion) → just leave **drains**

        If pancreatic duct involved →

            Distal pancreatic duct injury

                Tx: Distal pancreatectomy (can take 80% of gland)

                Through lesser sac

                Usually perform **splenectomy** w/ trauma distal
                    pancreatectomy

                Splenic vein is directly posterior to pancreas

                Splenic artery is superior and posterior

                Leave drains

            Pancreatic head duct injury

                Tx: Place drains initially, possible **delayed Whipple**
                    (mortality too high w/ trauma Whipple → 50%)

            Whipple vs. distal pancreatectomy

                Based on duct injury in relation to **SMV**

    Intra-op methods for assessing whether or not the duct is injured:

        1) **Look** for leaking duct

        2) Intra-op **ERCP**

        3) **Intra-op cholangiogram** (IOC) through gallbladder (hope for
            retrograde filling; can use **contrast** or **methylene blue** to find
            leak); use morphine to contract sphincter of Oddi w/ this

        4) Can also **transect tail of pancreas** and inject there

        5) Can also **open duodenum** and inject directly into ampulla of Vater

Persistent abdominal pain (or persistent amylase elevation)

    May indicate missed (delayed) pancreatic injury.

    CT scans poor at diagnosing pancreatic injuries initially

        Delayed signs – fluid, edema, necrosis around the pancreas

    Dx: ERCP good at picking up delayed duct injuries (MRCP if ERCP not
        available; exploratory laparotomy if neither are available)

    Tx:

        Early finding of duct injury (< 24 hrs) → go to OR

        Late finding of duct injury → **percutaneous drain**

            (cures 90% in 6-8 weeks); ERCP for failure of conservative Tx

Vascular trauma

In general, **vascular repair** performed before orthopaedic repair

Use **interposition greater saphenous vein graft** for repair if a $\geq$ **2 cm segment**
is missing or damaged (use contra-lateral leg vein if leg injury)

If < 2 cm segment missing, can attempt primary repair

Check for associated **nerve injury**

Major signs of vascular injury (hard signs):

1) **Active hemorrhage**
2) **Pulse deficit**
3) **Expanding or pulsatile hematoma**
4) **Distal ischemia**
5) **Bruit or thrill**

Tx for above: go to OR for exploration

Prep both legs and **harvest vein from other side** if injury in leg

Go through injury site clearing hematoma

Vascular control proximal and distal w/ vessel loops and fogarty
clamps

Can cut down at proximal femoral artery or brachial artery for control

Repair - **primary repair** (< 2 cm missing) or **saphenous vein
interposition graft** (> 2 cm missing)

Completion a-gram

After revascularization:

Feel **pulse** to make sure you got it back

Follow **extremity for swelling** and consider **fasciotomy**
(ischemia > 4-6 hours) for **compartment syndrome**

Check **urine myoglobin** (alkalinize urine if necessary)

Check **K and H** → watch for washout electrolyte problems and
hypotension

ASA post-op

Moderate signs of vascular injury (soft signs):

1) **History of hemorrhage**
2) **Deficit of anatomically related nerve**
3) **Large stable/non-pulsatile hematoma**
4) **Close to major artery** (ie GSW to medial thigh, arm)
5) **ABI < 0.9**
6) **Unequal pulses**

Dx: Any of above, go to angio

a.) **Small injuries that are <u>not</u> flow limiting** (small intimal flaps,
small segmental stenosis, small pseudoaneurysms, AVF's,
small focal narrowings, and dissections)

Tx: heparin, then coumadin

Careful F/U during admission and after discharge w/ duplex
studies

If there is any doubt, just operate

b.) **Flow limitation** →

Tx: operate w/ primary repair or interposition graft

Special issues:

Lower extremity clot – can cut down at trifurcation or even the posterior
tibial artery and dorsalis pedis at the ankle if needed to clear clot

Vein injuries that require repair – femoral, popliteal, innominate,
subclavian, axillary

Single artery transection in calf in o/w healthy patient → ligate

Anastomoses and repair sites should be **covered w/ viable tissue** (muscle
preferred)

Consider prophylactic fasciotomy if ischemia >4-6 hours – prevents
compartment syndrome

Compartment syndrome

> **Reperfusion** after **prolonged ischemia** (4-6 hrs) – occurs **soon post-op**
> **1st finding** – *pain w/ passive motion*; Others: *swelling* → paresthesias
> → anesthesia → paralysis → poikiothermia → pulseless (late)
>
> **Pressures > 30 mmHg** or if **exam** suggests (this is a clinical diagnosis)
> Can occur in any muscle compartment
> Caused by **reperfusion injury** (PMN mediated)
> **MC after:**
>> **Supracondylar humeral Fx's** (Volkmann's contracture)
>> **Tibial Fx's**
>> **Crush injuries**
>> Other injuries that result in an **interruption and then restoration of blood flow**
>
> Undiagnosed compartment syndrome can present as **renal failure** (myoglobin release) or **hyperkalemia**
>
> **Tx:** <u>fasciotomy</u>; dead muscle debrided to prevent **myoglobin** release

IVC Injury

> **Cattel maneuver** for exposure (see liver section above for retrohepatic IVC bleeding)
> IVC bleeding best controlled w/ **proximal + distal pressure** (sponge on a stick) <u>not</u> clamps (can tear it); can place **vessel loops** *(best control)*
> Primary repair is OK if residual diameter is > 50% of original diameter o/w place saphenous vein or Gortex patch
> **Posterior wall injury** – open anterior wall after vascular control and repair posterior wall through IVC; can also try to **IVC roll-over** maneuver
> **Infra-renal IVC ligation**
>> Can be performed if necessary w/ <u>little morbidity</u>
>> Consider lower extremity **fasciotomy** w/ this move
>
> **Supra-renal IVC ligation** (below hepatic veins) – <u>*not recommended*</u>
>> Will result in **renal failure**
>> If performed, consider returning to OR if pt stabilizes for IVC reconstruction

Superior Mesenteric Vein – ligation of SMV associated w/ 10% mortality
Portal Vein – ligation of portal vein associated w/ 50% mortality

Leg compartments:

> **Anterior** – <u>anterior tibial artery</u>, deep peroneal nerve
> **Lateral** – superficial peroneal nerve
> **Deep posterior** – <u>posterior tibial artery, peroneal artery</u>, tibial nerve
> **Superficial posterior** – sural nerve
> Arteries: 1) anterior tibial artery, 2) posterior tibial artery, 3) peroneal artery
> Nerves: 1) tibial, 2) superficial peroneal, 3) deep peroneal

Exposure for lower leg:

> 1) **Above knee popliteal**
>> Medial lower thigh incision (between quadriceps and hamstrings)
>> Posterolateral retraction of **sartorius** muscle
>> Popliteal artery **directly behind femur** (popliteal vein and tibial nerve nearby)
>
> 2) **Below knee popliteal**
>> Medial incision in proximal calf directly over greater saphenous vein
>> Try to protect vein
>> Medial head of **gastrocnemius** reflected posterio-laterally
>> Need to enter the posterior compartment
>> Incision carried through the deep muscular fascia
>> Popliteal artery dissected away from popliteal vein (lateral) and tibial nerve (posterior) **behind tibia**
>> Can gain access to trifurcation vessels (anterior tibial artery, posterior tibial, peroneal artery) by going distally through this incision
>
> 3) **Posterior tibial and dorsalis pedis** – can be accessed at foot w/ retrograde Fogarty balloon if needed to clear clot

Angiogram

> **Anterior tibial artery** branches off 1st laterally
> **Peroneal artery** is in middle; **Posterior tibial artery** is medial branch

Orthopaedic Trauma and Associated Injuries
Upper Extremity

Anterior Humerus dislocation	Axillary nerve
Posterior Humerus dislocation	Axillary artery
Proximal Humerus Fx	Axillary nerve
Midshaft Humerus Fx (spiral Fx)	Radial nerve
Distal (supra-condylar) Humeral Fx	Brachial artery
Elbow (Ulnar) dislocation	Brachial artery
Distal Radial Fx	Median nerve

Lower Extremity

Anterior Femur (hip) dislocation	Femoral artery
Posterior Femur (hip) dislocation	Sciatic nerve
Distal Femur (supra-condylar) Fx	Popliteal artery
Posterior (MC) Knee dislocation	Popliteal artery
Fibula neck Fx	Common peroneal nerve

Orthopaedic trauma (also see Orthopaedics chp for specific injuries)

Can loose 2 L of blood w/ a femur fx (class IV shock)

Long bone fx or dislocations w/ loss of pulse (or weak pulse)

1) **Immediate reduction** of Fx or dislocation and **re-assess pulse + ABI**:

    a. **If pulse does not return** → go to OR for vascular bypass or repair
Intra-op a-gram if not sure of location (± angio intervention), o/w
place incision at location of fx or dislocation

    b. **If pulse is weak or ABI < 0.9** → angiogram

2) ****All knee dislocations** → angiogram after reduction (all pts unless
pulse is absent, in which case you would just go to OR)

Crush Injury

Make sure you have a **distal pulse** if extremity

Check for **compartment syndrome** (ie pain w/ passive motion, swollen
extremity; see above vascular section)

Check for **myoglobinuria**

    Tx: HCO3⁻ drip, make sure volume resuscitated; lasix if poor UOP
(prevent oliguric renal failure); *if not making urine* → switch from
Lactated Ringers to normal saline to avoid K

Check K^+ and H^+ - released w/ muscle injury or poor perfusion
(see Fluids and Electrolytes chp for Tx)

Monitor for **DIC** (D-dimer, FDPs, PT/PTT) - Tx: FFP, cryo, plts, and warm pt

Hand injury

Abx's, washout, tetanus shot

1) **Tendon injuries** – 4-0 Tevdek core suture 1 cm back on both ends of
the tendon; 5-0 Tevdek interrupted sutures 1/2 cm back
If flexor injury, splint hand in flexor position
If extensor injury, splint hand in extensor position

2) **Nerve injuries** – 10-0 prolenes just through epineurium

3) **Vascular injuries** – can probably just ligate ulnar or radial artery in adult
If going to repair (probably indicated in child) → 8-0 prolene

Median nerve

    Sensory – 1ˢᵗ 3 1/2 fingers (palmer side)

    Motor – finger flexors, thumb flexion

Ulnar nerve

    Sensory – all of the 5ᵗʰ and 1/2 4ᵗʰ digits

    Motor – wrist flexion, intrinsic muscle of the hand

Radial nerve

    Sensory – 1ˢᵗ 3 1/2 finger and back of the hand

    Motor – wrist and finger extensors

Axillary nerve – deltoid

Orthopaedic emergencies

Pelvic fractures in unstable pts

Spine injury with neuro deficit

Open fractures

Dislocations or fractures with vascular compromise

Compartment syndrome

Avascular Necrosis – femoral neck fractures at high risk: Tx: hip replacement
Femoral nerve (L2 - 4)
>   **L3 nerve** – weak hip flexion
>   **L4 nerve** – weak knee extension (quadriceps), weak patellar reflex
Sciatic nerve (L4 - S3)
>   Splits into the **common peroneal** and **tibial nerves**
>   **L5 nerve** (deep peroneal nerve) – weak dorsiflexion (foot drop);
>   ↓ed sensation big toe web
>   **S1 nerve** (tibial nerve) – weak plantarflexion, weak Achilles reflex,
>   ↓ed sensation lateral foot
>   **Sciatic nerve** also controls **knee flexion** and **hip extension**
>   **Superficial peroneal nerve** – foot eversion

Ureteral trauma
>   **MCC** – penetrating injury
>   ****Hematuria <u>NOT</u> reliable sx**
>   Blood supply is **medial** to upper 2/3 of ureter and **lateral** to lower 1/3 of ureter
>   **Dx:**
>   >   **Multiple shot IVPs** (*best test*, looking for leak)
>   >   >   Get this for penetrating wounds to lower quadrants (or worried about
>   >   >   ureteral injury)
>   >   >   Will identify injury and presence of 2 functional kidney's
>   >   >   IV contrast, then plain film after 15 min
>   >   **Retrograde cystogram** – can also help identify leak
>   **Tx: Cattel or Mattox** maneuver or exposure
>
>   1) **If large ureteral segment is missing** (>2 cm; cannot perform re-
>   anastomosis):
>   >   **Upper 1/3 injuries** and **middle 1/3 injuries** won't reach bladder w/ bladder
>   >   psoas hitch (injuries above pelvic brim)
>   >   >   → **temporize with percutaneous nephrostomy**
>   >   >   >   Tie off both ends of ureter
>   >   >   Can go with **ileal interposition** or **trans-ureteroureterostomy** later
>   >   >   If pt stable, could perform <u>trans-ureteroureterostomy</u> at time of Dx
>   >   **Lower 1/3 injuries**
>   >   >   → **Reimplant in bladder**
>   >   >   5-0 PDS (use absorbable suture) for ureteral to bladder mucosa
>   >   >   anastomosis
>   >   >   Fold bladder muscle over ureter so you don't get **vesico-ureteral
>   >   >   reflux** (3-0 silks)
>   >   >   May need **bladder** (psoas) **hitch** procedure so that ureter can reach
>
>   2) **If small ureteral segment is missing** (<2 cm):
>   >   **Upper 1/3 or middle 1/3 area**
>   >   >   → **primary repair** (spatulate ends, 6-0 PDS sutures, use absorbable
>   >   >   suture); Repair over a ureteral stent
>   >   **For lower 1/3**
>   >   >   → ****Still re-implant in bladder**
>   >   >   Cysto-ureteral anastomosis has higher success rate than uretero-
>   >   >   ureteral
>   >   >   5-0 PDS (use absorbable suture) for ureteral to bladder mucosa
>   >   >   anastomosis
>   >   >   Fold bladder muscle over ureter so you don't get **vesico-ureteral
>   >   >   reflux** (3-0 silks)
>   >   >   May need **bladder** (psoas) **hitch** procedure so that ureter can reach
>
>   3) **Partial transections** can be repaired over stent
>
>   **Intravenous** **indigo carmine** or **methylene blue** to check for **leaks** after repair
>   Avoid stripping the ureters in order to preserve blood supply
>   **Leave drains for all ureteral injuries**
>   These injuries can also occur w/ pelvic **tumor resections, APRs** and **LARs**

Renal trauma

MCC – blunt trauma

Penetrating injuries have ↑ed concomitant abdominal injury (esp GSW)

95% of renal injuries are treated **non-operatively** (esp. blunt trauma)

Hematuria – *best indicator of renal trauma*; all of these pts need a **CT scan**

Hematuria highly sensitive but not specific

Anatomy

Gerota's Fascia covers kidney

Anterior to posterior renal hilum structures (VAP)

Renal Vein

Renal Artery

Renal Pelvis

Right renal artery is **posterior to IVC** (MC)

Left **renal vein** is **anterior to aorta** (MC) - need to watch for retro-aortic left renal vein when placing clamp for open AAA repair

Left renal vein

Can be ligated near IVC in emergency situation (has **adrenal vein and **gonadal vein** collaterals)

Right does not have these collaterals (plugs directly into IVC) – need repair or nephrectomy

Flank trauma and **pre-op IVP has no uptake on that side**

(ie no blood flow to kidney) →

Dx and Tx: **immediate angiogram**; can stent if intimal flap present

Urine extravasation on CT scan – not all injuries require operation

(conservative Tx for vast majority of these)

Indications for operation w/ blunt renal trauma:

1) **Acute ongoing renal hemorrhage w/ instability**

2) **After acute phase:**

a.) Major collecting system disruption

b.) Unresolving urine extravasation

c.) Massive hematuria

Finding injuries

1) **Single shot IVP** (intra-op; can also be done pre-op for certain injuries)

Get this for penetrating wounds to lower quadrants (or worried about ureteral or renal injury)

Will identify injury and presence of 2 functional kidney's

Give contrast, take a plain film after 15 min

2) **Intravenous methylene blue** can also be used to help find leak intra-op

Intra-op

1) **Expanding peri-renal hematomas or free hemorrhage** (blunt or penetrating injury) → **Exploration** (see below)

If considering nephrectomy, IVP to confirm contra-lateral kidney

2) **Non-expanding, stable, peri-renal hematomas** (blunt or penetrating injury) → **Get IVP**

If vascular injury, open and repair, o/w leave

Penetrating more likely requires exploration than blunt (60% vs. 1%)

Exploration

Left side → Mattox maneuver

Right side → Cattel maneuver

Get control of **vascular hilum 1st**

Dissect through **Gerota's fascia**, get proximal and distal control

Can use SVG if not enough length for renal artery or renal vein repair

Place **drains**, especially if collecting system is injured

Intravenous methylene blue can be used at the end of the case to check for leak (as above)

Kidney cortical injuries (> 95% non-operative) – when you do have to repair these, just perform **primary closure**

Bladder trauma

Hematuria – *best indicator of bladder trauma* (although not specific)
MC associated injury – pelvic fx (95%)
Sx's: hematuria, meatus blood, sacral or scrotal hematoma
Dx: cystogram *(best)*
***Extra*-peritoneal bladder rupture** – MC with pelvic fractures
    Cystogram - **starbursts**
    Tx: urinary catheter 1-2 weeks
***Intra*-peritoneal bladder rupture**
    Cystogram - **leak**
    Tx: operation and repair of defect (3-0 chromics), followed by urinary
        catheter 1-2 weeks

Urethral and Genital trauma

Sx's: hematuria or **blood at meatus** (*best indicator*), free-floating prostate
    ↑ed males
MC associated injury – pelvic fx
No Foley if urethral injury suspected (membranous portion of urethra at risk for
    dissection)
Dx: RUG (retrograde urethrogram) - *best test for urethral injury*
Tx:
    1) **Significant tears** (*most injuries treated this way*);
        Suprapubic cystostomy tube and **repair in 2–3 months** *(delayed
        repair)*
        There is a **high stricture** and **impotence rate** if repaired early
    2) **Small, partial tears**
        Tx: bridging urethral catheter across tear for 3 weeks (usually
        definitive)
    3) **Genital trauma** – need repair of **tunica albuginea** and Buck's fascia if
        injured
    4) **Testicular trauma** – U/S to see if **tunica albuginea** is injured, repair if
        necessary

Pregnancy and Trauma

First Rule – at all costs, **save mother**

Pregnant pts can lose 1/3 of blood volume w/o signs

Start w/ ABC's as usual – do w/u as if baby didn't exist (both blunt and penetrating) w/ exception of:

1) **Keeping pt on left side** (prevent compression of IVC)
2) Place a **fetal monitor**
3) Place a **uterine tocodynometer**
4) **FAST scan if hypotensive** (if you use DPL, needs to be sub-xyphoid)
5) Avoid CT scan and radiologic studies if possible w/ early pregnancy

Selective radiologic studies

> **Severe trauma** → get appropriate W/U
>
> _**No evidence**_ that exposure to < 5-10 rads has any adverse impact on fetal CA, growth retardation, premature labor or birth defects
>
> **Abd/pelvic CT scan** – 2.6 rads to fetus (no pelvic XR, use CT)
>
> **CXR** – < 0.0007 rads to fetus
>
> **Head CT** – < 0.05 rads to fetus
>
> *__Full trauma W/U is ≤ 3 rads__* (_excludes_ PXR but _includes_ pelvic CT)
>
> Use uterine shielding when possible
>
> Highest risk of radiation induced birth defects is in **1st trimester**

Estimate pregnancy – use fundal height (20 cm = 20 wk = umbilicus)

> Fetus needs to be at least **24 weeks** to survive

Vaginal Exam – discharge, blood, amnion; look for effacement, dilation, fetal station

Premature labor

Sx's: contractions, vaginal bleeding, water breaks

Use tocolytic agents only if **onset of premature labor** is confirmed or **uterine irritability** (<u>not</u> used prophylactically)

Tx:

1) **Magnesium sulfate** 2-4 gm/hr (want serum level 4-9 mg/dl) respiratory depression occurs at 13 mg/dl
2) **Indomethacin enemas**
3) **Terbutaline**

Indications for C-section during laparotomy for trauma:

1) **Risk of fetal distress exceeds risk of immaturity** (fetus needs to be > 24 weeks) - mother usually w/ **persistent shock**
2) **Pregnancy threat to mother's life** (eg uncontrolled hemorrhage, DIC)
3) **Mechanical limitation** (ie uterus in way) for a life-threatening vessel injury
4) **Pregnancy near term** (≥34 weeks) and mother has severe injuries (ie likelihood of child survival better w/ delivery)
5) **Direct uterine trauma** – through entire uterine wall
   Tangential injury to uterus (not through it) – just fix wall w/ chromics

Estimating fetal maturity (amniotic fluid)

> **Lecithin:sphingomyelin (LS) ratio > 2:1**
>
> Positive **phosphatidylcholine**

Placental abruption after trauma

MCC – shock (#2 - mechanical disruption)

Placental lining separates from the uterus

Placental abruption - 50% fetal demise

> Separation of 50% almost 100% fetal death rate

Sx's: vaginal bleeding, uterine tenderness, contractions, fetal HR <120

Kleihauer-Betke test – detects and measures fetal blood in maternal circulation → **sign of placental abruption (can also estimate amount of fetal-maternal hemorrhage)

Uterine rupture

MC site – posterior fundus

Uterine rupture after childbirth – aggressive fluid resuscitation indicated even w/ shock (best outcome compared to going to surgery). Uterus eventually clamps down after delivery

Hypothermia

Trauma W/U – ABCDE's

2 IV's , warm fluid resuscitation

T and C for 6 units

Lateral c-spine, CXR, PXR

1) **If in shock →**
- Need to r/o **traumatic causes of shock before going w/ hypothermia as cause**
- R/O bleeding in chest, abdomen, pelvis, or from extremity (also consider neurogenic shock)
- Exam, Hct, PXR and CXR, FAST scan (or DPL) → all needed to R/O other causes of shock

2) **Monitor for VF and PEA**
- **VF or PEA →** Prolonged CPR if this occurs until **pt warm**
  - Drugs likely to be ineffective until pt warm
- **Assess for potential causes of VF or PEA that could occur w/ trauma**
  - Hyperkalemia, hydrogen ion, hypotension (from associated trauma), **hypothermia**
  - **Hyperkalemia** and **metabolic acidosis** can occur if **underwater** for prolonged time
  - Continue CPR and tx these associated problems

3) **Start Warming Pt:**
- Warm humidified air for ET tube
- Remove wet clothing
- Dry warm blankets
- Warming lights and pads
- Warm IVF's (Max IV temp - **65.0 C**)
- Warm lavage – NGT, chest tubes, peritoneal lavage (through DPL catheter if present)
- Bair hugger (warm air conduction, Max temp - **43.3 C**)
- **Extreme measures** (temp < 27.0 C) – cardiopulmonary bypass (*highest rate of heat transfer*)
- **Rewarming shock** – peripheral dilatation from external warming (Tx: fluid)

4) *DO not stop CPR until warm and dead*

Electrical Injuries

These pt's are at risk for **rhabdomyolysis** and **compartment syndrome**

Do not put IV's into affected limbs

All need **significant volume resuscitation** (cell necrosis inside body)

Other injuries – quadriplegia, liver necrosis, intestinal or GB perforation, pancreatic necrosis

Evaluate for compartment syndrome → would need fasciotomy
- All extremities susceptible
- If muscle is dead (cadaveric), you need to debride it to prevent **myoglobin release**

EKG and **telemetry for 24 hours**

Renal issues – **hyperkalemia** and **myoglobinuria** causing renal failure can occur

Electrical burns to mouth in children (electrical cord) – wait 6-9 months before repair unless child cannot eat

MCC immediate death – cardiac arrest
- **Lightning strike** – MCC death is electrical paralysis of the brainstem

MCC death overall and late – infection

AC current more damaging the DC current
- **AC –** entrance and exit wound **same**;
- **DC – separate** entrance and exit wounds

Highest resistance - bone

<u>Hematomas</u> (Intra-op; **> 2 cm** considered significant)

Location	Penetrating	Blunt
Pelvic	explore	leave
Paraduodenal	explore	explore
Portal triad	explore	explore
Retrohepatic	leave if stable	leave
Midline^	explore	explore
Pericolonic	explore	explore
Peri-renal	explore *	leave†

*Unless preoperative CT scan or IVP shows no injury and hematoma is not
expanding.

†Unless preoperative CT scan or IVP shows injury or hematoma is
expanding

^Explore both supra-mesocolic and infra-mesocolic

Zone I Central Hematoma (medial to psoas)
→ open (potential for great vessel injury)
If more to the right → Cattel
If more to the left → Mattox
Supra-celiac hematomas
Hard to control w/ just Mattox or Cattel maneuver
Need **left thoracotomy** or **infra-diaphragmatic** and **aortic
clamping** (go through gastro-hepatic ligament) for vascular
control before exposure
Infra-celiac hematomas
Can usually control w/ Mattox or Cattel

Zone II Lateral Hematomas (lateral to psoas)
→ open (safest answer); potential for colon, duodenal, kidney injury
If blunt trauma w/ no obvious colon or duodenum injury, IVP is OK and
hematoma not expanding → observe
If on right → Cattel
If on left → Mattox

Zone III Pelvic Hematoma
→ leave if blunt; open if penetrating
w/ penetrating – may end up just packing and going to angio for
embolization after opening

Blood transfusion
Type O Blood (Universal donor) – contains no A or B antigens
Males can receive Rh positive blood
Females who are pre-pubescent or of child-bearing age should receive Rh
negative blood (O negative blood)
Type specific blood (non-screened, non-crossmatched) – can be administered
relatively safely but there may be affects from antibodies to minor antigens
in donated blood
Type and screen looks for **preformed antibodies** to **minor antigens**
Massive blood transfusion can result in
Dilution of coagulation factors → coagulopathy
Hypocalcemia (manifested as hypotension)
Hypothermia (manifested as coagulopathy)

Shock Class

	I	II	III	IV
Blood loss (cc)	<750	750-1500	1500-2000	> 2000
(~750 increments)				
Blood loss %	<15%	25 ± 5%	35 ± 5%	> 40%
Heart rate	<100	100-120	120-140	> 140
Blood pressure	normal	normal	↓ed	↓ed
Pulse pressure	normal	↓ed	↓ed	↓ed

Respiratory rate progressively ↑s w/ shock
Shock = inadequate tissue oxygenation
1st response to hemorrhagic shock – ↑ diastolic pressure (vasoconstriction)

Pediatric trauma

Best indicators of shock in children – HR, RR, mental status, clinical exam
Blood pressure <u>NOT</u> a good indicator for blood loss in children – last thing to go
Children are at high risk for **hypothermia** and **head injury**

Normal vital signs for pediatric patients

Age	HR	SBP	RR
Infants (< 1 yr)	120-150	70 ± 10	40
Preschool (1-5 yr)	100-120	90	30
Adolescent (> 10 yr)	90-100	100	20

Trauma Statistics
Trauma deaths
1st peak (0 to 30 min) – deaths due to lacerations of heart, aorta and brain
    Can't save these pts
2nd peak (30 min to 4 hrs) – deaths due to **head injury** (MC) and
    hemorrhage (#2, pts you can <u>save</u> w/ rapid assessment golden hour)
3rd peak (days to weeks) – deaths due to **MSOF** and **sepsis**
1) **Hemorrhage** – MCC of death in 1st hour
2) **Head injury** – MCC death after reaching the ER alive
3) **Infection** – MCC death in long term
Blunt injury – 80% of all trauma
    Kinetic energy = ½ MV², where M = mass, V = velocity
    Falls – age and body orientation biggest predictors of survival
        LD_{50} is 4 stories (50% die)
Penetrating injury – **small bowel** MC injured
Blunt Injury – **spleen** MC injured (some say liver)
Blood pressure is usually OK until 30% of total blood volume is lost
Tongue – MCC of upper airway obstruction → perform jaw thrust
Seat belts – can get small bowel perforations, lumbar spine fractures, sternal
    fractures
Saphenous vein at ankle – best site for cut-down access
Catecholamines – peak 24–48 hours after injury
ADH, ACTH, and glucagon – also ↑ after trauma (fight or flight response)
Pneumatic antishock garment – controversial; use in pre-hospital pts w/ SBP
    <50 and no thoracic injury. Release compartments one at a time

Injuries that can present late - pancreatic injuries, small bowel tears, duodenal
    injuries and diaphragmatic injuries
Snake bites (sx's depend on type of snake)
    Shock, bradycardia, and arrhythmias can result
    Neuro symptoms leading to respiratory failure
    Tx: stabilize patient, antivenin, tetanus shot
Brown recluse spider bite – Tx: Dapsone
Drains required for pancreatic, liver, biliary system, urinary, duodenal injuries
Septic shock w/ trauma → look for bowel perforation or early wound infection (re-
    explore abdomen)

CRITICAL CARE

Hemodynamics
Mean arterial pressure = CO x SVR
> Mean and diastolic aortic pressures slightly greater than radial
> Systolic radial pressures slightly higher than aortic

Cardiac output (C.O.) = HR x stroke volume
Cardiac index (C.I.) = CO / BSA
Systemic vascular resistance (SVR) = 80 x [(MAP – CVP) / CO]
Cardiac Output
> Kidney gets 25%
> Brain gets15%
> Heart gets 5%
> **Diastolic filling time** – C.O. increases w/ HR up to 120-130, then goes down (ventricle is not give enough time to fill w/ fast HR)

Preload – pressure stretching the ventricle of the heart
> Linearly related to left ventricular end-diastolic pressure (**L**VEDP) which is linearly related to left ventricular end-diastolic volume (**L**VEDV)
> > MC refers to **L**eft ventricle
> **Atrial contraction** (atrial kick) – ↑s LVEDV 25% (needed for sick hearts)
> **Wedge pressure** – used as a measurement of preload

Afterload – tension produced by the heart in order to contract
> Related to the resistance (SVR) against the ventricle contracting
> **High SVR** – hard for the ventricle to contract
> **Low SVR** – easier for the heart to contract

Stroke volume = LVEDV – LVESV
> Determined by LVEDV, contractility of the heart, and afterload
> **Anrep effect** – automatic ↑ in **myocardial contractility** w/ ↑ed **afterload**
> **Bowditch effect** – automatic ↑ in **myocardial contractility** w/ ↑ed HR
> **LVEDV** – determined by preload and distensibility of ventricle
> **LVESV** (LV end-systolic volume) – determined by contractility and afterload
> **Starling's Law** – the greater volume of blood entering the heart (LVEDV), the greater the ejection (stroke volume or ejection fraction)
> > Termed **right shift along curve** – at some point along curve, ↑ed volume no longer ↑s ejection and can worsen it
> > > (overdistension → **extreme right shift on Starling curve**)

Ejection fraction = stroke volume / LVEDV
Oxygen delivery and consumption
> O_2 **delivery**
> > = C.O. x arterial O_2 content (CaO_2) x 10
> > = C.O. x [Hgb x 1.34 x O_2 saturation + (pO_2 x 0.003)] x 10
> O_2 **consumption** (VO_2)
> > = C.O. x (CaO_2 – CvO_2); CvO_2 = venous O_2 content (mmHg)
> Normal O_2 delivery to O_2 consumption ratio is 4:1 (25% utilized; **SvO_2 75%**)
> > Thus there is 4 x more oxygen delivered then used
> > C.O. will increase to keep ratio constant
> > O_2 consumption is normally **supply independent**

Oxygen-Hgb dissociation curve
> 1) **Right Shift** (O_2 unloading) – ↑ CO_2 (Bohr effect), ↑ temp, ATP, 2,3-DPG, ↓ pH, methemoglobinemia (see below)
> 2) **Left shift** (hangs on to O_2) – opposite above, fetal Hgb, carbon monoxide poisoning
> **p50** (O_2 at which 50% of O_2 receptors are saturated) = 27mmHg

Mixed Venous Saturation (SvO_2 pulmonary artery catheter)
> Oxygen saturation of mixed venous blood (nl 75% ± 5), measurement taken in PA (allows mixing), assesses tissue oxygenation
> 1) **Elevated SvO_2** – shunting of blood or decreased O_2 extraction (eg septic shock, cirrhosis, cyanide toxicity, hyperbaric O_2, hypothermia, paralysis, coma, sedation)
> 2) **Decreased SvO_2** – occurs with:
> > ↑ed O_2 **extraction** (eg malignant hyperthermia) *or;*
> > ↓ed O_2 **delivery** (eg hypoxia, cardiogenic shock, low Hct)

Most impt determinant of myocardial O_2 consumption – <u>wall tension</u>
(followed by heart rate)

Bronchial blood flow – becomes unsaturated after delivery to bronchus
and lung tissue, then empties into pulmonary veins
Thus, LV blood pO_2 is 5 mmHg lower than pulmonary capillaries

Normal Alveolar:arterial gradient (A-a gradient): 10–15 mmHg
(non-ventilated pt)

Coronary sinus blood (ie coronary venous blood) – has lowest venous
oxygen saturation in body (**30%**)

Renal veins – has highest venous oxygen saturation in body (**80%**);
receives 25% of C.O. but does not have high oxygen expenditure

Pulse oximeter – reads Hgb-O2 as **red** and unbound Hgb as **infrared**
(Red / Red + Infrared) x 100 = % sat
Pulse oximeter mis-reads - nail polish, dark skin, low cardiac
output, ambient light, low Hct, hypothermia, carbon monoxide

During hypoxia, blood is shunted to the heart and brain

Shock = inadequate tissue oxygenation

<u>Pulmonary artery catheters</u> (PA catheter)

Inaccurate measurements can be caused by:
1) **PA catheter not in lung zone III** (lower lobes)
2) **Wedge pressure > LA pressure** (mediastinal fibrosis, pulm vein
obstruction, pulmonary HTN, high PEEP – compresses pulm veins)
3) **LA pressure > LV end diastolic pressure** (mitral regurgitation, mitral
stenosis)
PA diastolic pressure usually 1-2 mmHg higher than wedge

PA catheter distances to wedge (apx):

R SCV	45 cm
R IJ	50 cm
L SCV	55 cm
L IJ	60 cm

If distance much longer/shorter than expected (ie 8 cm) → in wrong place
or have loop

Optimal lung placement for PA catheter – zone III (lower lobes)
Has **less respiratory influence** on measurements

Wedge measurements are taken at **end-expiration**

You have gone from the **right ventricle** to the **pulmonary artery** w/ appearance
of the **dicrotic notch** and an **↑ in diastolic pressure**

Contraindications
Absolute – right sided endocarditis, right sided thrombus, or right
mechanical heart valve
Relative – coagulopathy (reverse), recent ICD or pacemaker (can use
fluoro), left bundle branch block (can cause complete heart block)

High PEEP:
1) can affect wedge measurements
Subtract 1/2 the PEEP from wedge value if PEEP > 10
2) can cause **↓ed CO** from **↓ed right atrial filling** *(main mechanism)*
Compresses SVC, IVC, and right atrium
Also compresses pulmonary capillaries, ↓left atrial filling → ↓ CO
**Causes poor UOP

Use C.O. wedge pressure, and SVR to guide therapy:
1) **Optimize pre-load** (wedge 15-20 usually) – give volume (5% albumin,
RBCs if low Hct); higher preload may be necessary w/ left ventricular
hypertrophy
2) **Optimize afterload**
SVR too high – vasodilators (NTG, nipride, ACE inhibitor)
SVR too low – vasopressor (norepinephrine, phenylephrine,
vasopressin)
3) **Optimize contractility** – inotropes (dopamine, dobutamine, milrinone)

Pulmonary vascular resistance (PVR) can be measured <u>only</u> using a PA
catheter (<u>not</u> measured w/ ECHO)

Diabetics – have ↑ed SVR from arteriopathy

Swan Numbers (normal)	
Cardiac output (C.O.)	4–8 L/min
Cardiac index (C.I.)	2.5–4 L/min
Systemic vascular resistance (SVR)	800-1400 (**1100**)
Pulmonary capillary wedge pressure (wedge)	7-**11**
Central venous pressure (CVP)	3-**7**
Mixed venous oxygen saturation (SvO$_2$)	**75%** ± 5

Types of Shock	CVP and wedge	C.I.	SVR	SvO$_2$
1) Hemorrhagic	↓	↓	↑	↓
2) Septic (hyperdynamic)	↓ (MC)	↑	↓	↑
3) Cardiogenic (eg MI)	↑	↓	↑	↓
4) Cardiac Tamponade	↑	↓	↑	↓
5) Neurogenic	↓	↓	↓	↑
6) Adrenal Insufficiency	↓ (MC)	↓	↓	↓
7) Pulmonary Embolus	↑	↓	↑	↓

1) **Hemorrhagic shock** – <u>initial response</u> is ↑ **in diastolic pressure**
   Tx: volume (LR, then blood in trauma pts)
2) **Septic shock**
   Sx's:
        Initial sepsis (early) – **mental status changes** (eg confusion)
              hyperventilation (resp alkalosis) and **hypotension** *(classic)*
        **Hyperglycemia – common early sign just before clinical sepsis
              Early sepsis – ↓ insulin, ↑ glucose (from impaired utilization)
              Late sepsis – ↑ insulin, ↑ glucose (from insulin resistance)
   Tx:
        1) Place PA catheter (Keep CVP 8-12, wedge 16-18, MAP 60-65; SvO$_2$ > 70%)
        2) **Give volume** to get wedge up (5% albumin, PRBCs if Hct low)
        3) **Levophed** *(best pressor Tx for septic shock)* for MAP 60-65
        4) **Vasopressin** as a 2nd line pressor if resistant to levophed
        5) **Broad spectrum abx's** until sensitivities known
        6) Consider testing for **adrenal insufficiency** if refractory to pressors
        7) Consider **activated protein C** (→ fibrinolysis; cx's - bleeding)
3) **Cardiogenic Shock** (eg shock from acute MI, CHF exacerbation)
   Sx's:
        Pulmonary edema; **chest pain** if myocardial infarction
        Heart can't contract effectively → **pulmonary congestion**
        Heart also becomes **over-distended** → further worsens contractility
   Tx:
        1) Place PA catheter
        2) Start **inotrope** *(best Tx,* Dobutamine) and bring C.I. ≥ 2
        3) Start **pressor** (Levophed) if MAP < 60
            If MAP > 70 → give **lasix** (↓s preload → ↓s pulmonary congestion and ↓s heart overdistension)
        4) **Morphine** (venodilator to ↓ pre-load)
        5) **NTG** (venodilator to ↓ preload; ↑s coronary perfusion w/ MI)
        6) Call cardiologist for cardiac catheterization if acute MI
        7) Keep Hct ≥ 30
        8) Intubate if necessary
        9) **Intra-aortic balloon pump** if necessary to stabilize (see below)

4) **Cardiac tamponade**

> Fluid around heart causes ↓ **ventricular filling** in diastole → hypotension
> **Sx's:** hypotension, jugular venous distention, and muffled heart sounds
>> (Beck's triad, complete triad present in *minority* of cases)
> **Dx: Initial ECHO sign of early cardiac tamponade** *(1ˢᵗ sign)* →
>> ***impaired diastolic filling of right atrium*** (from compression)
> **Tx:**
>> **Drain pericardial fluid** (eg pericardiocentesis or pericardial window)
>> Fluid resuscitation to temporize until definitive Tx above
>> Pericardiocentesis blood does not form clot

5) **Neurogenic shock**

> Neuro injury results in loss of sympathetic tone and decreased SVR
> **Sx's:** low HR, low BP, warm extremities (loss of autonomic tone)
> **Tx:**
>> 1) **Volume 1ˢᵗ** (CVP 8-12, wedge 16-18)
>> 2) **Phenylephrine** after resuscitated to raise SVR (MAP ≥ 65)

6) **Acute Adrenal Insufficiency**

> **Sx's: fever, N/V, abd pain** and **hypotension** (unresponsive to fluid/pressors)
>> Causes – **withdrawal of exogenous steroids** (MCC), *bilateral adrenal*
>>> *hemorrhage* (MC related to sepsis, eg Waterhouse-Friedrichsen
>>> syndrome), *adrenalectomy*
> **Dx:**
>> ↑ **ACTH** and ↓ **cortisol**
>> **Cosyntropin test** (*best test*, ACTH given and cortisol measured)
>>> **Baseline cortisol < 15** or **change < 9** ug/dl after stimulation
>>>> test = adrenal insufficiency
> **Tx:**
>> 1) **Dexamethasone** (2 mg IV Q 6) + **fludrocortisone** (50 ug/d)
>>> Give prior to ACTH stimulation test (dexamethasone does NOT
>>>> interfere w/ ACTH stimulation test)
>>> Do not wait on test results if clinically suspected
>> 2) **Volume** to temporize while waiting for steroids to take effect
>> Hydrocortisone after above
> **Relative potency of steroids**
>> 1 x – cortisone, hydrocortisone
>> 5 x – prednisone, prednisolone, methyl-prednisolone
>> 30 x – dexamethasone

7) **Pulmonary Embolism**

> **Sx's:** tachypnea, chest pain; **hypoxia + hypocarbia**; ↓**BP** + ↑**HR**
>> **MC EKG finding** – SVT
>> PA systolic pressures > 40 w/ significant PE
>> Respiratory alkalosis (from hyperventilation)
>> **Intubated pt** – ↓ ET-CO2 initial finding
>>> (sudden ↓ in ET-CO2 + hypotension)
>> Blood can't get to left side of heart due to PE
> **MC source** - iliofemoral DVT
> **Dx:** chest CT angio
>> 1/3 have negative lower extremity duplex
> **Tx:**
>> 1) Place PA catheter (if completely stable, may skip)
>> 2) **Give volume** acutely for hypotension
>> 3) **Inotropes** (dobutamine) to keep C.I ≥ 2.0
>> 4) **Pressors** (phenylephrine or levophed) for MAP < 60
>> 5) **Heparin bolus** 80 units/Kg, drip at 18 units/Kg/hr
>>> (*Do not wait* on chest CT for heparin – once suspected and
>>>> other causes of shock ruled out, give heparin)
>> 6) **Chest CT** to confirm diagnosis if pt stable
>>> **ECHO** may show right ventricular heart strain
>> 7) For refractory hypotension despite inotropes and pressors,
>>> consider **suction catheter embolectomy** or **open removal on**
>>> **cardiopulmonary bypass**

Cardiac Drugs

Receptors
> **Alpha-1** (phospholipase activation → ↑s intracellular Ca^{++})
>> Arterial and venous vasoconstrictor
>> Gluconeogenesis and glycogenolysis
>
> **Alpha-2** (↓s cAMP → ↓s Ca^{++}) – venous vasoconstrictor
> **Beta-1** (↑s cAMP → ↑s Ca^{++}) – ↑ contractility + HR
> **Beta-2** (↑s cAMP → ↑s Ca^{++})
>> Vasodilator
>> Bronchodilator
>> Increases glucagon and renin
>
> **Dopamine** (DA)
>> Relaxes renal blood vessels (↑ed blood flow to kidney)
>> Relaxes splanchnic smooth muscle
>
> **Vasopressin**
>> **V-1 receptor** – vascular smooth muscle constriction
>> **V-2 receptor** – water resorption from the collecting ducts
>> **V-3 receptor** – VIII and vWF release from endothelium
>
> **Soluble Guanylate Cyclase**
>> Nitric oxide (NO) synthesized by *nitric oxide synthetase* (**Arginine precursor**)
>> NO then acts on soluble **guanylate cyclase** (↑ cGMP) to dilate blood vessels
>
> **Angiotensin converting enzyme**
>> *Inhibition* blocks formation of angiotensin II
>> *Inhibition* results in ↓ed blood pressure, ↓ed aldosterone release, and ↓ed vasopressin release
>
> **Angiotensin II receptor** – *antagonists* (ARBs) cause arterial vasodilation, ↓ed aldosterone release and ↓ed vasopressin release
> **Prostacyclin receptor** – pulmonary vasodilation
> **Endothelin receptor** – pulmonary vasoconstriction

> **Inotropes that directly ↑cAMP**
>> Dopamine
>> Dobutamine
>> Epinephrine (mostly an inotrope, some pressor activity)
>> Isoproterenol
>
> **Inotropes that inhibit cAMP phosphodiesterase** (indirectly ↑ cAMP)
>> Milrinone
>
> **Inotropes that inhibit Na/K transporter**
>> Digoxin

Inotropes (↑ cardiac output)
> 1) **Dopamine** (1-20 µg/kg/min)

Low (1-5)	**DA receptors**
Moderate (6-10)	**Beta-1** and **Beta-2** (↑ contractility + HR)
High (>10)	**Alpha-1** (vasoconstriction, ↑ MAP)

> 2) **Dobutamine** (1-20 µg/kg/min)
>> **Beta-1** (contractility mostly)
>> *some* beta-2 (vasodilation) at higher doses (> 15)
>
> 3) **Milrinone**
>> **cAMP phosphodiesterase inhibitor** (results in ↑ed cAMP)
>> Ca^{++} influx ↑s **myocardial contractility**
>>> Also a **vasodilator** (relaxes vascular smooth muscle)
>>
>> ***Not* subject to beta-receptor down-regulation like other inotropes** (good for long-term use; eg pts awaiting heart TXP)
>>> Other drugs lose potency w/ time
>
> 4) **Isoproterenol**
>> **Beta-1** and **Beta-2** → ↑ HR and contractility, vasodilates
>> **S/Es**: arrhythmogenic; ↑ heart metabolic demand (rarely used) may actually ↓ BP (beta-2)

Pressors (↑SVR and ↑MAP; NE and Epi also inotropic)
  1) **Phenylephrine** (10-300 µg/min)
     Alpha-1 (vasoconstriction)
  2) **Norepinephrine** (NE, Levophed; 1-40 µg/min)
     Predominantly **Alpha-1** and **Alpha-2** (vasoconstriction); some Beta-1
     Acts as a potent **splanchnic vasoconstrictor**
  3) **Epinephrine** (1-20 µg/min)
     Low Dose (1-5)   **Beta-1** and **Beta-2** (can ↓ MAP at low dose)
     High Dose (> 5)   **Alpha-1** and **Alpha-2**
     Can *lower* blood pressure at low doses (Beta-2 > Beta-1)
     S/Es: 1) **arrhythmogenic** *and*
               2) creates **high oxygen demand** at higher doses
  4) **Vasopressin** (0.01 - 0.1 U/min)
     V-1 receptor – vasoconstriction

Vasodilators
  1) **Nipride** (0.1-10 µg/kg/min)
     NO mediated; predominantly arterial dilatation, some venodilatation
     Cyanide toxicity (at risk if >3 µg/kg/min for 72 hours)
         Check for **metabolic acidosis** and **thiocyanate** level
         Cyanide binds to cytochrome c in mitochondria and **disrupts
             electron transport chain**
         Cell cannot use oxygen so you get a **left to right shunt**
             (↑ SvO_2)
     Tx: amyl nitrite 1st, followed by **sodium nitrite**
  2) **Nitroglycerin** (10-1000 µg/min)
     NO mediated; predominantly venodilation, some arterial
     ↓s myocardial wall tension by decreasing pre-load
  3) **ACE inhibitor**
     ↓s angiotensin II (results in vasodilation, ↓ aldosterone, ↓ ADH)
     ACEI's 1) reduce mortality post-MI and 2) prevent CHF post-MI
     Absolute contraindications – previous angioedema, renal artery
         stenosis
     Relative contraindications – impaired renal function, hypovolemia,
         aortic stenosis
  4) **Angiotensin II receptor blocker** (ARB)
     Results in vasodilation, ↓ aldosterone, ↓ ADH
  5) **Hydralazine** – arterial vasodilator (? mech)
  6) **Fenoldopam** – arterial vasodilator (DA-1A receptor)
     S/Es reflex tachycardia
  7) **Labetalol** (has 2 active isomers)
     1st – **Alpha-1 blocker**
     2nd – **Beta-1 blocker** and <u>**Beta-2 agonist**</u>
     Decreases MAP w/o altering HR or cardiac output
  8) **Prostacyclin** (epoprostenol) – vasodilator (prostacyclin receptor)
     Can be given inhaled or IV (good pulmonary vasodilator)
  9) *Inhaled* **NO** - pulmonary vasodilator (soluble guanylate cyclase receptor)
     Also called **endothelium-derived relaxing factor** (EDRF)
  10) **Sildenafil** – pulmonary vasodilator (NO mediated)
  11) **Bosentan** – pulmonary vasodilator (blocks endothelin receptor)

<u>Intra-aortic balloon pump</u> (IABP)
  Sequence:
     Inflation – on **T wave** (diastole)
     Deflation – on **P wave or start of Q wave** (systole)
  Tip of balloon should be just distal to left subclavian (1-2 cm below top of arch)
  Effects:
     Improves MAP (inflation w/ ventricular diastole)
     Improves coronary perfusion (coronaries fill in diastole and ↑ed diastolic
         MAP improves coronary perfusion)
     Decreases afterload (deflation w/ ventricular systole)

IABP Indications:
1) **Cardiogenic shock** post-MI
2) **Ventricular septal rupture** post-MI
3) **Acute mitral regurgitation** (eg ruptured papillary muscle either spontaneously or post-MI)
4) **Unstable angina** (improves coronary flow)
5) Pre-op before cardiac surgery in pts w/ low EF

Has ↑ed survival following 1) ventricular septal rupture and 2) acute mitral regurgitation

Absolute contraindications – aortic regurgitation, aortic dissection, severe aorto-iliac occlusive DZ

Relative contraindications – vascular grafts in aorta; aortic aneurysms

Prolonged QT interval
Occurs w/ certain **drugs** (amiodarone, fluoroquinolones) or **hypomagnesemia**

An ***early after de-polarization*** (or premature ventricular complex) can occur within the QT interval precipitating ventricular tachycardia (torsades de pointes)

Stopping precipitating drugs or correcting hypomagnesemia shortens QT interval and lessens the likelihood of this happening.

Magnesium can be used to treat torsades de pointes

Acute Atrial Fibrillation (AF)
Chemical cardioversion – diltiazem, metoprolol, or amiodarone
> *Avoid combining 3 drugs* (S/Es – hypotension, complete heart block)
> *Don't use above w/ Wolf Parkinson White (WPW syndrome or pre-excitation syndrome)*

Digoxin does <u>not</u> convert pts out of AF but does slow ventricular response

Electrical Cardioversion if unstable (100, 150, 200)

AF lasting ≥ 24 hours:
> **Anticoagulate** – heparin, then coumadin
> **Consider cardioversion →**
>> If < 48 hours and low risk of stroke – cardioversion
>> If > 48 hours or high stroke risk – ECHO 1st to R/O thrombus in left atrium, then cardioversion

> 90% of cardiac surgery pts suffering from new peri-operative AF will be in normal sinus rhythm at 6 weeks

****Atrial fibrillation is the MCC of delayed discharge after cardiac surgery***

Ventricular Fibrillation Intra-op (VF)
Look at monitor and **feel aortic pressure** at hiatus (R/O monitor problem)
> **Shock** 200, 300 then 360; check rhythm, then **CPR** for 2 min, check rhythm again (then follow below)
> 1) **Shock x 1**
> 2) **Vasopressor** (epi 1 mg or vasopressin 40 units), then **CPR** 2 min
> 3) **Shock X 1,** then **CPR** for 2 min
> 4) **Anti-arrhythmic** (amiodarone, lidocaine, or magnesium), **CPR** for 2 min, back to top

Figure out cause:
> **Look at diaphragms** and see if they are **bulging → tension PTX** or **hemothorax** from central line placement (↑ airway pressures)
>> **Tx:** chest tube (or just open diaphragm from abdomen)
> **JVD** – pericardial tamponade from central line placement
>> Tx: open the pericardial sac (pericardial window)

Other possibilities:
> **Hypoxia** (have anesthesia listen for breath sounds)
> **Hyperkalemia** (check K level; one rhythm back look for peaked T waves)
> **Hemorrhage**
> **Myocardial infarction** (check EKG once rhythm back → ST changes)
> **PE** (ECHO to look for right heart strain once you get pt back; start heparin)

After you get rhythm back, take pt to ICU for diagnostics and support

Pulseless Electrical Activity Intra-op (PEA)

Look at monitor and **feel aorta** at hiatus (R/O <u>a-line</u> problem)
1) **Start CPR** when you feel no pulse
2) **Vasopressor** (epi 1 mg or vasopressin 40 units)
3) **Atropine** (1 mg) if HR is slow or asystole
4) **Give volume** – good initial maneuver in **vast majority** (many causes of PEA code can be treated or temporized w/ volume)

Figure out cause (H's and T's):

Hypoxia – have anesthesia listen for breath sounds
Hypovolemia
> Check for bulging diaphragms (hemothorax from central line)
> Check **CVP** if CTL is in
> Tx: Volume resuscitation

Hyperkalemia and **Hypokalemia** – check K
> Look at monitor or EKG for **peaked T waves** (hyperkalemia) or **flattened T waves** (hypokalemia)

Hydrogen ion – check ABG
Hypothermia
Hypoglycemia – check glucose

Tamponade (cardiac) – look for JVD
> Open pericardium from abdomen
> **Clinical sign** of this is **no pulse w/ CPR**

Tension PTX – look for JVD, tracheal shift, decreased breath sounds
> Open the diaphragm from the abdomen or place a chest tube

Thrombosis, coronary (MI) – check EKG, CK-MBs, and troponins
Thrombosis, pulmonary (PE) – CTL will have high filling pressures; ECHO for RV strain and dilatation
Toxins and **Tablets**

Asystole protocol is the same as PEA except try and use transcutaneous pacing if available

EKG findings

ST elevation – acute myocardial infarction
ST depression – ischemia
Q waves – old infarct

Pacemakers (temporary, after cardiac surgery)

3 letter designation, most common setting – **DDD**
1st letter is **chamber paced** (D = atrium and ventricle)
2nd letter is **chamber sensed** (D = atrium and ventricle)
3rd letter is **response to sensed beat** (D = inhibits or triggers the next beat; I = just inhibits the next beat)

1) **Not pacing → potential problems:**
a) **Increased pacing threshold due to local injury** –
> **Tx:** ↑ voltage through pacer (↑ mAmps)
b) **Low battery** – Tx: change batteries
c) **Lead dislodgement** – Tx: switch lead polarity to the device (may help) o/w need to replace lead
d) **Myopotential inhibition** (sensitivity is *too high*; pacer is picking up background noise, such as breathing and movement, thinking these are p waves + QRS) → Tx: turn sensitivity down (avoids background noise)

2) **Pacing too much** (pacing when it shouldn't) →
Sensitivity is *too low* (not sensing p waves + QRS) – Tx: turn sensitivity up

Kidneys (renal system)

Renin-angiotensin System

Glomerular filtration rate (GFR) is controlled by the **efferent limb**

Renin *(released from kidney)*

Release caused by:

↓**ed pressure** sensed by **juxta-glomerular apparatus**

↑**ed sodium** concentration sensed by **macula densa**

Additional releasing factors – Beta-2 stimulation, hyperkalemia

Inhibition of release – hypokalemia

Renin converts **angiotensinogen** *(synthesized in liver)* to **angiotensin I**

Angiotensin converting enzyme (ACE, in **lung**)

Converts angiotensin I to angiotensin II

ACE inhibitors work here; ACE also breaks down bradykinin

Angiotensin II effects (binds AG II receptor):

Primary effect – release of **aldosterone** from **adrenal cortex**

Secondary effects:

1) **Vasoconstrictor** (potent, ↓s renal blood flow) → ↑s BP

2) ↑**ed sympathetic tone** (↑ed HR and contractility)

3) **Release of ADH** (vasopressin, posterior pituitary gland)

Aldosterone

Activates **Na⁺/K⁺ ATPase** on cell membrane in *distal convoluted tubule* → Na⁺ and **water reabsorption**; K⁺ **excretion**

Also activates **Na⁺/H⁺ exchanger**→ H⁺ excretion (metabolic alkalosis)

Anti-diuretic hormone (ADH; vasopressin)

Released by posterior pituitary gland when osmolality is high

Acts on *collecting ducts* for water resorption

Also a **vasoconstrictor**

Atrial natriuretic peptide (ANP)

Atrial distension (ie volume overload) causes release from **atrial wall**

Mechanisms:

1) **Inhibits Na⁺** and **water resorption** in renal collecting ducts

2) **Vasodilator**

3) **Inhibits renin and aldosterone production**

Drugs toxic to kidneys

NSAIDs – **Inhibit prostaglandin synthesis**, causes renal arteriole vasoconstriction

Aminoglycosides – directly injure renal tubules

Contrast dyes – directly injure renal tubules

Myoglobin – directly injure renal tubules (see Tx below)

Electrolyte abnormalities w/ renal failure:

Volume overload

↓ed Na⁺ and Ca⁺⁺

↑ed K⁺, PO4⁻, Mg⁺⁺, and urea

Indications for dialysis:

1) Fluid overload

2) ↑ed K⁺, Mg⁺⁺, PO4⁻, or BUN

3) Metabolic acidosis

4) Uremic encephalopathy

5) Uremic coagulopathy

6) Poisoning

Hemodialysis – can cause **hypotension** from large volume shifts

CVVH – slower then HD, good for sick pts that cannot tolerate volume shifts

Hct increases 5–8 for each liter taken off

Elevated creatinine in pt needing contrast dye (eg CT scan or angiogram)

1) **Pre-op hydration** – *most renal protective measure*

2) **N-acetylcysteine** next best (600 mg PO BID day before and day of)

3) **HCO3⁻ drip** is also effective (1 hour before and for 6 hours after)

4) **Hold ACEI, ARBs, NSAIDs** and **diuretics**

5) **Minimize contrast volume** and use **isosmolar agents**

Note - gadolinium for MRI can cause contrast induced renal failure

Can use **CO₂ angiogram** (contrast not as good, less renal toxic)

Myoglobinuria
  Released from muscle after trauma or compartment syndrome
  Myoglobin is converted to **ferrihemate** in acidic environment (renal toxic)
  Tx: **HCO3⁻** drip to alkalinize urine (prevent conversion) + **fluid hydration**
Intra-op and Post-op management in pts w/ renal disease
  Hemodialysis (HD) day before surgery (schedule OR around HD)
  Swan, a-line, and foley → optimize fluid status (if renal insufficiency,
    maximize renal perfusion)
  Renal adjustment for post-op meds (especially Abx's)
  Use normal saline w/ chronic renal failure (stage 5 chronic kidney
    disease) – No K in IVF's (*avoid* Lactated Ringer's)
  Frequent electrolyte checks

<u>Poor urine output post-op</u> (oliguria; acute renal failure pathway)
  Check foley catheter (check to make sure its working; insert if not present)
  Check abdomen (eg abdominal compartment syndrome or bladder distension)
  Try **fluid challenge (1-2 L LR or NS) and/or **lasix challenge** (up to 100 mg,
    used if thought to have adequate volume or fluid overloaded)
  If above fail, get dx studies below
Dx studies:
  1) **Labs** - serum electrolytes, urine electrolytes
      FeNa – fractional excretion of Na
        ***Best test for acute renal failure* (azotemia)
      FeNa = (urine Na/Cr) / (plasma Na/Cr)
        Prerenal:
            FeNa < 1%
            Urine Na < 20
            BUN/Cr ratio > 20
            Urine osmolality > 500 mOsm (concentrated)
        Renal (ie ATN): FeNa > 2% and opposite above
  2) **PA catheter** (make sure pt has a good filling pressures)
  3) **Renal U/S** if potential for obstruction (eg kidney stones,
      clipped/transected ureter after APR, LAR, or pelvic mass resection)
  ARF (acute renal failure, ↑ Cr ≥ 0.5)
      70% of renal mass must be damaged before ↑ Cr and BUN
Use above to figure out cause:
  1) **Pre-renal oliguria / ARF** (poor perfusion; DDx – hypovolemia, any form
      of shock, high PEEP, abdominal compartment syndrome)
      Tx:
          Optimize **preload w/ volume** (CVP 10-15)
          Optimize **C.O.** (C.I. ≥ 2.2, dopamine, dobutamine)
  2) **Renal oliguria / ARF** (ATN, acute tubular necrosis)
      MCC renal ATN – hypotension intra-op
      Make sure pt not on any renal toxic drugs; adjust meds
      Tx:
          Diuretic trial (Lasix and Mannitol)
          Dopamine drip 3 ug/kg/hr
          Try to make **non-oliguric**
          (Tx above assumes pt has appropriate filling pressure)
  3) **Post-renal oliguria / ARF** (ureteral obstruction)
      Renal U/S shows **hydronephrosis**
      Tx: relieve obstruction
  MCC post-op <u>poor UOP</u> – hypovolemia
  MCC post-op <u>ARF</u> – hypotension, resulting in ATN
      (hypotension usually occurs intra-op)
With ARF →
  Check **electrolytes** frequently, adjust Abx's and meds, **D/C K** in IVF's
      (<u>No</u> Lactated Ringers, contains K)
  Dialysis if indicated (see previous for criteria)

Pulmonary Function Tests (PFTs)
Lung Measurements
Total lung capacity (TLC)
> Lung volume after maximal inspiration
> TLC = FVC + RV

Forced vital capacity (FVC)
> Volume of air w/ maximal exhalation after maximal inhalation

Residual volume (RV)
> Lung volume after maximal expiration (comprises 20% of TLC)

Tidal volume (TV)
> Volume of air w/ a normal inspiration and expiration

Functional residual capacity (FRC)
> Lung volume after normal exhalation
> FRC = ERV + RV
> Surgery (atelectasis), sepsis (ARDS), and trauma (contusion, atelectasis, ARDS) – all ↓ FRC

Expiratory reserve volume (ERV)
> Volume of air forcefully expired after normal expiration

Inspiratory capacity
> Maximum amount of air breathed in after normal exhalation

FEV_1 – forced expiratory volume in 1 second (after maximal inhalation)

Minute ventilation = tidal volume x resp rate

Compliance = (change in lung volume) / (change in lung pressure)
> **High compliance** - lungs easy to ventilate (eg COPD)
> **Low compliance** - lungs hard to ventilate (eg ARDS, fibrotic lung diseases, reperfusion injury, pulmonary edema)

Ventilation to perfusion ratio (V/Q ratio)
> Normally highest in upper lobes, lowest in lower lobes

Dead space
> Part of lung that is ventilated but <u>not</u> perfused
> Normally, dead space is the airway to level of the bronchiole (comprises 150 ml; conductive airways)
> **Causes of increased dead space** – ↓ed C.O. (capillary collapse), PE, pulmonary HTN, ARDS (edema compresses capillaries), excessive PEEP (capillary compression)
> Increased dead space leads to ↑ed pCO_2

V/Q mismatch (poor ventilation but good perfusion)
> **MCC** – atelectasis; others – ARDS

Chronic Pathology:
Restrictive lung disease – ↓ TLC, ↓ RV, and ↓ FVC
Obstructive lung disease (or aging) – ↑ TLC, ↑ RV, and ↓ FEV_1
Obesity – ↓ FVC, ↓ FEV-1 and ↓ FRC

Pulmonary vasodilators – prostacyclin (inhaled or IV), nitric oxide (inhaled or IV), bradykinin, prostaglandin, alkalosis

Pulmonary vasoconstrictors – hypoxia (very potent), acidosis, histamine, serotonin, thromboxane, epinephrine, norepinephrine

Pulmonary shunting can be caused by – nipride, nitroglycerin, nifedipine
> Manifests as **hypoxia**

Normal inspiratory time to expiratory time ratio (I:E ratio) – 1:3
> May need to ↑ inspiratory time in pts w/ ARDS to improve oxygenation

Atelectasis
Bronchial obstruction and ↓ed respiratory effort main causes
***MCC of fever in 1st 48 hours after operation**
Increased in pts w/ COPD, upper abdominal surgery, obesity
Sx's: fever, tachycardia
> **Fever** caused by release of **IL-1** (acts at hypothalamus) from **pulmonary macrophages**

Tx: incentive spirometer, pain control

Ventilator
Initial vent settings (TV 8 cc/kg, RR 12-14, FiO2 100%, PEEP 5)
Improving Oxygenation →
- ↑ PEEP – improves functional residual capacity (FRC; *best initial method to* ↑ pO_2); causes alveolar recruitment and keeps alveoli open during expiratory phase so oxygen exchange can continue
- ↑ FIO$_2$ – NOT as effective as ↑ed PEEP
  Keep FIO$_2$ ≤ 60% to prevent O_2 radical toxicity
- Excessive PEEP Cx's:
  - ↓ed right atrial filling → ↓ed C.O. → ↓ renal blood flow→ ↓ UOP (*main mechanism of ↓ed UOP w/ ↑ed PEEP*)
    - ↑PEEP also ↑s renal vein pressure → ↓ renal blood flow
  - ↑ed pulmonary vascular resistance → ↓left atrial filling → ↓C.O.

Improving ventilation (removing CO_2) →
- ↑ respiratory rate
- ↑ tidal volume

Pressure support – decreases work of breathing (inspiratory pressure held constant until minimum tidal volume is achieved)
Barotrauma – prevent by keeping pressure plateaus < 30 (*most important*) and peaks < 50
Normal extubation parameters:
- Negative inspiratory force (NIF) > 20
- FiO$_2$ ≤ 40%
- PEEP 5 (physiologic)
- Pressure support 5
- Others - RR<24, HR<120, pO2>60, pCO2<50, pH 7.35–7.45, O2 sat >92%, TV >5 cc/kg, off pressors, follows commands, protects airway
  Consider spontaneous breathing trial w/ T-piece or CPAP
- Rapid shallow breathing index (RR / TV) > 105 → 95% fail extubation

High-frequency ventilation – used a lot in children; tracheoesophageal fistula (TEF) bronchopleural fistula (BPF; maintains low airway pressures)
Laryngeal Edema – methylprednisilone 20 mg IV Q 12 before extubation (make sure pt has a cuff leak prior to pulling ET tube)
Mechanical ventilation in pts w/ hypovolemia – inspiration ↓s blood pressure
- ↓s venous return (SVC and IVC compression ↓s return to right ventricle and pulmonary capillary compression ↓s return to left ventricle))
  The opposite occurs w/ non-mechanical inspiration

COPD
Two components:
1) Parenchymal damage → small airway collapse/narrowing (lung trapping)
2) Chronic bronchitis

Oxygen – only tx found to ↑survival in COPD pts long-term
Auto-PEEP – Interruption of expiration before alveolar pressure falls to atmospheric; Keeps alveoli open
Right ventricular hypertrophy and dysfunction can occur w/ COPD (cor pulmonale → ascites, LE edema)
Work of breathing ↑ed due to prolonged expiratory phase (alveolar collapse)
Normally, work of breathing is 2% of total body VO_2
COPD exacerbation Tx:
- Oxygen
- Albuterol (beta-adrenergic agonist) + Atrovent nebulizer (anti-cholinergic)
- Inhaled Steroids (Advair Discus, fluticasone + salmeterol)
- Amoxicillin for wet cough (bronchitis)
- Oral or IV steroids if refractory to above
- BiPAP (non-invasive positive airway pressure; contraindicated w/ inability to cooperate or clear secretions, hemodynamic instability, UGI bleed)
- Intubation

Intra-op and post-op management of pts w/ COPD
- Swan, a-line and foley – minimize volume overload; use swan to help
- Epidural catheter to control post-op pain (very effective)
- Esophagectomy – if marginal PFT's, go w/ trans-hiatal as opposed to thoracotomy (thoracotomy restricts pulmonary function)

<u>ARDS</u> (Acute Respiratory Distress Syndrome)

Direct causes – **pneumonia** (MCC overall, 40%), aspiration (15%), inhalational injury, lung contusion

Indirect causes – sepsis (25%), shock, DIC, pancreatitis, trauma, transfusion related (TRALI)

Criteria *(need all 4):*
  1) **Acute onset**
  2) **Bilateral diffuse patchy air space disease** (CXR)
  3) **Wedge < 18** (<u>no</u> atrial hypertension, normal filling pressures)
  4) **PO_2 / FiO_2 < 300**

PMN's have a prominent role in ARDS w/ **inflammation of lung parenchyma**
Have **proteinaceous exudate** on bronchoalveolar lavage (BAL, *Not* diagnostic)
Impaired gas exchange + **inflammatory mediator release** can lead to **MSOF**
CXR findings can **lag behind** clinical findings

Tx:
  1) **Initial vent settings** *(applies to all ventilated patients in general)*
      TV 8 cc/kg
      RR 12-14
      FiO2 100% (wean this)
      PEEP 5
  2) **Sedate** and **paralyze**
  3) **Low tidal volume**
      (goal of 6 cc/kg to reduce barotrauma, start at 8 cc/kg)
  4) **Maintain plateau pressure < 30 cm H_2O**
  5) **Permissive hypercapnea** (allowing pCO_2 to rise)
      Increase the **inspiratory time** (to improve oxygenation) at the expense of expiratory time (causes pCO2 to rise)
          Although always want inspiratory time $\leq$ expiratory time
      Correct pH to > 7.30 (give HCO3⁻, may be able to ↑ RR)
  6) **Increase PEEP to sat $\geq$ 92%** and **$PO_2 \geq$ 60 mmHg**
      (try to keep FiO2 $\leq$ 60% - *prevents O_2 radical injury to lung*)
  7) **Keep CVP 4-6** – diuretics (Lasix) if needed
  8) **Optimize Hct** if necessary

  Specific ventilator modes have not made a difference (pressure control vs. volume control)
  Other options (none really shown to change mortality)
      Pressure control ventilation (have to <u>paralyze</u> for this)
      Prone and supine positioning
      Pneumothorax – high risk if plateau pressure >30 or peak pressure >50 → consider **prophylactic chest tubes**
  Avoid FiO_2 > 60 for > 24 hours → causes oxygen radical damage to lung

DDx: ARDS vs VAP vs PE

Ventilator Associated Pneumonia Criteria (VAP, see Infection chp for Tx)
  1) New unilateral infiltrate
  2) Fever
  3) Purulent sputum (consider bronchoalveolar lavage)
  4) > 48 hours on ventilator

Pulmonary Embolus Findings (see above for Tx)
  1) Normal CXR (sometimes have wedge shaped infarct)
  2) Hypoxemia *and* hypocarbia
  3) Sudden onset
  4) Predisposing condition

ARDS
  1) Acute onset
  2) Bilateral diffuse patchy air space disease (CXR)
  3) Wedge < 18 (<u>no</u> atrial hypertension, normal filling pressures)
  4) PO2/FiO2 < 300

<u>SIRS</u> (Systemic Inflammatory Response Syndrome)

MC etiology – infection (eg bacteremia, PNA)

Non-infectious etiologies – severe trauma, shock (any form), anaphylaxis, burns, acute pancreatitis

All mediated by **massive TNF-alpha** and **IL-1** cytokine release

Most potent stimulant for SIRS – GNR endotoxin (lipopolysaccharide – lipid A portion)

Criteria (need $\geq$ 2):

Temp	> 38°C or <36°C
HR	> 90 (or on pressors)
RR	> 20 (or requiring intubation)
pCO$_2$	< 32 mmHg
WBC	> 12 or < 4

Can lead to hypotension, shock, MSOF (eg ARDS, ARF, liver failure, cardiac failure) and **death**

Tx:

Identify and **treat underlying cause**

ICU care depending on organ dysfunction

Sepsis = SIRS + infection

Hyperglycemia – often occurs just before pt becomes clinically septic

Optimal glucose level in septic pts – 100-120

Sepsis triad – inflammation, hypercoaguability, and decreased fibrinolysis

Development of microthrombi results in relative hypoperfusion of organs and eventual organ failure

Theoretically, agents that ↓ microthrombi (eg Xigris – activated protein C) would ↓ MSOF and death (however, only specific circumstances does this actually hold true – see Antibiotics chp, Xigris)

<u>Gram-negative sepsis</u>

MC organism – E. coli

Endotoxin (LPS – lipopolysaccharide, **lipid A** portion) is released

Lipid A is the most potent trigger of **TNF-alpha** release

Triggers release of **TNF-alpha** (from macrophages) → activates **inflammatory- complement- coagulation-** cascades (microthrombi)

Septic shock - up to 30% mortality

Early GNR sepsis: ↓ insulin, ↑ glucose (impaired utilization)

Late GNR sepsis: ↑ insulin, ↑ glucose (due to insulin resistance)

<u>Air embolus</u> (CO_2 embolus similar)

MC occurs w/ sucking air through **central line or central line site**

CO_2 embolus can occur w/ **laparoscopic procedures** (eg laparoscopic cholecystectomy)

Sx's: sudden ↓ in ET-CO2, hypotension and **tachycardia** (*classic*)

May have 'mill wheel' murmur

Can lodge in RA, RV, and/or pulmonary arteries causing **air lock,** which **prevents venous return**

Tx:

1st step – *Stop insufflation* if laparoscopic procedure

Trendelenburg (head down)

Left lateral decubitus position (keeps air in RA and RV)

100% oxygen (comes into equilibrium w/ embolus and is reabsorbed faster); also improves oxygenation of ischemic tissue

Hyperventilation (↑ minute ventilation, RR x TV)

↓s blood pCO2, which ↑s gradient for CO2 or air to diffuse

Prolonged CPR if needed to allow embolus to be absorbed

Aspirate central line if present (gets air out of RA)

Intubate if necessary

Fluid, pressors and **inotropes** to maintain BP

Consider hyperbaric oxygen chamber

Tension PTX during a laparoscopic procedure appears as a bulging diaphragm tracheal deviation, absent ipsilateral breath sounds, and hypotension

Fat emboli

Sx's: petechiae, hypoxia, and **mental status changes** (eg confusion) - *classic*
other sx's similar to PE
Sudan red stain – fat in sputum and urine
MCC – lower extremity (hip and femur) fx's or ortho procedures

ETOH withdrawal

Sx's: hypertension, tachycardia, mental status changes (delirium), seizures after
48 hours; can be deadly
Tx:
Thiamine, folate, B-12, Mg^{++} and K^+
PRN **Ativan** for agitation and **Clonidine** for HTN
R/O other causes for change in neuro status

ICU psychosis

MC after **third post-op day**
Often preceded by lucid interval
Usually self-terminating but need to R/O other causes (ETOH withdrawal,
hypoglycemia, stroke, electrolyte imbalance, hypoxia, hypercarbia)

Brain death

The following preclude diagnosis (ie if present, can't make Dx of brain death):
Uremia
Temp < 32°C
BP < 70/40
Desaturation w/ apnea test
Drugs (eg phenol- or pento-barbital, ETOH, sedatives)
Metabolic issues (hypoglycemia, hyperglycemia, hepatic encephalopathy,
uremia, severe electrolyte D/O)
Requires neuro exam **by 2 physicians**
Following must exist for **6–12 hours**:
1) Unresponsive to pain
2) Absent cold caloric oculovestibular reflexes (cold water)
3) Absent oculocephalic reflex (ie has dolls eyes)
4) Positive apnea test (see below)
5) No corneal reflex
6) No gag reflex
7) Fixed and dilated pupils
EEG – should show electrical silence
MRA or angiogram – if used should show no blood flow to brain
Apnea test
Pt is **disconnected from ventilator** after pre-oxygenation (FiO2 100%)
→ pCO_2 > 60 mmHg or ↑in CO_2 by 20 is a **positive test for apnea**
If arterial pressure drops to < 60 or pt desaturates, test is terminated
(negative test for apnea)
**Impt - can still have deep tendon reflexes (DTRs) w/ brain death

Abdominal compartment syndrome

Sx's:
1) **Distended abdomen**
1) ↓ed UOP (↓ed C.O. is biggest factor, also renal vein compression)
2) ↑ed vent pressures (upward displacement of diaphragm)
Occurs w/ **hypotension** and **massive blood / fluid resuscitation** due to trauma
(esp w/ prolonged transport time) or abd surgery → abdominal contents
become swollen and compress IVC
IVC compression is the final common pathway for ↓ed **cardiac output
Dx: bladder pressure >20 (hook foley up to CVP monitor)
Cx's: gut malperfusion, poor ventilation
Tx: decompressive laparotomy, sterile cover for abdominal contents
Can't get abdomen closed after operation because of swollen bowel
→ cut sterile IV bag and sew to skin; ioban over that; bring back in 48
hours and close abdomen when visceral swelling goes down

THE COMPREHENSIVE ABSITE REVIEW

Stroke
Sx's: hemiplegia, slurred speech (if after CEA, see vascular chp):
1) Assess ABC's – intubate if necessary
2) Control blood pressure (want systolic < 185 mmHg, diastolic < 110 mmHg)
3) Get a head CT to R/O hemorrhagic stroke
4) Check or send off for a recent platelet count + coag's (PT, PTT)
5) If it is a **non-hemorrhagic stroke, start intra-venous tPA**
6) If the pt has a contraindication to intra-venous tPA (eg recent surgery), consider direct **intra-arterial tPA** - involves placing a catheter in the occluded vessel and giving tPA directly into thrombus or embolus
7) Control hyperglycemia

Acute Gout Flare
Sx's: painful arthritis, esp MTP of great toe (podagra), warm, tense
Dx: needle shaped **negatively birifringent crystals**, ↑ WBCs in joint tap
Tx:
>**Acute attacks** – indomethacin, colchicines, naproxen, steroids
>**Allopurinol** (xanthine oxidase inhibitor) – inhibits uric acid synthesis
>>Contraindicated in pts taking azathioprine (Imuran)
>**Probenecid** – inhibits renal reabsorption of uric acid

Carbon monoxide poisoning
MCC fatal poisoning (from suicide)
Binds hemoglobin and creates **carboxyhemoglobin** → O_2 can't bind anymore
Has a greater affinity for hemoglobin than oxygen (250 x)
**Results in a *left shift* in the oxygen dissociation curve
>Hgb will not let go of bound O_2
>Additionally O2 has to compete w/ CO for binding sites

Sx's: ↑ HR, HTN, mental status changes (headache, seizures)
Dx:
>**Falsely elevates oxygen saturation reading on pulse oximeter**
>**Abnormal carboxyhemoglobin**
>>**Non-smokers** > 10%
>>**Smokers** > 20%

Tx: Usually corrected w/ **100% oxygen on ventilator** (displaces carbon monoxide); may need hyperbaric O_2 if really high

Methemoglobinemia
Oxygen carrying **ferrous ion** (Fe2+) of heme group is **oxidized** to **ferric ion** (Fe3+) → forming **methemoglobin**, which cannot bind oxygen
**Results in a *right shift* is oxygen dissociation curve
Causes – topical anesthetics for EGD [benzocaine (Hurricaine spray)], dapsone, fertilizers (nitrates) – **all act as oxidizing drugs**
Sx's: ↑ RR, dyspnea; metabolic lactic acidosis (anaerobic metabolism)
>O_2 **saturation reads 85%**

Tx: oxygen + methylene blue (1%; 1 mg/kg <u>IV</u>, restores Fe to reduced state)

Critical illness polyneuropathy and myopathy
Usually motor > sensory w/ polyneuropathy (Dx electromyelography, EMG)
RFs – ARDS, sepsis, steroids, SIRS, paralytics, ↑ glucose
Can lead to failure to wean from ventilation; no good tx

Reperfusion injury
Critical role of **PMNs**
Xanthine oxidase (endothelial cells)
>Forms **toxic oxygen radicals** after reperfusion
>Normally metabolizes purines into uric acid

CO2 pneumoperitoneum (normal 10-15)

Cardiopulmonary dysfunction can occur w/ intra-abdominal pressure **> 20**

Increased w/ pneumoperitoneum:
- Pulmonary artery pressure
- Pulmonary vascular resistance
- HR
- Systemic vascular resistance
- Central venous pressure
- Mean airway pressure
- Peak inspiratory pressure
- CO_2

Decreased w/ pneumoperitoneum:
- pH
- Venous return (IVC compression)
- Renal flow primarily due to decreased cardiac output, some from renal vein compression, will increase renin production
- Cardiac output

Hypovolemia lowers pressure necessary to cause compromise

CO_2 can ↓ in **myocardial contractility**

Surgical technologies

Harmonic scalpel
- Cost-effective for medium vessels (short gastric arteries)
- Disrupts the **protein hydrogen bonds**, causes coagulation of vessels

Ultrasound
- **B-mode MC used** (B = brightness; assesses relative density of structures)
  - Forms 2 dimensional structure
  - **Shadowing** – dark area posterior to object indicates mass (eg gallstone, breast fibroadenoma)
  - **Enhancement** – brighter area posterior to object, indicates fluid-filled cyst or structure (eg gallbladder, breast cyst)
  - **Lower frequencies** – good for deep structures, less resolution
  - **Higher frequencies** – good for superficial structures, more resolution
  - **Breast CA** – jagged contour, heterogeneous
  - **Fibroadenoma** – smooth, rounded
- **Duplex ultrasound** combines **B** mode and **doppler**
  - Looks at how sound waves bounce off moving objects like blood
  - Gives colored visual description of blood flow (can see stenosis and direction)

Argon beam – energy transferred across argon gas
- Depth of necrosis related to power setting (2 mm usual)
- Good for **superficial coagulation**
- Is **non-contact** – good for hemostasis for liver and spleen

CO_2 Laser – return of electrons to ground state releases energy as heat
- Coagulates and vaporizes (eg condylomata accuminata - wear mask)
- **Max depth – 0.5 mm**

Nd:YAG Laser – good for deep tissue penetration like bronchial lesions
- **Size of the laser spot dictates effect**

1–2 mm	cuts (concentrated energy, **max depth - 5 mm**)
3–10 mm	vaporizes
1–2 cm	coagulates (energy spread out)

Gortex (PTFE) – smooth and <u>cannot</u> get fibroblast in-growth
- Good for AV fistulas and lower extremity bypass above the knee

Dacron (polyethylene terephthalate) – woven polyester graft allows fibroblast in-growth (good for big vessels like aorta)

Marlex Mesh (polypropylene mesh) – non-absorbable permanent mesh (used for hernias)

Vicryl Mesh – absorbable (90 d) mesh for temporary wound or organ support (good temporary coverage of large defects, eg necrotizing fasciitis and have to resect abdominal wall preventing closure → use vicryl mesh to cover defect, it will dissolve, then place skin grafts); **resistant to infection**

Incidence of vascular or bowel injury w/ Veress needle or trocar – 0.1%

Burns

Burn Wounds	
1st degree	Sunburn (epidermis)
2nd degree	
Superficial dermis (papillary)	Painful; blebs and blisters; hair follicles intact; blanches to touch (heals in 2 weeks)
Deep dermis (reticular)	Decreased sensation; loss of hair follicles (need skin grafts)
3rd degree	Leathery; down to subcutaneous fat (sub-dermal) (need skin grafts)
4th degree	Down to bone, adipose, or muscle

1st and superficial 2nd degree burns heal by **epithelialization**
    Epithelial cells come from hair follicles (primary site) and edges of wound

Initial burn wound management:
    1st Trauma W/U
        ABCDEs IV x 2, fluid resuscitation, CXR, PXR, C-spine
        Need to R/O other life-threatening trauma injures (may have fell from a
            height or had MVA)
        Start Volume resuscitation
            Parkland formula: 4 cc/kg x % burn over 24 hours
                Give **1/2 volume in 1st 8 hours,** next **1/2 over 16 hours**
                Calculate only for $\geq 2^{nd}$ degree burns that are ≥ 20% BSA
            Use **lactated Ringer's** (LR) in first 24 hours (switch to D5 1/2 NS
                after 24 hours)
            UOP best measure of resuscitation: Adults - 0.5 cc/kg/hr
                Child - 1 cc/kg/hr, Infant (< 6 mos) - 2 cc/kg/hr
            Parkland can grossly underestimate requirements w/ inhalational
                injury, ETOH, electrical injury or post-escharotomy
            Children need **Ca^{++}** and **glucose** in 1st 24 hours
            Use of albumin early in resuscitation after severe burns may ↑
                pneumonia
    2nd Finish trauma w/u as appropriate
        Head/Abd/Pelvic CT if appropriate
        Check trauma labs (including myoglobin)
    3rd Eschar and compartment syndrome evaluation:
        Escharotomy indications (within 4–6 hours to prevent myonecrosis):
            1) **Circumferential** deep burns w/ decreased temp, pulse, capillary
                refill, pain sensation, or neurologic function in extremity (may
                need **fasciotomy** if compartment syndrome suspected)
            2) **Trouble ventilating pt's** w/ significant chest torso burns
        Escharotomy (fasciotomy) **types:**
            1) **Medial and lateral sides of limbs** (*except* fingers, see below)
            2) **Dorsum of hand** (*avoid palm*)
            3) **Fingers** – mid-axial incision (*avoid lateral incisions → nerves there*)
            4) **Chest** – lateral chest wall, sub-clavicular and above costal margin
        If compartment syndrome → fasciotomy (all extremities susceptible)
        If muscle is dead (cadaveric) → debride it to prevent **myoglobin release**
    4th Renal issues:
        Hyperkalemia (released from dead tissue, see Critical Care chp for Tx)
        Myoglobinuria (released from dead muscle)
            Tx: volume resuscitation and HCO_3^- to alkalinize urine
        Renal failure (from volume loss, myoglobin; see Critical Care chp)
    5th Prevent heat loss (keep pt warm)
    6th Check carboxyhemoglobin (carbonaceous sputum, long extrication time)

Management after initial trauma phase:

Wash off and clean burns (warm water/soap)

Silvadene (or Neosporin) over area, telfa, wrap loosely w/ gauze

Sulfamylon for cartilaginous areas

Tetanus shot

Cardiac output initially decreased (24-48 hours) after burn then increases along w/ oxygen consumption; also get ↑ed temp late (↑ed catecholamines)

1st week: 1) **excise burned areas** and 2) **start nutrition**

1) **Early excision of burned areas** (48-72 hours after burn)

Use **dermatome** for deep 2nd degree and 3rd degree wounds

Residual skin viability based on **color, texture,** and **punctate bleeding** after eschar removal

Thrombin or epinephrine soaked pads to help control bleeding

Infected areas

1) excise, 2) place allograft, 3) then re-excise later (don't use auto-graft for infected areas)

Biopsy suspected burn wound infections *(best method of Dx)*

Auto-grafts contraindicated if culture positive for **beta-hemolytic strep** or **bacteria >10^5**

STSG donor site

Hemostasis w/ **epinephrine soaked gauzes**

Covered w/ **Op-site** *(semi-occlusive best)* → heals in **3 weeks**

Can use as a **donor site** *again* (w/ STSG, epithelium migrates from **hair follicles** primarily, also from wound edges; these are termed **epithelial appendages**)

Donor site **healing time** *inversely* proportional to **thickness of graft** harvested

FTSG donor site – need primary closure

Skin grafts need to be compressed down w/ xeroform gauze and cotton balls

Don't want seroma or hematoma to form which prevents graft from attaching

For each burn wound excision session:

< 1 L blood loss

< 20% of skin excised

< 2 hours in OR

Blood loss is to be expected

Pts can get extremely sick if too much time spent in OR

Types of Grafts

Autografts [split-thickness (STSG) or full-thickness (FTSG)]

Best overall

Split-thickness grafts should be 0.012 - 0.015 cm (includes **epidermis** and **part of dermis**)

Meshed grafts (large area) – back, trunk, arms, legs

STSG – *more likely to survive* compared to FTSG (graft not as thick, easier imbibition and subsequent re-vascularization)

FTSG – *less wound contraction* than STSG

Not as many donor sites

Can get better skin color match

Donor site must be closed primarily

Good for face, palms back of hands, genitals

Not good for large areas

FTSG can be harvested from **behind ear**, above **clavicle**, or **groin** (loose skin areas – **primary closure**)

Homografts (allografts; cadaveric skin; **xenografts** - porcine)

Not as beneficial as autografts

Good temporizing material (lasts 2 weeks); may be good for infected burn wounds

No allograft in **pregnant women** (reported fetal deaths from HLA mismatch)

Eventually allografts become **vascularized, undergo rejection, thrombosis, and then **require removal**

Graft survival:
    Imbibition (days 0-3) – osmotic nutrient and oxygen supply to graft for 1st 3 days
    Neovascularization (day 3+) new blood vessel growth to graft
    Areas w/ poor vascular supply will likely NOT support skin grafting → tendons, bone w/o periosteum, radiated skin
    Unusual areas that can support grafts – omentum, bowel wall, bone w/ periosteum intact
MCC skin graft loss → seroma or hematoma formation under graft
Reasons to delay autografting:
    Infection
    Not enough skin donor sites
    Pt septic or unstable
    Don't want any more donor sites with concomitant blood loss
    Wounds to **face, palms, soles,** and **genitals** *deferred 1st week*

2) **Nutrition**
    **Burn wounds must use <u>glucose</u> in an obligatory fashion
    Place **feeding tube**
    Caloric need – 25 kcal/kg/day + (30 kcal/d x % burn)
        – don't exceed 3000 kcal/d
    Protein need – 1 g/kg/day + (3 g/d x % burn)
    Glucose – best source calories (non-protein) for burns

2nd week
    Hands, feet, face, and **genital areas treated**
    Allograft replaced w/ autograft
    Face – topical abx's for 1 week, FTSG (non-meshed) for unhealed areas
    Hands – immobilize in functional position
        Abx's for 1 week
        Then FTSG and immobilize in functional position for another week
        Then physical therapy
        May need wire fixation of joints if unstable or open.
    Palms
        Preserve specialized palmar aponeurosis (avoid palmar fasciotomy or escharotomy – go on dorsal surface)
        Splint hand in **extension** for 1 week; FTSG in 2nd week
    Genitals – topical abx's for 1 week; FTSG in 2nd week

Admission criteria

1) 2nd and 3rd degree burns
    > 10% BSA in pts aged < 10 or > 50 years
    > 20% BSA in all other pts
    Significant portions of **special areas** (hands, face, feet, genitalia, perineum, or skin overlying major joints)
2) 3rd degree burns > 5% (any age group)
3) **Electrical and chemical burns**
4) Concomitant **inhalational** injury, mechanical **trauma** or medical comorbidities
5) Pts w/ special needs (social, emotional or long-term rehabilitation)
6) **Child abuse** or neglect (or suspected; accounts for 15% of burns in children)

Rule of 9's – assessing % of body surface burned
    Head = 9, arms = 18, chest = 18, back = 18, legs = 36, perineum = 1
    Patient's palm = 1% BSA (can use to measure size of burn)
Highest deaths – children and elderly (can't get away)
MC burn – scald burn (eg stove)
MC burn to present to hospital and be admitted – flame burn

Items that suggest child abuse

Delayed care	Lack of splash marks
Conflicting histories	Stocking or glove pattern
Previous burns or injuries	Flexor area sparing
Sharp demarcation	Dorsal area of hands
Uniform depth of burn	Deep and localized

Inhalational injury

From **carbonaceous materials** and **smoke**, <u>NOT</u> a heat or thermal injury

RFs – ETOH, trauma, closed space, rapid combustion, age > 10 or < 50, delayed extrication

Sx's of possible inhalational injury – stridor, facial burns, wheezing, carbonaceous sputum

Cx's of inhalational injury:
1) **Upper airway obstruction (MC HD #1**; can occur up to 24 hours after burn); **massive volume resuscitation** worsens obstruction **(edema)**
2) **Bronchospasm**
3) **Atelectasis**
4) **Carbon monoxide poisoning**

Dx: fiberoptic bronchoscopy *(best test)* – look for soot

Intubation criteria – upper airway stridor or obstruction, worsening hypoxemia, massive volume resuscitation (often w/ very large burns)

MC infection in pts w/ significant burns (> 30% BSA) → **pneumonia**
Etiology – inhalation injury, ↓ed immunity, fluid resuscitation causing pulmonary edema, requirement for mechanical ventilation

MCC death after significant burn – infection (#1 pneumonia)

Burn wound infections

<u>No</u> role for prophylactic IV antibiotics

Sx's of burn wound infection:
1) **Rapid eschar separation**
2) **Edema**
3) **2nd to 3rd degree conversion** (partial thickness → full thickness)
4) **Hemorrhage** in wound
5) **Erythema gangrenosum**
6) **Green** discoloration of fat (or other color changes)
7) **Black skin** around the wound
8) **Pseudomonas smell**

Dx burn wound infection (differentiate from colonization) →
Biopsy of burn wound (*best method*; > 10^5 organisms = infection)

Path

MC organism in burn wound infection – pseudomonas
others – staph, E. coli; **MC fungal infection** – candida
MCC burn wound sepsis – pseudomonas
MC viral infection of burn wound – HSV
The larger the burn, the greater risk of infection
Cell mediated immunity ↓ed in burn wound (↓ granulocyte chemotaxis)

Tx:

Burn wound excision w/ <u>allograft</u> (*best Tx*) + **systemic abx's**
Do <u>not</u> use autograft when excising infected burn wounds
If just cellulitis around burn wound → systemic and topical abx's

Prevention

Topical abx's ↓ incidence of burn wound infections (candida infections have ↑ed as a consequence)

Silvadene (silver sulfadiazine)
Limited eschar penetration (bacteriostatic)
Contraindicated w/ sulfa allergy
S/Es: neutropenia and **thrombocytopenia**

Silver nitrate
Limited eschar penetration
S/Es: Electrolyte imbalances (↓Na^+, ↓Cl^-, ↓Ca^{++}, ↓K^+)
Methemoglobinemia → contraindicated w/ G6PD deficiency
Discoloration

Sulfamylon (mafenide sodium)
Painful application
Good **eschar penetration**, good for **cartilage**
Good for **pseudomonas**
S/Es: Metabolic acidosis due to carbonic anhydrase inhibition
Hypersensitivity reactions

Carbon monoxide poisoning (carboxyhemoglobin levels)

Normal level	10%
Normal level in Smokers	20%
Coma	50%
Death	70%

Tx: 100% O2, hyperbaric O2

Complications after burns

Seizures – MC iatrogenic (related to Na^+ concentration and resuscitation)
> Also benzodiazepine withdrawal

Ectopia –contraction of burned adnexae and can't see out of eye.
> Tx: surgical eyelid release

Eyes – fluorescein staining to Dx injury; Tx: topical fluoroquinolone ointment
Corneal abrasion – Tx: topical fluoroquinolones ointment
Symblepharon – eyelid stuck to underlying conjunctiva
> Tx: release with glass rod and amniotic tissue transplantation

Fractures – Tx: may need external fixation to allow for treatment of burns
Curling's ulcer – duodenal ulcer w/ burns
Marjolin's ulcer – highly malignant, ulcerative, **squamous cell CA** in chronic
> non-healing burn wounds or in chronic healing unstable scars
> (osteomyelitis, venous ulcers, post-XRT → latency period 30 years)

Acalculous cholecystitis
Hypertrophic scar (does not go beyond original border of scar like keloids)
> Usually occurs 3–4 months after injury
> Secondary to increased **neovascularity**
> MC w/ deep thermal injuries that take > 3 weeks to heal, heal by
> contraction and epithelial spread, or heal across flexor surfaces
> Tx: steroids, silicone injection, compression, grafting, scar excision w/
> primary closure and steroid injections
> Wait 1–2 years before surgery

Special burns

Acid and alkali burns
> Need vigorous water irrigation (30-60 min)
> **Alkalis** deeper than acid due to **liquefaction necrosis**
> **Acid burns** result in **coagulation necrosis**

Hydrofluoric acid burns – **calcium** spread over the wound (neutralizes burn)
Powder burns – wipe off before irrigation
Tar burns – cool, wipe off w/ lipophyllic solvent (eg **glycerol**)
Phenol burns – are not water soluble; use lipophyllic solvent (eg **glycerol**)
Burn scar hypopigmentation – improved w/ **dermal abrasion** or thin STSGs

Serious Skin Injuries

Toxic Epidermal Necrolysis (TEN, variant of erythema multiforme major)
Stevens-Johnson Syndrome (less severe then TEN)
Staph Scalded Skin Syndrome
Multiple etiologies for above: Drugs (MCC; phenytoin, bactrim, PCN); Viruses
Involves **detachment of epidermis from dermis**
Tx:
> Remove offending agent if drug related
> **Topical antimicrobial** (<u>no</u> silvadene if thought to be sulfa related)
> **Topical Allografts** to prevent wound desiccation and super-infection
> **Wrap area w/ Telfa gauze**
> **Fluid resuscitation**
> **Abx's** if due to staph aureus
> **NO steroids**

Frostbite

> Rapid re-warming of part in circulating warm water 40-42°
> Pain control, Tetanus shot
> Silvadene over blistered areas
> Abx's for signs of infection
> May need amputation or skin graft later

HEAD and NECK

Normal Neck Anatomy

Anterior neck triangle
Anterior border of sternocleidomastoid muscle
Sternal notch
Inferior border of digastric muscle, and trachea
Contains **carotid artery, internal jugular vein, vagus nerve**

Posterior neck triangle
Posterior border of sternocleidomastoid muscle
Trapezius muscle
Clavicle
Contains **spinal accessory nerve and brachial plexus**

Nerves

Phrenic nerve – on anterior scalene muscle, controls diaphragm
Vagus nerve – runs between IJ and carotid arteries; recurrent laryngeal branch innervates larynx
Trigeminal nerve – ophthalmic, maxillary, mandibular branches
Sensation for most of face
Mandibular branch – taste for anterior ⅔ of tongue, floor of mouth, and gingiva
Facial nerve – temporal, zygomatic, buccal, marginal mandibular, and cervical branches; motor to face; runs through the parotid gland
Found between **upper ½ of mastoid** and **tympanomastoid fissure** (level of the digastric muscle)
Glossopharyngeal nerve
Sensory to posterior 1/3 tongue
Motor to stylopharyngeus and pharynx
Injury – trouble swallowing
Hypoglossal nerve
Motor to all of tongue except palatoglossus
Tongue deviates to **ipsilateral side** w/ injury
Recurrent laryngeal nerve (see Thyroid chp)
Innervates all of larynx except cricothyroid muscle
Injury causes hoarseness
Superior laryngeal nerve (see Thyroid chp)
Innervates cricothyroid muscle
Injury causes loss of voice pitch
Frey's syndrome – after parotidectomy; injury of **auriculotemporal nerve** that cross-innervates w/ **sympathetic fibers** to skin sweat glands
Sx's: gustatory sweating (sweating over cheek while eating)

Parotid glands – mostly serous fluid
Sublingual glands – mostly mucin
Submandibular glands – 50% serous, 50% mucin

False vocal cords superior to true vocal cords
Trachea – U-shaped cartilage w/ membranous posterior portion
Has longitudinal intra-mucosal blood supply (cartilage supplied by mucosa)
Thyrocervical trunk – "STAT":
Suprascapular artery
Transverse cervical artery
Ascending cervical artery
Inferior Thyroid artery
External carotid artery – 1st branch is the **superior thyroid artery**
Trapezius muscle flap (spinal accessory nerve, allows shoulder shrug) – flap based on **transverse cervical artery**
Pectoralis major muscle flap – flap based on **thoracoacromial artery**
Torus palatini – benign congenital bony mass on upper palate of mouth
Tx: nothing
Torus mandibular – as above but on anterior lingual surface of mandible
Waldeyer's Tonsillar Ring – lingual, palatine ("the tonsils"), tubal, and pharyngeal tonsils; in pharynx and back of oral cavity; **lymph node** ring

Neck mass (Enlarged lymph node)
- **DDx:**
  - 1) **Lymph node** (usually along cervical chain, anterior to sternocleidomastoid)
    - **Mets** – ENT tumor, lung, esophagus, thyroid or parathyroid, melanoma, distant site (breast or gastric CA)
      - **MC cell type** – squamous cell CA
    - **Other causes of enlarged LN** – lymphoma, TB, URI (viral), sarcoid
  - 2) **Thyroid nodule** (near midline mass)
  - 3) **Parathyroid adenoma** (*rarely* palpable, need to worry about parathyroid CA if palpable)
- **Exam:**
  - **Bruit** (carotid body sinus tumor)
  - **Bimanual oral exam + Fiberoptic laryngoscopy**
  - Look for **skin CA or other cervical adenopathy**
- **Dx** (for lymph node):
  - **If inflammatory** (tender, URI sx's), can tx w/ **abx's and F/U in 2 weeks**
    - Make sure getting **smaller**
  - **1st – FNA** (*best initial Dx test*, or core needle Bx) + **CXR** (in office, that day)
    - If core needle → send FS and permanent
    - If it shows malignant cells, base w/u on what type of cells it shows
    - If work-up and biopsy indeterminate, go to 2nd below
  - **2nd – Bronch / EGD** (w/ random Bx's if no lesion found)
    - **Neck/chest/abd CT** (neck CT picks up carotid body tumor)
    - **Mammogram** in women
    - All above looking for *primary lesion*
  - **3rd** – still can't figure it out → **perform excisional biopsy** → send FS
    - Need to be prepared for MRND

  - **Core needle Bx or excisional Bx shows →**
    - **SCCA w/ lung** (Stage IIIb) **or esophagus** (Stage IV) **primary →** unresectable (palliative chemo-XRT)
    - **SCCA w/ ENT tumor →** MRND; resect ENT tumor
    - **SCCA** (ie epidermoid) found in **cervical node *w/o* known primary**
      - Tx: **ipsilateral MRND, ipsilateral tonsillectomy** (25% of occult primaries eventually found here), **bilateral neck XRT** (to nodal region + potential head and neck primary sites)
      - Pt should be followed and re-examined periodically for primary
    - **Salivary gland tumor** – see Parotid Gland below
    - **Adenocarcinoma** – from esophagus (stage IV) or lung primary (stage IIIB) → unresectable (palliative chemo-XRT)
    - **Breast CA** – unresectable, stage IIIc
    - **Melanoma** (see Skin and Soft Tissue chp) → need MRND, find skin primary
    - **Lymphoma** (see Spleen chp for Tx) → just excisional Bx
      - Stage w/ neck/chest/abd CT and Bone marrow Bx
    - **Inflammatory cells→** Abx's, back in 2 weeks to make sure getting smaller
    - **Thyroid CA →** follow appropriate tx (see Thyroid chp)
    - **Find normal thyroid tissue in lymph node** (this is metastatic papillary thyroid CA) – Tx: total thyroidectomy, MRND, postop I-131 (see Thyroid chp)

- **Posterior neck masses** – Hodgkin's lymphoma until proved o/w
  - R/O epithelial ENT tumors
  - Resect Lymph Node for biopsy (need 1 cm^3 of tissue for Dx of lymphoma)

<u>Oral cavity cancer</u> (oro-pharyngeal, above larynx)
- **MC site for oral cavity CA** - lower lip
- **RFs** – ETOH and tobacco
- **Exam**
  - **Bimanual oral exam + Fiberoptic laryngoscopy**
  - **Look for adenopathy** (cervical, supra-clavicular, axillary)
- **Dx:**
  - **FNA** (or core needle Bx) of lesion *(best initial Dx step)*
  - **Head/Neck/Chest CT** – look for met's or a primary
  - **EGD** and **Bronch**
- **Path**
  - **MC type** – vast majority **squamous cell CA** (ie epidermoid)
  - **CA risk** – **erythroplakia** > leukoplakia
  - **Division of anterior oral cavity** and **posterior oral cavity** marked by:
    - Tonsilar pillars
    - Junction between the hard and soft palates
    - Tongue papilla
  - **Lip CA** and **Tonsilar CA** considered anterior oral cavity CA
  - **Anterior oral cavity CA→ submental + submandibular chain** 1st (level I)
    - *Exception* **Tongue CA** goes to cervical chain nodes (early)
  - **Posterior oral cavity CA → cervical chain nodes** 1st (levels II, III + IV)
    - 1) **Nasopharyngeal SCCA**: Sx's – epistaxis or obstruction
      - EBV associated; Chinese
      - ***Very responsive to XRT*** (different from other pharyngeal CA)
    - 2) **Oropharyngeal SCCA**; Sx's – neck mass, sore throat
    - 3) **Hypopharyngeal SCCA**; Sx's – hoarseness (**early LN spread**)
  - **Location w/ lowest survival rate** – hard palate (hard to resect)
  - Need **1 cm margin** for all *except* tongue (**2 cm margin** required)
- **Tx:**

  - **Stage I + II anterior tumors** (< 4 cm, no nodal or bone invasion) →
    - *Resection + prophylactic **supra-omohyoid LND*** (majority, 80%)
      - → If < 3 mm *or* risk of mets < 15%→ <u>no</u> prophylactic LND
      - **Areas w/ mets < 15%** → alveolus, hard palate. and lip CA
      - **Tongue CA gets extended supra-omohyoid LND**
    - **Positive nodes** found w/ supra-omohyoid LND → **formal MRND**

  - **Stage I + II posterior tumors** (< 4 cm, no nodal or bone invasion) →
    - **XRT** <u>only</u>
      - Hard to get at these tumors w/ surgery
      - If does not resolve w/ XRT, consider surgery →
        - *Exception* is **nasopharyngeal CA** → give **chemo + XRT**
    - Include **neck in XRT field** (want to get **neck nodes**)

  - **Stage III anterior or posterior tumors** (> 4 cm *or;* nodal or bone invasion)
    - ***All get:*** 1) *Resection,* 2) *LND* (see below),*and* 3) *postop **chemoXRT***
      - **N-0 anterior oral cavity** → **supra-omohyoid LND**
        - (*except* tongue → extended supra-omohyoid LND)
      - **N-0 posterior oral cavity**
        - **Oropharynx** → **anterolateral LND**
          - *Bilateral* LND if tumor **crosses midline**
        - **Hypopharynx**– *bilateral* **anterolateral** LND(early spread)
      - **N-1** (clinically positive nodes, anterior or posterior) → **MRND**
      - ***Exception*** – **nasopharyngeal CA** (either **N0** or **N1**) → all get
        chemo-XRT *only* (<u>no resection</u>; include neck nodes in XRT
        field)
  - **Stage IV** (mets)- palliative chemo-XRT

  - **Chemo** – **5-FU + cisplatin** (most effective for nasopharyngeal CA)
  - **Supra-omohyoid LND** (lymph node dissection) – level I, II, + III nodes
  - **Extended supra-omohyoid LND** – level I, II, III, + IV nodes
  - **Anterolateral LND** (anterior cervical chain) – level II, III, + IV nodes
  - **MRND** – level I, II, III, IV + V nodes; (V = posterior chain; posterior to SCM)

Special Issues

Lip CA

Lower lip CA MC than upper due to sun exposure

Lesions at commissure (angle of mouth) are **most aggressive**

Needs to involve **mucosa** or its <u>not</u> lip CA

Flaps needed if more than 1/3 of lip is removed

Tongue CA – jaw invasion still operable

Commando procedure – removes portion of the mandible

Early nodal invasion (cervical chain)

Verrucous ulcer (carcinoma) – often presents as **leukoplakia on cheek

Associated w/ **chewing tobacco**

<u>Very low grade,</u> well-differentiated squamous cell CA

Locally aggressive but <u>very rare</u> nodal or systemic mets

Often on **inner cheek** but can be anywhere in mouth

Tx: full cheek resection ± flap; <u>***No***</u> *lymph node dissection*

(even w/ palpable nodes – most likely inflammatory)

Maxillary sinus CA Tx: maxillectomy

Tonsillar CA: Sx's – asymptomatic until large; **RFs** - ETOH, tobacco

MC type – SCCA

Considered **anterior oral cavity CA**

80% have lymph node spread at time of dx

Tx: tonsillectomy (best way to get Dx and Tx lesion)

Therapy then same as above for anterior tumors

<u>Parotid tumors</u> can invade the oral cavity and **deviate the**

ipsilateral tonsil (see parotid mass below)

Other nasopharynx tumors

MC benign tumor of nasopharynx – papilloma

MC tumor of nasopharynx in children – <u>lymphoma</u> Tx: chemo

Nasopharyngeal angiofibroma

Benign, **extremely vascular**

Males < 20 years (obstruction or epistaxis)

Tx: **Angio embolization** (MC internal maxillary artery), then

resection; XRT for inaccessible tumors

Plummer-Vinson Syndrome – oral cavity CA, glossitis, cervical dysphagia

(esophageal web), spoon fingernails, Fe-deficient anemia (microcytic)

Laryngeal Cancer

Sx's: Hoarseness, aspiration, dyspnea, dysphagia

Exam: Bimanual oral exam + Fiberoptic laryngoscopy

Dx

FNA or **Bx** of lesion

Head/Neck/Chest CT – look for met's or a primary

EGD and Bronch (the vocal cords lie behind **thyroid cartilage**)

Tx (primarily XRT or chemo-XRT, not surgery)

Try to <u>***preserve***</u> *larynx*

1) **Tumor on vocal cord** *only* →

Cords <u>not</u> fixed → XRT *only*, re-assess (want <u>larynx preservation</u>)

Chemo-XRT if that fails

Endoscopic removal or partial laryngectomy if that fails

Cords fixed → **chemo-XRT**

Endoscopic removal or partial laryngectomy if that fails

2) **Vocal cord tumor and invasion of surrounding structures**

→ **chemo-XRT**, then re-assess

Partial laryngectomy if still present

3) **Not involving vocal cord but surrounding structures**

→ **Chemo-XRT,** then re-assess

If tumor still present → partial laryngectomy or surgical preservation

of vocal cords altogether if possible

XRT – spread field to get **ipsilateral neck nodes** (tumors go to **cervical chain**)

If tumor **crosses midline** → **bilateral neck XRT**

Stage III (positive nodes) → need above + MRND (take **ipsilateral thyroid lobe**)

MC benign tumor of larynx – papilloma

Parotid Mass

Pre-auricular mass just above angle of mandible, anterior to ear
   All are parotid tumors until proved otherwise
   Dx usually made after superficial lobectomy
DDx:
   Malignant – mucoepidermoid CA, adenoid cystic CA; lymphoma;
      melanoma met or skin SCCA met
   Benign – pleomorphic adenoma (5% malignant degeneration), Warthin's
Sx's: painless mass; **pain or facial nerve paralysis** suggests malignancy
Exam
   Bimanual exam + Fiberoptic laryngoscopy
   Look for **skin CA** (frequent skin CA mets site), **cervical adenopathy**
   Try to role lesion beneath mandible to assess attachment to parotid
   Assess for **facial nerve paralysis** (facial muscle function)
Dx:
   Head/Neck/Chest CT (assess for mets or synchronous lesions)
   EGD and **Bronch** (assess for mets or synchronous lesions)
   FNA (occasionally obtained)
      NO FNA if parotid mass is mobile, discrete and confined to superficial
         lobe (perform **superficial parotidectomy** – this is your biopsy)
      If the mass is in **deep parotid gland**, the pt is **poor operative risk**,
         or the mass is felt to be **metastatic** in nature (eg melanoma),
         then FNA useful
Path
   80% of all salivary tumors in parotid
   80% of parotid tumors benign
   80% of benign parotid tumors are pleomorphic adenomas
   Malignant parotid tumors metastasize to **lung**
Malignant parotid tumors
   Mucoepidermoid CA – MC malignant tumor of salivary glands
   Adenoid cystic CA – #2 malignant tumor of salivary glands
      Long, indolent course → propensity to **invade nerve roots**
      Can just give **XRT** if extensive _(very sensitive)_
   SCCA – _rare_ primary tumor of parotid
   Tx:
      Total parotidectomy + prophylactic MRND + Postop XRT
      Only exception is low grade mucoepidermoid CA → just total
         parotidectomy (no MRND or XRT)
      No paralytics w/ dissection; can use a nerve stimulator to help find
         the facial nerve branches
      **Try to preserve facial nerve (even if you have to peel tumor off)
         Unless that branch of facial nerve is already out (**pre-op exam**)
         XRT to that **area post-op**
Benign parotid tumors – often presents as a painless mass
   Pleomorphic adenoma (mixed tumor)
      MC benign tumor of salivary glands; **Malignant degeneration in 5%**
   Warthin's tumor (papillary cystadenoma lymphomatosum)
      #2 benign tumor of salivary glands; bilateral in 10%
   Tx: superficial parotidectomy (total parotidectomy if deep gland involved)
Technical considerations
   MC injured nerve w/ parotid surgery – greater auricular nerve
      (numbness over lower portion of ear auricle)
   Deep parotid tumor extending to parapharyngeal space (eg – _pushing
      tonsil towards midline_); **Tx – median mandibulotomy** for exposure
      (need mandibulectomy if bone involved)
   Frey's syndrome – cross innervation of the **auriculotemporal nerve** w/
      sympathetic fibers in skin sweat glands
      Sx's: gustatory sweating (sweating on cheek while eating)
      Tx: usually self limiting (use roll-on anti-perspirants) → If refractory,
         can place _alloderm skin graft_ between skin flap and nerve

Salivary gland cancers (other than parotid)

    Parotid (see above), submandibular, sublingual, and minor salivary glands

    Mass in large salivary gland → MC benign

    Mass in small salivary gland → MC malignant

        Although parotid gland is MC site for a malignant tumor

    Sx's: submandibular, sublingual, and minor salivary tumors → **neck mass or swelling in mouth floor**; lymphadenopathy

    1) **Malignant tumors**

        Mucoepidermoid CA (MC malignant salivary gland tumor)

            Wide range of aggressiveness

        Adenoid cystic CA (MC malignant salivary tumor of minor salivary glands)

            Often have a long, indolent course - Increased nerve root invasion

        Lymphatic spread to **intra-parotid nodes** and **cervical chain**

        Tx:

            Resection of salivary gland, prophylactic ipsilateral MRND (including parotid gland) and **postop XRT**

            Exception – low grade mucoepidermoid CA (**no MRND or XRT**)

    2) **Benign tumors**

        Pleomorphic adenoma (mixed tumor; MC benign tumor of salivary glands)

            Malignant degeneration occurs in 5% (mucoepidermoid CA)

            Tx: gland resection

            If there is malignant degeneration, need MRND and post-op XRT unless low grade mucoepidermoid

        Warthin's tumor (MC in males)

            Tx: gland resection

    Submandibular gland resection – find mandibular branch of facial nerve, lingual nerve, hypoglossal nerve

    MC injured nerve w/ submandibular resection – marginal mandibular nerve

        Supplies lower lip and chin

    MC salivary gland tumor in children – hemangiomas

Modified radical neck dissection (MRND)

    Takes omohyoid, submandibular gland, sensory nerves C2–C5, cervical branch of facial nerve, and cervical chain LN's

    No real mortality difference compared to RND

Radical neck dissection (not really used anymore)

    Takes **accessory nerve (CN XII)**, **sternocleidomastoid**, and **internal jugular**

    Also takes omohyoid, submandibular gland, sensory nerves C2-C5, cervical branch of facial nerve, cervical chain LN's

    Most morbidity w/ **accessory nerve resection** (muscles of neck including sternocleidomastoid; trapezius)

Ear Disorders (ear = pinna)

Cauliflower ear (ie boxers ear) – undrained hematomas that organize and
calcify; Tx: drain hematomas to avoid this

Glomus tumors (glomus skin tumor)

Tumor has **blood vessels** and **nerves**

Benign but *very painful*

MC site – tip of digits (often subungual – under nail)

Middle ear – reddish bulge behind intact ear drum; blanches w/ pressure to
external ear canal w/ pneumatic ear speculum

Glomus tympanicum – tinnitus (in 80%) and hearing loss (in 60%)

Glomus jugulare – cranial nerves of jugular foramen compressed,
resulting swallowing difficulty

Tx: tumor excision

Acoustic neuroma (vestibular schwannoma, CN VIII, vestibulocochlear)

Benign, slow growth

Association w/ neurofibromatosis (von Recklinghausen's DZ)

Almost always occurs on the **vestibular branch**

Sx's:

Tinnitus, hearing loss, unsteadiness, vertigo, N/V

Can compress cerebellopontine angle and brainstem affecting other
cranial nerves (facial, trigeminal, glossopharyngeal, vagus)

Dx: MRI *(best test)*

Tx:

Craniotomy and resection of tumor and superior/inferior vestibular
nerves; **facial nerve** at risk w/ surgery

XRT is alternative to surgery

Advanced age and **minor sx's** (eg age > 70) – can follow w/ MRI to
see if it's getting bigger (50% no growth over 5 years)

Cholesteatoma

Epidermal inclusion cyst of ear

Slow growing but erode as they grow

Can damage the middle ear bones (malleus, incus and stapes)

Can erode into mastoid

Sx's: hearing loss and brown/yellow drainage from ear, possibly bloody

Tx: surgical excision ± mastoidectomy

Pinna lacerations (ear) – sutures need to go full thickness through involved
cartilage

Ear Infections need to be treated promptly to avoid **cartilage necrosis**

MC childhood aural CA – rhabdomyosarcoma of middle or external ear

Head and neck melanoma (including ear) – see Skin and Soft Tissue chp

Head and neck skin SCCA (including ear) – see Skin and Soft Tissue chp

Nasal Disorders

Nasal fractures – wait for the swelling to go down before setting these

Septal hematoma – drain these to avoid infection and necrosis of septum

CSF rhinorrhea – MC from cribriform plate fracture (CSF has **tau protein** and
beta transferrin; see trauma section)

Epistaxis

90% anterior → 95% controlled w/ **packing** (Kiesselbach's plexus)

Posterior – pack, can use balloon tamponade (place Foley in back of
nose)

Refractory bleeding – internal maxillary artery or ethmoidal artery **angio
embolization** (or open ligation if that fails)

Keep on abx's while packing is in place

Neck and jaw Disorders
Thyroglossal duct cyst
From descent of thyroid from **foramen cecum**
Possible that this is only thyroid tissue pt has
Goes through the hyoid bone
Sx's: midline cervical mass, can get **infected**, may cause **dysphagia**
Tx: excision of **cyst, tract,** and **hyoid bone** through lateral neck incision
Branchial cleft cyst – can lead to sinus tracts, fistulas, and infection
1st Branchial Cleft Cyst – angle of mandible
Can connect with **external auditory canal**
Very often associated w/ facial nerve
2nd Branchial Cleft Cyst *(MC location)* – anterior border of SCM muscle
Goes through **carotid bifurcation** and into **tonsillar pillar**
3rd Branchial Cleft Cyst – deep in SCM, emerges in **pyriform sinus**
Tx for all cysts: resection
Cystic hygroma
Classically found in **lateral posterior neck triangle** (posterior to SCM)
MC on left; swollen area under skin; can form sinuses and get infected
Tx: resection
Branchial cleft cysts – are either anterior or through the SCM
Thyroglossal duct cysts – midline
Radicular cyst
Stratified squamous epithelium without keratin formation
Benign but can transform to CA (SCCA)
Lucent on x-ray
Tx: local excision or curettage
Ameloblastoma – tumor from tooth elements
Slow-growing malignancy
X-ray – 'soap bubble appearance'; can have mets
Tx: wide local excision
Osteogenic sarcoma – poor prognosis; (see Skin and Soft Tissue chp)
TMJ dislocations tx: closed reduction
Lower lip numbness – from inferior alveolar nerve damage
Stenson's duct laceration (ie parotid duct)
Opens into vestibule of mouth opposite upper 2nd molar
Primary repair over catheter stent
Ligation causes painful parotid atrophy and facial asymmetry
Suppurative parotitis
MC in elderly patients w/ dehydration
MC organism – staph
Tx: fluids, salivation, abx's; drainage if abscess develops or pt not
improving; Can be a life-threatening problem
Sialoadenitis
Acute inflammation of salivary gland related to stone in duct
Most calculi near orifice
Recurrent sialoadenitis from ascending infection from oral cavity
80% involves submandibular or sublingual glands
Tx:
Incise duct and remove stone
Gland excision may be necessary for recurrent disease
Paraganglioma
MC ENT site – carotid body (**carotid body tumor**, at bifurcation)
Can secrete **norepinephrine** ($\uparrow$ HR + HTN; palpations, HA's)
Highly vascular
Sx's: **neck mass w/ bruit**
Dx: angio, MIBG
Tx: surgical excision

Abscesses

Peritonsillar abscess (ie quinsy)

Older children (age > 10) and adults

Tonsillitis precipitating event

Sx's: sore throat, odynophagia; usually does <u>not</u> obstruct airway

Tx: **needle aspiration 1st + abx's**

Drainage through tonsillar bed if no relief in 24 hours

± intubation to drain; will self-drain w/ swallowing once opened

Retropharyngeal abscess

Young kids (< 10 years)

Bacterial infection originates in nasopharynx, tonsils, sinuses, adenoids or middle ear

Sx's: fever, odynophagia, drool; is an ***airway emergency***

Pott's disease – retropharyngeal abscess in elderly

Tx:

**Intubate pt in a calm setting

Drainage through posterior pharyngeal wall

Self-drains w/ swallowing once opened

Abx's

Parapharyngeal abscess

Even age distribution (children to adults)

MC w/ dental infections, tonsillitis, pharyngitis

Morbidity from **vascular invasion** and **mediastinal spread** via prevertebral and retropharyngeal spaces

Tx:

Drain through lateral neck (incision anterior to sternocleidomastoid) to avoid damaging carotid and internal jugular; leave drains

Mediastinal spread – right VATS or thoracotomy to wash out mediastinum

Abx's

Ludwig's angina

Acute infection and cellulitis of mouth floor

Involves **myelohyoid muscle**

Sx's: pain, swelling, raising of mouth floor, **can obstruct airway**

MCC – dental infection of mandibular teeth

MC organism – *Actinomyces israelii*

Can rapidly spread to deeper structures and cause airway obstruction

Tx: airway control, surgical drainage, antibiotics

Sleep apnea

Pt rarely aware of problem (spouse brings them in)

Pauses in breathing w/ sleep (**> 10 second interval** between breaths w/ either EEG changes or ↓ **O$_2$ sat 3-4%**

Types

1) **Obstructive** (85%) – breathing interrupted by a physical block

RFs – obesity, micrognathia, retrognathia

Have snoring and excessive daytime somnolence

2) **Central** (0.5%) – breathing interrupted by **lack of respiratory effort** (cycles between apnea and hyperventilation; **Cheyne-Stokes respiration**)

3) **Complex** (15%, or "mixed") – there is a transition from central to obstructive during the event

Cx's: cor pulmonale, MI's, arrhythmias, and death

Tx:

CPAP (or BiPAP) at night *(best Tx, works only for obstructive)*

Laying on side *(works for all types)*

Uvulopalatopharyngoplasty, hyoid suspension, or permanent tracheostomy

Congenital sleep apnea – need permanent tracheostomy, ventilator at night

Other Disorders

Esophageal foreign body
> **Sx's:** dysphagia, drooling, pain
> MC site – just below cricopharyngeous muscle (95%)
> **Dx: rigid EGD** under anesthesia (see Esophageal chp)
> **Perforation risk ↑s w/ length of time in esophagus**

Fever and pain after removal of foreign body
> **Dx:** CXR and gastrograffin (followed by barium) swallow to R/O perforation

Laryngeal foreign body
> **Sx's:** coughing
> **Tx:** emergent cricothyroidotomy if needed; secure airway, remove w/
> laryngoscope

Prolonged oral intubation – can lead to **subglottic stenosis**
> **Tx:** tracheal resection and reconstruction *(best Tx)*; can dilate temporarily

Tracheostomy – consider if pt requires intubation for > 7–14 days
> Benefits – ↓ secretions, easier ventilation, ↓ PNA risk

Median rhomboid glossitis – failure of fusion of the tongue. Tx: none required

Cleft lip (primary palate)
> **Highest prevalence** – Native Americans
> Failure of fusion of **maxillary** and **medial nasal processes**
> Involves lip, alveolus, or both structures
> May have poor feeding
> Repair at **10 weeks of age, 10 pounds,** and a **Hgb 10**
> Tx: **Millard procedure** (Z plasty); repair nasal deformities at same time

Cleft palate (secondary palate)
> The two plates of hard palate are not completely joined; also involves soft
> palate
> **Hole in roof of mouth** connects directly w/ **nasal cavity**
> Can affect **speech** and **swallowing** if not closed soon enough; can affect
> **maxillofacial growth** if closed too early → **repair at 12 months**
> **Palatal obturator** used to temporarily close hole before surgery
> **Latham appliance** – placed w/ pins and is gradually tightened w/ time to
> help bring plates together
> 80% require ≥ 2 surgeries

Hemangioma – MC benign head and neck tumor in adults
> **MC tumor overall of childhood**

Mastoiditis
> Infection of the mastoid cells; can destroy bone; rare
> From **untreated acute supportive otitis media**
> **MC organism** – strep pneumoniae
> Ear is pushed forward
> Tx: **abx's initially**, if condition does not improve quickly w/ abx's, may need
> **myringotomy** (small incision in tympanic membrane) or insertion of a
> **tympanostomy tube** to drain pus from middle ear;
> possible emergency mastoidectomy if above fails

Epiglottitis
> Rare since immunization started against *H. influenzae* type B
> Mostly children ages 3–5
> **Sx's: stridor**, drooling, leaning forward position, fever, throat pain
> Can cause airway obstruction
> **Dx:** lateral neck x-ray - thumbprint
> **Tx:** early control of the airway; abx's

ADRENAL GLAND

Blood supply
Superior adrenal artery – off inferior phrenic artery
Middle adrenal artery – off aorta
Inferior adrenal artery – off renal artery
Left adrenal vein – goes to **left renal vein**
Right adrenal vein – goes to IVC

Adrenal Cortex
Perimeter of adrenal gland
Derived from **mesoderm** (Zones, GFR = salt, sugar, sex steroids)
    Glomerulosa – aldosterone
    Fasciculata – glucocorticoids
    Reticularis – androgens + estrogens (minor role usually)
    All zones have 21- and 11- beta hydroxylase
Steroid hormone production pathway:
    Cholesterol → progesterone → androgens / cortisol / aldosterone

Adrenal Cortex – <u>NO</u> innervation
Adrenal Medulla – innervation from splanchnic nerve
Lymphatics – drain to subdiaphragmatic and renal lymph nodes
Renin-Angiotensin System (see Critical Care chp)
Hypothalamic-pituitary-adrenal axis
    Hypothalamus releases **CRH** (corticotrophin releasing hormone), which
        goes to anterior pituitary gland
    Anterior pituitary gland then releases **ACTH**, which goes to adrenal
        cortex
    Adrenal cortex then releases **cortisol**
        Diurnal (high am, low pm) peak at 4-6 a.m; also ↑ed w/ **stress**
        Cortisol effects – amino acid breakdown, lipolysis, gluconeogenesis,
            increased blood glucose levels (partially from insulin
            resistance); inotropic effect on heart
Adrenal production of estrogen and androgens has a **minor role** *except* in **post-menopausal women**
Excess **estrogens** or **androgens** from adrenals → almost always CA (unless
    congenital)

Adrenal Medulla
Center of adrenal gland
Derived from **neural crest cells** (ectoderm)
Produces catecholamines (pathway):
    tyrosine → dopa → dopamine → norepinephrine → epinephrine

Tyrosine hydroxylase
    Rate-limiting step for above pathway (converts tyrosine to dopa)
Phenylethanolamine N-methyltransferase (PNMT)
    Enzyme that converts norepinephrine → epinephrine (requires methylation)
    Enzyme *only* found in **adrenal medulla** (exclusive producer of
        endogenous epinephrine)
    Only adrenal pheochromocytomas produce epinephrine
Monoamine oxidase (MAO)
    Converts norepinephrine to normetanephrine
    Converts epinephrine to metanephrine
    Vanillyl mandelic acid (VMA) produced from normetanephrine and
        metanephrine
MC extra-adrenal site of neural crest tissue – organ of Zuckerkandl (aortic
    bifurcation); can also be retroperitoneal

After bilateral adrenalectomy → need glucocorticoids and mineralocorticoids
    1) prevents **Addison's Disease** (adrenal insufficiency)
    2) prevents **Nelson's Syndrome** (pituitary enlargement compresses optic nerve)
        From chronic CRH stimulation of pituitary adenoma (see neurosurgery chp)

<u>Congenital adrenal hyperplasia</u> (CAH; Adrenogenital Syndrome)
>Enzyme defects involving cortisol synthesis
>**21-hydroxylase deficiency**
>>**MCC of CAH** (95%; autosomal recessive)
>>**MCC of ambiguous genitalia** (prenatal virilization of genetic female, XX)
>>↑ 17-OH progesterone leads to ↑ **testosterone**
>>**Sx's** (mild to severe):
>>>1) *Hypotension (salt wasting crisis*; 2nd to 3rd week of life)
>>>>↓ Na^+, ↑ K^+, cortisol insufficiency, and **shock**
>>>2) **Virilization** in females + **Precocious puberty** in males
>>**Tx:**
>>>**Salt wasting crisis**
>>>>**Normal saline bolus** (20 cc/kg bolus x 2)
>>>>**Hydrocortisone**
>>>>**Glucose** (D10 NS)
>>>**Long term Tx**: hydrocortisone, fludrocortisone, and possible
>>>>genitoplasty for females
>**11-hydroxylase deficiency**
>>↑ 11-deoxycortisone and ↑ testosterone
>>**Sx's:**
>>>1) *Hypertension* – is salt saving (deoxycortisone acts as a
>>>>mineralocorticoid)
>>>2) **Virilization** in females + **Precocious puberty** in males
>>**Tx:** hydrocortisone, possible genitoplasty for females, <u>NO</u> fludrocortisone
>**17-hydroxylase deficiency**
>>Increased progesterone and pregnenolone
>>**Sx's:**
>>>1) *Hypertension* – salt saving
>>>2) **Ambiguous genitalia in <u>males</u>** at birth
>>>>**Females miss puberty** – Tx: estrogen to induce puberty
>>**Tx:** hydrocortisone, possible genitoplasty for males, <u>NO</u> fludrocortisone

<u>Malignant HTN on office visit</u> (> 220/100)
>**Acute Tx:** Hydralazine and/or Prazosin
>Admit the pt until this is under control (safest answer) and for HTN W/U
>Risk of hemorrhagic stroke w/ BP this high
>**DDx**:
>>Pheochromocytoma
>>Cushing's syndrome
>>Aldosteronoma
>>Renal artery stenosis
>>Coarctation

>**Dx**
>>Check renal function (BUN and Cr)
>>**24 hour urine**
>>>Epi, NE, VMA, metanephrines and nor-metanephrines
>>>>(pheochromocytoma)
>>>Cortisol levels after overnight dexamethasone suppression test
>>>>(Cushing's Syndrome)
>>**Serum levels**
>>>Metanephrines and nor-metanephrines (pheochromocytoma)
>>>Serum cortisol levels (Cushing's Syndrome)
>>>Aldosterone, renin, K^+ and Na^+ (K^+ < 3 → very likely aldosteronoma)
>>**Renal** and **carotid U/S** (can check for murmurs 1st)
>>**Chest/Abd/Pelvic CT scan**
>>>Look for **aortic coarctation** (bilateral arm BP's)
>>>Look for **CA** (eg small cell lung CA releasing ACTH)

<u>Asymptomatic adrenal mass</u> (incidentaloma, > 1 cm)
>   1% of abd CT scans show incidentalomas in adrenal gland (↑ w/ age)
>   **MC benign cause** – non-functional adrenal adenomas
>   **MC malignant cause** – met from separate primary (MC lung CA)
>>   Adrenals common site for **mets** – ask about previous CA, weight loss
>>   **Common mets to adrenal** – lung (MC), breast, melanoma, renal CA
>   **DDx:**
>>   Pheochromocytoma (see below)
>>>   **24 hour urine** - Epi, NE, VMA, metanephrines nor-metanephrines
>>>   **Serum** - Metanephrines and nor-metanephrines
>>   **Cushing's Syndrome** (see below)
>>>   Serum cortisol and ACTH levels
>>>   **Urine cortisol** after overnight dexamethasone suppression test
>>   Aldosteronoma (see below)
>>>   Serum aldosterone, renin, K and Na (HTN w/ K < 3 → likely
>>>   aldosteronoma)
>>   **Need to R/O mets from separate primary** (MC malignant adrenal tumor):
>>>   **Chest/Abd/Pelvic CT scan or MRI** – Bx suspicious lesions
>>>   Make sure pt has had **breast CA** (ie mammogram + breast exam)
>>>   and **colon CA** screenings (ie FOBT, colonoscopy)
>>>   Check for **skin lesions** (melanoma)
>>   **Adrenocortical CA** – look at CT and MRI characteristics
>>>   **50% are functional** (cortisol, aldosterone, sex steroids → virilization,
>>>   feminization)
>   **Dx: chest/abd/pelvic CT scan or MRI** (T2 images); above studies
>>   **Hypodense** (< 10 hounsfield units, lipid based) and **well circumscribed** →
>>   more likely benign
>   *FNA* **indicated for:**
>>   1) **CT > 10 hounsfield units** or **CT contrast washout < 50%** at 10 min
>>   2) **Previous CA** or if you think it is **a met from a separate primary**
>>   3) **Young age** (*less likely* benign adrenal adenoma)
>   *Surgery* **indicated for:**
>>   1) **≥ 5 cm**
>>   2) **Ominous characteristics** (complex, hemorrhagic areas, irregular
>>   margins, heterogeneous, dense, vascular appearance)
>>   3) **Functional tumor**
>>   4) **Is enlarging**
>>   5) **Significant FNA finding** (eg adrenocortical CA)
>>   <u>Anterior approach</u> for adrenal CA resection
>   **If going to follow** – repeat Abd CT every 3 months for 1 year, then yearly
>   **Adrenal cysts** → aspirate
>>   **Clear fluid** → follow, resection if it recurs
>>   **Bloody fluid** → resection
>   **Angiomyolipomas** (on Bx) – benign, leave

<u>Hypercortisolism</u> (Cushing's Syndrome)
>   MC **iatrogenic**
>   **Sx's:** abdominal striae, moon face, obesity, buffalo hump, depression, insomnia,
>   acne, weakness, hyperglycemia, diastolic HTN
>   **Dx:**
>>   **1st: 24-hour urine free cortisol** (*most sensitive test*) + **serum ACTH**
>>>   If ACTH is low (and cortisol high) → have a cortisol secreting lesion
>>>   (**adrenal hyperplasia** or **adrenal adenoma** → get abd CT)
>>>   If ACTH is high (and cortisol high) → have either a **pituitary**
>>>   **adenoma** or **ectopic source** (need to go to 2nd below)
>>   **2nd: If ACTH is high**→ give high dose **dexamethasone suppression test**
>>>   (will suppress pituitary adenomas) and **measure urine cortisol:**
>>>   If urine cortisol suppressed → **pituitary adenoma**
>>>   If urine cortisol not suppressed → **ectopic** producer (lung CA, etc)
>>   **Abd CT** and **MRI** useful for localizing adrenal tumors and differentiating
>>   adenoma vs. hyperplasia

NP-59 scintigraphy (iodo-cholesterol) taken up by **adrenal adenomas**
    (helps DDx hyperplasia vs. adenoma; _not_ taken up by adrenal CA)
If ectopic source suspected → chest/abd/pelvic CT scan
If pituitary source suspected → brain MRI

Pituitary adenoma (Cushing's Disease)
    MCC non-iatrogenic Cushing's Syndrome (70% of cases)
    High ACTH
    Cortisol suppressed with high-dose dexamethasone suppression test
    MRI and **petrosal sampling** to localize → mostly **micro-adenomas**
    Tx:
        Most tumors removed **trans-sphenoidal**
        Unresectable or residual tumor tx'd w/ XRT
        Possible bilateral adrenalectomy (medical w/ **mitotane** or surgical) for
            pituitary adenoma that can't be found
        Need glucocorticoids for up to 3 years after trans-sphenoid surgery
        Lifelong glucocorticoid + mineralocorticoid Tx for bilateral
            adrenalectomy

Ectopic ACTH
    #2 non-iatrogenic cause of Cushing's syndrome (15%)
    MC source of extra-pituitary ACTH – small cell lung CA
    High ACTH
    Cortisol _not_ suppressed with high-dose dexamethasone suppression test
    Chest/Abd/Pelvic CT or MRI can help localize
    Somatostatin scan can help to localize
    Tx: rsxn of primary if possible
    Medical suppression or bilateral adrenalectomy for in-operable lesions
        (would need to be a slow growing tumor to justify operating on pt)

Adrenal adenoma
    #3 non-iatrogenic cause of Cushing's syndrome (10%)
    Low ACTH
    Abd CT or MRI to localize (**NP-59 scintigraphy** if that fails)
    Tx: adrenalectomy

Diffuse adrenal hyperplasia
    Low ACTH
    Tx: medical Tx (see below); **bilateral adrenalectomy if that fails**

Adrenocortical Carcinoma
    Rare cause of Cushing's syndrome; usually advanced
    Bimodal distribution (before age 5 and in 5th decade)
    50% are functioning tumors (cortisol, aldosterone, sex steroids)
    80% advanced at time of Dx
    Sx's:
        Children display **virilization in 90%** (precocious puberty in males,
            virilization in females)
        Feminization in men; **masculinization** in women may occur
        HTN, abd pain, weight loss, weakness
    Tx:
        Radical adrenalectomy (take the kidney)
        Debulking can help pts and prolong survival
        Mitotane post-op ↑s disease-free interval
    5-YS – 20%

Medical Tx (for diffuse adrenal hyperplasia, unresectable ectopic ACTH
    production or adrenocortical CA w/ mets or if unresectable):
    1) **Metyrapone** (inhibits steroid formation)
    2) **Aminoglutethimide** (inhibits cholesterol conversion)
    3) **Ketoconazole** (inhibits steroid formation)
    4) **Mitotane** (Op-DDD) – adrenal-lytic, used for **adrenocortical CA**

Indications for Bilateral adrenalectomy
    Ectopic ACTH from tumor that is unresectable (rare, must be slow growing)
    Pituitary adenoma that can't be found (unusual)
    Bilateral adrenal hyperplasia (try medical Tx 1st)

Give glucocorticoids (+ mineralocorticoid if bilateral) after adrenalectomy

Pheochromocytoma

Chromaffin cells, usually slow growing, from **sympathetic ganglia or ectopic neural crest cells**

MC location – adrenal gland (**MC right side**; adrenal medulla)

10% rule – malignant, bilateral, in children, familial, extra-adrenal, MEN

Extra-adrenal tumors more likely **malignant** (25%)

Only adrenal pheochromocytomas produce **epinephrine** from NE (have **PNMT enzyme**)

Genetic Syndromes w/ pheochromocytoma – MEN 2A/B, von Hippel-Landau syndrome, Neurofibromatosis type 1, familial paraganglioma, tuberous sclerosis, Sturge-Weber disease

Sx's: HTN (often episodic, eg weight-lifting), HA, diaphoresis, palpitations, hyperglycemia

Dx:

> **24 hour urine** (*best test for Dx*, highest specificity, 98%) – Epi, NE, VMA, metanephrines and nor-metanephrines (**VMA most specific**)
>
> **Serum** – VMA, metanephrines, nor-metanephrines
>
> **Clonidine suppression test** – tumor will not respond, keeps catecholamines high
>
> **CT scan** (or MRI) can help localize tumors
>
> **MIBG scan** (*best test for localizing tumor*)
>> 131-meta-iodobenzylguanidine (MIBG; norepinephrine analogue)
>> Can help locate if not on CT scan
>
> <u>No</u> **venography** → will cause hypertensive crisis
>
> **Not able to localize** (rare) → still proceed w/ exploratory laparotomy

Preop

> **Alpha-blocker first**
>> **Phenoxybenzamine** (ramp up) or **prazosin** (ramp up)
>>> *Avoid* hypertensive crisis by starting the alpha-blocker 1st
>>
>> Start **2 weeks before surgery**, ↑ dose until slight orthostatic hypotension
>>
>> **Give volume replacement** during this time (have them fill a milk jug w/ urine QD – should **gain weight** during this time period)
>
> **Beta-blocker** if pt has tachycardia or arrhythmias while on alpha blocker (consider combined beta/alpha agent such as **labetalol**)
>
> *Careful* w/ beta-blocker and give after alpha blocker → avoids
>> **hypertensive crisis** (unopposed alpha stimulation→CHF, MI, stroke)

Tx:

> **Resection** (trans-abdominal approach if malignant)
>
> Have **nipride, esmolol, dopamine,** and **phenylephrine** at time of surgery
>
> **Ligate adrenal vein 1**[st] to avoid spilling catecholamines w/ manipulation
>
> **Debulking** helps sx's w/ unresectable DZ
>
> **Other sites of pheochromocytomas:**
>> Proximal to **aortic bifurcation** (**MC ectopic location**) – organ of Zuckerkandl
>>
>> Vertebral bodies
>>
>> Sympathetic chain ganglia (paravertebral)
>>
>> Opposite adrenal gland
>>
>> Bladder
>
> **Hypertension during removal** → esmolol, nipride
>
> **Persistent hypertension after removal**
>> Check for other sites of pheochromocytoma as above
>>
>> Check the contra-lateral adrenal (10% bilateral)
>
> **Hypotension after removal** – volume 1st , phenylephrine
>
> **Bronchospasm after removal** – albuterol, epinephrine
>
> **Metyrosine** – inhibits **tyrosine hydroxylase**, resulting in ↓ed synthesis of catecholamines (used for mets or pre-op prep)

False positive VMA – caffeine, fruits, vanilla, iodine, alpha- and beta-blockers

MC site of extra-medullary tissue - organ of Zuckerkandl (above aortic bifurcation)

Extra-medullary tissue – can cause **medullary CA of thyroid** and **extra-adrenal pheochromocytoma**

Hyperaldosteronism

Primary Disease (↓ renin and ↑ aldosterone; **Conn's Syndrome**)
    Adenoma (80%, **MCC primary hyperaldosteronism**)
    Adrenal hyperplasia (20%)
    Adrenocortical CA (<1%)
    Ovarian Tumors (< 1%)
    <u>Cushing's syndrome</u> can mimic hyperaldosteronism

Secondary Disease (↑ renin and ↑ aldosterone)
    More common than primary DZ
    1) **Primary reninism** – renin secreting tumor (Bartter's Syndrome)
    2) **Secondary reninism** – many causes; renal artery stenosis, CHF
        cirrhosis, nephrotic syndrome, liver failure, pregnancy, diuretics –
        need to tx underlying cause

Sx's (primary hyperaldosteronism):
    HTN from sodium retention <u>*without*</u> **edema**
    Hypokalemia, polydipsia, polyuria, weakness
    Need to check for hyperaldosteronism w/ **HTN** + (**↓K^+, adrenal mass,** or
        refractory to medical Tx)

Dx of primary hyperaldosteronism:
    Serum [usual findings, but not diagnostic; need both 1) + 2) below for Dx]:
        ↓renin and **↑aldosterone**
        ↓K^+ (usually < 3) and **↑Na^+**; **metabolic alkalosis**
        Urine: **↑K^+, ↓Na^+**
    1) **Plasma Aldosterone to renin ratio > 20** (w/ aldosterone level > 15-20,
        done in a.m.; then get salt suppression test below)
    2) **Salt Suppression test**
        24-hour urine aldosterone level obtained after 3 days of salt loading
        Need to be normokalemic at time of test
        Urine aldosterone > 14 mcg (w/ 24-h urine sodium >200 mEq) →
            primary hyperaldosteronism
        Alpha-blockers do not interfere w/ testing (eg doxazosin) and should
            be used for hypertension while testing (all other BP meds
            including beta-blockers can interfere w/ test)

Localizing studies (DDx - adenoma vs hyperplasia):
    Abd CT or MRI
    Selective adrenal venous sampling for aldosterone (if trouble localizing)

Tx:
    Adenoma (or <u>rare</u> single side hyperplasia) - adrenalectomy
    Diffuse hyperplasia
        Medical Tx
            Spironolactone, calcium channel blockers, eplerenone
                (aldosterone antagonist), other anti-HTN agents
            Potassium
        Bilateral adrenalectomy if above fails:
            MC indication – refractory hypokalemia
            Will need **fludrocortisone** and **hydrocortisone** post-op

Hypoaldosteronism
Etiologies
MCC – renal dysfunction from diabetic nephropathy ($\downarrow$ed renin, see below)

1) **Hypo-reninemic hypoaldosteronism** (ie Type IV renal tubular acidosis)
From **renal dysfunction** (MC; **diabetic nephropathy** MC subtype)
Many others contribute – HIV, ACE inhibitors, NSAIDs, CSA, etc

2) **Primary aldosterone deficiency** (*rare; $\uparrow$ renin*) – primary adrenal insufficiency, congenital adrenal hyperplasia (CAH), aldosterone synthase deficiency

3) **Aldosterone resistance** – Drugs (eg spironolactone, amiloride)

Sx's:
1) **Hypo-reninemic hypoaldosteronism** – *hallmark of disease is hyperkalemia,* also **hypertension + edema** (eg diabetic nephropathy)

2) **Primary aldosterone Deficiency** – **hyperkalemia**
Can get *hypotension* from salt wasting

3) **Aldosterone resistance** – **hyperkalemia**
Hypotension from volume loss possible

All of the above may have metabolic acidosis

Tx:
1) **Hypo-reninemic hypoaldosteronism** – fludrocortisone, control HTN, lasix for edema and hyperkalemia

2) **Primary aldosterone deficiency** – fludrocortisone, hydrocortisone if adrenal insufficiency, volume if salt wasting (CAH)

3) **Aldosterone resistance** – stop diuretic

Hypocortisolism (adrenal insufficiency, Addison's disease)
1) **Acute Adrenal Insufficiency** (Addisonian Crisis, adrenal crisis)
Sx's: fever, N/V, abd pain + hypotension (unresponsive to fluids / pressors)
Confusion, hypoglycemia, N/V, diarrhea

Causes
Withdrawal of exogenous steroids (MCC overall, acute and chronic)
Bilateral adrenal hemorrhage (rare; MCC - sepsis, ie Waterhouse-Friedrichsen syndrome)
Adrenalectomy
Severe stress (trauma, sepsis)
(see Critical Care chp for acute Dx and Tx)

2) **Chronic Adrenal Insufficiency** (Addison's disease)
Sx's: weakness, weight loss, abd complaints
Hyperpigmentation from MSH (melanocyte stimulating hormone, breakdown product of ACTH)
MC primary adrenal disease – autoimmune DZ
Other causes – TB, fungal, adrenal mets, pituitary disease
Dx (chronic): $\uparrow$ **ACTH, $\downarrow$ cortisol** and $\downarrow$ **aldosterone**
$\uparrow$K$^+$, $\downarrow$Na$^+$, $\downarrow$glucose

Tx:
Fluids (if acute), **hydrocortisone** and **fludrocortisone**
If testing for adrenal insufficiency, use **dexamethasone** instead and perform **ACTH stimulation test** (measure serum cortisol)

Waterhouse-Friedrichsen syndrome
MC organism – N. meningitides (others – strep, staph)
Overwhelming bacterial sepsis, shock, DIC, widespread purpura, and rapidly developing adrenal insufficiency from bilateral **adrenal gland hemorrhage**
Tx: abx's, cortisol

Von Hippel-Lindau Disease (VHL tumor supressor)
Hemangioblastomas in cerebellum, spinal cord and retina
Renal angioma and **renal cell carcinoma**
Pheochromocytoma

Carney complex (PR-KAR tumor suppressor)
Myxomas of heart and skin + skin hyperpigmentation (lentiginosis)
Endocrine over-activity (eg Cushing's Syndrome)

PITUITARY GLAND

Hypothalamus
> Releases **TRH, CRH, GnRH, GHRH,** and **dopamine** into median eminence
> Hormones then pass through the posterior pituitary (neurohypophysis) on
> > their way to the anterior pituitary (adenohypophysis)
> **Dopamine** – inhibits prolactin secretion (constitutive inhibitor)

Posterior pituitary (neurohypophysis)
> Consists of axons extending from **supraoptic** and **paraventricular nuclei**
> > of hypothalamus into the posterior pituitary gland
> **Secrete 2 hormones** into capillaries of the hypophyseal circulation:
> > 1) **ADH** (ie vasopressin)
> > > Release controlled by **supraoptic nuclei** mostly
> > > Regulated by **osmolar receptors** in hypothalamus
> > > > Released in response to **high plasma osmolarity**
> > > Causes increased **water absorption in collecting ducts**
> > 2) **Oxytocin** – release controlled by **paraventricular nuclei** mostly
> Posterior pituitary does <u>NOT</u> contain cell bodies

Diabetes insipidus ($\downarrow$ ADH)
> **Sx's:** N/V, diarrhea, dehydration
> **Dx:** $\uparrow$ UOP, $\downarrow$ urine specific gravity, $\uparrow$ serum Na^+ and osmolality
> Can occur w/ ETOH, head injury
> **Tx:** DDAVP, free water (correct Na^+ slowly to avoid brain swelling)

SIADH ($\uparrow$ ADH; syndrome of inappropriate anti-diuretic hormone)
> **Sx's**: N/V, delirium, seizures, coma; no edema despite fluid overload
> **Dx:** $\downarrow$ UOP, concentrated urine, $\downarrow$ serum Na^+ and osmolality
> Can occur w/ head injury
> **Tx:**
> > **Water restriction** (1st line), *then* **diuresis,** *then* **hypertonic
> > saline**
> > Correct Na^+ slowly to avoid **central pontine myelinosis**
> > ****If symptomatic,** skip diuresis and give **hypertonic saline**

> > **Conivaptan** - inhibitor of ADH (vasopressin)
> > > Blocks V1 and V2 receptors
> > > Result in removal of water *without* electrolyte loss (**aguaresis**)
> > > Used for chronic SIADH
> > **Demeclocycline** - inhibitor of ADH on collecting duct
> > > Used for chronic SIADH

Anterior pituitary (80% of gland, adenohypophysis)
> **ACTH, TSH, GH, LH, FSH,** and **prolactin** released
> *NO direct blood supply*; has **portal system** w/ blood passing through
> > neurohypophysis 1st

Bitemporal hemianopia (visual problems w/ pituitary mass) – from a pituitary
> mass compressing optic nerve (CN II) at the chiasm
Nonfunctional Pituitary Tumors – MC macro-adenomas (almost always)
> **Sx's:** mass effect and decreased ACTH, TSH, GH, LH, FSH
> **Tx:** trans-sphenoid resection
Contraindications to **trans-sphenoid resection of tumors** – supra-cellar
> (dumbbell-shaped tumor) extension, massive lateral extension
Bromocriptine – can be used reduce all endocrine secreting pituitary tumors
> *except* ACTH secreting
Pituitary gland found in **sella turcica**

Pituitary tumors
Prolactinoma
MC pituitary tumor
MC *micro*-adenomas
Sx's: amenorrhea, galactorrhea, infertility, poor libido, visual problems
Dx: ↑ **prolactin** (> 150 usual)
    MRI and visual field testing if MRI shows tumor
Tx:
    Most prolactinomas do __NOT__ need surgery
    1) **Asymptomatic** and **microadenoma** (≤ 10 mm) – follow w/ MRI
    2) **Symptomatic** or **macroadenoma** (> 10 mm):
        Bromocriptine (dopa agonist) – 85% successful (safe w/ pregnancy)
        Trans-sphenoid surgery (for failed medical tx, hemorrhage, visual loss, wants pregnancy, CSF leak) – 85% successful (15% recurrence)
    XRT if above not successful

Acromegaly (excessive growth hormone)
Growth hormone stimulates secretion of **insulin-like growth factor-1**
MC *macro*-adenomas
Higher remission rate for micro-adenomas
Sx's: jaw enlargement, HA, ↑ soft tissue, HTN, macroglossia, amenorrhea, DM, giganticism; visual problems related to size
    Can be **life-threatening** from **cardiac issues** (valve dysfunction, cardiomyopathy)
Dx:
    ↑ **IGF-1 level** (random growth hormone level __not__ useful)
    Oral glucose tolerance test (growth hormone not suppressed to < 2 ng/ml by 2 hours)
    MRI to look for tumor
Tx:
    Surgery 1st choice if not invading surrounding tissues (→ trans-sphenoid resection)
    Octreotide and **bromocriptine** can shrink tumor and relieve sx's (used pre-op to shrink tumor, for refractory DZ after surgery, or unresectable macro-adenoma – both drugs ↓ GH production)
    Pegvisomant (GH receptor antagonist)
    XRT
    Without tx – 3 x mortality risk, pituitary insufficiency, and colon CA

Other conditions
Sheehan's syndrome
Pituitary insufficiency in mother after childbirth
From hypovolemia or shock following childbirth causing pituitary ischemia
1st sign – postpartum **trouble lactating;** can also have amenorrhea, adrenal insufficiency, hypothyroidism
Affects anterior pituitary (portal venous blood supply), posterior pituitary usually not affected (direct arterial blood supply)
Craniopharyngioma
Benign
MC children aged 5-10 years
Calcified cyst near anterior pituitary, remnants of Rathke's pouch
Sx's: headaches, growth failure, bi-temporal hemianopia, endocrine abnormalities, hydrocephalus
Tx: surgery, XRT; **Diabetes insipidus** – frequent cx postop
Bilateral pituitary masses – if non-endocrine producing → probably metastases
Nelson's syndrome
After **bilateral adrenalectomy**, ↑ CRH causes **pituitary enlargement** (usually have pre-existing pituitary adenoma)
Sx's: amenorrhea, bi-temporal hemianopia, hyperpigmentation from **MSH** (melanocyte-stimulating hormone, peptide byproduct of ACTH), and muscle weakness; Tx: prevent w/ prednisone long term

THYROID

Thyroid Anatomy and Function
General
Derived from the 1st and 2nd pharyngeal pouches

Ligament of Berry – posterior medial suspensory ligament
Very close to RLNs; need careful dissection

Tubercles of Zuckerkandl – most lateral, posterior extension of thyroid
These are rotated medially in order to find RLNs
Are left behind w/ **subtotal thyroidectomy** due to proximity of RLN's

Post-thyroidectomy stridor due to hematoma – open neck and remove hematoma *emergently* → can result in airway compromise

Thyroidectomy indications: 1) CA, 2) large glands w/ compressive Sx's: 3) cold nodules; 4) toxic multinodular, toxic adenomas or Grave's not responsive to medical Tx, 4) pregnant pts not controlled medical Tx

Subtotal thyroidectomy – can leave pt euthyroid

Vascular supply
Superior thyroid artery – 1st branch off external carotid artery
At superior pole of thyroid

Inferior thyroid artery – off thyrocervical trunk (inferior)
Supplies **both inferior and superior parathyroids**
W/ thyroidectomy, need ligation of inferior thyroid arteries close to thyroid gland to avoid injury to parathyroid glands

Ima artery (1%), from innominate or aorta; goes to isthmus

Superior and **middle thyroid veins** – internal jugular vein drainage

Inferior thyroid vein – innominate vein drainage

Nerves
Recurrent laryngeal nerves (RLNs)
Motor to entire larynx <u>*except*</u> cricothyroid muscle (superior laryngeal nerve); injury *intra-op* should undergo immediate repair

In **tracheoesophageal groove** (posterior to thyroid)

Can track w/ inferior thyroid artery

Left RLN – loops around aorta

Right RLN – loops around right subclavian (or innominate) artery

1) **Unilateral injury** – **hoarseness** (if vocal cord abducts, ie paramedian location) **or nothing** (if vocal cord adducts, ie median location);
Hoarse – may get better (wait 6 mos.), **medialize vocal cord** w/ silicone wedge or injection if persistent sx's *(<u>not</u> reop repair of nerve)*
Asymptomatic – leave alone

2) **Bilateral injury**
Can **obstruct airway acutely** (vocal cords adducted, Sx's-severe stridor) → need *emergency* **tracheostomy**
Can't intubate due to cords blocking airway
Can **cause profound aspiration** (vocal cords abducted) → will need **tracheostomy**

Right RLN can run a little more **lateral** (and thus more vulnerable to injury) – why surgeries like cricopharyngomyotomy for Zenker's is performed on left

Non-recurrent laryngeal nerve (1%)
MC side – right (associated w/ aberrant right subclavian artery off the descending thoracic aorta)
Risk of non-recurrent laryngeal nerve injury during thyroid surgery

Superior laryngeal nerve (external branch)
External branch – motor to **cricothyroid muscle**
Runs superior and lateral to thyroid lobes
Can track w/ **superior thyroid artery** at upper pole of thyroid
Injury causes in **loss of projection** (or pitch) and **easy voice fatigability** (eg opera singers)
Ligating the superior thyroid artery branches at the level of the thyroid capsule may help avoid this injury

Function

Hypothalamus – releases **thyrotropin-releasing factor** (TRF) → goes to anterior pituitary gland

Anterior pituitary gland – releases **thyroid-stimulating hormone** (TSH) → goes to thyroid gland

Thyroid Gland – releases T4 and T3 (mechanism involves ↑ cAMP)

T4 and **T3** then bind the **thyroid hormone receptor** in the **nucleus**

Thyroid Hormone Function - ↑ cardiac output, HR, RR, basal metabolic rate and potentates effects of catecholamines
Although not involved in flight or fight response

TRF and **TSH** release controlled by T4 and T3 negative feedback loop

Only **free T4** and **T3** are active (protein bound not active) –
Free hormone represents < 1% of total serum T4 and T3

T4:T3 serum ratio is **20:1**

Most T3 produced in **periphery** from T4 to T3 conversion (**deiodinases**)

**T3 is the more active form (4x more potent than T4)

Thyroglobulin – stores T4 and T3 in **colloid**

Peroxidases links tyrosine and iodine

Forms mono-iodotyrosine (MIT) and di-iodotyrosine (DIT)

MIT + DIT → triiodothyronine (T3)

DIT + DIT → thyroxine (T4)

Deiodinases – separate iodine ions (eg T4 to T3 conversion)

Serum thyroid hormone binding proteins (all bind T4 and T3):

1) **Thyroxin-binding globulin** (TBG) – carries majority of T4 and T3

2) **Transthyretin** (pre-albumin)

3) **Albumin**

Tests of thyroid function

TSH – is the most sensitive indicator of gland function

T4 and **T3 levels**

Resin T3 uptake – measures free T3 by having it bind resin

↑ resin uptake → hyperthyroidism or ↓ TBG

↓ uptake → hypothyroidism or ↑ TBG

Thyroxine treatment – TSH levels should fall to 50%

S/Es – osteoporosis long-term

Abnormalities in thyroid descent

Pyramidal lobe (10%) – extends from isthmus toward the thymus

Lingual thyroid

Thyroid tissue that persists in area of foramen cecum at **base of tongue**

The only thyroid tissue in 70% of pts who have it

1% malignancy risk

Sx's: dysphagia, dyspnea, dysphonia

Tx:

Thyroxine suppression for sx's

Abolish w/ **I-131** or **resection** if it does not shrink after thyroxine

Resection if worried about CA

Thyroglossal duct cyst

From descent of thyroid from **foramen cecum**

Possible that this is only thyroid tissue the pt has

Risk of **infection**; 1% **malignancy** risk

Sx's:

Midline cervical mass, MC between hyoid and thyroid isthmus

Classically moves upward with swallowing

May cause dysphagia, susceptible to infection

Tx: excision of entire **cyst, tract,** and **hyoid bone** (midportion) through lateral neck incision (Sistrunk procedure)

Thyroid Nodule w/u

Check for **attachment to trachea** and for **cervical adenopathy**
MC in females

1) Get **FNA** *(best initial Dx test)* and **U/S**
2) **TFTs** (T3, T4, TSH), **PTH , Ca**, and **Calcitonin**
3) **If T3/T4 elevated** and **FNA shows thyroid tissue** - likely a toxic nodule
   Tx: see hyperthyroidism section below
4) **If T3/T4 are not elevated** and **FNA + U/S are →**

     a.   **Determinant** (85%) → follow appropriate tx below
   Shows **just follicular cells** (5% malignant) → lobectomy, **send FS**
   and **permanent**, follow appropriate tx if CA
   Shows **thyroid CA** → lobectomy (possible total thyroidectomy).
   Follow tx for CA
   Shows **simple cyst** → drain fluid and send for cytology
      If recurs → lobectomy, send FS and permanent, follow
      appropriate tx if CA
   Shows **complex cyst** → lobectomy, **send FS** and **permanent**, follow
   appropriate Tx:
      papillary thyroid CA can present as complex cyst
   Shows **colloid tissue** (repeat x 3 to be sure)→ most likely **colloid
   goiter**
   Low chance of malignancy (< 1%)
   Follow lesion serially, lobectomy if it grows
   Tx for toxic multi-nodular goiter if appropriate (see below)

     b.   **Indeterminate** (15%)→ get radionuclide study (technetium 99, 99-Tc)
   Hot nodule → thyroxin for 6 weeks
      This will ↓ TSH and nodule should go away
      If size does not decrease → **lobectomy, send FS,** follow
      appropriate tx if CA
   Cold nodule → lobectomy, send FS and permanent, follow
   appropriate tx if CA

Thyroid Lymphoma
MC Non-Hodgkins lymphoma
Frequently associated w/ Hashimoto's thyroiditis
MC in women
LDH and **beta-2 microglobulin** predict worse prognosis
Tx: chemo ± XRT

Thyroid cancer
MC endocrine malignancy in US – thyroid CA
MC type – papillary thyroid CA (85%)
Sx's: painless mass, voice changes, dysphagia
Follicular cells only on FNA – *cannot* differentiate follicular cell adenoma,
   follicular cell hyperplasia, normal thyroid tissue, and follicular cell CA; 5-
   10% will be malignant
↑ed malignancy risk – solid on U/S, solitary, cold on radionuclide, slow
   growing, hard; males, age > 50, previous neck XRT, MEN IIa/IIb
Previous XRT associated w/ 10% of all thyroid CA (esp. if XRT exposure at age
   < 15)
Sudden growth – likely hemorrhage into undetected nodule or CA
Thyroid adenomas – need to be differentiated from carcinomas → *requires
   lobectomy*
Follicular adenomas – colloid, embryonal, and fetal subtypes; all have no
   increase in CA risk, although **still need lobectomy** to prove it is adenoma

__Papillary thyroid carcinoma__ (MC type-__85%__, psammoma bodies, orphan annie nuclei)
> __MC Thyroid CA__ to present as a __complex cyst__
> __MC Thyroid CA w/ previous XRT__
> Path
>> Least aggressive, slow growing, best prognosis
>> Usually in young women, children
>> __Older age__ has worse prognosis (> 50 years)
>> __Lymphatic spread 1st__ although this is __*not*__ __prognostic__
>>> __Positive nodes – children__ (75%) > adults (15%); large + firm
>> Prognosis based on __local invasion__ (MCC death)
>> Often __multicentric__
> Perform __lobectomy__ initially, send for FS and permanent
> Indications for __total__ thyroidectomy:
>> __Tumor > 1 cm__
>> __Extra-thyroidal DZ__ (capsular invasion, clinical / positive nodal DZ, or mets)
>> __Multicentric or bilateral lesions__
>> __Previous XRT__
> Indications for __MRND:__
>> __Extra-thyroidal DZ__ (capsule invasion, clinical or positive nodal DZ or mets)
> Indications for ^{131}I (6 weeks after surgery):
>> __Tumor > 1cm__
>> __Extra-thyroidal DZ__ (capsule invasion, positive nodal DZ or mets)
> Do not give thyroid replacement until __after__ Tx w/ ^{131}I to avoid suppressing ^{131}I
> uptake (want TSH level 3 x normal before tx w/ ^{131}I)
> __XRT__ only for unresectable DZ not responsive to ^{131}I
> Follow __thyroglobulin level__ post-op for tumor recurrence (if total thyroidectomy)
> ^{123}I can be used to look for recurrence late after total thyroidectomy
> After tx w/ ^{131}I, __give synthroid__ to keep TSH levels low
>> Want TSH $\leq$ 0.03 and pt mildly thyrotoxic
>> This is __very effective__ for metastatic DZ
> Met's go to __Lung__ (__rarely__ occur)
> __Overall 5-year survival__ – 95% (__MCC death__ – local invasion)
> __Enlarged lateral neck lymph node__ w/ normal thyroid tissue = __papillary thyroid
>> CA__ w/ lymphatic spread.
>> Tx: __total thyroidectomy, ipsilateral MRND,__ and ^{131}I

__Follicular thyroid carcinoma__
> More aggressive than papillary
> Older women (> 50); some association w/ __iodine deficiency__
> __Follicular cells on FNA__ – 10% chance of malignancy; need lobectomy
>> → perform __lobectomy__ initially, send for FS and permanent, if path shows
>>> __adenoma or follicular cell hyperplasia__, nothing else needed
> Indications for __total thyroidectomy:__
>> __Tumor > 1 cm__
>> __Extra-thyroidal DZ__ (capsular invasion, clinical/positive nodal DZ, or mets)
>> __Multicentric or bilateral lesions__
>> __Previous XRT__
> Indications for __MRND:__
>> __Extra-thyroidal DZ__ (capsule invasion, clinical or positive nodal DZ or mets)
> Indications for ^{131}I (6 weeks after surgery):
>> __Tumor > 1cm__
>> __Extra-thyroidal DZ__ (capsule invasion, positive nodal DZ or mets)
> Do not give thyroid replacement until __after__ Tx with ^{131}I to avoid suppressing ^{131}I
> uptake (want TSH level 3 x normal before tx w/ ^{131}I)
> __XRT__ only for unresectable DZ not responsive to ^{131}I
> Follow __thyroglobulin level__ post-op for tumor recurrence (if total thyroidectomy)
> ^{123}I can be used to look for recurrence late after total thyroidectomy
> After tx w/ ^{131}I, __give synthroid__ to keep TSH levels low
>> Want TSH $\leq$ 0.03 and pt mildly thyrotoxic
>> This is __very effective__ for metastatic DZ
> Met's go to __Bone__ (hematogenous) → 50% have mets at time of dx
> __Overall 5-year survival__– 70% (prognosis based on hematogenous + LN spread)

RFs for mets or recurrence w/ papillary and follicular thyroid CA (GAMES)

> **Grade** – poorly differentiated
> **Age** < 20 or > 50
> **Metastasis** or **Male gender**
> **Extra-thyroidal disease**
> **Size** > 1 cm

Medullary thyroid carcinoma (MTC)

> Associated with:
>> 1) **MEN IIa** (see MEN section below)
>> 2) **MEN IIb**
>> 3) **Familial MTC only**
>> 4) **Sporadic Form** (non-syndrome associated; accounts for **80% of MTC**)
>
> **Worse prognosis** – MEN IIb and sporadic forms
> Usually is **1st manifestation of MEN IIa** and **MEN IIb** (sx's - diarrhea, flushing)
> **Path**
>> From **parafollicular C cells** which secrete **calcitonin** (diarrhea, flushing)
>> Considered **neural crest cells**
>> **C-cell hyperplasia** considered pre-malignant
>> More aggressive than follicular and papillary CA
>> **Gastrin** test for medullary thyroid CA → causes ↑ed **calcitonin**
>> Screen for **pheochromocytoma** and **hyperparathyroidism** (MEN IIa + IIb)
>> Path shows **amyloid**
>
> **Early spread** – pts who present w/ MTC as **palpable thyroid mass** →
>> 20% already have **distant mets** (liver, lung, or bone)
>> 70% already have **nodal DZ**
>
> **Pre-op w/u**
>> **Neck/Chest/Abd CT scan**
>> **Bone scan**
>> **LFTs**
>> → needed for all pts w/ MTC presenting as a **palpable thyroid mass**
>> **Liver** and **bone mets** prevent attempt at cure
>
> **Tx:**
>> Pts w/ MTC as a **palpable thyroid mass:**
>>> **Total thyroidectomy**
>>> **Central neck node dissection**
>>> **MRND on side of tumor** (bilateral if both lobes have tumor)
>>
>> Pts w/ **Fam Hx** and **RET proto-oncogene** _w/o_ a mass:
>>> **MEN IIa** → prophylactic total thyroidectomy and central LN dissection at age **6 years**
>>> **MEN IIb** → prophylactic total thyroidectomy and central LN dissection at age **2 years**
>>> Not done earlier due to difficulty in finding the recurrent laryngeal nerves in children (too small); high risk of injury (including bilateral injury and need for **permanent tracheostomy**)
>>
>> **XRT** may be useful for unresectable local and distant metastatic disease
> Monitor **calcitonin levels** for disease recurrence
> **5-year survival** for pts who present w/ **palpable thyroid mass**
>> **MEN IIa** – 50% (prognosis based on **distant mets**)
>> **MEN-IIb** – 10%
>
> **Central LN neck dissection** (removing all lymphatic tissue)
>> From internal jugular vein to internal jugular vein
>> Up to hyoid
>> Down to innominate vein (as low as you can go)

Hurthle cell carcinoma
MC benign (80%, adenoma); older patients
Path – Ashkenazi cells; <u>cannot DDx benign vs malignant based on FNA</u>
Need lobectomy to make diagnosis →
> **If benign** – Tx: lobectomy
> **If malignant** – Tx: total thyroidectomy; MRND for clinically positive nodes

Anaplastic thyroid cancer
Elderly pts, long-standing goiters
**Most aggressive thyroid CA – propensity to invade other structures (eg trachea) – rapidly lethal
Path – vesicular appearance of nuclei
Tx:
> Total thyroidectomy for rare resectable lesion (possible tracheal resection)
> Palliative thyroidectomy for compressive symptoms or chemo-XRT
> Rapidly lethal (5-YS - 5%); usually beyond surgical management at time of Dx

XRT and hormonal therapy for various thyroid CA
XRT – effective for papillary, follicular, medullary, and Hurthle cell thyroid CA
^{131}I – effective for papillary and follicular thyroid CA <u>only</u> (<u>not</u> Hurthle, MTC, or anaplastic)
Can cure bone and lung mets
Indications (**6 weeks** after surgery, want **TSH high** for maximal uptake):
> **Tumor > 1 cm**
> **Extra-thyroidal DZ** (capsule invasion, positive nodal DZ or mets)
> **Recurrence**

Pts w/ papillary or follicular cell CA w/ mets → need to perform total thyroidectomy to facilitate uptake of I^{131} to metastatic lesions
S/Es: sialoadenitis, GI symptoms, infertility, parathyroid dysfunction, bone marrow suppression (rare), leukemia (rare)
> ^{131}I should <u>not</u> be used in **children** (CA risk)**, during pregnancy** (cretinism, can traverse placenta) or **lactating mothers** (in milk)

Thyroxine – suppresses TSH and slows metastatic disease
Administered after ^{131}I therapy has finished
Hold for 6 weeks prior to ^{131}I to get TSH high (want maximal uptake)
TSH levels highest 6 weeks after thyroidectomy – good time for ^{131}I Tx
Lymphoma and squamous cell CA – are <u>very</u> rare causes of thyroid CA

Hyperthyroidism
MCC hyperthyroidism – Grave's Disease (80%)
DDx Hyperthyroidism:
> **Grave's Disease** (autoimmune, **IgG** Ab's to TSH receptor)
> > Usually older women
> > **IgG Abs** – long acting thyroid stimulator (LATS) and thyroid stimulating immunoglobulin (TSI)
>
> **Toxic adenoma** (single; usually needs to be 2 cm to cause sx's)
> > Usually young women
>
> **Toxic multinodular goiter**
> **Thyroiditis** (thyrotoxic phase specifically)
> **TSH secreting pituitary tumor** (rare) – TSH will be high and T4 high
> **Struma ovarii** (3% of ovarian dermoid tumors)
> **Amiodarone** (can cause hyper- or hypo-thyroidism)

Sx's: goiter (Grave's and multi-nodular toxic goiter), heat intolerance, thirst, ↑ed appetite, weight loss, sweating, palpitations, atrial fibrillation
> **Sx's only w/ Grave's disease** – exophthalmos and pre-tibial edema
> Sx's can worsen w/ **contrast dyes**

Dx:
> **TFTs** (thyroid function tests)
> > ↑ed T3 and T4
> > ↓ed TSH

Thyroid scan (RAIU, radio-active iodide uptake)

↑ed ^{123}I uptake **homogenously** and **diffusely** – Grave's

↑ed ^{123}I uptake **heterogeneously** and **diffusely** – toxic multinodular goiter

↑ed ^{123}I uptake **localized** – hot nodule

U/S – look for solitary adenoma (hot nodule)

Tx for hyperthyroidism (Grave's, toxic adenoma, or toxic multinodular goiter):

Medical Tx manages hyperthyroidism in **95%** (*unusual* to have to operate)

PTU or **methimazole** (50% recurrence; 0.5% risk of agranulocytosis)

^{131}**I**: 5% recurrence w/ Grave's and toxic adenoma

↑ed recurrence w/ toxic multinodular goiter- due to inhomogenous uptake

Beta-blocker helps w/ sx's

Indications for surgery:

1) **Suspicious nodule** (MC indication for operation)
2) **Failed medical Tx**
3) **Non-compliance**
4) **Children** and **pregnant women w/ refractory hyperthyroidism** (if PTU fails, *cannot use* ^{131}I)
5) **Obstructive Goiter**

Preop preparation

Make sure **euthyroid** before operating

PTU until euthyroid (4 weeks prior to surgery)

Beta-blocker, 2 week prior to surgery or if still having sx's on PTU

Lugol's solution 2 weeks prior to surgery to ↓ friability and vascularity (start after euthyroid)

Surgical options

Subtotal thyroidectomy (5% recurrence; good for multinodular goiters)

Total thyroidectomy with thyroxin replacement

Pregnancy

Tx hyperthyroidism w/ **PTU** until 2nd trimester

If pt still having sx's despite PTU, **add beta-blocker**

Cannot use ^{131}I (will destroy fetal thyroid tissue → cretinism)

If PTU has effectively treated the problem → *no surgery*

If PTU has not effectively treated the problem (ie still requiring beta-blocker to control sx's) →

Operate in 2nd trimester (best time, ↓ risk of teratogenic events and premature labor)

Total thyroidectomy or sub-total thyroidectomy

↑ed still birth if you let hyperthyroidism go into 3rd trimester

Avoid beta-blockers in 3rd trimester (potential for fetal growth retardation)

Children – there is general concern for the development of malignancy in young children treated w/ ^{131}I so it is *not used*

^{131}I should **NOT** be used in **children** (malignancy risk), **during pregnancy** (cretinism, can traverse placenta) or **lactating mothers** (in milk)

Methimazole should NOT be used **during pregnancy** (cretinism)

Exophthalmos can get worse after ^{131}I

Tx: steroids, XRT, or surgical decompression of orbits

PTU (propylthiouracil)

Inhibits peroxidases, which connects iodine to tyrosine to form di-iodo-tyrosine (T4) and mono-iodo-tyrosine (T3) – less T3 and T4 released

Also blocks conversion of T4 to T3 in periphery (also deiodinases)

S/Es – aplastic anemia or **agranulocytosis** (rare)

**Can be used in pregnancy (does not cross the placenta)

Methimazole

Inhibits peroxidases and prevents DIT and MIT coupling

S/Es – cretinism in newborns (crosses placenta)

Aplastic anemia or **agranulocytosis** (rare)

**Do NOT use in pregnancy

Thyroid storm
Sx's: ↑ HR, fever, numbness, irritability, N/V, diarrhea, HTN, diaphoresis
  High output cardiac failure (MCC of death)
MC occurrence – after surgery in pt w/ **undiagnosed Grave's Disease**
  Other precipitants – anxiety, excessive gland palpation, adrenergic agents
ABC's, IV x 2 , fluid resuscitation (normal saline)
Tx:
  Beta-blockers (esmolol drip)
  PTU (propylthiouracil)
  **Lugol's *(best therapy*, potassium iodide, give 1 hr after PTU)
  Cooling blankets
  Oxygen
  Glucose
  Steroids (cortisol 100 mg Q 8)
  Emergent thyroidectomy <u>rarely</u> indicated

Wolff-Chaikoff effect
  High doses of iodine (eg Lugol's solution, potassium iodide), inhibit TSH
    action on thyroid and inhibits organic coupling of iodide, resulting in
    less T3 and T4 release
  Very effective for pts in thyroid storm

Goiter = any abnormal thyroid enlargement
MC type of goiter – non-toxic multinodular colloid goiter
MC identifiable cause of goiter – iodine deficiency
Substernal goiter (almost always multinodular goiter w/ mediastinal extension)
  Almost always **secondary** (vessels from superior and inferior thyroid
    arteries); goiter grew into mediastinum from a normally placed gland
  Primary substernal goiter – very rare; vessels originate from innominate
    artery

Multi-nodular goiter (can be toxic or non-toxic)
Unusual to have to operate unless in setting of:
  1) **suspicious nodule** *or;*
  2) **cosmesis issues** *or;*
  3) **compression of neck structures** (eg airway obstruction w/ stridor)
These pts usually become only mildly thyroid toxic
Causes: iodine deficiency (MC worldwide), chronic low-grade TSH stimulation
  (MC US)

Dx
  Check **TFT's** [can be toxic or non-toxic (MC)]
  U/S and **FNA** if any suspicious lesions are present
Path – shows colloid
Tx for multi-nodular goiter (either for <u>hyperthyroidism or large size</u>)
  PTU (50% rate of failure or recurrence)
  ¹³¹I (can be less effective in these pts due to inhomogenous uptake)
  Beta-blocker helps w/ sx's
  Medical Tx usually manages hyperthyroidism
  Subtotal thyroidectomy **if medical treatment ineffective**
Preop preparation for hyperthyroidism if present (see hyperthyroidism section
  above)

Thyroiditis
Hashimoto's disease
MCC hypothyroidism in adults
MCC thyroiditis
Sx's: enlarged gland (goiter), painless, chronic thyroiditis
    Women; often Hx of childhood XRT
    Usually euthyroid or hypothyroid
Dx: ↑ **thyroid peroxidase** and **anti-thyroglobulin Ab's**
Path
    Autoimmune destruction of thyroid (humeral and cell-mediated)
    Lymphocytic infiltrate
    May cause transient **thyrotoxicosis** in acute early stage
    Goiter – from **lack of organification** of **trapped iodide** inside gland
    Unusual to have to operate unless in setting of suspicious nodule
Tx:
    Thyroxine 1st line (treats vast majority)
    Beta-blocker if hyperthyroid sx's (transient)
    Partial thyroidectomy (unusual) - if continued growth despite
        thyroxine, if nodules appear, or compression sx's

Bacterial thyroiditis (acute suppurative thyroiditis; rare)
MC from **contiguous spread** (pharynx)
Sx's: MC starts w/ **pharyngitis**,(**MC strep**), then dysphagia, tenderness
Dx: have normal TFT's; FNA should show **WBCs, bacteria**
Tx:
    Abx's, may need percutaneous drainage of **abscess**
    Possible **lobectomy** to R/O cancer in pts w/ unilateral swelling and
        tenderness
    Possible total thyroidectomy for **persistent inflammation**

DeQuervain's thyroiditis (acute viral thyroiditis)
May have transient hyperthyroidism initially
Sx's: starts w/ **viral URI** (sore throat, fatigue, rhinorrhea), then tender
    thyroid, mass
MC in women
Dx: ↑ed **ESR** can help
Tx:
    NSAID's, possible **steroids;** beta-blocker if hyperthyroid sx's
    Possible **lobectomy** to R/O cancer in pts w/ unilateral swelling and
        tenderness
    Possible total thyroidectomy for **persistent inflammation**

Riedel's fibrous struma (rare)
Replacement of the thyroid tissue w/ **woody, fibrous component**
Can involve adjacent strap muscles and carotid sheath
May resemble thyroid CA or lymphoma (get Bx)
Sx's: **hypothyroidism** and **compression**
Associations – sclerosing cholangitis, fibrotic diseases, methysergide Tx
    (for migraines), retroperitoneal fibrosis
Tx:
    Steroids and **Thyroxine**
    Possible isthmectomy or **tracheostomy** for compression
    Can be hard to find RLN's w/ resection.

PARATHYROID

Normal Parathyroid Function and Anatomy
Superior parathyroids
Posterior surface of superior portion of gland, often lateral to RLN's
Above inferior thyroid artery
Derived from **4th pouch** (associated w/ **thyroid complex**)
Can migrate to **posterior mediastinum**
Inferior parathyroids
More anterior, often medal to RLN's
Below inferior thyroid artery
Derived from **3rd pouch** (associated w/ **thymus**)
Inferior parathyroids have more variable location and are more likely to be **ectopic (aberrant)
Occasionally in **tail of thymus** (MC ectopic site)
Can migrate to **anterior mediastinum**
Inferior thyroid artery – blood supply to both **superior** and **inferior parathyroid glands**
95% of population has 4 glands
MCC hypo-parathyroidism – previous thyroid surgery
PTH – increases serum Ca by 3 mechanisms:
1) **Kidney Ca reabsorption** in distal tubules, also ↓s kidney PO_4 absorption (all mediated by **cAMP**)
2) **Osteoclast release of Ca in bone** (also releases PO_4)
3) **Vitamin D production in kidney** (↑s 1-alpha hydroxylation of Vit D)
Net serum PO_4 ↓s due to PTH
Vit D (1,25-dihydroxy-cholecalciferol)
Vit D synthesis: 7-dehydrocholesterol → **UV light** → Vit D3 → **liver** (*25-hydroxylation*) → Vit D3-25OH → **kidney** (*1-hydroxylation*) → **Vit D**
Active Vit D ↑s intestinal Ca and PO_4 absorption by increasing **calcium binding protein**
Calcitonin - ↓s serum Ca by 2 mechanisms:
1) **Bone Ca resorption** (osteoclast inhibition)
2) **Kidney Ca and PO_4 excretion**
Normal Values
Normal Ca:	2.2 - 2.6 mmol/L (8.5 -10.5 mg/dL)
Normal Ionized Ca (1/2 above)	1.1 - 1.5 mmol/L (4.5 - 5.5 mg/dL)
Normal PTH:	10 - 60 (pg/ml)
Normal PO_4:	2.5 - 5.0
Normal Cl$^-$:	98 - 107
Parathyroid weight	60 - 80 gm

DDx for hypercalcemia (90% from hyperparathyroidism or CA):
Hyperparathyroidism (MCC overall; primary and tertiary)
CA (*only* 25% related to osteolysis by tumor)
1) **PTH-rp** [lung CA and breast CA (tied for #1), renal cell CA]
↑ Urine cAMP w/ PTH-rp excess (acts on kidney PTH receptor)
2) **Cytokines + excess Vit D precursors** (hematologic malignancies)
3) **Osteolysis** (MC-myeloma) – only causes 25% of hypercalcemia from malignancy (75% from PTH-rp or ↑cytokines + Vit D precursors)
CA w/ *highest risk* of hypercalcemia – small cell lung CA
Familial Hypercalcemia Hypocalciuria
Vit D excess
Milk-alkali syndrome – massive dairy consumption or Ca antacids
Thiazide diuretics
Immobilization
Paget's
Hyperthyroidism
Vitamin A overdose
Granulomatous DZ (eg sarcoid, TB, histoplasmosis, Wegener's)
Acute presentation – more likely CA
Chronic or asymptomatic – more likely hyperparathyroidism

Primary Hyperparathyroidism

PRAD-1 oncogene increases risk for parathyroid adenomas

Genetic Syndromes w/ hyperparathyroidism – MEN I and IIA, familial hyperparathyroidism

MC in women

Sx:

Muscle weakness, nephrolithiasis, pancreatitis, GI ulcers, depression, bone pain, pathologic fx's, bone loss on densitometry scan

Most asymptomatic – ↑ed Ca found on routine lab work

Osteitis fibrosa cystica (ie brown tumor) – bone lesion from Ca resorption

Hypertension can result from renal impairment

Dx:

↑ **PTH** and ↑ **Ca** (*ionized* best test)

Other abnormalities:

↓ phos

Cl⁻ to phos ratio >33 (**hyperchloremic metabolic acidosis**)

↑ **renal cAMP** (action of PTH on PTH receptor)

↑ **urine Ca**

Check CXR for granulomas (eg sarcoid) or CA (eg small cell lung CA)

Check UA for Ca (if low urine Ca → Dx is FHH, see below)

Check TFTs (R/O hyperthyroidism)

PTH-rp (rp = related peptide) **related to breast CA** (or other CA) has:

Low to normal PTH (PTH-rp does not cross react w/ assay)

↑ **serum Ca**

High urine cAMP

High Cl:PO4 ratio

Small cell lung CA and other non-hematologic CA can have PTH-rp

Familial hypercalcemic hypocalciuria

Caused by ↑ed binding of PTH to PTH receptor (**defect in PTH receptor**) in kidney

Normal PTH (or slightly elevated)

↑ **serum Ca** (only to 11 or so, never symptomatic)

**Low urine Ca (*this is the key finding*)

NO parathyroidectomy in these pts

Sestamibi scan (controversial; most endocrine surgeons would not get this unless re-op)

Helps **localize adenomas**

Can detect **multiple adenomas**

Can suggest **diffuse hyperplasia** as cause (all glands are big and light up)

Possibly could suggest pt has **abnormal number of glands** (3 or 5)

If pt has a big adenoma, all the sestamibi may be taken up there and you won't see the other glands

Can detect **mediastinal gland**

Path

Single adenoma (80%)

Diffuse hyperplasia (15%)

Pts w/ MEN I or MEN IIa have 4-gland hyperplasia

Multiple adenomas (4%)

Parathyroid adenocarcinoma (< 1%, very rare), can get very ↑ Ca levels

Indications for surgery:

1) **Symptomatic DZ:**

(pancreatitis, ulcers, joint or bone pain, Fx, weakness, kidney stones)

2) **Asymptomatic DZ w/:**

Ca > 13

↓ Cr clearance (> 30%; from chronic Ca overload)

↓ed bone mass (densitometry **t-score < −2.5** at any site)

24-h urinary calcium > 400 mg

Age < 50 (↓ lifetime risk of problems)

Pt preference

Tx:

Adenoma – resection

Inspect other glands; R/O hyperplasia and multiple adenomas

Parathyroid hyperplasia:

Do <u>NOT</u> biopsy all glands → risks hemorrhage and hypoparathyroidism

Resect 3 1/2 glands (<u>form the 1/2 gland 1st</u>) or total para-thyroidectomy and auto-implantation (in SCM or forearm)

Parathyroid CA – radical parathyroidectomy (take **ipsilateral thyroid**)

Pregnancy – surgery in 2nd trimester; ↑ **stillbirth** if not resected

Get intra-op frozen section of specimen – don't want to resect piece of fat; confirm tissue taken was **parathyroid**

Get intra-op PTH level:

Determines if causative gland is removed (*peripheral* blood draw)

**PTH should go to 50% of the pre-op value in 10 minutes

Missing Gland locations:

Thymus tissue (MC ectopic location for parathyroid gland)

Near **carotid bifurcation** (open carotid sheath)

Anterior to **vertebral bodies**

Superior and **posterior to pharynx**

Tracheo-esophageal groove

Intra-thyroid (use U/S)

Anterior and **posterior mediastinum** are possibilities *(can't really reach these from the neck)*

Perform thymectomy if you can't find gland (can do this through neck incision; ligate thymic vein)

If you find 3 fairly big glands (ie you have **hyperplasia** and are missing a gland or you have hyperplasia and pt was born w/ 3 glands)

Check missing gland locations above

Take **2 ½ glands** (or 3 glands w/ auto-implantation)

Check PTH:

1) If decreased > 50% in 10 min → you're done

2) If still ↑ed PTH → close, post-op parathyroid scan to localize missing gland

If you find 3 totally normal sized glands (ie you can't find the adenoma)

Check the missing gland locations above + **thymectomy**

Ipsilateral thyroidectomy if still not found

Still not found, close, get sestamibi scan

At reoperation for missing gland, MC location for gland → normal anatomic position; others – **thymus, thyroid,** anterior / posterior mediastinum (always re-check Ca and PTH before reop)

Follow Ca post-op

Post-op hypocalcemia etiology

Bone hunger (early) – normal PTH, decreased HCO3-

Graft/Remnant failure – decreased PTH, normal HCO3-

Hypomagnesemia

Remember to give Ca post-op

Persistent hyperparathyroidism post-op (1%)

MCC – missed adenoma in neck

Sestamibi scan to localize, re-operate

Recurrent hyperparathyroidism

Occurs after a period of hypo- or normo-calcemia:

Possible **new adenoma** formation

Possible **tumor implants** at original operation have now grown

Possible recurrent **parathyroid CA**

Reoperation – ↑ recurrent laryngeal nerve injury and permanent hypoparathyroidism

MEN – total parathyroidectomy w/ auto-implantation (**forearm** flexor compartment usual)

Do not want to re-implant in neck w/ high chance of recurrent parathyroid hyperplasia in the re-implanted parathyroid tissue (risk injury to recurrent laryngeal nerve)

Secondary hyperparathyroidism

MCC – chronic renal failure (can also occur w/ malabsorption of Vit D in gut)

Dx:

    ↑ **PTH** and ↓ **serum Ca** (may be near normal)

    ↑ed **urine Ca**

    ↑ed **serum PO$_4$**

Path

    Low Ca due to:

        1) ↓ **Ca reabsorption in kidney** (due to renal failure)

        2) ↓ **active vitamin D** (↓ 1-OH hydroxylation due to renal failure) →

            ↓ Ca reabsorption from gut (from ↓ calcium binding protein)

    Increased PTH in response to low Ca

    Failing kidneys do NOT excrete PO$_4$ →

        Insoluble **calcium phosphate** forms in body (get <u>ectopic</u>

            <u>calcifications</u>)

Most do <u>not</u> need surgery (95%)

Indications for Surgery:

    1) **Refractory Bone Pain** (MC indication for surgery) – 85% get relief

    2) **Refractory Pruritis** – 85% get relief

    3) **Fractures**

Tx:

    Control diet PO$_4$

    PO4 binder - sevelamer chloride (Renagel), calcium acetate (Phoslo),

        lanthanum carbonate (Fosrenol), calcium carbonate (Tums)

    Calcium and **Vit D** (also calcium in dialysate)

    Cinacalcet (mimics action of Ca)

        Activates calcium-sensing receptor in parathyroid and ↓s PTH

        Used for secondary hyperparathyroidism and parathyroid CA w/ mets

    Surgery (rarely needed, 5%) – subtotal (3 1/2 glands) or total

        parathyroidectomy w/ auto-implantation

Renal osteodystrophy

    Defective bone mineralization due to chronic **secondary**

        hyperparathyroidism

    Causes osteopenia and chondrocalcinosis

    Tx:

        Dialysis (more frequent may be beneficial)

        Calcium and **Vit D** (↑ Ca)

        Restrict dietary PO4

        PO4 binders (see above)

        Cinacalcet (↓s PTH)

Calciphylaxis (calcific uremic arteriopathy)

    Associated w/ **chronic renal failure**

    Calcification and **thrombosis** of small to medium sized blood vessels

        Can occur in all tissues of body

        1st manifestation usually is **skin ischemia** and **necrosis**

    Dx: skin Bx

    Tx:

        Dialysis (may need to increase frequency)

        Aggressive wound care

        Keep Ca and **PO4 low (want Ca x PO4 product < 55)

            Avoid Vit D and Ca supplementation

            Non-calcium containing **PO4 binding gel** [sevelamer chloride

                (Renagel) or lanthanum carbonate (Fosrenol)]

            Restrict dietary phosphate

        Sodium thiosulfate (↑s solubility of Ca deposits)

        Cinacalcet (↓s PTH)

        Parathyroidectomy controversial

        Poor prognosis overall

Tertiary hyperparathyroidism

Renal DZ now corrected w/ **kidney TXP** but still have overproduction of PTH
Lab values same as primary hyperparathyroidism (ie ↑ **PTH** and ↑ **Ca**)
Same indications as primary hyperparathyroidism
Tx: subtotal (3 1/2 glands) or total parathyroidectomy w/ auto-implantation

Familial hypercalcemic hypocalciuria (FHH)

High serum Ca and *low urine Ca* (would be high if hyperparathyroidism)
Defect in **PTH receptor in distal convoluted tubule of kidney** that ↑'s
resorption of Ca
Dx:
> **Ca 9–11**
> **PTH is normal** (5-40)
> ***Urine Ca is low** (key to Dx)*
Tx: **nothing** (Ca not that high); <u>no</u> **parathyroidectomy**

Pseudo-hypoparathyroidism

Low serum Ca and high serum PO4; high PTH
Defect in **PTH receptor in distal convoluted tubule of kidney** that ↓'s
resorption of Ca (receptor does <u>not</u> respond to PTH; G protein problem)
Defect in **Albright's hereditary osteodystrophy** – founded facies, short 4th and
5th metacarpals
Tx: calcium

Parathyroid cancer (Rare)

Mortality is due to **hypercalcemia** – can have extremely high Ca levels (> 15)
Increased Ca, PTH, and alkaline phosphatase
MC site for mets – lung
Tx wide en bloc excision (**parathyroidectomy** and **ipsilateral thyroidectomy**)
Recurrence rate – 50%
Overall 5-year survival – 50%

Hypercalcemic Crisis (also see Fluids and Electrolytes chp)

Ca usually **>13** (ionized >6) w/ symptoms
MCC hypercalcemic crisis – previous primary hyperparathyroidism undergoing
another procedure
MC malignant cause – breast CA
Sx's: lethargy, oliguria, hypotension, arrhythmias
Tx:
> **Rapid volume Infusion** – normal saline at 200-300 cc/hr – <u>NO lactated
> ringers</u> (contains Ca)
> **Lasix** (do <u>not</u> use thiazide diuretics which cause Ca resorption)
> **Dialysis** if refractory to above
> **Chronic Tx in malignancy →**
> > **Bisphosphonates** [eg alendronate (Fosamax)]
> > > Inhibits osteoclast bone resorption
> > **Calcitonin** - inhibits osteoclast bone resorption
> > > **S/Es** – quick onset of tachyphylaxis
> > **Glucocorticoids**
> > **Mithramycin** - inhibits osteoclast bone resorption
> > > **S/Es** -liver, renal, hematologic
Just to re-state: **lactated ringers** and **thiazide diuretics** are *contraindicated* in
pts w/ hypercalcemia

Hypocalcemia (also see Fluids and Electrolytes chp)

Ca usually < 8 (ionized < 4) w/ symptoms
Sx's:
> **Perioral tingling** – 1st symptom
> Chvostek's sign (tapping face causes twitching)
> Trousseau's sign (carpopedal spasm after blood pressure cuff)
> Hyper-reflexia
> Prolonged QT on EKG

THE COMPREHENSIVE ABSITE REVIEW

Multiple Endocrine Neoplasia Syndromes

From APUD cells

Neoplasms develop individually, synchronously or metachronously

Autosomal dominant w/ 100% penetrance, has variable expressivity

MENIN – tumor suppressor (in nucleus)

RET – proto-oncogene; receptor tyrosine kinase (TGF-beta receptor)

MEN I (MENIN inactivation)

Parathyroid hyperplasia

Usually first part to become **symptomatic**; (kidney stones)

Tx: four-gland resection w/ auto-transplantation in forearm

Don't leave gland in neck – hard reop if recurrence

Pancreatic islet cell tumors

Gastrinoma MC (50% multiple, 50% malignant)

MCC death in these pts (also MCC morbidity)

Pituitary adenoma

Prolactinoma MC

Simultaneous tumors - need to correct **hyperparathyroidism 1st**

MEN IIa (RET proto-oncogene)

Parathyroid hyperplasia

Tx: four-gland resection w/ auto-transplantation in forearm

Don't leave gland in neck – hard reop if recurrence

Medullary CA of thyroid

Usually 1st part to be **symptomatic** (MC sx - <u>diarrhea</u>)

Nearly all pts w/ MEN IIa get this (95%); often bilateral

MCC death in these pts

Pheochromocytoma

Often bilateral, nearly always benign

Simultaneous tumors - need to correct **pheochromocytoma 1st**

MEN IIb (RET proto-oncogene)

-

Medullary CA of thyroid

Usually 1st part to be **symptomatic** (MC sx - <u>diarrhea</u>)

Nearly all patients w/ MEN IIb get this (95%); often bilateral

MCC of **death** in these pts

More aggressive than MEN IIa

Pheochromocytoma

Often bilateral, nearly always benign

Mucosal ganglioneuromas (anywhere in GI tract)

Marfan's habitus, musculoskeletal abnormalities

Simultaneous tumors - need to correct **pheochromocytoma 1st**

BREAST

Normal Breast Anatomy

Breast development
Breasts are formed from the ectoderm milk streak – ducts are double layered columnar cells
Estrogen – duct development
Progesterone – lobular development
Prolactin – synergizes both estrogen and progesterone
Cyclical Changes of Breast Tissue
Estrogen – causes breast swelling from glandular tissue growth
Progesterone – causes maturation of glandular tissue; withdrawal of progesterone results in menses
FSH and LH surge – result in ovum release
Following menopause, lack of estrogen and progesterone results in atrophy of breast tissue

Nerves
Long thoracic nerve – innervates **serratus anterior**
Injury results in winged scapula; may have trouble lifting arm above head
Lateral thoracic artery goes to serratus anterior
Thoracodorsal nerve – innervates **latissimus dorsi**
Injury results in weak pull-ups and weak arm adduction
Thoracodorsal artery goes to latissimus dorsi
Medial pectoral nerve – goes to pectoralis major and pectoralis minor
Lateral pectoral nerve – goes to pectoralis major only
Intercostobrachial nerve – lateral cutaneous branch of 2nd intercostal nerve
Provides sensation to medial arm and axilla
Found just below axillary vein w/ axillary lymph node dissection
Can transect without serious consequences (can get numbness)
MC injured nerve w/ mastectomy or axillary node dissection

Arterial supply to breast
Branches of internal mammary (internal thoracic) artery, intercostal arteries, thoracoacromial artery, and lateral thoracic artery

Batson's plexus
Valveless vein plexus that extends from pelvic region up to dura of brain;
Allows **direct hematogenous metastasis** of breast CA, prostate CA, and rectal CA to **spine**

Lymphatic drainage
97% - axillary nodes
2% - internal mammary nodes; any quadrant can drain to internal mammary nodes
< 1% - supraclavicular nodes (M1 disease in breast CA)
MCC of malignant axillary adenopathy – lymphoma

Cooper's ligaments – suspensory ligaments of breast; act to divide breast into segments; breast CA involving these strands can cause dimpling of skin

Benign Breast Disease
Infectious mastitis
MC w/ breastfeeding

MC organism – staph aureus

Tx lactation associated – abx's for staph/strep
> Avoid tetracycline, chloramphenicol, and fluoroquinolones (released in breast milk)

> **Breast feeding** (or breast pump) should be continued to facilitate drainage of engorged area

Tx non-lactation associated – abx's for aerobic and anaerobic
> **RF** – smoking

Failure to resolve w/ abx's (2 weeks) – mammogram and incisional biopsy (including skin) to R/O necrotic CA

Breast Abscesses
MC w/ breastfeeding

MC organism – staph aureus

Tx lactation associated
> **Skin intact** – repeated aspiration w/ abx's; incision and drainage if that fails

> **Skin thinned out** – incision and drainage, abx's

> **Breast feeding** (or breast pump) should be continued to facilitate drainage of engorged area

> **Failure to resolve** (2 weeks; esp. older pts) – excisional Bx (including skin) to R/O necrotic CA

Tx non-lactation associated
> **Periareolar** – can get pus in nipple discharge (duct fistula)
>> **RF** – smoking

>> Tx: aspiration; abx's; terminal duct excision if that fails

> **Lateral** – aspiration or incision and drainage, abx's

> **Failure to resolve** (2 weeks; esp. older pts) – excisional Bx (including skin) to R/O necrotic CA

Mammary duct ectasia (ie plasma cells mastitis)
From obstruction of lactiferous duct

May have history of difficulty breastfeeding

Sx's:
> Non-cyclical mastodynia, nipple retraction, creamy discharge from nipple; possible sterile subareolar abscess

> Dilated mammary ducts, inspisated secretions, marked periductal inflammation

Tx:
> **Typical creamy discharge only and no nipple retraction** – reassure; excisional Bx if fails to resolve

> **Non-creamy or nipple retraction** – excisional Bx

Galactocele
Breast cysts filled w/ milk; occurs w/ breastfeeding

Tx: aspiration, incision and drainage if that fails

Galactorrhea
Etiologies – ↑ prolactin (prolactinoma), OCPs, TCAs, phenothiazines, metoclopramide, alpha-methyl dopa, reserpine

Often associated w/ amenorrhea

Gynecomastia (2 cm pinch)
Neonatal – circulating female hormones from mother; regresses

Adolescence – often **obesity**
> **Leave alone in adolescence** - will usually regress in 1-2 years (no further W/U needed)

> **If obesity-** possible ↓ resect if cosmetically disforming / social problems

Adults (Elderly – likely ↓ed testosterone)
> Most idiopathic – can be from adipose tissue or breast tissue

> Should be **bilateral** (if not, think breast CA)

> **R/O specific etiologies**
>> **Chronic DZ** – cirrhosis, renal failure

>> **Drugs** – cimetidine, omeprazole, spironolactone, finasteride

CA – testicular or adrenal tumors

Unilateral and **adult** – need to R/O breast CA

Accessory breast tissue – MC in axilla

Accessory nipples (polythelia) – anywhere from axilla to groin (MC breast anomaly)

Breast asymmetry – common finding in women

Breast reduction – ability to lactate usually <u>not</u> compromised

Poland's syndrome

>Hypoplasia of chest wall w/ amastia and no pectoralis muscle
>
>Hypoplastic shoulder
>
>Webbing of fingers (syndactyly)

Mondor's disease

>Sclerosing superficial vein thrombophlebitis of breast from trauma or strenuous exercise; Cordlike, can be painful
>
>**MC location** – lower outer quadrant
>
>Tx: NSAIDs

Mastodynia (pain in breast)

Rarely this is breast CA

>5% of breast CA has mastodynia associated w/ initial sx
>
>However, < 1% of pts w/ mastodynia have breast CA

Cyclic mastodynia – pain before menstrual period

>**MCC** – fibrocystic disease

Continuous mastodynia – continuous pain

>**MC defined etiology** – acute or subacute infection
>
>Etiology often not found for continuous mastodynia
>
>Continuous mastodynia more refractory to tx than cyclic mastodynia

Dx

>**Breast exam**
>
>**Bilateral mammogram**
>
>**U/S**

Tx:

>Danazol, OCP's, NSAID's, evening primrose oil, bromocriptine, thyroxine, Vit E, low fat diet
>
>***Avoid*** **nicotine** and **methylxanthines** (caffeine, theophyllin)
>
>Abx's if thought to be infectious (see infectious mastitis above)
>
>If truly disabling and refractory to all Tx's (rare) → consider mastectomy
>
>**Suspicious lumps or lesions on mammogram** need appropriate w/u

Fibroadenoma

MC breast lesion in adolescent and **young women**

Can **change in size** w/ menstrual cycle and **enlarge** w/ pregnancy

Can have large, **coarse calcifications** (popcorns lesions) on mammography from degeneration

10% multiple

Sx's: usually painless, slow-growing, well circumscribed, firm, rubbery

Dx and Tx:

>**Pts aged < 30 → need U/S**
>
>>1. Mass needs to **feel clinically benign** (firm, rubbery, rolls, not fixed)
>>2. **U/S** needs to be consistent w/ fibroadenoma (distinct borders, homogenous, hyper-echoic)
>>3. **Need FNA or core needle biopsy** demonstrating the fibroadenoma (not just normal breast tissue)
>>
>>Need all 3 of the above to be able to follow the mass
>>
>>If above 3 criteria not full-filled → excisional Bx
>>
>>**Avoid resection in teenagers and younger** → can affect breast development
>>
>>**Path** – prominent fibrous tissue compressing epithelial cells
>
>**Pts aged ≥ 30 → bilateral mammogram** and **U/S**
>
>>Tx: **excisional biopsy** to ensure diagnosis

Nipple discharge

Majority of nipple discharge **benign**

Dx (all need following):

Breast exam (look for discharge **trigger point** - potential subareolar rsxn in that area)

Bilateral mammogram

U/S

If discharge was bloody:

Ductogram to identify likely papilloma

Place a wire in appropriate duct and resect that area

Tx:

Non-spontaneous and **Yellow-Green Discharge**

Usually due to fibrocystic disease

Should also have lumpy tissue c/w fibrocystic DZ

Should be cyclical and non-spontaneous

Tx: reassure patient

If there is any doubt → excisional Bx

Any other type of discharge (spontaneous or another color) → needs some sort of **resection:**

Place a probe in responsible duct so you get the right gland or area (3 x 3 x 3 cm rsxn area)

If you cannot localize (ie on physical exam, mammogram, or ductogram) → need complete subareolar rsxn

Bloody nipple discharge

MCC – intraductal papilloma; occasionally ductal CA

Tx: resection (usually curative) of ductal quadrant and any associated mass (use wire localization for responsible duct based on **ductogram → will show papilloma;** if papilloma not seen on ductogram, wire localization of duct w/ bloody discharge)

Place probe in responsible duct so you get the right gland or area (3 x 3 x 3 cm rsxn)

Can start w/ FNA if you find a mass initially (eventually will need rsxn of the mass)

May have to do **complete subareolar rsxn** if you cannot localize

Serous nipple discharge

Worrisome for CA

Tx: Excisional Bx of that ductal area and any associated mass

Place probe in responsible duct so you get the right gland or area (3 x 3 x 3 cm rsxn)

Can start w/ FNA if you find a mass initially (eventually will need rsxn of the mass)

May have to do **complete subareolar rsxn** if you cannot localize

Spontaneous nipple discharge

Worrisome for CA

Tx: Excisional Bx of that ductal area and any associated mass

Place probe in responsible duct so you get the right gland or area (3 x 3 x 3 cm rsxn)

Can start w/ FNA if you find a mass initially (eventually will need rsxn of the mass)

May have to do **complete subareolar rsxn** if you cannot localize

Fibrocystic Disease

Lots of types – fibromatosis, sclerosing adenosis (can have cluster calcifications resembling breast CA), apocrine metaplasia, duct adenosis, epithelial hyperplasia, ductal hyperplasia, lobular hyperplasia

Only **significant** breast CA risk is in **atypical ductal hyperplasia** or **atypical lobular hyperplasia** (unusual findings, **relative risk 4-5**)

Sx's: breast pain, nipple discharge (yellow to brown), masses, lumpy tissue
Often varies w/ hormonal cycle

Dx: Breast exam + Bilateral mammogram + U/S

Tx:

Reassurance unless suspicious breast exam, mammogram, or U/S
Repeat in studies in 3 months to make sure finding not worse

If breast Bx shows atypical ductal or lobular hyperplasia →
1) need to resect suspicious area (on exam or mammogram
2) Do <u>not</u> need negative margins but do need following:

→ you must **remove all of the mass** if one is present
The mass can harbor CA separate from atypical hyperplasia
Example: FNA of mass shows atypical hyperplasia → still need excisional Bx of the residual mass

→ you must also **remove all of the suspicious area** on mammogram if present (ie **BIRAD 4 or 5 lesions**)
Avoids sampling error (CA next to area of atypical hyperplasia)
Example: stereotactic needle Bx for BIRAD 4 lesion comes back atypical ductal hyperplasia → still need needle localization and excisional biopsy of the area

Lobular Carcinoma In Situ (LCIS)

Path

30% lifetime risk for breast CA (<u>both breasts </u>have same risk; **1%/year**)
Considered **marker** for breast CA → *NOT pre-malignant itself*
No invasion of basement membrane
No calcifications
Not usually palpable
Not usually seen on mammography
Multifocal DZ is common
MC in **pre-menopausal women**
Usually an **incidental finding**
Pts that develop breast CA are more likely to develop a **ductal CA** (70%)
5% risk of **synchronous breast CA** at time of dx of LCIS (**MC ductal CA**)

Tx:

1) **Need to resect original suspicious area**
2) **Do <u>not </u>need negative margins for LCIS** (not pre-malignant) but do need following:

→ important that you must **remove all of the mass** if one is present;
The mass can harbor CA separate from LCIS (need to avoid sampling error)
· **Example:** FNA of a mass shows LCIS → still need excisional Bx of residual mass

→ important that you **remove all of the suspicious area** on mammogram (ie **BIRAD 4 or 5 lesions**)
CA can be next to area of LCIS (need to avoid sampling error)
Example: stereotactic needle Bx for BIRAD 4 lesion shows LCIS → still need needle localization, resection of area

Tx Options for LCIS:

1) **Nothing** and **careful F/U**
2) **Hormonal Therapy**
Pre-menopausal – Tamoxifen and careful F/U (5 years maximum)
Post-menopausal – Raloxifene and careful F/U
Above have 50% reduction in risk of breast CA
3) **Bilateral simple mastectomy** (<u>No</u> *ALND*)

THE COMPREHENSIVE ABSITE REVIEW

Ductal Carcinoma In Situ (DCIS)

Usually <u>not</u> palpable - presents as a **cluster of calcifications** on mammography

Calcifications can be **linear** or **branching**

Path

No invasion of basement membrane

Malignant cells of ductal epithelium

50% get CA if not resected **(*ipsilateral breast at risk*)**

Considered **pre-malignant**

Variants – solid, cribriform, papillary, and comedo

Comedo subtype – most aggressive

High risk of multicentricity, microinvasion, and recurrence

Tx: total mastectomy (see below)

Recurrence risk – increased w/ comedo type and lesions > 2.5 cm

Tx: 2 options

1) **Lumpectomy + XRT→** rsxn usually done by needle localization

Take X-ray of lesion you took out (oriented) to make sure you got all of the calcifications

Send to path for permanent (oriented) to make sure you got the margins (want 1 cm margin); Need to perform re-resection if you did not get appropriate margins

XRT ↓s local recurrence for DCIS, <u>no</u> change in survival

2) **Simple mastectomy** (indications below)

Diffuse malignant appearing calcifications that are hard to follow

Multi-centric or multi-focal DCIS

Inability to get **margins** despite re-resection

Inability to get **good cosmetic result**

Pt preference

Previous XRT that would result in excessive total XRT dose

Comedo necrosis

High grade

DCIS recurrence

DCIS in male pts

**<u>*NO axillary lymph node dissection w/ lumpectomy or mastectomy*</u>

Consider **SLNBx** at time of surgery if **total mastectomy**

(<u>*controversial*</u> 1-2% have nodal CA)

Subcutaneous mastectomy (eg simple or total mastectomy)

Leaves 1% of breast tissue; **preserves nipple-areolar complex**

<u>**NOT**</u> **indicated for breast CA treatment →** used for DCIS and LCIS

Tamoxifen for 5 years for resected DCIS (optional)

↓'s risk of CA by 45%

0.1% risk of endometrial CA, 1% risk DVT

Only for ER or PR positive lesions

DCIS w/ small focus microinvasion of basement membrane (< 10% of total DCIS area)

Tx: lumpectomy + XRT or simple mastectomy

Need negative margins, <u>no</u> **ALND**

If > 10% invasion → Tx like breast CA

Intraductal papilloma

MCC bloody discharge from nipple

Papilloma usually small, non-palpable, and close to nipple

Benign lesion – NOT pre-malignant

Dx: contrast **ductogram** best way to localize – leave wire in responsible duct and resect (see nipple discharge section above for resection)

Diffuse papillomatosis (Juvenile papillomatosis)

Papillary intraductal hyperplasia

Affects **multiple ducts**; can affect **both breasts,** usually **serous discharge**

MC presentation – mass

Papillomas larger than when they occur solitarily – block ducts and form cysts

Mammogram – Swiss cheese appearance

*↑ed breast CA risk (40% eventually get breast CA) – <u>not</u> w/ solitary papilloma

Tx: excision of area

Breast Cancer

1) Epidemiology and RFs

MC CA in women in US (Japan has lowest rate in the world)

2nd MCC of cancer related death in women (lung CA 1st)

1 in 8 women get breast CA (12%), only 4% in women w/o RFs

↓ed incidence in economically poor areas

Screening ↓s mortality by 25%

10% of breast CA has <u>negative</u> U/S and <u>negative</u> mammography

Median survival for untreated breast CA – 2.5 years

First-degree relative w/ bilateral, premenopausal breast CA increases breast CA risk to 50%

Gail risk assessment

Age (need to be 35 or older)

Race

Age at menarche (early menarche increased risk)

Age at 1st live birth (> 35 and nulliparity increased risk)

Number of 1st degree relative /w breast CA

Number of previous breast Bx's

Any Bx's w/ atypical ductal hyperplasia?

Computer program calculates Breast CA risk (**next 5 yrs + lifetime**)

If calculated risk in next 5 years > 10% → offer **BRCA** genetic testing

Pts w/ either DCIS (risk of CA in same breast) or LCIS (risk of CA in both breasts) should <u>NOT</u> use Gail

RFs not in Gail – late menopause, previous **XRT**, menopausal hormone replacement therapy (OCP's <u>NOT</u> a RF), obesity

Genetic screening for BRCA should be performed for the following:

Family Hx of **BRCA gene**

1° relative w/ **bilateral** breast CA

1° relative w/ **pre-menopausal** breast CA

1° relative w/ **both breast** and **ovarian CA**

1° relative w/ **ovarian CA at age < 60**

3 or more 1° relatives w/ breast CA

Ashkenazi Jews w/ 1° relative w/ breast CA

Gail Risk assessment > 10%

BRCA I and II (+ family history of breast CA)

BRCA I

Female breast CA	60% lifetime risk
Ovarian CA	40% lifetime risk
Male Breast CA	1% lifetime risk

BRCA II

Female breast CA	60% lifetime risk
Ovarian CA	10% lifetime risk
Male Breast CA	10% lifetime risk

50% will get CA in the other breast w/ CA in the 1st breast

BRCA I and II found in < 5% of all breast CA

Screening in pts w/ BRCA

Yearly mammograms + MRI starting age 25

Yearly pelvic exam, pelvic U/S, and CA-125 starting age 25

Prophylaxis

TAH and BSO w/ BRCA gene → ↓'s risk of breast CA 70%

Bilateral prophylactic mastectomy w/ BRCA gene → ↓'s risk of breast CA 90%

Bilateral prophylactic mastectomy and **TAH and BSO** w/ BRCA gene → ↓'s risk of breast CA 95%

Tx options

a) **Careful F/U** (± Tamoxifen) *or;*

b) **Prophylactic mastectomy** (± TAH and BSO)

Consideration for prophylactic mastectomy:

a. Family history + BRCA gene <u>*or:*</u>

b. LCIS

Also need either 1) high pt anxiety, 2) poor access for F/U, 3) difficult lesion to follow w/ exam, mammo., or U/S, *or* 4) pt preference

2) **Screening**
  a) **Self breast exam** – no proven benefit
  b) **Clinical breast exam** (CBE) – no proven benefit independent of mammography
  c) **Annual mammography + CBE** starting at **age 40** (general population)
    Earlier screening for:

BRCA	Age 25
Family Hx breast CA	5-10 yrs before earliest case
Thoracic XRT	8-10 yrs after XRT
Benign lesion w/ ↑ risk	upon diagnosis

  Mammography
    ↓s breast CA mortality by 25%
    Has a 90% sensitivity and specificity
      Sensitivity ↑s w/ age as dense parenchymal tissue is replaced w/ fat
      Mass needs to be **≥5 mm** for detection
      5% of cancers have sharp margin
    Abnormal findings
      Irregular borders
      Spiculated, multiple clustered, small, thin, linear, and/or branching micro-calcifications
      Crushed calcification appearance
      Asymmetry compared to other breast - density, ducts, architecture, borders
      Radial scar
      Enlarging mass
      Skin or nipple tethering, distortion or retraction
  Breast MRI – if > 20% risk (2 family members, BRCA, prior chest XRT); performed in addition to mammogram
    MRI detects contralateral CA in 3% of women w/ recently diagnosed breast CA and negative contralateral mammogram
  BRCA – largest RF for breast CA

3) **Diagnostic Evaluation**
  Mammography - BIRAD lesions
    1 – normal exam → routine F/U
    2 – benign finding → routine screening
    3 – **probably benign finding** → 6 month F/U imaging
    4 – **suspicious abnormality** → stereotactic core needle Bx
      F/U needle localization and excisional Bx if indeterminate or if it shows only benign tissue → this area will eventually be resected in some fashion in all scenarios
    5 – **highly suspicious finding** → needle localization and excisional Bx

    Suspicious lesion on mammogram (BIRAD 4 and 5 lesions)
      Tx: stereotactic core needle Bx (BIRAD 4) or needle localization excisional biopsy (BIRAD 5)

      Stereotactic core needle Bx → if it comes back benign or indeterminate → still need to proceed w/ **excisional Bx** (avoids sampling error)

      Needle localization excisional Bx
        Need to remove all of the suspicious area
        Get XR of lesion after excision to make sure you got it all
        Review **permanent sections**, will have to come back if CA and margins are positive

Palpable breast mass
> **< 30 years old** – U/S and core needle Bx (CNBx)

>> **If malignant on CNBx** → follow appropriate tx
>> **If indeterminate on CNBx** → **excisional Bx** of mass
>> **If benign on CNBx** but **indeterminate/suspicious on U/S** →
>> **excisional Bx** of mass
>> **If benign on CNBx** but **indeterminate/suspicious on exam** →
>> **excisional Bx** of mass
>> **If benign on CNBx** and **mass does not feel or look**
>> **suspicious on exam or U/S** (i.e. is a fibroadenoma) →
>> F/U exam in 3 months
>> **If pt desires excision** → **excisional Bx** of mass
>> **Any doubt** → **excisional Bx** of mass

>> These pts most commonly have **fibroadenomas** and can leave
>> alone if CNBx is diagnostic, U/S looks like fibroadenoma,
>> and exam looks/feels like fibroadenoma
>> However, if the fibroadenoma enlarges, need excisional biopsy

> **≥ 30 years old** – bilateral mammograms, U/S and CNBx

>> **If malignant on CNBx** → follow appropriate tx
>> **If indeterminate on CNBx** → **excisional Bx** of mass
>> **If benign on CNBx** but **mass feels suspicious/indeterminate**
>> → **excisional Bx** of mass
>> **If benign on CNBx** but **mass suspicious on mammo or U/S**
>> → **excisional Bx** of mass
>> **If benign** on CNBx and **mass does not feel or look**
>> **suspicious on mammo, U/S, or exam** (ie is fibrocystic
>> DZ) → F/U exam in 3 months
>> **If pt desires excision** → **excisional Bx** of mass
>> **Any doubt** → **excisional Bx** of mass

> **If U/S shows cyst fluid, aspirate it:**
>> If **bloody**, need cyst excisional Bx
>> If **complex** cyst on U/S, need cyst excisional Bx
>> If **clear and recurs**, need cyst excisional Bx

> **Core needle biopsy** (CNBx) – gives architecture
> **Fine needle aspiration** (FNA) – gives cytology (just cells)

4) Staging

> 1) **CXR** and **LFT's** if CA diagnosis has been made (mets w/u)
> 2) **Chest/abd/pelvic CT scan** for advanced DZ or elevated LFT's
>> **Advanced DZ:**
>>> Inflammatory breast CA
>>> Skin involvement
>>> Chest wall involvement
>>> > 5 cm
>>> N2 or N3 nodal disease
> 3) **Bone scan** – for bone pain or elevated alkaline phosphatase
> 4) **Brain MRI** – for HA's

TNM

Tis – LCIS, DCIS, Paget's DZ of nipple w/o tumor
T1 mic: micro-invasion 0.1 cm or less
T1: < 2 cm
T2: 2–5 cm
T3: > 5 cm
T4:

    T4a – chest wall involvement (does <u>not</u> include pectoral muscles)
    T4b – skin (edema, ulceration, or satellite nodules)
        Includes peau d'orange
    T4c – both above
    T4d – inflammatory breast CA (erythema)

N1: ipsilateral movable axillary nodes
N2:

    N2a – fixed ipsilateral axillary nodes
    N2b – clinically positive internal mammary nodes in absence of
        axillary nodes

N3

    N3a – ipsilateral infraclavicular nodes
    N3b – ipsilateral axillary and internal mammary nodes
    N3c – ipsilateral supraclavicular nodes

M1: distant metastasis

Stages

Stage I	T1, N0, M0
Stage IIa	T0-1, N1, M0 or T2, N0, M0
Stage IIb	T2, N1, M0 or T3, N0, M0
Stage IIIa	T0-3, N2, M0 or T3, N1, M0
Stage IIIb	T4, N0-2, M0
Stage IIIc	N3
Stage IV	M1

**Node status– single most impt prognostic factor in pts w/o systemic mets
    Survival directly related to number of positive nodes

0 positive nodes	80% 5-year survival
1–3 positive nodes	60% 5-year survival
$\geq$ 4 positive nodes	40% 5-year survival

    Tumor size related to **positive nodes** [(size x 10) + 20%]

1 cm	**30%**
2 cm	**40%**
3 cm	**50%**
4 cm	**60%**
> 5 cm	**70%**

    Non-palpable nodes – 30% are positive at surgery
    Other prognostic factors – tumor size, tumor grade, progesterone
        and estrogen receptor status

Receptors

    Positive PR and **ER receptors** – better overall prognosis
        Better response to hormones, chemo, surgery, and better
            overall prognosis
        Receptor-positive tumors are MC in **postmenopausal women**.
        PR–positive tumors better prognosis than ER–positive
        Tumor that is both PR and ER–positive has best prognosis
        10% of breast CA is *negative* for both receptors
    HER2/neu receptor – worse prognosis
        Trastuzumab (Herceptin) blocks this receptor

MC site breast CA mets – bone (axial skeleton)
MC type of breast CA – ductal CA (85%)
Central and **subareolar tumors** have increased risk of <u>multicentricity</u>
Takes **5–7 years** to go from single malignant cell to 1-cm tumor
Adenocarcinoma in axillary node in woman w/ no identifiable source
    Check for **ER and PR** receptors → if positive → ipsilateral MRM (70%
        will have ipsilateral breast CA)

5) **Surgical Treatment**
  a. **Lumpectomy** (*plus* SLNB or ALND) and **XRT** – need <u>1 cm margin</u>
   Results of lumpectomy (breast conserving therapy, BCT) **w/ XRT**
      Need to have **negative margins** before starting XRT
      No real difference in **survival** compared to MRM
      Can be done under local; Need good F/U
      2% risk of **local recurrence** →
         Usually occurs within 2 years of 1st operation
         Often have **distant DZ** w/ recurrence
         These pts have **advanced DZ** and need **complete re-
            staging** (eg mammogram, chest/abd/pelvic CT)
         Need **salvage MRM** for **local recurrence**
         If mets detected, chemo-XRT only
         5-YS after recurrence – 5%
   Absolute *contraindications* to BCT
      1) **2 or more primaries** in separate quadrants
      2) **Positive margins despite re-resection** (can re-resect x 1
         for negative margins) – need negative margins
      3) **Pregnancy** (1st trimester + early 2nd trimester) – see below
      4) **Previous XRT** that would result in excessive total XRT dose
      5) **Multi-focal or multi-centric DZ**
      6) **Diffuse malignant appearing calcifications**
   Relative *contraindications* to BCT
      1) **Unacceptable cosmetic result** from large tumor (eg T3/T4)
         If neoadjuvant Tx shrinks T3/T4 down → can go w/ BCT
      2) **Scleroderma** or **SLE**
      3) **Inflammatory breast CA**
   SLNBx (sentinel lymph node biopsy)
      Fewer cx's than ALND
      Indicated only for malignant tumors **> 1 cm**
         Possible exception is **DCIS** and performing **total
            mastectomy** (2% have CA in nodes)
      <u>Not</u> indicated in pts w/ **clinically positive nodes**→ need ALND
      Accuracy best when **primary tumor is present** (finds correct
         lymphatic channels)
      Lymphazurin blue dye and **technetium labeled sulfur
         colloid radiotracer** used (injected around tumor area):
         Need 1-4 hours for technetium uptake
         Type I hypersensitivity reactions (1%) have been
            reported w/ lymphazurin blue dye
      Usually find 1-3 nodes (in 95% sentinel node found)
      Can't find dye or tracer in OR → **formal ALND**
      Tumor found in LN's on path → **formal ALND**
      If **positive** for tumor → **formal ALND**
      Contraindications to SLNBx:
         1) **Pregnancy** (see below)
         2) **Multi-centric DZ**
         3) **Neoadjuvant therapy**
         4) **Advanced Disease** (eg inflammatory breast CA, T4)
         5) **Palpable nodes** (clinically positive)
         6) **Previous axillary dissection**
         7) **Large tumor** (> 5 cm, T3) – blocks lymphatics
         8) **Tumor already taken out** (relative)
      ***Can perform SLNBx even if planning on mastectomy**
   ALND (axillary lymph node dissection)
      For **clinically positive nodes, positive SLNBx** or
         contraindication to SLNBx
      Superior border – axillary vein
      Medial border – chest wall (watch for the long thoracic nerve)
      Lateral border – skin flap
      Anterior border – pectoralis minor muscle
      Posterior border – latissimus dorsi (find thoracodorsal nerve)

THE COMPREHENSIVE ABSITE REVIEW

Node levels
> I – lateral to pectoralis minor muscle
> II – beneath pectoralis minor muscle
> III – medial to pectoralis minor muscle, extends to
> > thoracic inlet (Halstedt's ligament)
> Rotter's nodes – between the pectoralis major and
> > pectoralis minor muscles
> Remove **Level I and II nodes** en bloc w/ ALND for breast
> > CA (borders outlined above)
> Level III nodes are removed only if grossly involved
> Lymphedema and other cx's ↑ed w/ level III dissection
> Node dissection does <u>not</u> improve survival
> **Long thoracic nerve** – innervates serratus anterior muscle
> > Injury results in a winged scapula
> **Thoracodorsal nerve** – innervates latissimus dorsi muscle
> > Injury results in poor adduction and inability to do pull-up

b. Modified radical mastectomy
> Removes all breast tissue, muscle fascia, nipple-areolar complex, and level
> I and II nodes (ALND) en bloc
> **Radical mastectomy** – <u>rarely</u> performed anymore; includes MRM and
> > overlying skin, pectoralis major and minor muscles, level I/II/III nodes
> Can perform mastectomy + SLNBx (must remove nipple-areolar complex
> > as above, but substitute SLNBx for ALND)

c. Complications (Cx's)
> **Cx's of mastectomy** – infection, flap necrosis, seromas
> **Cx's of ALND** – infection, lymphedema, lymphangiosarcoma
> **Cx's of XRT** – edema, erythema, ulceration, rib fractures, pneumonitis,
> > sarcoma, contralateral breast CA
> **Axillary vein thrombosis** – early, sudden onset, post-op swelling
> **Lymphatic fibrosis** – slow swelling over 1-2 years
> **Intercostal brachiocutaneous nerve**
> > MC injured nerve after mastectomy; no significant sequelae
> > Hyperesthesia and numbness of inner arm and lateral chest wall
> **Drains** – should leave in until drainage < 30-40 cc/day

6) Systemic therapy and XRT
Systemic Therapy
> **Stage I, II, IIIa,** and **IIIc** (N3a *or* N3b)
> > **Surgery 1st**
> > **Adjuvant chemo** (TAC, see below) – for tumors > 1 cm, positive
> > > nodes, or ER/PR negative tumors
> > **Trastuzumab** – if HER2 positive and tumor > 1 cm or positive nodes
> > **Hormonal Tx** – for ER or PR positive tumor (or unknown status)
> > > **Pre-menopausal** – *Tamoxifen* (2-3 years)
> > > **Post-menopausal** – *Aromatase inhibitor* (5 years)
> > **XRT** after chemo if needed (eg w/ lumpectomy *or* if indicated after
> > > MRM, see below)
> **Stage IIIb**
> > **Neoadjuvant chemo** → then **surgery** (usually MRM)** → then
> > > **adjuvant chemo-XRT**(MC scenario)
> > **Trastuzumab –** if HER2 positive
> > **Hormonal therapy** - for ER or PR positive tumor (or unknown status)
> > > **Pre-menopausal** – Tamoxifen (2-3 years)
> > > **Post-menopausal** – aromatase inhibitor (5 years)
> > ***MRM <u>not</u> always required after neoadjuvant chemo*
> **Stage IIIc** (N3c) and **Stage IV** (both non-operable disease)
> > **ER or PR positive** – hormonal therapy (as above) ± chemo
> > **ER/PR negative, HER positive** – chemo + trastuzumab
> > **ER/PR negative, HER negative** – chemo
> > **Bony mets** – bisphosphonates (eg alendronate) → ↓ skeletal cx's
> > Can consider MRM for **palliation** (eg ulcerative, fungating lesion)
> > N3 DZ w/ good response to chemo-XRT – consider MRM

Chemo
- **TAC** (A + C → 3 times weekly for 6 cycles)
  - **Taxanes** (Docetaxel or Paclitaxel, weekly, 12 cycles)
    - S/E - neuropathy
  - **Adriamycin** (S/Es - cardiomyopathy)
    - Max dose – 500 mg/cm^2 body surface area
  - **Cyclophosphamide** (S/Es - hemorrhagic cystitis)
- Chemo given before XRT
- Tumors < 1 cm, negative nodes and positive ER/PR receptors – <u>no</u> chemo (**hormonal therapy only**)

Trastuzumab
- (Herceptin, anti-HER2/neu monoclonal Ab)
- **50% ↓ in recurrence** for HER positive tumors
- **Blocks HER2/neu receptor** (erbB2) – human epidermal growth factor receptor 2 (receptor tyrosine kinase)
- **S/Es** – cardiac DZ
- **Duration of Tx** – 1 year
- **Given after chemo** – ↑ cardiotoxicity if given w/ Adriamycin
- *Contraindications* – previous cardiac DZ

Hormonal
- **Tamoxifen**
  - **For pre-menopausal breast CA**
  - **50%↓ in recurrence** and **35% ↓ in breast CA mortality**
  - Need positive ER or PR receptors for benefit
  - **Mechanism** – blocks receptors
  - **↓ed osteoporosis**
  - **S/Es** - 1% risk of **blood clots,** 0.1% risk of **endometrial CA**
    - Post-menopausal pts highest risk
  - **Duration of Tx** – Dose is 20 mg/d for 2-3 years
  - *Raloxifene <u>not</u> approved for adjuvant breast CA Tx*
- **Aromatase inhibitors** (anastrozole, letrozole, exemestane)
  - **For post-menopausal breast CA**
  - **50% ↓ in recurrence**
  - Need positive ER or PR receptors for benefit
  - **Mechanism** - blocks conversion of testosterone to estrogen in peripheral tissues
  - **↓ed stroke, endometrial CA,** and **blood clots** compared to Tamoxifen
  - **S/Es** – fractures
  - **Duration of Tx** – 5 years
- **Oophrectomy** also an option instead of oral agents

XRT – 6 weeks, 10 minutes/d, **5000 rads total**
- **↓s local recurrence; small ↑survival** after lumpectomy
- **Indications for XRT after <u>MRM:</u>**
  - **Skin or chest wall involvement** (not pectoral muscle)
  - **Positive margins**
  - **Tumor > 5 cm** (T3)
  - **Inflammatory CA**
  - **Advanced Nodal Disease** (XRT to nodal area)
    - ≥ 4 nodes positive
    - Extracapsular invasion
    - N2 or N3
- *Contraindications* to XRT:
  - **Scleroderma or collagen vascular DZ**(get severe fibrosis, necrosis)
  - **Previous XRT**
  - **Pregnancy**
  - **SLE** (Lupus, relative)
  - **Active rheumatoid arthritis** (relative)

5-YS:

Stage I	90%
Stage II	75%
Stage III	50%
Stage IV	15%

Almost all women w/ recurrence die of disease
F/U after resection of breast CA – annual mammograms + breast exams

7) Prevention - Selective Estrogen Receptor Modulators (SERMs)
    Tamoxifen
        ↓ risk of contralateral breast CA 50% when given as adjuvant tx
        S/Es – 1% DVT or PE and 0.1% uterine CA
            S/E risks are higher in **post-menopausal women**
            Some have questioned all-cause mortality benefit
        Indications:
            1) **Pre-menopausal** pts at high risk for breast CA
            2) **↓ recurrence after breast CA**
        Contraindications – previous thromboembolic events, coumadin tx,
            pregnancy
    Raloxifene
        Estrogen effects on **bone; Anti-estrogen** on **uterus and breast**
        Compared to Tamoxifen
            Same ↓ in breast CA
            ↓ed PE/DVT and **↓ed cataracts** compared to Tamoxifen
            ↓ risk of fractures
        Indications:
            1) **Post-menopausal pts** at high risk for breast CA (preferred)
            2) **Post-menopausal pts** w/ osteoporosis for ↓ breast CA risk
        Contraindications – previous thromboembolic events, pregnancy

8) Breast CA types
    Ductal CA (85% of breast CA)
        Subtypes
            Medullary breast CA – ↑ lymphocytes, smooth borders, bizarre
                cells; vast majority ER and PR positive
            Tubular CA – small tubule formations
            Mucinous CA (colloid) – produces **mucin**
            Scirrhotic CA – worse prognosis of all subtypes
    Lobular CA (10% of all breast CA)
        Does not form calcifications
        Extensively **infiltrative** w/ increased **bilateral, multifocal,** and
            multicentric disease
        Signet ring cells – worse prognosis
    Metaplastic adenocarcinoma
        Appearance of non-glandular cells
        MC subtypes → squamous and pseudosarcomatous
        Prognosis same as tumor cell line from which it was derived
    Adenoid cystic carcinoma
        Large and often well-circumscribed lesions
        Better prognosis than other types of breast CA
    Cystosarcoma phyllodes (1% of breast CA)
        Can be very fast growing, and can increase in size in just a few weeks
        10% malignant – based on mitoses per high-power field (> 5-10)
        No nodal spread; hematogenous spread in any (although rare)
        Resembles giant fibroadenoma
        Path – has stromal and epithelial elements (mesenchymal tissue)
        Can be large
        Considered a sarcoma if malignant
        Tx: WLE w/ 1 cm margins; *No ALND*

9) Special Issues

Metastatic flare – pain, swelling, erythema in mets areas
- **Tx**: XRT (eg bone mets)

Occult breast CA presenting in axillary node
- Breast CA that presents as an axillary node w/ unknown primary
- 70% are found to have breast CA at mastectomy
- Tx: MRM

Recurrence along mastectomy scar
- **1st Mammogram and exam** of remaining breast
- **2nd Metastatic w/u**
    - Chest/abd/pelvic CT and LFT's
    - Consider bone scan and brain MRI
- **3rd Resection** if no other DZ (need 1 cm margin)
- **4th Salvage chemo** and **XRT** after resection
- If pt has **metastatic DZ**, no resection and just follow stage IV systemic therapy and XRT (if XRT total dose not exceeded) although can consider palliative resection of the recurrence

Inflammatory breast CA (T4d)
- **Very aggressive**
    - **Median survival** – 36 months (much worse than other breast CA)
- **Dermal lymphatic invasion**, which causes peau d'orange lymphedema appearance but is also **erythematous and warm** (T4d)
- **Sx's:** pain, erythema, warmth
- **Dx:**
    - **Bilateral mammogram**
    - U/S
    - ****Full thickness incisional biopsy including skin**
    - **Need full pre-op w/u** for metastatic DZ
        - Although would likely still do mastectomy for comfort measures
        - **Chest/abd/pelvic CT** and **LFT's**
        - Consider bone scan and brain MRI
- **Tx:**
    - **1st give chemo** (4 cycles)
        - If the tumor responds – go to step 2
        - If the tumor does not respond – give XRT, then step 2
    - **2nd MRM** (send skin margins for FS, may need to raise skin flaps)
        - BCT not really an option here because you should take the skin w/ resection (*inflammatory breast CA considered relative contraindication to BCT*)
    - **3rd chemo-XRT** (follow stage III systemic Tx)

Chest wall attachment w/ breast CA (T4a)
- **Dx:**
    - **Bilateral mammogram**
    - U/S
    - **Need full pre-op w/u** for metastatic DZ
        - **Chest/abd/pelvic CT** and **LFT's**
        - Consider bone scan and brain MRI
- **No metastatic DZ →**
    - **1st give chemo** (4 cycles)
    - **2nd MRM** (usual) and **chest wall resection**
        - Will need thoracotomy for this
        - Outline area of resection on chest wall
        - Try to remove the lesion en bloc (rib cutters)
        - Can remove associated lung if necessary
        - If > 5 cm (3 or more ribs) of chest wall taken, you will need to place a marlex mesh to reconstruct chest wall
        - If neo-adjuvant chemo shrank tumor way down, *may not need chest wall resection or MRM* → could potentially perform BCT for negative margins
    - **3rd chemo-XRT** (follow Stage III systemic therapy)
- **Metastatic DZ →** just go w/ **chemo-XRT**

Male breast CA (<1% of all breast CA)

    Almost always **ductal**

    Poorer prognosis due to **late presentation**

    ↑ed **pectoral muscle** involvement

    Males do <u>not</u> get – lobular CA, multi-centric CA, or contra-lateral breast CA

    Need to R/O gynecomastia (bilateral)

    RFs – steroids, XRT, family history, Klinefelter's Syndrome

    90% **estrogen receptor positive → 80% respond to Tamoxifen**

    Tx: MRM and tamoxifen; post-op systemic therapy as previously described

        Can consider mastectomy + SLNBx as opposed to MRM

Paget's Disease of Breast

    Sx's: scaly, weepy skin lesion on nipple (areolar)

    Dx: **Breast Exam**

        Bilateral mammogram (look for underlying mass or suspicious

            calcification – *all pts* have either underlying DCIS or ductal CA)

        U/S

        Incisional breast Bx – shows **Paget's cells in skin**, may show

            DCIS or CA cells (pts have either DCIS or ductal CA)

    Tx:

        1) **If mass present →** core needle Bx

            Underlying CA → need **MRM**

            Underlying DCIS → simple mastectomy

                (*not* lumpectomy, *need to* **include** *nipple areolar*

                    complex for Paget's)

                Need to confirm on FS and permanent that no CA is

                    present → MRM if present

                Typically, a simple mastectomy leaves the nipple-areolar

                    complex but w/ Paget's, the nipple areolar complex

                    is involved in the disease and **needs resection**

        2) **If no mass or core needle indeterminate →** simple mastectomy

            (need to include nipple-areolar complex), send for FS, MRM if

            CA present

Stewart-Treves syndrome

    Lymphangiosarcoma from chronic lymphedema after **axillary dissection**

    Dark purple nodule or lesion on arm 5–10 years after surgery

    Tx: sarcoma w/u and resection

Radial scar

    Can present as a stellate, irregular, spiculated mass lesion

    Consists of fibroelastic core with entrapped ducts (<u>not</u> really a scar)

    These pts have small ↑ risk of breast CA (2x normal risk)

Benign conditions that look malignant

    Fibromatosis – benign, locally invasive **fibroblast spindle cells**; can have

        skin retraction and dimpling

    Granular cell tumors – benign, slow growing, neural tumor; can have skin

        retraction and dimpling

    Fat necrosis – poorly defined borders, skin retraction; fibrosis causes

        findings; related to trauma; path shows **macrophages laden with fat**

        or foreign body giant cells (FNA or core needle biopsy)

Malignant tumors that look benign (eg smooth, rounded masses) – mucinous

    CA, medullary CA, cystosarcoma phyllodes

Most masses that contain fat are benign – nodes, posttraumatic oil cyst,

    hamartomas, fibrolipoadenomas

TRAM Flap (transverse rectus abdominal myoplasty) for breast reconstruction

    Should be performed **months after XRT** for best cosmetic result

    Should <u>not</u> be used on side of CABG w/ previous left internal mammary

        artery takedown (superior epigastric off this)

    Best indicator of flap survival – good peri-umbilical muscle perforators

    Compromised vascular supply can also result in **flap contracture**

    Previous laparoscopic cholecystectomy is <u>not</u> a contraindication

    Contraindications – smoking, transverse laparotomy incision

        (compromised superior epigastric artery), ipsilateral CABG-IMA use

    Felt to give **better cosmetic result** compared to implant

Pregnancy with mass
Often presents late, leading to worse prognosis
Mammography and U/S don't work as well during pregnancy
Dx

Breast Exam
Mammography w/ lead shielding to avoid radiation
Ultrasound
Get **core needle Bx** or **excisional Bx** under local
If **cyst**, drain it and send FNA for cytology
If **solid** →

If **fibroadenoma** on core needle Bx and **pt < 30** → follow (must feel like fibroadenoma; mammogram and U/S must look like fibroadenoma; if not need **excisional Bx** under local)
If **benign** on core needle Bx (other than fibroadenoma) but **mass suspicious on U/S, mammogram, or exam** → **excisional Bx** under local
If **indeterminate** → **excisional Bx** under local

If DCIS → **Lumpectomy under local** + *post-partum* XRT
Consider completion mastectomy after delivery if high risk DCIS
If breast CA →

1st trimester options:
1) **MRM** (post-partum chemo if needed)
2) Therapeutic abortion, lump (ALND or SLNBx) + XRT
3) Tumor < 1 cm → perform lumpectomy w/ ALND
(if nodes negative, you're done until after pregnancy)

2nd and 3rd trimester options:
If less then 20 weeks → options same as 1st trimester
If after 20 weeks →
1) **above options**
2) can perform **lumpectomy, ALND** (<u>NO</u> SLNB) and give **chemo** for 12 weeks while pregnant
Have to accept 2% incidence of teratogenic effects for 2nd and 3rd trimesters
Wait 6 weeks after chemo
Deliver child
Then XRT after delivery
< 6 weeks until delivery →
1) **MRM**
2) **Lumpectomy** w/ **ALND** (<u>NO SLNBx</u>) and give postpartum XRT (+ chemo if indicated)

<u>*No*</u> *XRT* while pregnant (**main issue** dictating pathway above – need to control primary w/ either MRM or lumpectomy + XRT)
Chemotx – risk of malformation in $1^{st}, 2^{nd}, 3^{rd}$ trimesters is 40%,2%,2%
Need discussion w/ pt on **case by case** basis
No breastfeeding after delivery w/ CA

Bloody nipple discharge in 2nd or 3rd trimester → <u>vast majority benign</u> (from ductal irritation relating to milk production in glands
Dx: check cytology of nipple discharge and look for mass (exam, U/S, mammogram w/ uterine shielding) → if neither present, follow; o/w need W/U as above

Lung Anatomy and Physiology

Airways (trachea to level of terminal bronchiole)
>> **Conducting airways** – 150 cc of anatomic dead space
>> Left mainstem bronchi longer than right
>> Right pulmonary artery longer than left before 1st branch
>> **Single most impt predictor of difficult intubation** – CXR (gives body
>>> habitus, airway anomalies. etc)

Blood supply
>> **Upper 2/3 trachea** – inferior thyroid arteries
>> **Lower 1/3 trachea** – bronchial arteries
>> **Lung parenchyma** – bronchial arteries

Mediastinal Structures
>> **Azygous vein** runs along right side and dumps into **superior vena cava**
>> **Thoracic duct** runs along right side, **crosses midline at T4-T5**, goes into
>>> left neck, turns around and dumps into **left subclavian vein** at
>>> junction w/ internal jugular vein
>> **Phrenic nerve** – runs anterior to hilum
>> **Vagus nerve** – runs posterior to hilum
>> Suprasternal notch T2; angle of Louis T4, xyphoid T10

Lung
>> **Right lung volume**   55% (3 lobes: RUL, RML, and RLL)
>> **Left lung volume**   45% (2 lobes: LUL and LLL; lingula)
>> **Quiet inspiration** – diaphragm 80%, intercostals 20%
>> **Greatest change in dimension** – superior and inferior (diaphragm)
>> **Accessory muscles** – sternocleidomastoid muscle (SCM), levators,
>>> serratus posterior, scalenes
>> **Type I pneumocytes** – gas exchange (diffusion in **alveoli**)
>> **Type II pneumocytes** – surfactant production
>> **Surfactant** – **phosphatidylcholine** main surface active agent; 80%
>>> phospholipids; ↓s **alveolar surface tension, keeps alveoli open**
>> **Pores of Kahn** – direct air exchange between alveoli
>> **Lung zones in upright person** (P = pressure)
>>> **Zone I** (apex) – Palveolar > Parterial > Pvenous (no pulmonary artery
>>>> blood flow at lung apex under nl conditions)
>>> **Zone II** (middle) – Part > Palv > Pven (flow only w/ inspiration)
>>> **Zone III** (lower) – Part > Pven > Palv (flow continuous)
>> Normal pulmonary artery pressure = 25/10 (mean 15)

Pulmonary function tests before pulmonary resection

Need predicted post-op FEV_1 > 0.8 L (> 40% of predicted value)
>> If close →
>>> Get **split function V/Q scan** (use perfusion measurement)
>>> Find the contribution of that portion of lung to overall FEV_1 and the
>>> predicted FEV_1 after resection
>> **FEV_1 single best predictor of being able to wean off ventilator after
>> pulmonary resection**

Need following pre-op values
>> DLCO > 11-12 ml/min/mmHg CO (> 50% of predicted value)
>>> **DLCO – carbon monoxide diffusion capacity**
>>> Measure of lung's ability to **transfer gases**
>>> Affected by pulmonary capillary surface area, Hgb, alveolar
>>>> architecture, dead space, low C.O., pulmonary hypertension
>>> Some use **predicted post-op > 40%**
>> pCO_2 < 45 (at rest)
>> pO_2 > 60 (at rest, not on oxygen)
>> **VO_2 max > 10** ml/kg/min (maximum oxygen consumption
>>> (10-15 intermediate risk, need pt discussion)

Pulmonary Resection Complications

Pulm cx's account for **most deaths** after pulm surgery (eg resp failure)
MCC hypoxemia – V/Q mismatch from **atelectasis** (shunt) MC
MCC hypercarbia – alveolar **hypoventilation** (poor minute ventilation)
Brachial plexus injuries – dependent arm (MC nerve injury)
Common Peroneal Nerve Injury– dependent leg (flex dependent leg to avoid)
MC resection resulting in:
>   **Persistent air leak** – segmentectomy/wedge
>   **Atelectasis** – lobectomy (**MC Cx following lobectomy**)
>   **Arrhythmias** – pneumonectomy
>   Post-op **tracheoesophageal fistula** – pneumonectomy (right MC)
>   Post-op **bronchopleural fistula** – pneumonectomy (right MC)
>   **Mortality** – pneumonectomy (right MC)
>   **Post-pneumonectomy syndrome** – right pneumonectomy
>>   Mediastinal shift after pneumonectomy →main bronchial compression
>>   **Sx's: stridor**; Tx: tissue expanders (silicone implants) on
>>   pneumonectomy side to shift mediastinum back
>   **Cardiac herniation** through pericardium – pneumonectomy (right MC)
>>   **Sx's:** hypotension, **cyanosis**, tachycardia, displaced heart on CXR
>>   **Tx** and **prevention** – pericardial Gortex patch after pneumonectomy
>   **Long bronchial stump syndrome** – pneumonectomy (left MC)
>>   Secretions pool; get recurrent infection or bronchial stump blowout
>>   Tx: shorten bronchus; cover w/ flap; keep bronchus short to prevent
Mortality w/ resection – wedge 1%, lobectomy 3%, pneumonectomy 6% (R > L)

Persistent air leak

Make sure **chest tube on suction** and **check system** → **repeat CXR**
Place 2nd chest tube anteriorly
Bronch if still having a problem w/ re-expansion [look for foreign body or
>   bronchus problem (eg BPF, mucus plug)]
Consider chest CT
Wait it out if lung re-expanded and just simple air-leak (7 days)
Not resolved →
>   **If after spontaneous PTX** – OR for staple bleb, possible mechanical
>   pleurodesis
>   **If after pulmonary resection** – mechanical pleurodesis

Atelectasis (lung collapse)

MC Cx following lung resection
MCC hypoxemia following lung resection
Results in **hypoxemia** and **pulmonary shunting**
Tx: incentive spirometer, cough, pain control, walk pt, consider early epidural
>   If refractory consider bronch to look for **mucus plugging**
>   If already on the ventilator, may need to ↑ TV's

Adult Tracheo-esophageal Fistula

Sx's: pulmonary aspiration w/ swallowing, cough
MCC – esophageal CA eroding into trachea; Tx: stent esophagus
Can also occur post-op (MC after pneumonectomy)
Post-op TEF
>   Repair esophagus primarily
>   Close hole in trachea or bronchus
>   Interpose tissue so TEF won't come back (eg pericardial fat pad or
>   intercostal muscle)

Post-pneumonectomy pulmonary edema (can also occur after lobectomy)

ARDS picture after pneumonectomy or lobectomy
>   Primary cause – **inflammatory reaction** (PMNs, O2 radical, cytokines) ↑s
>   **vascular permeability**
>   May also be related to ↑ **perfusion** to remaining lung
Is **non-cardiogenic** w/ **normal filling pressures** (wedge is normal)
Tx: follow ARDS protocol

Empyema

MCC empyema – pneumonia w/ subsequent infection of parapneumonic
effusion; can also occur after thoracic surgery (pulmonary, esophageal)
Sx's: pleuritic chest pain, fever, cough, SOB
Pleural fluid – WBCs >500 cells/cc, bacteria, positive Gram stain
Has 3 stages:
1) **Exudative** - swelling of pleura (low protein and cell count)
   Tx: chest tube + Abx's (send drainage for culture and cytology)
2) **Fibrinopurulent** (transitional) - fibrin deposits, purulent fluid; ↑PMNs
   Tx: chest tube + Abx's (send drainage for cultures and cytology)
   Failure to re-expand the lung → VATS deloculation
3) **Organizing** (chronic phase) - occurs in 3-4 week period
   In-growth of fibroblasts and capillaries w/ **lung trapping** by collagen
   Lung no longer able to be expanded → pus and thick fibrous peel
   Tx:
> **Decortication** (visceral + parietal peel removed) ± muscle flap;
> Send fluid for **cultures and cytology**; **Abx's, nutrition**
> *If can't tolerate decortication* → place **Eloesser flap** (open
> thoracic window - direct opening to external environment)
> In general, decortication seldom required → most tx'd before
> chronic organizing phase (reserve for obvious tx failures)

Broncho-pleural Fistula (BPF)

***Timing of post-op BPF important for Tx*

1) **Early post-op BPF** (< 7 days, usually 24-48 hrs post-op)
   MCC – technical complication
   Sx's: massive air-leak, resp compromise
   Dx: CXR – collapsed lung, PTX
   Tx: re-operation (if previous lobectomy, most likely need <u>completion
   pneumonectomy</u>); place **intercostal muscle flap** over bronchus

2) **Late post-op** (≥ 10 d) or **non-surgical BPF** (ie pneumonia→empyema→BPF)
   MCC – pressure from **empyema** makes hole in bronchus
   Sx's:
   > Abrupt serosanguinous or purulent sputum production
   > Can have resp distress
   ***Key issue* - protect contralateral lung** *from* **aspiration** *of empyema fluid*
   Dx: CXR (or chest CT)
   Findings after lobectomy or non-surgical cause
   > Fluid collection and PTX
   > If organized empyema present, will have **thick rind on CT**
   > May have contra-lateral infiltrate from aspiration
   Findings after pneumonectomy – lowering of air-fluid level on
   pneumonectomy side w/ new infiltrate on contra-lateral side (ie
   aspiration of the fluid, *classic*)
   Tx:
   > **1st step** place **chest tubes** - prevent contamination contralateral lung
   > **Place pt w/ affected side down**
   > **Bronch** to confirm Dx
   > **Broad spectrum abx's**
   > *If after lobectomy or spontaneous* →
   >> **Re-expand lung** (eg remove mucus plugs, VATS deloculation,
   >> CT drainage) → will likely heal
   >> **If organized empyema** → decortication or Eloesser flap
   > *If after pneumonectomy* → **Claggett procedure** (fills post-
   > pneumonectomy space w/ permanent abx solution + bronchus
   > coverage w/ intercostal muscle flap)
   > **High frequency ventilation** lowers airway pressures and may be
   > beneficial in pts w/ BPF

Hamartomas
MC benign adult lung tumor (represent 75% of all benign adult tumors)
10% of all solitary pulmonary nodules
Contain **fat, cartilage,** and **connective tissue** (eg muscle)
Calcifications can appear as **popcorn lesion** on chest CT
Dx: chest CT (can be diagnostic w/o need for Bx)
Do not require resection
Repeat chest CT in 3 months to confirm diagnosis

Upper airway tumors (trachea and main bronchi)
Children – 90% benign
    MC benign – hemangioma (usually resolves on its own)
    MC malignant – carcinoid
Adults – 90% malignant
    MC benign – papilloma (usually resolves on its own)
    MC malignant – SCCA (others-adenoid cystic, carcinoid, mucoepidermoid)

Carcinoid
    90% of bronchial gland tumors in adults
    Typical carcinoids (90%) – 5% mets; homogenous, 5-YS – 95%
    Atypical carcinoid (10%) – 50% mets; necrosis, disorganized, $\geq$ 1
        mitosis/2HPF, heterogenous, 5-YS – 50%
    Strongest RF for survival – atypical vs. typical
Adenoid cystic CA (cylindroma)
    Mucosa frequently intact
    Predilection to **peri-neural invasion**
    CA spread often **well beyond endoluminal component**
    **Very responsive to XRT
    Slow growing – can survive decades even w/ met's
    If you can't get complete rsxn – give XRT (very sensitive to XRT)
Mucoepidermoid CA – can be low or high grade
Bronchial gland tumors – carcinoid, mucoepidermoid and adenoid cystic CA
    MC slow growing and unusual to rare mets
Tx: resection (1 cm margin) for all if resectable primary and no distant mets

Trachea Complications
MC late Cx after tracheal surgery – granulation tissue formation
MC early Cx after tracheal surgery – laryngeal edema
    Tx: re-intubation, inhaled racemic epinephrine, steroids
Post-intubation stenosis
    MC at stoma site w/ tracheostomy; at balloon cuff site w/ ET tube
    May be able to treat w/ a few **serial dilatations** if mild
    Tracheal resection w/ end-to-end anastomosis if moderate or severe
    If emergent airway issue (severe stridor or resp difficulty), Dx and Tx –
        emergent rigid bronch, dilation, likely emergent tracheostomy
Tracheo-innominate artery fistula
    MC after tracheostomy
    Sx's: usually premonitory bleed, followed by no bleeding period, then
        massive hemorrhage (very lethal problem)
    Go to OR immediately if this is suspected
    Tx options (want to 1st control airway and 2nd stop bleeding):
        1) Blow-up trach balloon to see if it tamponades fistula or;
        2) Oral intubation + compress fistula w/ finger through trach hole or;
        3) Use rigid scope through mouth to push trach tube up against fistula
        After control of airway and bleeding →
            Median sternotomy
            Surgical ligation + partial innominate artery resection
                NO graft – will become infected
            Tracheal repair w/ strap muscle interposition between ligated
                innominate ends and trachea
            Very low stroke rate with this method
    This is avoided by keeping tracheostomy at **3rd tracheal ring or above**

Tracheo-esophageal fistula (generally in cervical portion of trachea)
  MC after tracheostomy
    Sx's: tracheal secretions that look like saliva **or** gastric distension if
      intubated; coughing w/ swallowing if extubated
    Dx: Bronch (*best test*) - pull tracheostomy tube or ETT back
      Usually a big hole 1-2 cm below tracheal stoma (balloon site)
    Tx: wait until extubated before repair (keep ET tube below fistula)
      Tracheal resection and re-anastomosis
      Primary repair esophagus; interpose strap muscle between
        esophagus and trachea so it does not recur

Want tracheostomy between the 2nd and 3rd tracheal rings
    Too high – vocal cord problems
    Too low – tracheo-innominate fistula

<u>**Hemoptysis with pulmonary artery catheter**</u>
  Main issue here is to get control of the airway *(pts die of asphyxiation*, <u>not</u>
    hemorrhage)
  Pull swan slightly back
  Increase PEEP which will help tamponade PA bleed
  Bronch (possibly rigid if in OR) and **mainstem intubate** non-affected side with
    single lumen tube and inflate balloon
  Keep bleeding side down
  Correct coagulation times
  T and S for 6 units of blood
  May need **lobectomy** (MC right lower lobe) if bleeding continues

<u>**Massive hemoptysis**</u> (> 600 cc / 24 hrs)
  Causes (US): **90% due to →**
      1) **TB** (MCC overall; bronchial arteries, pulmonary artery aneurysms)
      2) **Bronchiectasis** (MC from cystic fibrosis; dilated bronchial arteries)
      3) **Lung abscess** (bronchial arteries)
      Others – cyanotic congenital heart DZ, fungus ball, tumor, AVF
      MCC non-US → <u>infection</u> (MC mycetoma – chronic granuloma infection)
  MCC of death w/ massive hemoptysis – asphyxiation
  MC site of bleeding – high pressure <u>bronchial arteries</u>
  ***Pts die of asphyxiation*, <u>not</u> hemorrhage**
  Tx:
      Quick history – blood thinners, heart problems, lung problems
      Affected side down if known (prevent contralateral contamination)
      1st Emergent bronch (rigid)
          Clear blood to figure out which side the problem in on
          Place rigid bronch on **non-affected side, ventilate** through bronch
          Control bleeding on affected side – cold saline irrigation,
            epinephrine soaked gauzes, cautery, bronchial blockers
          Get to point of placing a **double lumen tube** or **mainstem single
            lumen tube** and **control of bleeding**
          Reverse anti-coagulation if on blood thinners
          Careful light sedation – inhalational anesthetic
          If still bleeding → mainstem intubate (or double lumen tube), pack
            bleeding side if pt tolerates, go to angio (see 2nd below)
      2nd bronchial arteriography + embolization
          (for TB, bronchiectasis, CA, uncorrectable cyanotic DZ)
      3rd PA angiography (< 10% need this, used if above does not find
          bleeding) and **embolization** – lung abscess, pulm AV malformations

  ***Almost <u>all</u> cases** of non-traumatic massive hemoptysis can be initially
      controlled w/o surgery
      Vast majority have **limited lung function** and **cannot tolerate resection**,
          makes angio + embolization preferred if bleeding not controlled in OR
      Exception → bleeding **carcinoid tumor** in o/w health pt – resect
      After angio, if W/U shows a resectable lesion in operable pt → resection

Lung Abscess
MCC – aspiration PNA
> **MC location** – superior segment of RLL; 2nd – posterior segment of RUL
> **MC organism** – staph aureus (usually polymicrobial)

RF's – ETOH
Dx: chest CT (*best test*)
Tx:
> **Abx's** → *main Tx for lung abscess, cures 95%*
> > **Therapeutic bronch** (to R/O obstruction and tumor; send BAL for
> > cultures and cytology – necrotic CA can present like this)
> > **Pulmonary Toilet + Nutritional support**
> > Clinical response usually within **2 weeks**
>
> **CT guided drainage** if the above fails
> **Surgery** if above fails or can't R/O necrotic CA (>6 cm, persistent after 6 wks)
> **Massive hemoptysis** or **rupture** into pleural space – **emergency lobectomy**
> > ****Key issue** - protection of contralateral lung from filling w/ blood or pus
> > *Pts die of asphyxiation*

Pleural effusions:
Exudative Effusion
> **Protein** > 3
> **Specific gravity** > 1.016
> **LDH ratio** (fluid:serum) > 0.6

Dx:
> **Thoracentesis + pleural Bx** – 80% accurate for diagnosis of problem
> causing effusion (Bad for mesothelioma)
> **VATS** – 95% accurate for diagnosis of problem causing effusion

Tx of recurrent pleural effusions → **VATS pleurodesis**
> Benign – mechanical pleurodesis
> Malignant – talc pleurodesis

Spontaneous Pneumothorax
Typical pt – tall, healthy, thin, young, males, smoking
Recurrence:

After 1st PTX	**20%**
After 2nd PTX	**60%**
After 3rd PTX	**80%**

Etiology – rupture of a **lung bleb**; MC in **upper lobe apex**; MC **right side**
Tx - chest tube
> **Surgery for:**
> > **Recurrence**
> > **Large blebs on CT scan**
> > **Air-leak > 7 days** despite 2 good chest tubes
> > **Non-reexpansion of lung** despite 2 good chest tubes
> > **Tension PTX**
> > **Bilateral PTX**
> > **Hemothorax**
> > **Previous pneumonectomy**
> > **High risk profession** → pilot, diver, mountain climber, or pts that live
> > in remote areas
>
> **Surgery** – thoracoscopy, blebectomy, and mechanical pleurodesis

Thoracic outlet syndrome (TOS)

Scalene triangle – anterior scalene, middle scalene, 1st rib

Subclavian vein is anterior to the anterior scalene

Subclavian artery + brachial plexus are between anterior and middle scalenes

Sx's:

Pain + paresthesias (present in 95%) in medial forearm and fingers; Also chest, shoulder, and neck

Motor weakness + atrophy of hypothenar muscles

Unable to use arm at work

Neurologic involvement – much more common than vascular

MC anatomic abnormality – cervical rib

MC cause of pain – brachial plexus irritation

Tinsel's test – tapping reproduces symptoms (neurogenic TOS)

Adson's test – ↓ radial pulse with head turned ipsilateral side

Subclavian artery compression – arterial TOS

Neurogenic (MC type)

Usually have **normal** neuro exam; sx's **worse w/ manipulation**

Dx:

1) **CXR** – look for cervical ribs, bony spurs, cervical space narrowing
2) **MRI** – look for cervical space narrowing (eg herniated disk, C5-C6)
3) **Nerve conduction velocity** (NCV)

Abnormal < 60 m/S at thoracic outlet

Path

MC nerve distribution – Ulnar Nerve (C8-T1)

Lower portion of brachial plexus

Weak 4th and 5th fingers; intrinsic muscles of hand

Weak wrist flexion

Triceps weakness and atrophy

Pain and paresthesias in medial forearm

Tx

Physiotherapy for 3 months *(all pts)*

Change jobs, PT, OT – *don't rush to operate on these pts*

If above fails and **NCV < 60 m/S →** **1st rib resection**, cervical rib resection if present, anterior and middle scalenes divided

Arterial (Subclavian Artery)

Compression usually secondary to **anterior scalene hypertrophy**

Can get **aneurysms** or **acute occlusion** (No pulse, arm **white + cold**)

Adson's, hyper-abduction, costoclavicular tests – all result in loss of radial pulse; hand cold and pale

Dx: angio

Tx

Emergent

Threatened (loss of sensation and motor) – brachial artery dissection and fogarty, 1st rib resection; may need prosthetic bypass

Non-threatened (intact motor and sensation) – catheter directed intra-arterial thrombolytics

Non-emergent

1st rib and cervical rib resection; possible bypass graft if artery too damaged or aneurysm present

Venous (Subclavian Vein; Paget Von Schrotter's)

Sx's: usually presents as **effort-induced thrombosis of subclavian vein** (eg baseball pitchers, excessive use of arm)

Arm **acutely swollen** and **blue**

Venous thrombosis – much more common than arterial

Dx: Duplex U/S (*venogram is Gold Standard but takes too long*)

Tx:

Acute occlusion – TPA 1st (intra-vein directed lysis of clot), heparin, then 1st rib resection during that hospital admission

Surgical approach
>   **Trans-axillary approach** – good for neurogenic and venous
>   **Supra-clavicular approach** – good for arterial
>   **Phrenic nerve** crosses anterior scalene from **lateral to medial**
>   **Long thoracic nerve** is posterior to middle scalene
>   **The scalene muscles** originate from **C2-C6 transverse processes**
>>   Anterior and middle scalenes insert on **1st rib**
>>   Posterior scalene inserts on **2nd rib**
>   **The thoracic duct** ascends into the scalene triangle before inserting into
>   the subclavian-IJ junction (can be injured w/ dissection)
> **Surgery 70-80% successful for neurogenic TOS**
>>   Much better success rate for arterial / venous
> **Recurrence** (1%) – either 1st rib was only partially resected and still have
>   compression or you took 2nd rib by mistake
> **Recurrence operation** – posterior high thoracoplasty

Solitary Pulmonary Nodule (coin lesion)
> **Definition, need all:**
>>   1) **Single**
>>   2) **< 3 cm**
>>   3) **Surrounded by normal lung**
>>   4) **No adenopathy**
>>   5) **No pleural effusion**
>>   *If does not meet solitary pulmonary nodule criteria – W/U as lung CA*

> → **Observation criteria:**
>>   1) Needs to meet definition of **solitary pulmonary nodule** above *and*
>>   2) **Low risk** - (place into general low, intermediate, and high risk groups)
>>>   Age < 45
>>>   Never smoked or quit > 7 years ago
>>>   Smooth lesion
>>>   Size < 1.5 cm
>>>   Popcorn calcification (hamartoma) or laminated calcification
>>>   (granuloma)
>>>   No change on CXR in 2 years if previous CXR available
>>>   ****Above are general criteria for low risk*
>>   **If following, need serial chest CTs** (q3 mos x 4, then Q6 mos x 2, shared
>>   decision w/ pt)

> → **Tissue Dx** if fails to meet **observation criteria** (eg intermediate, high risk)
>>   1) **Intermediate risk** (general criteria - age 45-60, size 1.5-2.2 cm,
>>   scalloped, current smoker or quit < 7 years ago)
>>   **Dx:**
>>>   **Trans-pleural** or **trans-bronchial needle Bx** (95% accurate for
>>>   Dx: trans-pleural Cx's → 10% PTX, 1% chest tube rate)
>>>   **VATS wedge resection** if above non-diagnostic or not
>>>   accessible to above
>>>   If Bx is diagnostic, still need to follow the lesion as above w/
>>>   serial CT scans, VATS wedge resection if any change
>>   2) **High risk** (age > 60, size > 2.2 cm, spiculated, current smoker)
>>   **Dx:**
>>>   **VATS wedge resection** if pt can tolerate (avoids 1% false
>>>   negative rate w/ needle Bx from sampling error – ie Bx
>>>   shows granuloma but scar contains focus of CA)

Overall 5-10% are malignant
>   Age < 50   < 5% malignant
>   Age > 50   > 50% malignant
>   **MC lesion overall** – granuloma (histoplasmosis MC, cocci, TB)
>   **MC tumor overall** – hamartoma (benign, 10% of all cases)
>   **MC malignant tumor** – bronchogenic CA (MC adenocarcinoma)
>>   **#2 mets** (breast CA MC)

Lung cancer

MC CA related death in US

> Risk proportional to smoking pack-years (biggest RF)
>
> Risk ↓s after quitting smoking but not back to baseline

Sx's:

> **Asymptomatic** (10%)
>
> **Cough, hemoptysis, wheezing** – suggests endobronchial central tumor
>
> **Chest pain**
>
> **Dyspnea** – pleural effusion or lung collapse
>
> **Pancoast Syndrome** (T4) – tumor invades apex of chest wall (superior sulcus) and pts have **Horner's syndrome** (invasion of sympathetic chain → ptosis, miosis, anhidrosis) and/or **ulnar** nerve sx's
>
> **Superior vena cava syndrome** – SVC compression from tumor (MC from involved nodes, can be from primary); HA, facial swelling, dyspnea

Path

> **MC type** – Adenocarcinoma (not squamous)
>
> **Nodal involvement** has strongest influence on survival in pts devoid of systemic mets
>
> **MC site of mets** – brain
>
> > **Resection of solitary brain met** → 5-YS 20%
>
> **Left sided tumors** have increased N3 rate
>
> **Overall 5-YS rate** – 10% (35% w/ rsxn for cure)
>
> 80% of recurrences occur within 1-2 yrs (MC w/ diffuse mets)
>
> **Small cell lung CA** – vast majority not resectable due to early spread

Dx and Evaluation for operability (for non-small cell CA, NSCC):

> 1) **CXR**
>
> > **Bloody pleural effusion** = malignant pleural effusion if known CA
> >
> > **Non-bloody pleural effusion** – send to cytology
>
> 2) **Chest/abd/pelvic CT**
>
> > Assess **primary lesion** and for **adenopathy** + **mets** (liver + adrenals)
> >
> > **Chest MRI** – best for assessing spinal cord invasion and superior sulcus tumors
> >
> > **Head MRI** – only if symptomatic (headaches)
> >
> > **Bone scan** – for bone pain or elevated alk phos
>
> 3) **Bronchoscopy** (mandatory w/ central tumors), brush + wash cytology
>
> 4) **Labs** – LFTs (liver mets)
>
> 5) **PET scan** (PET-CT most sensitive) – looking for mets
>
> > 5-10% **false positive rate** (inflammatory DZ)
> >
> > 5-10% **false negative rate** (bronchoalveolar CA, carcinoid)
>
> 6) **Assess patient operability**
>
> > **EKG** and **stress test** (if necessary)
> >
> > **PFT's, ABG,** and **DLCO**
> >
> > **Criteria used for lung resection include:**
> >
> > > Predicted post-op FEV-1 > 800 cc ($\geq$ 40% predicted)
> > >
> > > Pre-op DLCO > 10-12 ml/min/mmHg ($\geq$ 50% predicted)
> > >
> > > pO_2 > 60 mmHg (room air)
> > >
> > > pCO_2 < 45 mmHg
> > >
> > > VO2 max > 10-12 ml/min/kg (maximal exercise oxygen consumption)
> >
> > **Methods to improve pulmonary function pre-op include:**
> >
> > > **Albuterol/Atrovent inhalers** for wheezing
> > >
> > > **Abx's** for wet cough (amoxicillin/clavulanic acid)
> > >
> > > **D/C smoking**
> > >
> > > **Incentive spirometry** (send home w/ pt pre-op to practice)
> > >
> > > **Pulmonary rehab before operation** (chest PT; work of breathing exercises)
> >
> > **PA catheter, a-line,** and **foley** intra-op to minimize volume overload
> >
> > **Epidural catheters** are very effective after thoracotomy to control post-op pain and improve breathing dynamics

If w/u reveals suspected **mets**
→ need **Tissue dx** of suspected mets; if negative, proceed below
If w/u reveals **mediastinal adenopathy** (> 1.0 cm) or a **central mass** –
→ perform **Mediastinoscopy**
Assesses **ipsilateral** (N2) and **contralateral** (N3) **mediastinal nodes** – If positive, tumor unresectable
Looking into **middle mediastinum** w/ mediastinoscopy
Left-sided structures – RLN, esophagus, aorta, main PA
Right-sided structures – azygous and SVC
Anterior – innominate vein, innominate artery, right PA
If w/u reveals **para-aortic** or **AP** (aorto-pulmonary) **window adenopathy**
→ Perform **Chamberlain** (go through left 2nd rib cartilage) or VATS
Mediastinoscopy does not assess AP window nodes
If w/u reveals **supra-clavicular or scalene adenopathy** → **FNA** of node

No mets or **adenopathy** (or adenopathy is negative for tumor after Bx):
Some may want to **perform trans-thoracic or trans-bronchial needle biopsy** to get tissue diagnosis before going to OR:
Bx → **Lung CA** – proceed w/ resection
Bx → **Indeterminant** – proceed w/ resection
Bx → **Benign** but CT **suspicious for CA**–proceed w/ resection
Bx → **Benign** and **meets criteria for following a solitary pulmonary nodule** – can follow (see above)

Staging
Primary
TX cannot be evaluated
T0 – no evidence of primary tumor; (eg have met but can't find primary)
T1 (resectable)
< 3 cm, surrounded by **lung,** and **no invasion of main bronchus**
Also superficial tumors of main bronchus (limited to bronchial wall)
T2 (resectable)
> 3 cm or:
Invasion of **visceral pleura** or:
Atelectasis or PNA not involving whole lung or:
Main bronchial tumors ≥ **2 cm away from carina** (or invasion of bronchus intermedius)
T3 (resectable)
Direct invasion of **chest wall** (superior sulcus tumors), **diaphragm, mediastinal pleura** or **pericardium** (No extension into heart, great vessels (intrapericardial), trachea, esophagus, vertebral body or brachial plexus) or:
Main bronchial tumors **within 2 cm of carina** or:
Atelectasis or PNA involving the **whole lung**
T4 (usually considered unresectable)
Invasion of mediastinum, heart, trachea, esophagus, vertebra, neural foramina, carina, brachial plexus, SVC, subclavian artery, subclavian vein, aorta, or intra-pericardial PA or:
Malignant pleural or pericardial effusion or:
Satellite tumor nodules involving same lobe (different lobe is M1)
Nodes
N1 (resectable) – ipsilateral peri-bronchial or hilar
N2 (unresectable) – ipsilateral mediastinal or carinal
Esophageal and inferior pulm ligament; AP window and peri-aortic
N3 (unresectable) – contralateral mediastinal or hilar
supraclavicular or scalene nodes
Mets – M0 or M1 (MX – cannot assess)
Distant organ or lymph node (excludes supraclavicular and scalene LN which are N3 and Stage IIIB)
2nd lung CA not in primary lobe

Stage
> **Stage 0** – CIS
> **Stage I**
>> IA – T1,N0,M0
>> IB – T2,N0,M0
> **Stage II**
>> IIA – T1,N1,M0
>> IIB – T2,N1,M0 or T3,N0,M0
> **Stage III**
>> IIIA – T3,N1,M0, T1-3,N2,M0
>> IIIB – any T4 or N3
> **Stage IV** – M

Tx:

Stages I and II
> **Formal lung resection** (lobectomy or pneumonectomy)
>> If you don't have CA diagnosis → **wedge resection 1st**
> **Mediastinal lymph node dissection** (can skip if mediastinoscopy done)
> **Adjuvant chemo – carboplatin + paclitaxel** (<u>not</u> stage Ia)
>> Cisplatin + pemetrexed can be used for lung SCCA
> Stage I tumor in pt that cannot tolerate resection – potentially curable w/
>> just XRT

Stage III
> **IIIA** (some resectable)
>> **T3,N1,M0** – resectable, usually **neoadjuvant chemo-XRT**
>>> **Neoadjuvant chemo-XRT** can convert non-resectable into
>>>> resectable (shrinks primary, eg superior sulcus tumors)
>> **N2** – *unresectable*
>> **Chest wall invasion** – still resectable, use **PTFE for reconstruction**
>>> Posterior defects up to 10 cm require no chest wall
>>>> reconstruction (scapula covers it)
>>> Anterior defects up to 5 cm require no chest wall reconstruction
>> **Resectable** – diaphragm, pericardium, or mediastinal pleura invasion
> **IIIB** (usually unresectable)
>> **T4 tumors** (IIIB, usually unresectable)
>>> 20% 5-YS, often need **pneumonectomy**
>>> Should <u>not</u> have N2 DZ if contemplating resection
>>> Examples of resectable T4 tumors:
>>>> 2 primaries in same lobe
>>>> Minor heart invasion (pulmonary vein within pericardium
>>>>> or pulmonary artery)
>>>> Carinal or tracheal invasion
>>>> Cortical bone invasion (not calcenous bone), Dx - MRI
>>>> Subclavian artery/vein (as long as you can re-construct it)
>> **N3** – *unresectable*

Stage IV
> **Palliative chemo-XRT** usual (primary and mets)
> **Malignant pleural effusion** – talc pleurodesis (try bedside 1st, only 5 gm of
>> talc/side, one side per day); only Tx if symptomatic
> **Solitary brain met and o/w resectable lung CA** – surgical resection of
>> brain lesion 1st, lung resection, then chemo-XRT w/ whole brain XRT
> **5-YS after resection for cure** – 35%
> **XRT** – ↓s local recurrence; painful mets; no change in survival
> **Chemo-XRT** does not change 5-YS

Special Issues
- **Superior vena cava syndrome** (MCC SVC syndrome→ non-small cell lung CA)
  - **90% due to malignancy** (lung CA, lymphoma, germ cell tumors)
  - **MC benign cause** – mediastinal fibrosis (chronic problem)
  - **Sx's:** head and neck fullness, dyspnea, dizziness
  - **Tx: emergent XRT** (*best Tx:* effect in 12 hrs; raise head, O2, lasix, steroid)
  - **Chronic** (Non-CA source or slow growing CA) → **PTA + stent** to SVC
    - Other options – vascular reconstruction
- **Pancoast tumors** (superior sulcus tumors)
  - **Horner's Syndrome w/o gross mediastinal invasion or N2 DZ** -
    - neoadjuvant chemo-XRT, followed by resection
  - **Ulnar nerve sx's w/o N2 DZ** – can resect if just involvement of lower nerve roots (give neoadjuvant chemo-XRT 1st)
- **Paraneoplastic syndromes**
  - **Squamous cell CA** – PTH-related peptide
  - **Small cell CA** – ACTH, ADH
    - **MC paraneoplastic syndrome** – small cell ACTH
  - **Clubbing** – squamous and adenocarcinoma
  - **Hypertrophic pulmonary osteoarthropathy** (symmetric polyarthritis and proliferative periostitis of long bones) – adenocarcinoma
  - **Eaton Lambert** (peripheral neuropathy, cerebellar degeneration, weakness and fatigue) – small cell
- **Mesothelioma**
  - **RFs** – asbestos exposure (↑s risk 90x), males
  - **Most malignant thoracic tumor**
  - Aggressive local invasion, nodal invasion, and distant mets common
  - Takes 30 years to develop after exposure. Median survival after Dx - 1 year
- **Cell types**
  - **Non-small cell CA (NSCC)** – 80%
    - **Adenocarcinoma** (MC overall) – usually peripheral, gland formation
    - **Squamous cell CA** – usually central, necrosis, often obstructive PNA or bloody sputum, stratified squamous epithelium, keratin pearls
    - **Bronchoalveolar** – can look like pneumonia
  - **Small Cell** (neuroendocrine, Kulchitsky cells) – 20%
    - Usually **central**
    - Usually **unresectable** at time of dx (<5 % candidates for surgery)
    - Often **mets to mediastinum**, median survival 1-2 years
    - Surgery only for T1N0M0 - 5-YS 50% w/ stage I
    - **Chemo main tx:** Cisplatin and etoposide; add XRT for limited stage
    - **Prophylactic cranial XRT** ↑s median survival for limited stage DZ

- **Mets to lung** → if isolated may be resected for colon, renal cell CA, sarcoma, melanoma, ovarian, or endometrial CA
- In case of primary cancer with a resectable lung metastasis, MC take out primary 1st, then metastasis (in general metastases don't metastasize).
- **Solitary pulmonary nodule w/ PMHx of a previous cancer** (> 2 years):
  - **Sarcoma** or **melanoma** → nodule more likely mets
  - **Head, neck,** or **breast CA** → nodule more likely primary lung CA
  - **GI or GU CA**→ even chance for mets or new primary lung CA

Mediastinum
- **Normal Structures**
  - **Anterior** – thymus
  - **Middle** – heart, great vessels, phrenic and vagus nerves, trachea and main bronchi, SVC, IVC
  - **Posterior** – esophagus, descending aorta, vertebral bodies, thoracic duct, azygous vein, hemi-azygous
- **Mediastinal mass sx's** (any location can cause these sx's)
  - **Often asymptomatic**
  - **Respiratory insufficiency** (MC Sx), chest pain, and dysphagia
- **Tumors**

25% of mediastinal masses are **malignant**
Symptomatic (60%) more likely **malignant**
Asymptomatic (40%) more likely **benign**
MC mediastinal tumor in adults and **children**– neurogenic (MC posterior)
MC location for mediastinal tumor in adults and **children** – anterior
Adult solitary mediastinal mass

MC mediastinal overall	**neurogenic**
MC anterior	thymoma*
MC middle	cyst
MC posterior	neurogenic

Children solitary mediastinal mass

MC mediastinal overall	**neurogenic**
MC anterior	germ cell*
MC middle	cyst
MC posterior	neurogenic

Anterior (T's) – Thyroid, parathyroid, T-cell lymphoma, Thymoma,
Teratoma (and other germ cell), cystic hygroma
Middle – cysts (bronchogenic and pericardial), lymphoma, teratoma
Posterior – neurogenic, lymphoma, enteric duplication cysts
Thymoma (see Anesthesia chp for tx of myasthenia gravis)
All thymomas need resection
Thymus too big or associated w/ refractory myasthenia gravis→ resection
50% of thymomas are **malignant**
Epithelial type **worse prognosis**
50% of pts w/ thymomas are **symptomatic** (*almost never SVC syndrome*)
50% of pts w/ thymomas have **myasthenia gravis**.
10% of pts w/ myasthenia gravis have **thymomas**.
Children *almost never* get thymomas
Lymphoma (MCC mediastinal **adenopathy**)
NHL (MC lymphoma in mediastinum) and **Hodgkin's lymphoma**
Tx: (see Skin and Soft Tissue chp)
Germ cell tumors
Teratoma
MC germ cell tumor in mediastinum
Benign tumors are <u>marker negative</u>
Tx: resection; chemotherapy if malignant
Seminoma
MC primary malignant germ cell tumor in mediastinum
10% have beta-HCG
Tx: *XRT* (*primary Tx:* extremely sensitive); chemo for positive nodes
or residual disease; surgery for residual disease after that
Non-seminoma
90% have elevated **beta-HCG** and **alpha-fetoprotein** (AFP)
Tx: *cisplatin-based chemo* (*primary Tx*) and XRT
Surgery for residual disease after above
Chemo – **cisplatin, bleomycin,** and **etoposide** (for both seminoma and
non-seminoma)
LDH – independent prognostic value for malignant germ cell tumors

Cysts
Bronchogenic Cysts + Enteric Cysts – posterior to carina, Tx: resection
Can get infected and small malignancy risk
Pericardial Cyst– usually at right costophrenic angle, Tx: leave (no CA risk)
Neurogenic tumors – have pain, neurologic deficit. Tx: resection
10% have intra-spinal involvement requiring spinal surgery
Neurolemma (schwannoma, nerve sheath) – MC
Neurofibroma (nerve sheath) – assoc. w/ von Recklinghausen's disease
Can also get:
Ganglioneuroma (benign)
Ganglioneuroblastoma (malignant, children)
Neuroblastoma (very malignant, children, see Ped. Surgery chp)
<u>**Chylothorax**</u>

Milky white fluid – sudan red stains the TAG's
Has ↑ lymphocytes and TAGs (>110 ml/μl) - *Fluid is <u>resistant</u> to infection*
50% secondary to **trauma** or **iatrogenic injury**
50% secondary to **tumor** (MC – lymphoma, tumor burden in lymphatics)
Injury above T5–6 – left-sided chylothorax.
Injury below T5–6 – in right-sided chylothorax
**Thoracic duct crosses mediastinum at T5-6
Tx:

- 1-3 weeks of conservative Tx → chest tube, NPO TPN, octreotide
  1) If above fails, surgery w/ **ligation of thoracic duct** on right side low in mediastinum (80% successful) if secondary to **trauma or iatrogenic** injury (ligate area between esophagus and vertebral bodies)
  2) If above fails for **malignant causes of chylothorax** (lymphoma MC), perform mechanical or talc **pleurodesis** (less successful than above)

Scalene LN Bx
Borders of scalene triangle
Sternocleidomastoid anterior and Trapezius posterior
Subclavian vein inferior, Internal jugular medial, Omohyoid superior
Phrenic nerve and thoracic duct can be injured
Phrenic nerve – anterior to anterior scalene muscle
Long thoracic nerve – posterior to middle scalene muscle
Thoracic duct – travels in neck before subclavian vein insertion

Other conditions
Tension PTX – MCC of arrest after blunt trauma; impairs venous return
Catamenial PTX – occurs in temporal relation to menstrual cycle
Endometrial implants in the visceral lung pleura
Tx: **VATS resection** of endometrial implants + pleurodesis
Leuprolide (GnRH agonist) if too many or can't be found
Residual hemothorax despite 2 good chest tubes → OR for thoracoscopic drainage (need to prevent fibrothorax)
Clotted hemothorax – surgical drainage if 1) > 25% of lung, 2) there are air-fluid levels, <u>or</u> 3) sx's of infection (fever, ↑ WBCs)
Surgery in 1st week to avoid peel
Broncholiths – usually secondary to chronic granuloma (MCC – histoplasmosis)
Histoplasmosis infects lymph node, becomes calcified w/ time, then forms broncholith (erodes into bronchus)
Tx: thoracotomy and resection
Mediastinitis – MC occurs after cardiac surgery
White-out on chest x-ray →
Midline shift toward whiteout –likely collapse → need bronchoscopy to remove plug
No shift – CT scan to figure it out
Midline shift away from whiteout – likely effusion → place chest tube
Bronchiectasis – acquired from infection or tumor (MCC - **cystic fibrosis**)
Diffuse nature prevents surgery in most
Massive bleeding can occur (see Massive hemoptysis above)
Tuberculosis – lung apices; get calcifications, caseating granulomas
Gohn complex = parenchymal lesion + enlarged hilar nodes
Tx: INH, rifampin, pyrazinamide, streptomycin, ethambutol
Sarcoidosis – has non-caseating granulomas
Airway fires – MC associated with the laser and catching ET tube on fire
Tx: stop gas flow, remove ET tube, re-intubate for 24 hours; bronchoscopy
Pulmonary AVMs – between pulmonary arteries and pulmonary veins
MC site – lower lobes
Sx's: hemoptysis and SOB
Tx: embolization
Can occur w/ **Osler-Weber-Rendu Syndrome** (pulmonary AVMs + teleangiectasias → each can bleed; **MC sx** - epistaxis)
Chest wall tumors
MC Benign – osteochondroma; **MC Malignant** – chondrosarcoma

CARDIAC

Congenital heart disease
In utero circulation
Ductus arteriosus – connection between descending aorta and left
pulmonary artery (PA); blood shunted away from lungs
Ductus venosum – connection between portal vein and IVC
Blood shunted away from liver
Fetal circulation to placenta – 2 umbilical arteries
Fetal circulation from placenta – 1 umbilical vein

1) L→R shunts cause CHF
Sx's: 1st sign- **hepatomegaly**, others - failure to thrive (FTT), tachycardia,
tachypnea, recurrent pulmonary infections (from pulm edema)
L→R shunts
VSD *(MC congenital heart lesion)*
ASD
PDA
Initial Tx for CHF – Lasix + Digoxin; ACE inhibitor for afterload reduction

2) R→L shunts cause cyanosis
Children squat to ↑ SVRI and decrease R→L shunts (more blood to lungs)
Cyanosis cx's – polycythemia, strokes, brain abscess, endocarditis,
chronic cyanotic heart DZ
R→L shunts (T's)
Tetralogy of Fallot (MC cyanotic congenital heart lesion)
Transposition of the great vessels
Truncus arteriosus
Tricuspid atresia
Initial Tx of cyanosis – ensure appropriate **blood mixing** (of oxygenated
and de-oxygenated blood); **If severe cyanosis →**
1) **PGE**-1 keeps ductus arteriosus open (PA mixing) *or*;
2) **Balloon atrial septostomy** (mixing at atrial level)
Eisenmenger's syndrome – shunt shifts from L→R to R→L
Sign of ↑ing pulmonary vascular resistance (PVR)→ pulmonary HTN
This condition is generally *irreversible*

Ventricular septal defect (VSD)
MC congenital heart defect
L→R shunt
80% close spontaneously by age 1 year
Large VSD – usually cause sx's after 4–6 weeks of life; PVR ↓s, shunt ↑s
Sx's: CHF (FTT, ↑ HR, ↑ RR)
Medical Tx: Lasix, Digoxin and ACE inhibitor
Timing of repair
Large VSDs (shunt > 2.5) – *1 year*
Medium VSDs (shunt 2-2.5) – 5 years
Small VSDs usually left alone
Earlier repair if sx's not controlled w/ medical tx
FTT – MC reason for early repair
PVR > 8 Woods units contraindication for repair → use vasodilators
to see if it's reversible; if so, can repair

Atrial septal defect (ASD)
L→R shunt
90% close spontaneously by age 1 year
Ostium secundum (MC ASD) – centrally located, patent foramen ovale
Ostium primum (or atrioventricular septal defects or endocardial cushion
defects); associated w/ Downs Syndrome and mitral valve defects
Usually get sx's when shunt (Qp/Qs) >2 → CHF
Rare for ASD to ↑ PVR before adulthood
Can get paradoxical emboli and arrhythmias in adulthood
Medical Tx: Lasix, Digoxin and ACE inhibitor
Timing of repair (Ostium secundum and ostium primum) – *1-2 years*
Earlier if Sx's not controlled w/ medical tx
PVR > 8 Woods units contraindication for repair → use vasodilators
to see if it's reversible; if so, can repair

Patent ductus arteriosus (PDA)

> **L→R shunt**
> **Causes CHF**
> **Tx: Indomethacin** – closes PDA, rarely successful after neonatal period
> Requires **surgical ligation** through left thoracotomy if persists
> PGE-1 (ie prostaglandin)– keeps PDA open (used to tx congenital lesions
> w/ R→L shunt or if left ventricle not working well)

Tetralogy of Fallot

> *MC cyanotic congenital heart defect*
> **R→L shunt**
> **4 anomalies** – VSD, pulmonary stenosis, overriding aorta, right ventricular
> (RV) hypertrophy
> **Sx's: Tet spells** (cyanosis – child then squats to ↑ SVR and ↑ blood flow
> to lung – essentially ↓s blood flow through VSD)
> **Morphologic abnormality** – anterior displacement of infundibular septum
> **Medical Tx:** beta-blocker
> **Definitive repair:** RV outflow tract obstruction division, patch enlargement
> of outflow tract, and VSD repair
> Blalock-Taussig (BT) shunt can be used for palliation to delay repair
> **Timing of operation:** 3-6 months (earlier if ↑ cyanosis)

Transposition of the great vessels

> **R→L shunt**
> Mixing usually occurs through **ASD**
> **Medical Tx:** aimed at allowing appropriate mixing
> > 1) **Balloon atrial septostomy** (to allow mixing at atrial level)
> > 2) **PGE$_1$** (keeps PDA open and allows mixing)
> **Repair** – arterial switch with coronary re-implantation
> **Timing of repair**
> > **No VSD** – 1st 1-2 weeks
> > **VSD** – 1st 1-2 months

Truncus arteriosus

> **R→L shunt**
> Aorta and pulmonary artery form 1 vessel (LV + RV both eject into truncus)
> **Sx's:** CHF, has VSD that allows mixing
> **Medical Tx:** diuretics, Digoxin, fluid restriction, afterload reduction
> **Repair** – VSD closure, remove pulmonary arteries from aorta, and repair
> aorta; restore RV outflow tract w/ Dacron graft to pulmonary arteries
> **Timing of repair:** neonatal period

Tricuspid atresia (Univentricular heart)

> **R→ L shunt**
> Need eventual **Fontan procedure** to direct all vena cava blood to the PA
> Right atrium and SVC connected to PA directly (bypasses right ventricle)
> **Prerequisites** – nl. PA pressure (< 20 mmHg) + nl. PVR (< 4 Woods units)

Hypoplastic left heart

> Need **Norwood procedure**
> Main PA becomes the single outflow from the heart for what is to become
> single-ventricle physiology.
> Tx: Aorta is augmented w/ large piece of allograft artery and attached to
> main PA trunk
> Distal pulmonary arteries are separated and supplied through
> systemic-PA shunt (BT shunt).
> Palliative procedure - eventually need heart TXP

Vascular rings – double aortic arch most common

> May manifest as recurrent pulmonary infections or dysphagia
> Trachea most commonly affected
> Tx: divide smaller arch through left thoracotomy

Coarctation of the aorta

> MC occurs just **distal to the left subclavian artery**
> Associated w/ Turner's syndrome
> Rib notching from the IMA and intercostal collaterals
> Can present with profound CHF
> All pts should undergo repair to prevent CHF; Tx: rsxn and re-anastomosis

Coronary artery disease

MCC of death in US

RFs – smoking, HTN, males, family history, hyperlipidemia, diabetes

Medical Tx – nitrates, smoking cessation, weight loss, statin drugs, ASA

Anatomy

> **Right dominant circulation** (MC) – posterior descending artery comes off the right coronary artery
>
> **Left dominant circulation** (10%) – posterior descending artery comes off the circumflex coronary artery
>
> **Left main coronary artery** branches into left anterior descending and circumflex
>
> Most atherosclerotic lesions are **proximal**

Revascularization

> **PTCA and stent** – 90% patency at 1 year
>
> **Saphenous vein graft** – 80% 5-year patency
>
> **Internal mammary artery** (IMA) – off subclavian arteries
>
> > _Best conduit for CABG_ – 90% 20-year patency rate

CABG procedure

> **Potassium** and **cold** solution **cardioplegia**
>
> > Causes **arrest of heart** in diastole
> >
> > Keeps heart **protected** and **still** while grafts are placed
>
> **Indications** (stenosis needs to be ≥ 70%)
>
> > Left main disease
> >
> > Left main equivalent (LAD and proximal circumflex)
> >
> > 3-vessel disease
> >
> > 2-vessel disease w/ proximal LAD stenosis and either:
> >
> > > LVEF <50% _or;_
> > >
> > > Extensive ischemia on noninvasive imaging study
> >
> > 1- or 2-vessel disease with:
> >
> > > Large area of viable myocardium and high-risk criteria on noninvasive testing _or_
> > >
> > > Unstable angina, life threatening arrhythmias, or ongoing ischemia despite maximal nonsurgical therapy

High mortality RFs: <u>pre-op cardiogenic shock</u> (#1), emergency surgery, age, reoperation, and low EF

Allen's Test - test for adequate ulnar artery flow when considering use of radial artery for grafting; palmar blanch should occur within 7 sec of ulnar release

Mechanical complications from myocardial infarction

MC occur **3-7 days after myocardial infarction**

Sx's: hypotension 3-7 d after MI, if VSR or acute MR have new systolic murmur

DDx:

> 1. **Ventricular septal rupture** (VSR, holo-systolic murmur heard best at right sternal border)
> 2. **Papillary muscle rupture** [causes acute mitral regurgitation (MR), holo-systolic murmur heard best in axilla]
> 3. **Free wall rupture** (usually quickly fatal)

Dx:

> **ECHO** – best for DDx VSR vs. papillary muscle rupture
>
> **PA catheter** – **step-up in oxygen content** between right atrium and pulmonary artery secondary to L→R shunt will occur w/ VSR (not w/ papillary muscle rupture and acute MR)

Tx:

> **Intra-aortic balloon pumps** (IABP) have ↑ed survival for VSR and acute MR due to acute papillary muscle rupture following MI
>
> **VSR Tx** – patch
>
> **Papillary muscle rupture Tx** – replace valve
>
> **Free wall rupture Tx** – patch
>
> **LV aneurysm**
>
> > MC occurs late after large, transmural, anterior MI
> >
> > **Sx's**: CHF, arrhythmias, angina
> >
> > **Indications for surgery**: refractory sx's

<u>Valve disease</u>
Aortic stenosis
MC valve lesion

MCC – calcification of aortic valve (RFs – age, bicuspid aortic valve)

Path

Adequate CO and normal pressures maintained until late in disease

Eventually, LV (left ventricle) hypertrophy leads to ↓ compliance and pulmonary congestion; LV failure ultimately develops

Cardinal sx's:

Angina	5 year mean survival
Syncope	3 year mean survival
Dyspnea at rest (from heart failure)	2 year mean survival

Valve area < 1.0 cm^2 – considered severe

Indications for operation (only for severe AS):

1) **Symptomatic AS** or:

2) **Asymptomatic AS** and **valve area < 0.6 cm2**

Aortic insufficiency

MCC – annulo-aortic ectasia (aortic root dilatation makes valve incompetent)

Path

LV becomes dilated, wall tension ↑ (law of LaPlace)

LV failure eventually occurs

Indications for operation (only for severe AI)

1) **Symptomatic AI** (heart failure or angina not due to CAD) <u>*or*</u>

2) **Asymptomatic AI** w/ either:

EF < 50% *or*

LV dilatation (LV end diastolic dimension > 70 mm) *or*

Aortic root dilatation ($\geq$ 4.5)

Mitral stenosis

MCC – rheumatic fever

Leads to **pulmonary congestion;** atrial fibrillation common

High risk for **mural thrombi** – 50% go to cerebral circulation

These pts usually undergo **balloon commissurotomy** at least once before contemplating surgery

Indication for operation (only for severe MS) – symptomatic severe MS

Mitral regurgitation

MCC – myxomatous degeneration (ie mitral valve prolapse)

Path

LV becomes dilated, wall tension ↑s

Left atrium becomes less compliant → pulmonary congestion ensues, can lead to right-sided heart failure

Atrial fibrillation common

Indications for operation (only for severe MR)

1) **Symptomatic** ($\geq$ NYHA class II) <u>*or*</u>

2) **Asymptomatic** w/ either:

EF < 60% *or*

LV dilatation (end systolic dimension > 45 mm) *or*

Pulm HTN (PA systolic > 50) *or*

Atrial fibrillation

Tissue valves (do not require anticoagulation)

For pts who want pregnancy, have contraindication to anticoagulation, are older and unlikely to require another valve in their lifetime (age > 65), or have frequent falls

Not as durable as mechanical valves

Rapid calcification in **children** and **young pts occurs,** use of tissue valves is *contraindicated* in these populations

Chronic renal dialysis is also a relative contraindication (↑ed calcification)

Endocarditis

Sx's: fever (MC sx), chills, sweats; CHF; stroke
RFs – IVDA, indwelling catheters, dental procedures, HD, DM, abnormal valve
Dx studies
- **EKG** – look for conduction deficits (PR interval)
- **CXR** – look for heart failure
- **ECHO** – assess leakage, look for vegetations, abscess, LV function
- **Cardiac cath** if over 35 if considering surgery
- **Labs** – ↑ WBCs, blood cultures
- **Intubated** – get a head CT to R/O septic embolus

Dx Criteria for endocarditis (2 major, 1 major and 2 minor, or 3 minor)
- **Major criteria:**
  1) **Positive blood culture**
  2) **Positive ECHO finding** (vegetation, abscess, new regurgitation)
- **Minor criteria**
  1) New or changing **murmur**
  2) **Vascular sx's** – embolism, Janeway lesions (hemorrhagic, non-tender septic emboli to palms and soles), mycotic aneurysm
  3) **Progressive CHF**
  4) **Fever** (MC sx, 95%) – usually 1-2 hours after peak bacteremia
  5) **Predisposing RF** (see above)
  6) **Immune Sign** – **Osler's nodes** (tender nodes on pad of digits)
     Roth's spots (retinal hemorrhages)
- **Negative cultures ↑ed w/** PVE, previous abx's, mycoplasma, chlamydia

Path
- **MC organism overall** – strep bovis
  - **MC acute endocarditis** – staph
  - **MC chronic endocarditis** – strep bovis
- **MC on left side** except **IV drug abusers** (IVDA)
- **MC site overall** – aortic valve
- **MC iatrogenic organism** - staph (dialysis pts; sclerotic valves; MC left side)
- **MC IVDA organism** – pseudomonas; 50% TV

Initial Tx:
- Get **blood cultures** before Abx's
- **Vancomycin + gentamicin** (*add* rifampin if prosthetic valve), 4-6 weeks
- **Medical tx of heart failure**
  - Diuretics
  - Afterload reduction (Captopril)
  - Inotropes (Dopamine, Dobutamine)
- *Medical Tx fairly effective* – 80% do not require surgery

Surgical Indications
- Heart failure (moderate to severe)
- Severe regurgitation
- Major embolic events
- Important arrhythmias and conduction problems (heart block)
- Progressive renal failure
- Fungal valve infection
- Ongoing sepsis despite medical tx (> 1 week; fever, WBCs)
- Abscess
- Failure of medical tx or relapse while on abx's
- Valve thrombosis
- Large vegetations (> 1 cm) or enlarging vegetations (usually)

Pre-op CHF is most impt prognostic indicator for surgery on endocarditis
Survival after surgery
- **NVE** (native valve endocarditis) – 85%
- **PVE** (prosthetic valve endocarditis) – 75%
- **Survival worse for PVE due to** – reop, increased abscess, erosion, aneurysm, fastidious or fungal organisms, insidious
- Try to avoid operating on pts w/ **septic emboli to head** (bleeding risk)

Peri-procedural endocarditis prophylaxis:

Prosthetic valves or previous valve surgery
Rheumatic heart disease
Congenital heart disease
Mitral valve prolapse
Previous endocarditis
Tx: 1st generation cephalosporins starting 1 day prior to procedure

Acute Heart Failure Tx

Want MAP > 60, CI 2.2, SVR < 800, wedge 15-20
Initial Tx (LMNOP):
    Lasix (wedge 15-20)
    Morphine (venodilator and afterload reduction)
    Nitrate (venodilator)
    Oxygen
    Position – sitting position
Advanced Tx:
    IV vasodilators (NTG, nipride, ACEI)
    Cardiogenic shock
        Add pressor - norepinephrine
        Add Inotropes – dopamine, Dobutamine, Milrinone
    Consider ultrafiltration; IABP, Ventricular assist device, Heart TXP

Chronic Heart Failure Tx:

Beta-blocker (carvedilol specifically) – ↓s hospitalizations and mortality
    Carvedilol is both a <u>beta</u> and <u>alpha</u> adrenergic blocker
ACE inhibitor – improves blood flow, controls hypertension, and has a positive
    effect on cardiac remodeling; ↓s mortality
Spironolactone (aldosterone antagonists) – ↓s hospitalizations and mortality
Digoxin – slows heart and acts as an inotrope
Low sodium diet (< 2 gm/day) and **Fluid restriction** (1-2 L/day)
Other options
    Biventricular pacer – refractory CHF, EF < 35% and QRS > 120 msec
    AICD considered if EF < 30-35% (↓s arrhythmogenic deaths)
    Anticoagulation for atrial fibrillation, LV thrombus, or EF < 30%
    Atrial fibrillation – consider catheter ablation

Heart Block

SA node – is located at the right atrial-SVC junction (antero-lateral)
AV node – is located in the triangle of Koch (atrial septum near tricuspid valve)
First degree A-V block is a prolonged PR interval (>0.2 msec)
Second degree Type I A-V block is progressively lengthening PR intervals until
    a QRS is finally dropped
Second degree Type II A-V block is where the p wave is randomly not followed
    by a QRS complex
Third degree A-V block is where there is no association between P waves and
    QRS complexes
**Second degree type II A-V block is worrisome because it can degenerate into
    complete (third degree) heart block and if there is not a ventricular escape
    rhythm, the pt will become asystolic
**Third degree heart block is worrisome because asystole can occur or
    underlying ventricular escape rate may not support perfusion

** → *Second degree type II AV block* and *third degree AV block require
    permanent pacemakers*

Aortic Dissection

MC location for intimal tear – ascending aorta

Dissection occurs in **media layer** of blood vessel wall

Can be confused w/ myocardial infarction (<u>don't give tPA</u> w/ dissection)

Cx's of ascending aortic dissection:

Aortic insufficiency – from annular dilatation or aortic valve cusp tear

Coronary or aortic branch occlusion – from flap (eg myocardial infarction, stroke)

Death w/ ascending aortic dissections usually secondary to **cardiac failure** (from aortic insufficiency), **tamponade**, or **rupture**

Sx's:

Tearing anterior chest pain radiating to **back** (knife-like)

95% of pts have **severe HTN**

Other sx's – CVA, syncope

RFs – HTN, connective tissue disorders (Marfan's, Ehlers Danlos, annuloaortic ectasia), family Hx, bicuspid aortic valve, coarctation, aortitis (Takayasu's), pregnancy (3rd trimester), cardiac catheterization, cocaine, aneurysms, atherosclerosis

Dx:

Listen for **aortic insufficiency** murmur

Check for **extremity pulses** (can have unequal BP due to flap)

MC – normal right radial, weakened left radial (from flap)

May have **neuro deficits**

EKG – R/O MI (although can have coronary ischemia w/ dissection)

CXR (often normal) – may have widened mediastinum, left effusion

Chest CT *(best test)*

ECHO can also be used to diagnose dissections

Classifications

Stanford Type A – any involvement of the ascending aorta

Stanford Type B – not involving the ascending aorta

Cut-off between Type A and Type B is proximal **innominate artery**

Debakey Type I – ascending and descending aorta

Debakey Type II – ascending aorta only

Debakey Type III – descending aorta only

Initial medical Tx (stabilizing the dissection)

Esmolol *(best Tx*, beta-blocker)

Hydralazine (use after beta-blockade) or **Labetalol**

Morphine for pain

Right radial a-line

Type and cross for 6 units of blood

Tx:

Ascending Aortic Dissections – *all need repair*

Surgery aims at obliterating the false lumen and placing graft

Descending Aortic Dissection – *repair <u>only</u> if there is a complication→*

Rupture

Rapid expansion of an aneurysm

Limb ischemia

Organ ischemia

Uncontrolled HTN

Intractable pain

Extensive hemothorax

Need to follow these pts w/ **lifetime serial CT scans**

30% eventually get **aneurysm formation** requiring surgery

Postop cx's – MI, renal failure, paraplegia (esp. descending aortic dissection repairs)

Paraplegia caused by **spinal cord ischemia** due to occlusion or ligation of **intercostal arteries** and/or the **artery of Adamkiewicz** during repair

Thoracic Aortic aneurysms

1) Ascending aortic aneurysms

MCC – <u>cystic medial necrosis</u> (eg Marfan's syndrome, idiopathic)
Dx: chest CT *(best)*
Can get aortic insufficiency (can lead to CHF)
Often asymptomatic and picked up on routine CXR
Can get compression of → vertebra (back pain), RLN (voice changes),
    bronchi (dyspnea or PNA), or esophagus (swallowing trouble)
Indications for repair:
    Symptomatic
    Rapid ↑ in size (> 0.5 cm / yr)
    ≥ 5.5 cm

2) Transverse aortic arch aneurysms

MCC – <u>cystic medial necrosis</u> (eg Marfan's, idiopathic)
Pts will need to be **cooled down** (18 C) + **circulatory arrest** for repair
Indications for repair:
    Symptomatic
    Rapid ↑ in size (> 0.5 cm / yr)
    ≥ 5.5 cm

3) Descending aortic aneurysms (or thoracoabdominal aneurysms)

MCC – <u>atherosclerosis</u>
Risk of paraplegia – 10% w/ open techniques, 1% w/ aortic stent grafts
    Reimplant intercostal vessels below T8 to help prevent paraplegia
Indications for repair:
    Symptomatic
    Rapid ↑ in size (> 0.5 cm / yr)
    ≥ 6.5 cm

Repair indications

Ascending	**≥ 5.5 cm**
Aortic arch	**≥ 5.5 cm**
Descending Thoracic Aortic	**≥ 6.5 cm****
Abdominal Aortic Aneurysms (AAA)	**≥ 5.5 cm**

Marfan's pts get operated on 0.5-1.0 cm lower than above
RFs for aneurysms – cystic medial necrosis, atherosclerosis, age, family history
RFs for rupture – women, smoking, HTN
Medical Tx – beta-blockers, ACEI, no burst activity (exercise or valsalva
    maneuvers)

Indications for stand-alone MAZE (for atrial fibrillation)

1) Atrial fibrillation resistant to drug Tx
2) Intolerance to drug Tx
3) Six months of atrial fibrillation w/ enlarged atrium
4) High risk for thromboembolism (eg hypercoaguable state)
5) Contraindication to anticoagulation
6) Pts who have suffered stroke on coumadin
Key maneuver is **pulmonary vein isolation** (majority of atrial fibrillation foci
    located in pulmonary veins)
MAZE can be done **off cardiopulmonary bypass** (cryolesions, RF ablation)
Success rate – 70%

Internal mammary artery

Is a branch of the subclavian artery
It divides into the musculophrenic and superior epigastric arteries
Has branches to the intercostal arteries
LIMA to LAD (left anterior descending artery) – 90% patency at 20 years
Saphenous vein graft – 80% 5 year patency

Vasovagal episode – ↑ parasympathetic tone (which ↓s HR) and ↓ sympathetic
tone (which ↓s blood pressure); can lead to **syncope**
Tx: raise legs, can give **atropine**
Can occur w/ **carotid PTA** (distends carotid body) – body thinks BP is high, so ↑
    parasympathetic and ↓ sympathetic tone → ↓ HR, ↓ BP

Cardiac Tamponade Post-op

Sx's: classic is severe mediastinal tube drainage that suddenly stops, followed by ↑ed filling pressures (PA and CVP) and low BP

Can also have sudden ↓ in UOP

Dx: usually a clinical Dx, **CXR** w/ widened mediastinum; **ECHO** may help

Tx:

1) **Emergent re-exploration in operating room** – if pt still has a pulse

2) **Open pts chest at bedside** – if you can't feel a pulse

First sign of cardiac tamponade on ECHO – right atrial diastolic compression

Mechanism of tamponade – ↓ed ventricular filling due pericardial fluid (blood)

Other cardiac conditions

Cardiac Tumors

MC tumor (and MC benign tumor) – myxoma; 80% in left atrium

Can get mitral stenosis-type sx's

MC primary malignant tumor – angiosarcoma

MC metastatic tumor to heart – lung CA

MC primary pediatric cardiac tumor – rhabdomyoma

Idiopathic hypertrophic subaortic stenosis (IHSS)

Too much volume can lead to volume overload and CHF

Too little volume can lead to LV outflow tract collapse and CHF

Usually have associated **mitral regurgitation**

Tx:

Give sufficient volume

Slow HR to allow LV to fill and stretch LV outflow tract (use beta-blocker)

Avoid Inotropes *(will collapse LV outflow tract)*

Coming off cardiopulmonary bypass and aortic root vent blood is **dark** and aortic perfusion cannula blood is **red** → Tx: **ventilate lungs**

Coronary veins have lowest oxygen tension of any body tissue (30% sat, high oxygen extraction by myocardium)

Mediastinal bleeding – > 500 cc over 1st hour or >250 cc/hr over 4 hours → re-explore after cardiac procedure

RFs for mediastinitis – obesity, use of bilateral internal mammary arteries, diabetes, increased blood transfusion

Tx: debridement with pectoralis flaps; can also use omentum

Postpericardiotomy syndrome

Sx's: pericardial friction rub: fever, chest pain, SOB, left pleural effusion

EKG – diffuse ST segment elevation in all leads

From pericarditis – MC after CABG

Tx: **NSAIDs, steroids**

Severe carotid stenosis in pt needing CABG

Vast majority of data points towards ↑ed stroke rate for combined CABG/carotid procedure compared to staged (6% for combined *vs.* 3% for staged)

In general, the CEA should always be performed 1st in asymptomatic pts w/ stenosis > 80% or if symptomatic w/ stenosis > 70%. The CABG is done 4 weeks later. Exceptions to this rule include pts w/ USA or significant left main disease. Then combined CEA/CABG with the CEA 1st should be performed.

VASCULAR

Atherosclerosis stages
Normal arterial wall – intima, media, and adventitia
LDL cholesterol becomes **oxidized** in blood and **damages arterial wall**
Macrophages come to repair the damage, causing an **inflammatory reaction**
Macrophages cannot process cholesterol, so **cholesterol builds up** in wall,
    attracting more macrophages (macrophages become **foam cells** w/
    absorption of LDL)
Initially starts as a **fatty streak** and then cholesterol builds up
Smooth muscle proliferation in media occurs, further narrowing the arterial wall
    (causes HTN)
Thrombus can form on the damaged arterial wall, which if already narrowed, will
    completely **occlude the vessel** *(etiology of myocardial infarction)*
RFs: smoking, HTN, ↑ LDL or VLDL, DM, age, males, family Hx, ↑ cholesterol
Prevention and **Tx of atherosclerosis:**
    Statin drugs (eg simvastatin, *best preventive agent for atherosclerosis*)
    Dietary change – less fat and cholesterol; ↑omega 3 fatty acids
    D/C smoking
    Control HTN
    DM control
    ASA
    Progressive exercise program, weight loss if obese
Homocysteinemia can ↑ risk of atherosclerosis. **Tx: folate, B-6, B-12**

Cerebrovascular disease
Stroke 3rd MCC of death in US
Most important RF – <u>HTN</u> (others – smoking, DM)
Anatomy
    Carotids supply 85% of blood flow to brain
    Normal internal carotid artery has **continuous forward flow**
    Normal external carotid artery has **triphasic flow** (late-phase reverse flow)
    1st branch of external carotid artery (ECA) – superior thyroid artery
    1st branch of the internal carotid artery (ICA) – ophthalmic artery
    Communication between internal carotid artery and external carotid artery
        is through **ophthalmic artery** (off ICA) and **internal maxillary artery**
        (off ECA)
    MC diseased intracranial artery – middle cerebral artery
    MC site of stenosis – carotid bifurcation
Cerebral ischemic events
    Stroke usually from arterial **embolization** (not thrombosis) from ICA
    Can also occur from a **low-flow state** through a severely stenotic lesion
    Heart 2nd MC source of emboli
    Sx's: amaurosis fugax, aphasia, hemiparesis, paresthesias (tingling)
        Amaurosis fugax
            Occlusion of ophthalmic branch of ICA
            Get visual changes → shade coming down over pts eyes
                visual changes are <u>transient</u>
            Hollenhorst plaques on ophthalmologic exam
        Transient ischemia attacks (TIAs) → sx's for < 24 hours
        Anterior cerebral artery events – mental status changes, frontal
            release, slowing
        Middle cerebral artery events – contralateral motor and speech (if
            dominant side); contralateral facial droop
        Vertebral artery events – diplopia or binocular vision loss, vertigo,
            tinnitus, drop attacks, incoordination
Vertebral disease
    Stenosis usually at **origins** (subclavian arteries)
    Usually need bilateral disease to have sx's
    Can be caused by atherosclerosis, spurs, bands, or trauma
    Dx: duplex U/S, angiography
    Tx: PTA w/ stent *(best Tx)*, vertebral artery transposition to subclavian,
        trans-subclavian endarterectomy, rsxn of bands or osteophytes

Carotid Disease
MC occurs at **carotid bifurcation**
Dx: Carotid Duplex U/S every 6 months (measures carotid flow velocities; ICA/CCA ratio, want a certified lab), **angiography** *(best test; although many surgeons will operate just on U/S findings)*
Medical Therapy
   Modify RFs
      Smoking cessation (offer nicotine patch)
      HTN modification (beta-blocker)
      Cholesterol control (statin drug)
      DM → good glucose control
      Weight loss if indicated
   ASA
Recommendations for Surgery
   Asymptomatic ≥ 70% (little controversial for 70-80%)
   Symptomatic ≥ 60% (little controversial for 60-70%)
   Bilateral carotid stenosis
      Repair **tightest side** 1st
      If equally tight, repair **dominant side** 1st (hand dominance)
   Occluded internal carotid artery – do NOT repair (no benefit)
   Completed stroke → CEA 6 weeks later if stenosis meets criteria (**head CT** to confirm stroke)
   Crescendo TIA's (or fluctuating neuro sx's) → emergent CEA
   Carotid traumatic injury w/ major fixed deficit
      If occluded do not repair → can exacerbate injury with bleeding
      If not occluded → repair
Carotid endarterectomy
   Removing the **intima** and part of the **media**
   Most impt technical concern – *getting a good distal end-point* (want to avoid an intimal flap)
   Completion a-gram in OR if worried about an intimal flap
   Facial vein – can be routinely divided
Criteria for Shunting during CEA (some always shunt)
   Pressure < 40
   You are operating on pt awake and they have neuro changes
   EEG changes (slowing)
Nerve injuries
   Vagus
      MC injured nerve w/ CEA
      Between IJ and carotid
      Injury causes **hoarseness** (recurrent laryngeal nerve off vagus)
      MC from **vascular clamping** during endarterectomy
   Marginal mandibular branch of facial nerve
      Injury causes droop in corner of mouth
      Catch this w/ **retractor** at angle of jaw
      Often recovers in 3 weeks
   External branch of superior laryngeal nerve
      Goes behind external carotid just superior to the bifurcation (loss of pitch)
   Hypoglossal
      Near digastrics (2 cm above carotid bifurcation)
      Injury w/ high dissection
      Tongues deviation to side of injury
      Difficulty w/ speech and mastication
   Glossopharyngeal
      Superior to the hypoglossal (would be very high dissection)
      Usually from retraction
      Injury results in trouble swallowing (unlikely injury)
   Ansa cervicalis – strap muscles; no serious deficits

Other Complications:
Stroke Rate: 1-2%
HTN post-op
Tx: Nipride, esmolol, hydralazine
Likely from injury to the **carotid body**
Look for hematoma and breathing status – back to OR if stridor or expanding hematoma
Severe HTN (> 200) can cause stroke
Need to R/O **pain** as a cause of HTN
Neuro event early post-op (eg in PACU):
Back to OR (worried about flap or thrombosis / embolus here)
Heparinize pt
Re-open incision and **doppler** proximal and distal end of CEA:
1) **If you have good proximal and distal flow,** likely have <u>embolic problem</u>
Could have broken off plaque during operation or you may have a flap distal to suture line
Place clamps, open the carotid again, and shunt
Ensure you do not have an intimal flap somewhere along the CEA plane
Tack the flap up if one is present
Completion a-gram
2) **If you have poor flow, the arteriotomy is the problem** (<u>thrombotic problem</u>)
Place clamps, open the carotid again, and shunt
Re-do arteriotomy w/ patch enlargement and tack down any flaps
Completion a-gram
Head CT post-op
Keep drains in
Heparinize post-op if non-hemorrhagic infarct (keep drains)
Neuro event many days post-op:
Duplex – look for flow through repair (re-operate if no flow)
Angio to look for flap – possible stent if present
Head CT – to R/O hemorrhagic stroke
Heparinize if not hemorrhagic
Pseudoaneurysm – pulsatile, bleeding mass after CEA
Tx: drape and prep before intubation, intubate, then repair
Myocardial infarction – MCC mortality following CEA
Re-stenosis rate after CEA – 15%

Carotid stents – best indications →
1) Carotid stenosis after previous CEA
2) Previous neck XRT
3) Pt deemed medically unfit to undergo surgery

Carotid body tumor
Sx's: painless **neck mass** w/ **carotid bruit**
Usually near bifurcation
Is a **paraganglioma** and can release **norepinephrine** (→ HTN, tachycardia)
Tx: resection

Indication for external carotid endarterectomy – occluded internal carotid w/ ipsilateral cerebral or ocular sx's and tight external carotid artery (external carotid collateralized to ipsilateral cerebral vessels through the ophthalmic artery and is causing ischemia)

Peripheral Vascular Disease (PVD)

MCC – atherosclerosis

MC atherosclerotic occlusion in lower extremities – Hunter's canal (distal superficial femoral artery exits here); **sartorius muscle** covers Hunter's canal

Sx's of PVD

Cramping, pain w/ exercise (ie claudication); pallor, hair loss, abnormal nail growth, ↓ capillary refill

Severe Disease →

If leg is dependent → rubor + pain relieved

If leg is elevated → pallor + pain worsens (blood flow can't be sustained against gravity)

Sx's occur one level below occlusion

Buttock claudication – aortoiliac DZ

Mid-thigh claudication – external iliac DZ

Calf claudication – common femoral artery or proximal superficial femoral artery DZ

Foot claudication – distal superficial femoral or popliteal artery DZ

Leriche syndrome

1) **No femoral pulses**

2) **Buttock or thigh claudication**

3) **Impotence** (from hypogastric obstruction, ↓ flow in internal iliacs) Lesion at aortic bifurcation or above

Lumbar stenosis – can mimic claudication (but occurs after standing for long periods, not after walking).

Diabetic neuropathy – can mimic rest pain (numbness and tingling at night, but not ↑ed pain w/ exercise)

Dx:

ABI's (ankle-brachial index; normal 1-1.2)

Claudication	< 0.9 (**same distance** each time)
Rest pain	< 0.5 (usually starts across **distal foot/arch**)
Ulcers	< 0.4 (starts in **toes, non-healing**)
Gangrene	< 0.3 (starts in **toes**)

ABI's can be very **inaccurate w/ DM** secondary to **incompressibility of vessels**; have to go off PVRs and angio

W/ claudication, the ABI in affected extremity drops w/ walking (eg resting ABI is 0.8 but drops to <0.5 w/ exercise causing pain)

ABI based on return of systolic blood pressure after application of blood pressure cuff

PVRs (pulse volume recording) – finds occlusion and at what level

Arteriogram (*best test* for PVD)

Needed if PVRs and/or ABI's suggest significant disease

Can possibly intervene w/ angio as well

Anatomy and Path

Collateral circulation – forms from abnormal pressure gradients

Circumflex iliacs to subcostals

Circumflex femoral arteries to gluteal arteries

Geniculate arteries around the knee

Postnatal angiogenesis – budding from preexisting vessels; **angiogenin** involved

Leg compartments

Anterior

Deep peroneal nerve (dorsiflexion, sensation 1st and 2nd toes)

Anterior tibial artery

Lateral

Superficial peroneal nerve (eversion, lateral foot sensation)

Deep posterior

Tibial nerve (plantarflexion)

Posterior tibial artery and peroneal artery

Superficial posterior – sural nerve

Claudication (pain w/ exercise that is relieved by rest)

Gangrene risk – 2% per year; **Amputation risk** – 1% per year

Tx:

Medical Tx 1st for claudication:
> Statin drugs
> Smoking cessation (offer nicotine patch)
> Graded exercise program (until pain occurs; improves **collaterals**)
> HTN Tx
> DM Tx
> ASA
> Weight loss if needed
> Screen for hyperlipidemia problems

Revascularization procedure indications:
> 1) Significant **lifestyle limitation** despite maximal medical tx
> 2) **Rest pain** (implies threatened limb, ie ABI $\leq$ 0.5)
> 3) **Tissue loss, non-healing ulcers**, or **limb salvage**
> 4) Atheromatous **embolization**
> → **Get angio**, correct most proximal problem 1st

Guidelines for PTA (± stent) *vs.* **bypass procedures:**
> 1) Endovascular techniques best for lesions where the same level of
> symptomatic improvement will be obtained using open bypass
> procedures (ie same clinical result percutaneous versus open)
> 2) **In general:**
>> **PTA + stent** – best for **isolated, short** and **proximal lesions**
>> (eg isolated iliac disease)
>>> **Endovascular mortality** < 1%
>> **Open bypass** – best for long length, multiple, and distal lesions
>>> **Operative mortality**: 3-4%
> 3) **5-year patency rates:**

Iliac **PTA** + stent	80%
Iliac **PTA** *only*	60%
Femoral or popliteal **PTA** (± stent)	40%
Femoral to popliteal **bypass graft** (saphenous vein)	70%
(above or below knee bypass)	

> 4) **Summary**
>> **PTA + stent**- *best Tx* for **isolated iliac disease**(supra-inguinal)
>> **Open bypass** - *best Tx* for lesions **below knee** (only done for
>> **limb** or **tissue salvage**)
>> **Infra-inguinal but above knee** → can use either of above
>>> Many going w/ PTA + stent despite ↓ed patency
>>> **In high risk pts,** PTA + stent may be best option (↓
>>> mortality risk of procedure)

PTA
> Intima **ruptured** and media **stretched**
> Pushes plaque out
> Requires passage of wire 1st

PTFE (Gortex)
> ↓ed patency when crosses knee
> ***Have to use <u>saphenous vein graft</u> below knee**

Dacron – good for aorta and large vessels

Tx of Specific Lesions

Aortoiliac occlusive disease
> Most get aorto-bifemoral repair
> Abdominal and groin incisions
> **High-risk pts** – can perform axillary-femoral bypass w/ femoral-
> femoral crossover (keeps you out of the abdomen)

Isolated iliac or common femoral lesions
> **PTA + stent** *(best Tx)*
> If that fails can perform femoral-to-femoral crossover if iliac or cut
> down on common femoral artery w/ patch plasty of vessel

Femoro-popliteal grafts (above or below knee popliteal)
> 5-year patency – 70%
> ↑ed patency w/ surgery for **claudication** as opposed to **limb
> salvage**

Femoral-distal grafts (eg peroneal, anterior tibial or posterior tibial artery)
- **5-year patency** – 50% (even if not patent, may still get **limb salvage** through development of collaterals)
- Patency <u>not</u> influenced by level of distal anastomosis (can be below the ankle if necessary)
- **Need to have run-off below the ankle** (ie a native vessel needs to go past the ankle joint) for this to be effective
- Distal lesions more **limb threatening** because of lack of collaterals
- **Indications** – bypasses distal to knee only for **limb** or **tissue salvage** (eg non-healing ulcer)

Extra-anatomic grafts used if hostile conditions in abdomen (eg aortic graft infections – still need to resect graft, multiple previous surgeries)

Femoral-to-femoral crossover graft – doubles blood flow to donor artery; can get vascular steal in donor leg

Post-op need **81 mg ASA indefinitely** (↑s patency)
- **Statin drugs** may also improve patency

Best predictor of long term patency in extremity vein graft– vein quality

Cx's

In general, **patency is worse for limb salvage operations** compared to claudication or lifestyle limitation

Early **swelling** following lower extremity bypass – edema from *reperfusion injury* (can get compartment syndrome)

Late **swelling** following lower extremity bypass – likely *DVT,* get U/S

Cx's of reperfusion of ischemic tissue:
- **Lactic acidosis** (Tx: HCO3- to keep pH > 7.25)
- **Hyperkalemia** (Tx: see Critical care chp) – from injured muscle
- **Myoglobinuria** (Tx: see Critical care chp) – from injured muscle
- **Compartment syndrome** (Tx: fasciotomy, see below)

MCC early failure of reversed saphenous vein graft - technical problem

MCC late failure of reversed saphenous vein graft - vein atherosclerosis

Compartment syndrome
- Reperfusion injury (PMNs) of leg following prolonged (4-6 hrs) ischemia
- MC affects **anterior compartment** of leg (get foot-drop)
- **Sx's: 1st - *pain w/ passive motion*;** early post-op extremity **swelling,** paresthesias, paralysis; loss of pulse is a <u>late finding</u>
- **Dx:** based on **clinical suspicion**
  - Compartment pressure > 30 mmHg abnormal → fasciotomy
- **Tx: Fasciotomies** → leave open 5–10 days (skin graft after that)
  - Undiagnosed compartment syndrome can present as **renal failure** (from **myoglobin release** w/ muscle necrosis) or **hyperkalemia** (intra-cellular potassium release)
- With fasciotomy, you are through fascia when **muscle bulges**

Late hemorrhage or pseudoaneurysm (weeks to years) → *likely graft infection*; eroding into suture line (see Graft Infection below)

Popliteal entrapment syndrome
Sx's:
- ****Intermittent lower extremity claudication in young pts** (< 30)
- *Can be **bilateral**;* Loss of **pulse w/ plantar-flexion**

Dx: angiogram

Usually have medial deviation of popliteal artery around medial head of gastrocnemius muscle

Tx: rsxn of gastrocnemius muscle medial head; possible arterial reconstruction

Adventitial cystic disease
Sx's: intermittent claudication, usually middle aged males, 40-50

Changes in sx's w/ **knee flexion** and **extension**

MC area – **popliteal,** often bilateral

Ganglia from adjacent joint capsule or tendon sheath→ **compress artery**

Dx: angiogram

Tx: vein graft needed if vessel occluded; o/w just resection of cyst

Arterial autografts
Internal iliac artery for children requiring renal artery repair
Radial grafts for CABG
IMA for CABG

Lower Extremity Fasciotomy
Incise 2 cm posterior to the tibia medially
> Opens **superficial posterior** space
> > **Soleus muscle** then incised longitudinally (or retracted back) to open **deep posterior space**

2nd incision on anterior/lateral leg 2 cm anterior to fibula
> Going after anterior and lateral compartments
> > ***Watch for superficial peroneal nerve** (injury would cause decreased eversion of foot)

Muscle should **bulge** if you are in the right spot
Incision should be **length of leg**

Graft Infection
Late hemorrhage or **late pseudoaneurysm** after vascular bypass graft is most consistent w/ ***graft infection*** (breaks down suture line)

MCC of graft infection overall	staph epidermidis
MCC early (< 1 month)	staph aureus
MCC late	staph epidermidis

Sx's:
> Fever, chills; recent infection or procedure; can have **sepsis**
> **Late hemorrhage** or **late pseudoaneurysm** (wks, mos, or yrs out)
> **Incision site** may have **erythema** and **pus,** possible **exposed graft**
> Infections ↑ed in grafts going to **groin**

Dx:
> **Visual inspection** of wound(s)
> **CT scan w/ contrast** (micro-bubbles sign of infection)
> Consider **diagnostic tap of fluid** if unsure
> **Most sensitive test for Dx of graft infection** – tagged WBC scan

Tx:
> Start **abx's**
> **Excision of entire graft** + bypass through **non-infected planes** *(best Tx)*
> > Various modifications of above have been used w/ success (eg partial graft excision, placing new graft though previous plane)

Upper Extremity Occlusive Disease
Occlusive disease
> Proximal lesions usually asymptomatic secondary to ↑ collaterals
> **MC site of stenosis** – subclavian artery
> > Can cause coronary ischemia in pts w/ previous CABG w/ IMA graft
> Tx: PTA + stent *(best Tx)*; common carotid to subclavian bypass if that fails

Subclavian steal syndrome
> Proximal subclavian artery stenosis resulting in reversal of flow through ipsilateral vertebral artery into subclavian
> **Sx's** – pre-syncope, syncope, vertigo, falls, ocular problems, arm pain
> Repair with limb or neurologic sx's (MC Sx's – vertebrobasilar)
> Dx: angiogram
> Tx: PTA + stent *(best Tx)*; common carotid to subclavian bypass if that fails

Amputations
Criteria for amputation:
> 1) **Wet gangrene**
> 2) **Non-healing ulcers** not amenable to revascularization
> 3) **Unrelenting rest pain** not amenable to revascularization

Mortality rate 50% within 3 years of AKA or BKA
BKA (below knee) – 80% heal, 70% walk again, 5% mortality
AKA (above knee) – 90% heal, 30% walk again, 10% mortality
Emergency amputation for systemic cx's, extensive infection, failure of abx's

Diabetic foot ulcer w/ Dry Gangrene (non-infectious or mild cellulitis)

Diabetics can't feel feet, so **plantar ulcers** form at pressure areas

Usually at **metatarsal heads** and **heel**

General tx of Dry Gangrene

(eg superficial, no bone or joint involvement, not systemically toxic):

Admit pt

Plain X-ray to look for osteomyelitis

Aggressive wound care (heals from base up)

Debridement

Keep ulcer moist

Whirlpool therapy

Leg elevation and **non-weight bearing on area**

Broad spectrum abx's for cellulitis

Polymicrobial – GPCs (staph, strep), GNRs (includes pseudomonas), and anaerobes

Tx: Augmentin or (fluoroquinolone + clindamycin)

Better fitting shoes before discharge w/ **daily foot checks**

ABI's before discharge + **angio** if indicated to R/O occlusive disease

Non-healing ulcer

Get ABI's, if < 0.6 **get angiogram** to R/O occlusive DZ

(possible revascularization to prevent tissue or limb loss)

Diabetics may have non-compressible vessels, making ABI inaccurate

Consider angio w/o ABI

Non-healing ulcer (despite above Tx) and **non-revascularizable**

Non-infectious – can allow to auto-amputate if just toes

Larger lesions should be amputated

Special issues

Heel ulceration to bone (exposed calcaneus) → Tx: amputation

Malperforans ulcer (at **metatarsal heads**, MC **2nd MTP joint**)

Often have osteomyelitis

Tx: as above but also need cartilage debridement of metatarsal head if osteomyelitis present

Diabetic foot ulcer w/ Wet Gangrene (infectious)

Infectious – erythema, ± pus, ± red streaks, ± crepitus, ± clinical sepsis

General Tx of wet gangrene:

***Early, aggressive, and repeated debridement of ulcerated area → surgical emergency**

1) **May need early amputation if severe**

(eg toe amputation; guillotine foot or leg amputation)

2) **Open pus tracks**

3) **Wound Bx** (wound curettage to base of wound)– send for culture

Best Dx test for organism (also *best Dx test for osteomyelitis*)

Blood Cultures

X-rays to look for osteomyelitis

WTD dressing changes **TID**

Broad spectrum abx's

1) Unasyn + gentamicin or 2) fluoroquinolone + clindamycin

Osteomyelitis – requires debridement + abx's for 4-6 weeks or possible amputation of area

After infection clears, ABI's and possible angio before discharge

Severe cellulitis spreading past ulcerated area (red streaks, erythema + swollen toe or extremity, pus coming out of ulcer)

→ *early amputation at appropriate level*

Example – ulcer at 2nd MTP joint w/ pus coming out and **swollen, erythematous** toe) → Tx: toe amputation w/ resection of metatarsal head (ray amputation)

Foot or leg – consider guillotine amputation 1st, place flap later

Abdominal aortic aneurysms (AAA)

Normal aorta 2-3 cm

90% are infra-renal

MCC: atherosclerosis

Metal matrix metalloproteinases (MMP's, <u>zinc dependent</u>) have been implicated in aneurysm formation

Aneurysm results from degeneration of **medial layer**

Other RFs: HTN, male gender, smoking, elderly age

Screening recommendations: one-time screening U/S in men age 65 to 75 years who have smoked

Sx's: MC found incidentally; can present w/ rupture, distal embolization (lower extremity ischemic symptoms), or compression of adjacent organs

Rupture

MCC death without an operation

Sx's: back or abd pain; hypotension

Dx: *duplex U/S in ER best*

CT - fluid in retroperitoneal space, **extra-luminal contrast**

MC site of rupture – left posterolateral wall, 2–4 cm below renals

↑rupture risk w/ **diastolic HTN** or **COPD** (coughing→expansion)

50% mortality w/ rupture (if pt reaches hospital alive)

AAA repair criteria

1) **Size ≥ 5.5 cm**

> 6 cm → 20% risk of rupture over 5 year

> 8 cm → 100% risk of rupture over 5 years

2) **Infected AAA** (mycotic aneurysm)

3) **Symptomatic AAA**

4) **Growth > 0.5 cm/yr**

Open Repair Issues

1) **Re-implantation of inferior mesenteric artery criteria:**

Back pressure < 40 mmHg (poor back-bleeding)

Previous **colonic surgery**

SMA stenosis

If flow to left colon appears inadequate

2) **Ligate bleeding lumbar arteries**

3) **Re-implantation of internal iliac artery** (hypogastric)

Need to maintain at least one open internal iliac artery

Absence of retrograde internal iliac flow (ie absence of back-bleeding) → re-implant one of the internal iliacs arteries

Avoids potential **vasculogenic impotence, pelvic ischemia, spinal cord problems,** and **rectosigmoid ischemia**

Open Repair Cx's

Mortality with elective open repair – 3-4%

MCC death (and MCC of acute death) – MI

MCC late death – renal failure

Major vein injury w/ proximal cross-clamp – retro-aortic left renal vein

Impotence – 50% (disruption of autonomic nerves and blood flow to pelvis)

Graft infection – 1% (Dx: **U/S** w/ aspiration of fluid, **Tx:** see below)

Pseudoaneurysms – 1% (Dx: **duplex U/S**, *best test*; **Tx:** repair in OR)

Anastomotic Stenosis – <1% (Dx: **duplex U/S**, *best initial test*)

Diarrhea (esp. bloody) after AAA worrisome for **ischemic colitis**

IMA often sacrificed w/ AAA repair and can cause left colon ischemia

Dx: colonoscopy (*best test*, need to go to splenic flexure) – see Colon and Rectum chp

Chylous Ascites following ABF repair

Drainage catheter and **conservative Tx** for 2-3 weeks (same Tx as chylothorax)

If that fails, re-op to **ligate cisterna chili area**

Located to the **right of the aorta near the right renal artery**

MC late cx after aortic graft placement – atherosclerotic occlusion

Leg ischemia after ABF repair

    DDx: 1) technical problem w/ **thrombosis** (poor femoral pulse) *or;*

        2) **embolus** (good femoral pulse) *or;*

        3) **compartment syndrome** (tight, swollen calf)

    Heparinize (80 units/kg) and **go back to OR** (unless compartment
syndrome → Tx fasciotomy)

    Re-open incision and **doppler** proximal and distal to the
anastomosis to find the level of the obstruction:

        1) If **nothing wrong w/ anastomosis** → likely **embolic** problem

            Open anastomosis

            Fogarty back and forth **+ heparin flushes** to remove clot

            Want **2 consecutive passes w/o clot + good back flow**

        2) If **anastomosis is problem** → **thrombotic** problem

            Re-do anastomosis w/ possible enlargement w/ bovine
pericardium or saphenous vein patch

            Fogarty and heparin flush as above

    Completion angiogram in OR

    Feel pulse to make sure you got it back

    Feel calfs and consider **fasciotomy** (esp if ischemia > 4-6 hours)

    Check urine myoglobin

    Check K^+ and H^+ → watch for washout electrolyte changes and
hypotension

Aortic graft infections

    MCC overall – staph epidermidis

        MCC late – staph epidermidis

        MCC early – staph aureus

    MC w/ grafts going to **groin** (aorto-bifemoral grafts)

    Dx:

        CT scan – fluid, gas, thickening around graft

        Blood cultures negative in many pts

    Tx:

        Bypass through non-contaminated field (axillary-femoral
bypass w/ femoral to femoral crossover graft), **graft
excision**, and **aortic stump closure** *(standard Tx)*

        Other options for revascularization:

            Spiraled saphenous vein graft (Claggett procedure -
wind a split-open saphenous vein over a large chest
tube and sew it together) → in-situ graft replacement

            Homograft – in-situ graft replacement

Aortoenteric fistula (eg aortoduodenal fistula)

    Usually **> 6 months** after surgery

    Pt's have history of abdominal vascular surgery, now w/ UGI bleeding

    Sx's: herald bleed w/ **hematemesis**, then **blood per rectum**, then
exsanguination (*classic*)

    MC site – **duodenum** (3rd or 4th portion) erodes into **proximal suture
line** (vast majority) leading to **UGI bleed**

    Dx:

        EGD – possibly see graft if you make it to 3rd and 4th portions of
duodenum; often 1st study obtained in w/u of UGIB

        CT scan *(best test)* – fluid around graft, thickened bowel wall,
graft possibly in bowel lumen

    Tx: same as aortic graft infections above + duodenum closure

        If graft not grossly infected, some just replace graft

    Prevention - need to **cover proximal suture line w/ aortic
aneurysm sac** at time of original operation to prevent this cx

    Graft erosion into bowel can also occur w/o bleeding (sx's - chronic
anemia, fever and guaiac positive stools) Tx: as above

Ischemic colitis (see Colon and Rectum chp)

Suspected ruptured AAA – U/S in emergency room for quick Dx (would
not send pt off to CT scan)

Endo-Vascular Aneurysm Repair (EVAR)

Main advantages over open repair
Less peri-operative mortality (1%, but overall mortality unchanged)
Less time in ICU
Less time in hospital overall
Earlier return to normal activity

Disadvantages
More frequent, ongoing hospital reviews
Higher chance of further procedures being required

EVAR procedure doesn't offer any benefit to overall survival or quality of life compared to open surgery, although aneurysm repair related mortality is lower

EVAR probably better for **older, higher risk pts**

Criteria for EVAR
Proximal neck (landing zone) - $\geq$1.5 cm in length, $\leq$ 3 cm in diameter
Distal neck (landing zone) - $\geq$1.5 cm in length, $\leq$ 3 cm in diameter
Exclusion criteria – ruptured AAA, mycotic aneurysms, unfavorable anatomy

Endoleaks:
Type I endoleak – leak at **proximal** or **distal graft attachment sites**
Tx: re-balloon area; if that fails, you may need to place another graft more proximal or distal to seal the leak
Type II endoleak – retrograde flow from **collateral branch** into aneurysm sac (eg lumbar artery, testicular artery, IMA)
Tx: in general you can watch these for the first 6 months
If leak is persistent and aneurysm sac is getting larger, you need to try and thrombose the feeding vessel
If no change in aneurysm size or smaller - follow
Type III endoleak – leakage between **different parts of stent grafting** (leakage at the **junction** between components)
Tx: place another graft across the junction to seal it
Type IV endoleak – leakage **through stent graft wall**
Tx: place another graft inside the original graft

Inflammatory aneurysms
10% of AAAs, usually males
Sx's: weight loss, $\uparrow$ ESR
Thickened aortic wall peripheral to calcifications on CT scan
Adhesions to **3rd and 4th portions of duodenum**
Ureteral entrapment in 25%
Not secondary to infection
May need to place preop **ureteral stents** to avoid injury
Inflammatory process resolves after aortic graft placement

Mycotic aneurysms
Bacteria infect atherosclerotic plaque and cause aneurysm
MCC – salmonella (others – Staph)
Sx's: pain, fevers, positive blood cultures in 50%
Dx: CT scan – peri-aortic fluid, gas, retroperitoneal soft tissue edema, lymphadenopathy
Tx: extra-anatomic bypass (axillary bifemoral) and resection of infrarenal abdominal aorta to clear infection

Aneurysms of Extremities

MC cx of aneurysms above inguinal ligament – rupture
MC cx of aneurysms below inguinal ligament – thrombosis and emboli
Dx: Duplex U/S (*best test for all below*), angiogram, CT scan

Iliac

Intervention indications:
Symptomatic (thrombosis, emboli, compression, or rupture)
> 3.0 cm
Mycotic

Tx:
Percutaneous stent across aneurysm (*best option*) – do <u>not</u> use if mycotic; If that fails, bypass w/ exclusion
Ruptured – open exclusion and bypass

Femoral

Intervention indications:
Symptomatic (thrombosis, emboli, compression, or rupture)
> 2.5 cm
Mycotic

Tx: **bypass w/ exclusion** (*best option*)

Popliteal

MC peripheral aneurysm
MCC – atherosclerosis
Leg exam has prominent popliteal pulses
50% bilateral
50% have **another aneurysm elsewhere** (eg AAA, femoral)
Sx's:
Most likely to get **emboli** (MC) or **thrombosis** w/ **limb ischemia**
Can present w/ an **acutely threatened leg**
(<u>rare</u> rupture, < 5%)
Intervention indications:
Symptomatic
>2 cm
Mycotic
Tx: **bypass w/ exclusion of all popliteal aneurysms**; 25% have complication that requires amputation if not treated
↓ patency for repair of **symptomatic** popliteal aneurysm (eg thrombosis)

Femoral Pseudoaneurysm

Sx's: groin pain and swelling
Collection of blood in continuity w/ arterial system but not enclosed by all 3 layers of arterial wall
2 causes:
1) Disruption of a suture line between graft and artery <u>or</u>:
2) Percutaneous interventions
Dx: Duplex U/S (*best test*)
Tx:
1) **If from percutaneous intervention** →
U/S guided compression w/ thrombin injection → if flow remains, need surgical repair (stitch at puncture site)
Acutely expanding, nerve compression or compromising skin → operative repair
2) **From disrupted suture line** (eg technical error, not getting full thickness bites) → *emergent operative repair* (can have massive blood loss if this bursts)
3) **Late Pseudoaneuryms** → MC related to infection and suture line breakdown, *need resection of graft*

Visceral Artery Aneurysms

Repair all splanchnic aneurysms when diagnosed (50% rupture) *except*
splenic (< 2% rupture, see splenic artery aneurysms below)
Diameters > 2 cm considered aneurysmal (renal > 1.5 cm)
RFs: medial fibrodysplasia, portal HTN, inflammation (eg pancreatitis)

Visceral aneurysms can be treated w/:
1) **Stent graft** across lesion w/ intra-aneurysmal coil embolization (not for
emergency repairs) – *best option for most*
2) **Exclusion + bypass graft** (if spleen, just exclusion, no splenectomy)
3) For **intra-hepatic hepatic artery aneurysms,** standard **coil
embolization** *best option*
4) For **splenic artery aneurysm**, can also perform just coil embolization
Stent across aneurysm before coil embolization of aneurysm sac
preserves blood flow through the artery
Proximal common hepatic artery (ie proximal to GDA) and **splenic
artery aneurysms** can just be excluded w/o bypass graft (make sure
GDA is open)

Splenic artery aneurysm
MC visceral artery aneurysm (> 2 cm considered aneurysmal)
MC in women
Overall, **1-2% rupture risk** (*much lower* than other visceral aneurysms)
Need repair w/ any following criteria:
1) **Symptomatic**
2) **Pregnancy**
3) **Child Bearing Age**
4) **Aneurysms > 3-4 cm** (↑ed rupture risk)
Splenic artery aneurysms have a specific propensity to *rupture w/
pregnancy* (MC in 3rd trimester – *90% rupture rate in some reports*)

Hepatic artery aneurysm
Intra-hepatic – RUQ pain, jaundice, ± hemobilia; Tx: **coil embolization**
Extra-hepatic proximal to GDA – stent ± coils into aneurysm sac if GDA
open; can also perform open surgical ligation as a 2nd option (make
sure GDA open 1st – gives collateral flow to liver)
Extra-hepatic distal to GDA – stent ± coils into aneurysm sac or open
exclusion w/ bypass graft

Renal artery aneurysm
Tx: **stent** (not for emergency repairs) – *best option*
Other options – reconstruction w/ vein patch or vein interposition graft
Nephrectomy if rupture occurs

Acute Arterial Emboli (MCC of acute extremity ischemia)

Emboli more commonly have (DDx emboli *vs.* thrombosis) →

    1) **No collaterals** (often do have collaterals w/ thrombosis)

    2) **No signs of chronic limb ischemia** on either lower extremity

    3) **No history of claudication**

    4) **Contralateral leg** pulses that are *normal*

    5) **Arrhythmias**

MCC arterial emboli – **atrial fibrillation** (70%); other – myocardial infarction w/ LV thrombus (20%), endocarditis, cardiac tumor, paradoxical embolus from patent foramen ovale, atherosclerotic plaque, aneurysms (esp infrainguinal)

MC site of obstruction from arterial emboli – <u>common femoral artery</u>

Sx's: pain, paresthesias, paralysis, poikilothermia, pulseless

Leg Exam:

    Progression: *pallor* (white) → *cyanosis* (blue) → *marbling*

    Assess **motor function + sensation**; assess **pulses**; (start heparin early)

Tx:

    1) **Intact motor function** and **sensation**

        Most likely has a distal clot (eg trifurcation vessels)

        Best tx - catheter directed intra-arterial thrombolysis (**tPA + Heparin**)

            Infuse through catheter inside clot, run 8-12 hrs, repeat angio

        Need to get **guidewire through clot 1st**; only used for **distal clot**

        Thrombolytics better because its difficult to perform embolectomy for the trifurcation vessels and more effective to lyse clot w/ tPA

        If worsening exam while infusing → OR for embolectomy

        Contraindications – <u>common femoral artery or more proximal clot</u>

            (ie should be able to feel a femoral pulse before starting tPA)

            Also see contraindications to thrombolytics, Hematology chp

    2) **Loss of motor function** or **sensation**

        Most likely has a more proximal clot → ***leg is threatened***

        Best Tx – OR for **cut-down** and **balloon catheter embolectomy**

            Consider fasciotomy if ischemia > 4-6 hrs

        Also indicated for known common femoral or more proximal clot

        Thrombolysis would take too long and less likely to work

    3) **Need to work-up** <u>cause of embolus</u> after removing

Special Issues

    Saddle embolus – lodges at aortic bifurcation, bilateral femoral pulses lost

        Tx **bilateral** femoral artery **cut-downs + retrograde embolectomies**

            (breaks up embolus, remove through groins)

    Atheroma embolism (blue toe syndrome)

        Renals MC involved; cholesterol clefts in small arteries

        Sx's: fever, muscle aches, purple discoloration of toes

        Flaking atherosclerotic emboli off abdominal aorta or branches

        Pts typically have good distal pulses

        MC source – aortoiliac disease

        Usually occurs after procedure (eg cardiac cath, angio, AAA repair)

        Dx: 1) **chest/abd/pelvic CT scan** – look for aneurysmal source or atherosclerosis; 2) **ECHO**, and 3) consider **angio**

        Tx: aneurysm repair, endarterectomy, or arterial exclusion w/ bypass

Acute Arterial Thrombosis (Sx's – usually less than above; start heparin early)

Thrombosis more commonly has (DDx thrombosis *vs.* emboli) →

    1) **Chronic PVD** – no hair on legs, shiny surface

    2) **Hx of claudication** or previous bypass graft

    3) **No arrhythmias**

    4) **Weak contralateral pulse** (from diffuse atherosclerotic DZ)

Exam: usually have developed collaterals (so <u>less likely</u> leg will be threatened)

Tx:

    1) **Non-threatened leg** (motor + sensation intact)

        Mild sx's (good collateral perfusion) – heparin only

        Moderate sx's- catheter directed intraarterial tPA +heparin(as above)

        Can also tx any **stenoses** w/ PTA ± stent as same time

    2) **Threatened leg** (loss of motor or sensation) – OR for thrombectomy

<u>Renal vascular disease</u> (renal artery stenosis, renovascular hypertension)
>Right renal artery goes posterior to IVC
>Left renal vein MC anterior to aorta
>Accessory renal arteries occur in 25%
>**MC source of renal emboli** – heart
>**Suggestive of renovascular HTN:**
>>1) **Renal bruits**
>>2) **Diastolic blood pressure > 115**
>>3) **Worsening HTN w/:**
>>>**Children**
>>>**Premenopausal women**
>>>**Rapid onset after age 50**
>>>**Refractory to drug Tx**
>Need to R/O other HTN sources (eg pheochromocytoma, aldosteronoma)
>**Dx: ↑ renin** and **↑ aldosterone; angio** if suspected
>**Renal atherosclerosis** – left side MC, proximal ⅓ of artery, men
>>Tx: PTA w/ stent
>**Fibromuscular dysplasia** (FMD) – right side MC, distal ⅓ of artery, women
>>Tx: PTA w/ stent
>**Indications for nephrectomy w/ renal HTN** – atrophic kidney < 6 cm and
>>minimal collaterals w/ persistently high renin levels

<u>Other vascular diseases</u>
>**Fibromuscular dysplasia** (FMD)
>>Young females; HTN occurs if renal involved
>>**Medial fibrodysplasia** most common variant (85%)
>>**MC involved vessels** – <u>renals</u> (right side), followed by carotid and iliac
>>Causes **stenosis; 50% bilateral;** stenosis more **distal** then atherosclerosis
>>**Dx: angiogram** *(best for Dx)* – 'string of beads' appearance
>>>(can be <u>missed</u> on duplex U/S due to distal nature of DZ)
>>**Tx: PTA** ± stent *(best Tx,* <u>not</u> endarterectomy) or **bypass**
>**Buerger's disease** (from tobacco; *thromboangiitis obliterans*)
>>Young men, **smokers**, can also occur w/ smokeless tobacco
>>Severe **rest pain** w/ bilateral **ulceration + gangrene of digits** (esp fingers)
>>**Criteria:**
>>>**Age < 45 years**
>>>Current (or recent) history of **tobacco** use
>>>Distal extremity **ischemia** (claudication, rest pain, ulcers, gangrene)
>>>Consistent **angio findings** (see below)
>>>Exclusion of autoimmune diseases, hypercoaguable states, and DM
>>>Exclusion of a proximal source of emboli (ECHO and angiogram)
>>**Dx: angiogram**
>>>1) **corkscrew collaterals** w/ severe distal disease
>>>2) **normal arterial tree proximal to popliteal** and **brachial vessels**
>>>>(ie small vessel disease)
>>**Tx:** stop smoking or will require continued amputations
>**Cystic medial necrosis syndromes** (necrosis of medial layer of arterial wall)
>>**Marfan's disease**
>>>**Fibrillin defect** – connective tissue protein
>>>Marfanoid habitus, retinal detachment, ascending aortic aneurysms,
>>>>mitral valve prolapse, dissections
>>**Ehlers-Danlos syndrome**
>>>Many types of **collagen defects** identified
>>>Easy bruising, hypermobile joints, aneurysm formation and rupture
>>>>(esp abdominal vessels), uterine rupture w/ pregnancy,
>>>>dissections, mitral valve prolapse
>>>*Avoid angiograms* → risk of laceration to vessel
>>>Very often too difficult to repair and need vessel ligation to control
>>>>hemorrhage

Immune arteritis
Large arteries
Temporal arteritis
Giant cell inflammation of *large blood vessels*; granulomas
Women, age > 55;
MC involved artery – temporal
Sx's: fever, arthralgia, visual changes (risk of blindness)
Dx: arterial biopsy (*best test*); ↑ ESR
Long segments of **smooth stenosis** alternating w/ segments of
　　larger diameter (aneurysms)
Can affect **aorta**, its **branches**, or **pulmonary artery**
Tx: steroids, bypass of large vessels if needed;
　　<u>No</u> endarterectomy
Takayasu's arteritis (same pathology as above)
Affects **young Asian women** (15-35)
Stenosis, thrombosis, and aneurysms of aorta and its branches
Tx: **steroids**, bypass of large vessels if needed;
　　<u>No</u> endarterectomy
Medium arteries
Polyarteritis nodosa
MC Adults – fatigue, weakness, muscle aches, fever,
Dx: ↑ CBC, ↑ ESR, p-ANCA, arteritis on Bx, ↑ CRP
Get **aneurysms** that thrombose and cause ischemia
MC involved artery – renals
Tx: steroids
Kawasaki's disease
MC Children (80% < 5)
Dx: Five days of **fever** *plus* (need 4 of below):
　　1) **Erythema** of lips or oral cavity or cracking of lips
　　2) **Rash** on trunk
　　3) **Swelling or erythema** of hands or feet
　　4) **Red eyes** (conjunctival injection)
　　5) **Swollen lymph nodes** in neck of at least 15 mm
Get **coronary artery aneurysms** which can thrombose and
　　cause **myocardial infarction**
MCC death – arrhythmias
Tx:
　　IV **immunoglobulin** (IV-IG, *Best Tx*)
　　ASA
　　Steroids for refractory DZ
　　CABG for aneurysms
　　Early tx to prevent coronary aneurysms
Small arteries
Hypersensitivity angiitis
Often secondary to **drug / tumor antigens**
Sx's: rash, fever, petechiae, purpura, sx's of end-organ
　　dysfunction
Tx: stop offending agent, **antihistamines**
　　Steroids or **IV-IG** if end organ damage
Radiation arteritis

Early	**Sloughing + thrombosis** (obliterative endarteritis)
Late (1–10 years)	**Fibrosis + stenosis**
Very late (3–30 years)	**Accelerated atherosclerosis**

Raynaud's disease
Affects fingers, toes, nose and ears w/ stress or cold
Young women
R/O secondary Raynaud's – connective tissue D/Os (eg SLE,
　　scleroderma), carpal tunnel, obstructive arterial DZ, meds (eg beta-
　　blockers and ergotamine)
Classic findings in fingers: pallor (white) → cyanosis (blue) → rubor (red)
Tx: calcium channel blockers, warmth, *avoid* decongestants (eg
　　pseudoephedrine)

A-V Fistula for Dialysis

Access grafts

MCC of A-V graft failure – venous obstruction from **intimal hyperplasia**
Cimino fistula – radial artery to cephalic vein; wait 6 weeks to use →
    allows vein to mature (dilates venous system)
Interposition graft – wait 6 weeks to allow fibrous scar to form

W/U before A-V graft placement:

1) **Feel pulses** in hand for inflow
2) **Get duplex U/S of upper arm** venous system for outflow
    Vein needs to be at last **4 mm** and have no distal stenosis

Tx:

Start w/ Cimino if 1st graft
    (radial artery-cephalic vein graft near wrist; ligate distal cephalic vein)
Use A-V fistula grafts after 6 weeks:
    1) allows **PTFE to scar in w/ loop graft**
        Brachial, radial or ulnar artery to **cephalic vein** (lateral) or
            basilic vein (medial upper arm)
    2) allows **Cimino to develop large enough venous drainage** (radial
        artery to cephalic vein) → cannulate the veins that dilate

Cx's

Early failure – technical problem
Late failure – intimal hyperplasia on venous side
Early thrombosis → suspect technical problem
    De-clot and get a **fistulogram** to help figure out problem
    Fix venous problem w/ a PTFE patch hood or use interposition graft
        to go distal to vein stenosis

Problems w/ HD
    1) Poor flows (inflow or outflow problem)
    2) ↑ in **pressure in returning line** > 200 (outflow problem)
    3) ↑ in **re-circulation** (a sign of inefficient HD, outflow problem)
    → are all indications of impending graft failure – get U/S (or
        fistulogram) to figure out problem

Arm swelling after AV fistula
    Results from venous HTN
    Initial Tx: elevation, as collaterals develop the swelling goes down
    Persistence of major swelling suggests obstruction of a major
        outflow vein (axillary, subclavian, innominate) → **need**
        angiogram of shunt run-off
        Tx: 1) PTA of stenotic area *(best Tx),* 2) extend fistula to
            unobstructed vein, *or* 3) may need new site (last resort)

Extremity ischemia w/ AV fistula:
    Mild form
        Sx's: cool, numbness, pain in hand w/ HD
        Usually reverses in a few weeks after starting HD
    Severe form
        Sx's: can start immediately after placing graft, gross ischemia
            (mottling, cyanotic)
        Usually associated w/ upper arm graft
        Can be associated w/ **arterial obstruction proximal to graft**
            (eg subclavian stenosis)
        Dx: angiogram – check for arterial obstruction proximally
        Tx:
            Band venous end of graft (do this acutely if hand
                threatened, W/U cause later)
            Revascularize inflow problem if present
            Graft ligation (last resort)

Infection – early (MC from **contamination** at time of surgery)
    Superficial – Tx: local wound care and Abx's
    Deep – Sx's: pain, swelling, redness, pus drainage, cellulitis,
        excessive fluid around graft (↑ WBCs); Tx: **graft excision**
Infection – late (MC from **needle puncture** from HD); can often salvage
    graft w/ local Tx

Pseudoaneurysm - MC from a needle stick that failed to seal
> Tx: **U/S + thrombin injection** or open site and place stitch in hole

Seroma - MC along arterial side
> Tx: percutaneous drainage; consider pseudocapsule rsxn

Cardiac failure- can occur w/ traumatic AVF; rare after shunt
> High venous return to heart ↑s C.O. leads to high output CHF
> **↓ed heart rate** w/ compression of shunt suggests **CHF** from graft
> Tx: band around shunt to ↓ flow rate (if intentional AV fistula); if traumatic – repair (see below)

Acquired AV fistula
MC secondary to trauma

Sx's
> **Arterial insufficiency** (eg claudication)
> > **CHF** – high output cardiac failure due to **shunt** (CO will be <u>high)</u>
> > > Left ventricular hypertrophy, hypotension, tachycardia
> > > ↑ed mixed venous saturation (SVO2) from shunt
>
> **Aneurysm**
> **Limb-length discrepancy**
> **Prone to infections** (venous side – where jet hits)

Dx: Duplex U/S *(best test)* or angio; May feel **thrill** or hear **bruit** over area

Tx:
> **Open Repair** → lateral venous suture; patch arterial side (may need bypass graft), interpose sartorius muscle between artery and vein so that it does <u>not</u> recur
> **Endovascular stent** → also an option

Abdominal pain after CABG
DDx: Pancreatitis
> **Mesenteric ischemia**
> **Acalculous cholecystitis**
> **Ischemic colitis**
> **Ischemic liver injury**

RUQ pain – likely cholecystitis
Pain out of proportion to exam – mesenteric ischemia
Atrial fibrillation – mesenteric ischemia
Mid-epigastric pain – pancreatitis or ulcer
Bloody stools – ischemic colitis or mesenteric ischemia

Abdominal pain after cardiac cath
Mesenteric ischemia (Dx - angio)
Retroperitoneal bleed (Dx - abd CT scan; Tx: cut down on artery and repair or angio + stent for continued hypotension despite blood products)

<u>Normal Vein Anatomy</u>
Greater saphenous vein – joins femoral vein near groin; runs medially
Lesser saphenous vein – joins popliteal vein in lower leg; runs lateral at first

<u>Primary Venous Insufficiency</u>
Sx's: edema, ulceration, aching, heaviness, bleeding, thrombophlebitis
Brawny edema – suggests severe DZ
Ulceration occurs **above and posterior to malleoli**
Edema – secondary to incompetent perforators
Elevation brings relief
RFs – obesity, low activity, smoking
Dx:
Duplex U/S *(best Dx study)* w/ pt standing, look for:
1) **Sapheno-femoral** or **sapheno-popliteal valve incompetence**
2) **Incompetent perforator valves**
3) **DVT**
Need to make sure pt does **not** have a DVT
DVT is a contraindication to vein stripping and avulsion
Gives **location** and **size of veins** as well as **direction of blood flow**
Diagnosis of **valve incompetence** made if relief of muscle pressure distally (eg thigh) causes retrograde flow
Normal venous Duplex U/S – augmentation of flow with proximal compression (eg calf) or release of proximal compression (eg thigh)
ABI's to r/o arterial insufficiency (< 0.7 worrisome for Unna boot)
Medical tx 1st
Avoid prolonged standing
Weight loss
D/C smoking
Elevate legs at night
Elastic stockings
Unna Boot for severe DZ
Zinc oxide triple layer wrap
For severe ulcers or significant edema
Need snug graded compression to tibia for 1 week at a time
90% of ulcers cured this way – if this fails, try **endoscopic Linton procedure** below
Surgical tx (for failure of medical tx)
Fundamental of surgical tx of varicose veins is **ablation of reflux source** (escape point)
Dx: Duplex U/S will tell you where problem is (also make sure <u>no DVT</u>)
Tx:
Varicosities < 1 mm (eg varicose veins) – sclerotherapy
0.2% sodium tetradecyl
Fill the vein – no single vein injection should exceed 0.1 cc
Pressure dressing for 48 hours
3 weeks later open area and remove hematoma
Varicosities > 4 mm
1) If sapheno-femoral (GSV) + sapheno-popliteal (LSV) junctions are <u>**competent**</u> (just have **incompetent perforators**)
→ **stab avulsion technique** to remove varicosities (or **endoscopic Linton procedure** which ligates perforators → esp. good for non-healing ulcers)
Venous ligation unnecessary – hemostasis is achieved w/ compression during and after surgery
Mark varicosities you are going to take while pt standing
Wrap leg at end of procedure

2) If sapheno-femoral (GSV) and sapheno-popliteal (LSV) junctions are <u>**not competent**</u> → ***vein stripping***
Done from thigh downward w/ vein stripper; wrap leg

Superficial thrombophlebitis (nonbacterial inflammation)

    MC in setting of **previous peripheral IV**

    Tx: NSAIDs, warm packs, arm elevation

Suppurative thrombophlebitis – fever and ↑WBCs

    Sx's: erythema, red streaking up arm, and **fluctuance** at site

        Possible **palpable cord**

        MC in setting of **previous peripheral IV**

    MC organism – staph aureus

    Dx: U/S will show **cord**; blood cultures may show organism

    Tx:

        1) **Remove peripheral IV** and **abx's;** warm compress, elevation

        2) Need to **resect entire vein** for continued **purulence or bacteremia despite abx's**

Migrating thrombophlebitis – pancreatic CA, other CA (need CA w/u)

Lymphatics

Lymphatics do <u>not</u> contain a basement membrane

Lymphatics <u>not</u> found in bone, muscle, tendon, cartilage, brain, or cornea

Deep lymphatics have **valves**

Lymphedema

    Lymphatic fluid retention caused by a compromised lymphatic system

    Primary (congenital): L > R

    Secondary: MC in women after ALND

        Also caused by tumor burden in lymphatics

    Lymphatics obstructed, too few in number, or nonfunctional

    Sx's:

        Leads to **woody edema** secondary to fibrous tissue in subcutaneous tissue – toes, feet, ankle, leg

        Infection, cellulitis and **lymphangitis** secondary to minor trauma are a big problem w/ this

    MC infection – strep

    Tx: extremity elevation, compression, abx's for infection

Lymphangiosarcoma

    Raised nodule w/ blue/purple/red coloring in extremity w/ chronic lymphedema

    Early mets to lung

    Stewart-Treves syndrome – associated with breast ALND

Lymphangiectasia

    MCC – congenital

    others – CA, granulomatous DZ

    Sx's: numerous clear fluid-filled vesicles in a chronic lymphedematous area

    Dx: skin Bx

    Tx: compression, resection if refractory, keep clean to avoid infection

Lymphocele following surgery

    Usually after dissection in the groin (eg femoral to popliteal bypass)

    Leakage clear fluid; need to R/O an infectious source for the fluid (send cultures, get CT scan of area)

    Small lymphoceles can be observed (may reabsorb spontaneously)

    Dx: Duplex U/S

    Tx:

        Initial tx – percutaneous aspiration (can try a couple of times)

        If that fails:

            Inject **isosulfan blue dye** into foot to identify the lymphatic channels supplying the lymphocele

            Resect lymphocele and ligate supplying lymphatic channel

GASTROINTESTINAL HORMONES

Gastrin
>	Produced G cells in **antrum** and **duodenum**
>	**Secretion stimulated by** – protein, vagal input (acetylcholine), calcium, ETOH, antral distention, pH > 3.0
>	**Secretion inhibited by** – pH < 3.0, somatostatin, secretin, CCK, VIP, GIP, glucagon, calcitonin
>	**Target cells** – parietal cells (via enterochromaffin cells) and chief cells
>	**Response**
>>		Secretion of **HCl, intrinsic factor** and **pepsinogen** (*strongest stimulator for all*)
>>		↑ **gastric motility** (although ↓s motility for rest of GI tract)
>>		**Trophic effects** on gastric mucosa
>	**Proton pump inhibitors** (eg Omeprazole) block H^+/K^+ ATPase of parietal cell (final pathway for H^+ release).
>	**Parietal cells** – release HCl and Intrinsic Factor
>	**Chief cells** – release pepsinogen

Somatostatin
>	Produced by D cells in **antrum**
>	**Secretion stimulated by** – acid in duodenum
>	**Target cells** – many "the great inhibitor" (acts through G-protein linked somatostatin receptor)
>	**Response**:
>>		Inhibits gastrin and HCl release
>>		Inhibits release of insulin, glucagon, secretin, CCK, GIP, VIP, motilin
>>		↓s pancreatic and biliary output
>>		Slows gastric emptying
>	**Octreotide** (somatostatin analogue) – may be used to ↓ pancreatic fistula output

Glucose-dependent insulinotropic peptide (GIP)
>	Formerly called gastric inhibitory peptide (GIP)
>	Produced by K cells in **duodenum**
>	**Secretion stimulated by** – glucose in stomach *only*
>	**Target cells** – pancreatic beta cells
>	**Response** – ↑ insulin release
>	Once thought to have more functions but physiologically just does the above

CCK (cholecystokinin)
>	Produced by I cells of **duodenum** (MC site) and jejunum
>	**Secretion stimulated by** – protein and fat in duodenum
>	**Response**
>>		**Gallbladder contraction**
>>		**Relaxation of sphincter of Oddi**
>>		↑ **pancreatic acinar** enzyme **secretion** (acinar cells, zymogen granules)
>>		↑ **intestinal motility**
>>		Hepatic bile synthesis
>>		**Satiety** – receptor in hypothalamus

Secretin
>	Produced by S cells of **duodenum**
>	**Secretion stimulated by** – acid (pH < 4), fat, bile
>	**Secretion inhibited by** – pH > 4.0, gastrin
>	**Endocrine** (primarily) + **exocrine** effects
>	**Response**
>>		**Inhibits gastrin** (*reversed w/ gastrinoma*) and **HCl release** (*primary duty*)
>>		↑s pancreatic ductal $HCO3^-$ secretion
>>		↑s bile flow
>>		↑s $HCO3^-$ secretion from duodenal **Brunner Glands**
>>>			High pancreatic duct output has – ↑ $HCO3^-$, ↓ Cl^-
>>>			Slow pancreatic duct output has – ↓ $HCO3^-$, ↑ Cl^-
>>>			**Carbonic anhydrase** in duct exchanges $HCO3^-$ or Cl^-
>	Most important stimulant of pancreatic ductal cells

Vasoactive intestinal peptide (VIP)

    Produced by cells in **gut and pancreas**

    Secretion stimulated by – fat, acetylcholine

    Response

        ↑ **intestinal secretion** (water and electrolytes)

        ↑ **motility**

        ↓ **gastrin release**

Glucagon

    Released by alpha cells of the **pancreas** (also stomach, intestine)

    Secretion stimulated by – ↓ serum glucose, ↑ amino acids (to protect from hypoglycemia w/ all protein meal), acetylcholine (vagus), GRP, catecholamines (beta adrenergic)

    Secretion inhibited by – ↑ serum glucose, ↑ insulin, somatostatin, ketones, free fatty acids in blood

    Response

        Glycogenolysis and **gluconeogenesis**

        Lipolysis and **ketogenesis**

        Proteolysis

        All decreased → gastric acid secretion, pancreatic secretion, intestinal motility, stomach motility, myenteric motor complexes

        Increased LES tone

    Alpha and **beta cells** = G.I. (glucagon and insulin)

Insulin

    Released by beta cells of the **pancreas**

    Secretion stimulated by – serum glucose, glucagon, CCK, protein ingestion

    Secretion inhibited by – somatostatin

    Response

        Cellular glucose uptake

        Protein, glycogen, and **triacylglyceride** (ie fat) **synthesis** (<u>anabolic</u>)

    Type I diabetes – pancreatic beta islet cells destroyed

    Type II diabetes – insulin resistance

Pancreatic polypeptide

    Secreted by islet cells in **pancreas**

    Secretion stimulated by – fasting, exercise, and hypoglycemia

    Secretion inhibited by – serum glucose and somatostatin

    Response – ↓s pancreatic endocrine and exocrine function

Peptide YY

    Released from terminal ileum and colon

    Response

        Inhibits gastric emptying, gastric acid secretion, pancreatic function, and gallbladder contraction

        Increases water and electrolyte absorption from colon

        Suppresses appetite

Gastrin-releasing peptide (Bombesin)

    Release from post-ganglionic fibers of vagus nerve

    Response – ↑ gastric acid secretion, intestinal motor activity, and pancreatic enzyme secretion

Motilin

    Release by M cells primarily from **duodenum** (some jejunum)

    Highest concentration of motilin receptors – stomach antrum, duodenum, colon

    Secretion stimulated by – duodenal acid, vagus input

        Released during **fasting** *or* **inter-digestive phase** (not while eating)

    Secretion inhibited by – somatostatin, secretin, pancreatic polypeptide, duodenal fat

    Primary Response – ↑ed **antrum** and **duodenal motility** [initiates phase III (peristalsis) of the migrating motor complex (MMC)]

    Erythromycin acts on this receptor

Anorexia – mediated by hypothalamus (CCK, peptide YY)

Bowel recovery after surgery

    Small bowel recovers in 24 hours

    Stomach recovers in 48 hours

    Large bowel recovers in 3-5 days

Normal Anatomy and Function

Anatomy

Layers

Mucosa: squamous epithelium + basement membrane
Submucosa
Muscularis propria: inner circular + outer longitudinal muscle layers
No serosa
Upper esophagus– **striated muscle**
Lower esophagus– **smooth muscle**

Blood supply

Cervical – inferior thyroid artery
Thoracic – vessels directly off aorta (main supply to esophagus)
Abdominal – left gastric artery (primary); inferior phrenic artery

Lymphatics:

Upper 1/3 – cervical, thoracic
Middle 1/3 – thoracic
Lower 1/3 – abdominal, thoracic

Innervation

Right vagus nerve
Travels on posterior portion of stomach as it exits chest
Becomes **celiac plexus**
Has **criminal nerve of Grassi** → causes persistently high acid
levels post-op if left undivided w/ vagotomy

Left vagus nerve
On anterior portion of stomach; goes to **liver + biliary tree**

Thoracic duct
Runs along right side of lower mediastinum
Crosses midline at T4-T5 and now runs on left side of mediastinum
Goes into left neck for a ways, turns around, and dumps into left
subclavian vein at junction w/ internal jugular vein

Normal manometry

Pharyngeal contraction w/ food bolus	70-120 mmHg

Upper esophageal sphincter

At rest	60 mmHg
W/ food bolus	15 mmHg

Failure of pressure drop indicates <u>failure of cricopharyngeous</u> to relax

Lower esophageal sphincter

At rest	15 mmHg
W/ food bolus	0 mmHg

Resting LES pressure frequently ≤ 5 w/ <u>GERD</u>

Esophageal contraction w/ swallow	30-120 mmHg

Ineffective if < 10 mmHg throughout (ie burned out esophagus)

Normal Distances (anatomic areas of narrowing listed below, measurements
from incisors, esophagus is **30 cm total length**):

Cricopharyngeous	15 cm
Aortic arch indentation	25 cm
Diaphragmatic hiatus	45 cm

LES is <u>not</u> visible – is a manometric finding

Upper esophageal sphincter – cricopharyngeus muscle (circular muscle)
Prevents air swallowing
Recurrent laryngeal nerve innervation
MC site of esophageal perforation – near cricopharyngeus (MC w/ EGD)
MC site for foreign body – just above cricopharyngeous (Killian's triangle)
Aspiration w/ brainstem stroke – failure of UES to relax

Lower esophageal sphincter (40 cm from incisors) – relaxation mediated by
inhibitory neurons; normally contracted at rest → <u>prevents reflux</u>
1) LES is <u>not</u> an anatomical sphincter *and*; 2) LES is <u>not</u> seen on EGD
Is a physiologic zone (3-5 cm) of ↑ed pressure found w/ **manometry**

Swallowing stages

CNS initiates swallow
Primary peristalsis – occurs w/ food bolus and swallow initiation

Secondary peristalsis – occurs w/ incomplete emptying and esophageal distention, consists of propagating waves

Tertiary peristalsis – non-propagating, non-peristalsing (dysfunctional)

UES + LES are contracted between meals to avoid reflux + air swallowing

Swallowing mechanism

Soft palate occludes nasopharynx

Larynx rises and airway opening is blocked by epiglottis

Cricopharyngeus relaxes

Pharyngeal contraction moves food into esophagus

**LES relaxes soon after initiation of swallow (vagus induced relaxation)

Surgical approach to esophagus

Cervical esophagus	left neck (left sided course here)
Upper 2/3 thoracic	right (avoids the aorta)
Lower 1/3 thoracic	left (left-sided course here)

Hiccoughs

Etiologies – gastric distention, temp change, ETOH, tobacco

Reflex arc – vagus nerve, phrenic nerve, sympathetic chain T6–12

Esophageal dysfunction

Primary – achalasia, nutcracker, and diffuse spasm

Secondary – GERD (MC), scleroderma, polymyositis

Endoscopy

Procedure of choice for **heartburn**

Procedure of choice for **foreign body** (Dx and Tx)

Esophagogram (gastrograffin or barium)

Procedure of choice for **dysphagia** and **odynophagia**

Procedure of choice for **suspected perforation** (gastrograffin, then thin barium)

Pharyngoesophageal disorders

Sx's: trouble transferring food from mouth to esophagus

Liquids worse than solids

MC secondary to **neuromuscular disease** – myasthenia gravis, Parkinson's disease, polymyositis, muscular dystrophy, stroke, others - Zenker's

Plummer-Vinson syndrome – esophageal webs; Fe^{++}-deficient anemia

Tx: dilation, Fe^{++}; screen for oral CA

Dysphagia (difficulty swallowing) or Odynophagia (painful swallowing)

DDx

Primary esophageal motility D/Os (Achalasia, DES, nutcracker)

Secondary esophageal motility D/O (MC – GERD reflux causing esophageal damage and motility problems)

Esophageal CA

Peptic Stricture

Zenker's

Leiomyoma

Additional Sx's

Weight loss – CA

Halitosis – Zenker's

PNA, asthma, aspiration or **regurgitation** - GERD, achalasia, Zenker, CA

Heart burn – GERD

ETOH or tobacco – CA

Dysphagia usually **intermittent** w/ functional D/Os

Liquids only	more likely pharyngeal motor D/O
Solids and liquids	more likely esophageal motor D/O
Solids only	more likely CA or stricture

Dx:

1st **Barium swallow** *(Best initial test for dysphagia or odynophagia)*

Get this 1st so you don't perforate a potential Zenker's

2nd **EGD w/ Bx** – evaluate to level of duodenum

Manometry studies – may need depending on Barium Swallow, EGD

ph study – may need depending on Barium Swallow, EGD

Achalasia
1) **Inability of LES to relax**
2) **Loss of peristalsis**

Autoimmune destruction of myenteric plexus → **loss of neuronal ganglion cells** (Auerbach's myenteric plexus)

Sx's: **dysphagia** (both solids and liquids; in nearly <u>all</u> pts) and **regurgitation**
Chagas disease - similar mechanism, bite wound, caused by *T. cruzi*

Dx:

> **Esophagogram** *(initial test for dysphagia)*
> > Esophageal dilatation w/ tapering distally (bird's beak)
> > Can see tortuous, dilated, floppy esophagus if burned out
> > Occasionally have epiphrenic diverticula
>
> **EGD** – needed for all pts to R/O **malignancy**
> > If having difficulty in passing scope past EGJ → suspect **pseudoachalasia** (ie **GE junction malignancy**)
>
> ****Manometry Studies** *(best test for Dx of Achalasia)*
> > 1) **LES fails to relax** w/ swallowing (usually is > 25 mmHg)
> > 2) **Loss of peristalsis** (low amplitude and fails to progress)

Burned out esophagus
> \> 50% non-pulsatile contractions
> < 30 mmHg w/ each contraction
> Big and dilated esophagus
> If esophagus is burned out, medical tx and esophagocardiomyotomy are not going to be effective → consider esophagectomy

SCCA of esophagus
> ↑ed in pts w/ achalasia (15 x normal)
> Very concerning if pt has associated **weight loss**
> All pt's w/ achalasia need an **EGD** and **esophagogram** to R/O CA

Medical Tx:
> Primary goal is **relief of obstruction at LES**
> Try **balloon dilatation** x 2 (80% effective)
> **Calcium channel blocker**
> **Nitrates**

Surgical Tx
> **Esophago-cardiomyotomy** (Heller Myotomy, *definitive Tx*)
> > At time of operation, **EGD** used to **clean out esophagus** to avoid aspiration
> > Left thoracotomy or laparoscopic
> > Myotomy should extend **1-2 cm below EGJ** and **7 cm proximally on esophagus** or approximately to level of inferior pulmonary vein
> > Separate muscle layers from mucosa laterally for 1 cm (180° or 1/2 circumference of the esophagus) to **prevent re-healing**
> > <u>Partial</u> fundal wrap (↓s reflux + avoids dysphagia) then performed
> > POD#1 → **gastrograffin swallow** (then thin barium; **re-operate** if early leak), then **clears**
> >
> > **Cx's:**
> > > **Late leak** - make sure adequately drained (percutaneous drain or chest tube)
> > > Abx's for at least 1 week, NPO, TPN
> > > Chest/abd CT to R/O abscess
> > > Gastrograffin (then thin barium) swallow to R/O distal stenosis
> > > Wait it out
> > > Surgery if still not closed after 6-8 weeks
> >
> > **Pneumothorax**
> > **Splenic injury**

> **Esophagectomy** considered for Achalasia w/
> > 1) **burned out esophagus** that fails to empty
> > 2) repeated myotomies and now w/ **stricture**

Diffuse esophageal spasm

Sx's: dysphagia and **chest pain**; possible psych history

Dx:

EKG, CXR, Troponins, and CK-MB → *need to r/o myocardial ischemia*

Barium swallow – corkscrew esophagus; may see diverticulum

**Manometry *(best test for Dx DES)*

High amplitude, repetitive, *non-peristaltic*, contractions (long duration)

Peristalsis interspersed w/ these non-peristaltic contractions

> 30% non-peristaltic

LES relaxes normally

EGD – normal (r/o any other pathology)

Medical tx *(best Tx);*

1) **Calcium channel blocker** (Diltiazem, titrate to effect)

2) **Trazodone**

Decrease anxiety – psych assessment

Indications for surgery: reserved for pts w/ recurrent, incapacitating episodes of dysphagia ± chest pain who do not respond to medical tx (last resort)

Surgery Tx – long esophageal myotomy

Right thoracotomy or thoracoscopic approach MC

Myotomy whole length of thoracic esophagus (180 degrees around)

Carried 1-2 cm onto stomach

Anti-reflux procedure (eg Belsey intra-thoracic fundoplication – considered a partial wrap)

Surgery better at resolving dysphagia than pain

Treatment usually less effective than for achalasia

Nutcracker esophagus (MC primary esophageal D/O)

Sx's: chest pain (MCC of non-cardiac chest pain); ± dysphagia

Dx:

EKG, CXR, Troponins, and CK-MB → *need to r/o myocardial ischemia*

Esophagogram – not really diagnostic

**Manometry *(best test for Dx of nutcracker)*

Very **high amplitude *peristaltic* waves** (> 180 mmHg)

LES relaxes normally

EGD – normal (r/o any other pathology)

Medical tx *(best treatment, same as DES above);*

1) **Calcium channel blocker** (Diltiazem titrate to effect)

2) **Trazodone**

Decrease anxiety - Psych assessment

Indications for surgery: reserved for pts w/ recurrent, incapacitating episodes of dysphagia ± chest pain who do not respond to medical tx (last resort)

Surgery Tx – long esophageal myotomy

Right thoracotomy or thoracoscopic approach MC

Myotomy whole length of thoracic esophagus (180 degrees around)

Carried 1-2 cm onto stomach

Anti-reflux procedure (eg Belsey intra-thoracic fundoplication – considered a partial wrap)

Surgery better at resolving dysphagia than pain

Treatment usually less effective than for achalasia

Scleroderma

Sx's: Heartburn (massive reflux, much greater than GERD) and **dysphagia**

Get complete loss of LES tone and fibrous replacement of smooth muscle

CREST – Raynaud's, pulmonary DZ, renal DZ

Calcinosis

Raynaud's phenomenon,

Esophageal dysmotility

Sclerodactyly

Teleangiectasias

Dx:
>Esophagogram – need to R/O adenocarcinoma (2% of these pts)
>>Can get strictures
>**Manometry** *(best test for Dx)*
>>Aperistalsis and weak contractions
>>Low or absent resting LES pressure
>EGD – best to assess **damage**; also look for **adenocarcinoma**
>**24 hour pH probe** – most sensitive indicator of reflux

Path
>Sclerosis of small arteries w/ collagen and fibrous tissue deposition
>**Atrophy** and **fibrosis of smooth muscle** in distal 2/3 esophagus
>Can affect heart, lungs, kidney's – **esophagus MC affected organ**
>Can be localized or systemic
>**Raynaud's** – considered most impt clinical finding associated w/
>>esophageal dysfunction
>**MCC death w/ scleroderma** – pulmonary fibrosis
>5-YS – 80%

Medial tx:
>**Omeprazole**
>**Head of bed elevation**
>**Avoid large meals**
>**Reglan** (Prokinetics)
>**Nystatin** – prevent thrush
>**Balloon dilatation for strictures** (steroids do NOT work)
>These pts should have continued surveillance

Indications for operation:
>GERD sx's refractory to medical tx
>Development of refractory cx's – ulcers, strictures

Types of operations:
>1) **Partial wrap + Collis gastroplasty**- for normal size esophagus + GERD
>2) **Esophagectomy** (for Cx's of GERD) – many believe this is the best TX

Epiphrenic diverticula (rare)
>*Is a false diverticula* – usually in **distal** 1/3 of esophagus
>Presence is not an indication for operation although underlying problem may be
>**MCC** – primary esophageal motility D/O (**MC achalasia**)
>>others - hiatal hernia w/ peptic stricture
>Is a **pulsion diverticula** – distal narrowing (failure of LES to relax w/ achalasia,
>>peptic stricture) causes pressure → esophageal protrusion proximally
>**Sx's**: MC are **asymptomatic**; can have dysphagia and regurgitation
>**Dx**: esophagogram, manometry, EGD
>**Tx**:
>>**Fix underlying motility problem if present**
>>>(eg balloon dilatation for achalasia or peptic stricture)
>>>Diverticula does not necessarily need to be resected
>>**Refractory Achalasia**
>>>**Longitudinal myotomy** – perform on the opposite side of the
>>>>diverticula if you plan on resecting it
>>>**Diverticulum resection indications** – narrow neck (traps food),
>>>>inflammation, large size, or CA present; o/w can just suspend
>>>>(diverticula resection not necessary to fix underlying problem)

Traction diverticulum
>*Is a true diverticula* – usually lateral **middle** 1/3 of esophagus
>**MCC** – infection [chronic granulomatous DZ (eg histoplasmosis)]
>>others – inflammation, tumor
>Above processes pull esophagus out
>**Sx's**: regurgitation of undigested food, dysphagia
>**Dx**: esophagogram, chest CT, EGD
>**Tx**: ****Leave alone unless causing sx's**
>>Excision and primary closure if symptomatic
>>Palliative Tx (eg XRT, esophageal stent) if due to invasive lung CA

THE COMPREHENSIVE ABSITE REVIEW

Pharyngoesophageal Diverticulum (Zenker's)

Due to **ineffective relaxation of cricopharyngeous**

Pharyngeal constrictors push against this, creating high pressure

Diverticulum found **between cricopharyngeous** and **pharyngeal constrictors** (Killian's triangle)

Is a false diverticulum (not all layers; no muscle; pulsion diverticulum)

MC location – posterior

Sx's:

Dysphagia and **regurgitation of non-digested food** present in <u>almost all</u>

Halitosis, lump sensation, aspiration, noisy swallowing

Dx:

Barium swallow – midline protrusion at posterior hypopharyngeal wall above UES

**NO EGD → *avoided* due to risk of perforation; distal esophageal problems evaluated after Zenker's operation

Manometry studies – show lack of UES relaxation (not really necessary)

pH probe – unnecessary

Tx:

Cricopharyngeal myotomy *(Key Point of Tx, <u>not</u> resection of diverticulum)*

Performed over 180 degrees of esophagus

Left neck incision on anterior border of SCM (**inferior thyroid artery** and **middle thyroid vein** ligated for exposure) – left side has more predictable location of left recurrent laryngeal nerve (avoids injury)

Extend cricopharyngomyotomy 3 cm over hypopharynx and 3 cm over cervical esophagus

Usually staple off diverticula (**GIA 45 over a 54 Fr bougie** to avoid stenosis)

Can also <u>suspend diverticulum</u> if too hard to resect

(resection of diverticulum <u>not</u> necessary to fix problem)

Leave drains

Gastrograffin/Barium swallow POD #1 to r/o leak (**re-operate** for early leak); Pull drain after tolerating clears w/o leak

Cx's:

Late leak – make sure adequately drained

Abx's for at least 1 week, NPO, TPN

Chest and neck CT to R/O abscess

Gastrograffin (then thin barium) swallow to R/O distal stenosis

Wait it out

Surgery if still not closed after 6-8 weeks

Wound infection → open wound

Gastrograffin (then thin barium) swallow to R/O leak

If you find leak, tx as above

Stenosis (eg dysphagia post-op) → want to start dilating this area after 1 week; Can be a problem if you do not tx early

Esophageal Perforations

Sx's:

Chest pain and **dysphagia**

Subcutaneous emphysema, fever, resp distress, tachycardia (all suggest **free perforation**)

Often in setting of EGD

RFs – EGD, balloon dilatation, pre-existing esophageal DZ, foreign body

Dx:

CXR, AXR and **neck films** (initial studies) – PTX (80%), subcutaneous air (50%), fluid collection

Esophagogram *(Best Test,* gastrograffin followed by thin barium)

Get even w/ known perforation, want to identify level of perforation and multiple perforations *(No EGD for Dx)*

Path

MC site overall – near cricopharyngeous (UES, narrowest point)

Other sites – indentation of aortic arch, LES

MCC overall – EGD (50% iatrogenic)

Cervical – perforation of bucco-pharyngeal fascia allows access to **retrovisceral + pre-tracheal space** → can get **mediastinitis**

Initial Tx: ABC's, IV x 2, fluid resuscitation, Abx's

Contained Perforation (unusual, most need repair)

Needs to be self-draining back into esophagus, no systemic effects, no distal obstruction (eg achalasia, stricture, or CA)

Conservative Tx: TPN, NPO x 7 days, spit, broad-spectrum abx's

Repeat esophagogram after 7 days

Clears for 1 week, mechanical soft for 2 weeks after that

Free perforation of **cervical esophagus** – left neck incision

Primary repair and leave drains

If you can't repair - just **leave drains**, will heal

Usually No esophagectomy if just cervical and can't repair

Can't find cervical perforation – just **leave drains**, repeat contrast studies in 7 days; *Usually No esophagectomy if just cervical*, will heal

Free perforation of **thoracic esophagus**

Incision based on level of injury

Proximal thoracic esophagus – right thoracotomy

Distal thoracic esophagus – left thoracotomy

1) **< 24 hrs, minimal contamination, no mediastinitis**, and **not septic** → ****Primary repair***

Adequate **longitudinal myotomy** to see length of injury

2 layer closure of esophagus

Cover w/ viable tissue (intercostal muscle)

Need to **relieve any associated distal obstruction w/ repair** (eg achalasia or peptic stricture)

Leave CTs; NPO x 1 week; NGT past repair, abx's, TPN or J-tube feeds

After 1 week – esophagogram to R/O leak or stenosis, start clears

After 3 weeks – mechanical soft diet

Esophagectomy – may be needed in stable pts w/ perforation and intrinsic disease (eg burned out esophagus, CA, non-dilatable stricture)

24-48 hours – assess esophagus and mediastinum → if favorable, primary repair, if not, esophagectomy and diversion below

2) **> 48 hours, mediastinitis, gross contamination,** or **septic pts** → ****Esophagectomy** and diversion*

Cervical esophagostomy for spit diversion

Staple above GE junction

Esophagectomy

Washout mediastinum, place chest tubes, place feeding J tube

Later gastric pull-up (6-8 weeks)

If really sick, *can leave esophagus* at initial washout (still need diversion and washout procedure)

Special Issues

Perforation after dilation for **Achalasia** (Dx studies as above)

Contained perforation (unusual)

Make sure **LES was effectively dilated** prior to perforation before going w/ conservative Tx above (o/w pressure will build and won't be a contained perforation anymore)

Non-contained perforation

Esophageal Repair

Left thoracotomy (if perforation at LES)

After repair of perforation, also need **longitudinal myotomy** on opposite side of perforation to Tx achalasia (repair won't last if LES can't relax) → this is **definitive Tx for achalasia**

Burned out esophagus (non-functional) or **can't repair** (esophagus too badly damaged):

1) **No mediastinitis** → esophagectomy and gastric pull-up at the time of perforation

2) **Mediastinitis** → esophagectomy and diversion

Perforation of **Peptic Stricture**

Contained perforation (unusual)

Make sure **stricture was effectively dilated** prior to perforation before going w/ conservative Tx (o/w pressure will build and you won't have a contained perforation anymore)

Non-contained perforation

If long term problem w/ repeated dilatations, unlikely to be able to repair → likely need **esophagectomy** (gastric pull-up at same time if no mediastinitis)

If able to dilate stricture (relieve distal obstruction) → **primary repair**

Need partial wrap or PPI post-op

Perforation of **Esophageal CA**

1) **Resectable DZ and no mediastinitis** → esophagectomy and gastric pull-up at the time of perforation

2) **Resectable DZ but pt has mediastinitis** → esophagectomy and diversion

3) **If not resectable** (eg diffuse mets)→ **palliative stent** *(best option)*

Trans-esophageal ECHO (TEE) **induced esophageal dissection and intra-mural hematoma** (can create a dissection plane in esophagus)

Sx's – hematemesis, chest pain

Tx: conservative management unless free perforation, NPO for 7 days, abx's, etc.(most managed conservatively here)

Mediastinal abscess after foreign body removal – CT guided percutaneous drain if not systemically ill

Boerhaave's Syndrome

MC results in perforation in **lower left esophagus** (4 cm above EGJ; 80%)

Sx's: large meal + ETOH → **forceful vomiting** episode → **chest pain** *(classic)*, SOB and fever; *these are almost never contained perforations*

Dx:

CXR + AXR - free air, PTX, or pleural effusion (usually left); mediastinal emphysema

Esophagogram *(Best test;* gastrograffin then thin barium) – finds perforation area; if not available, get chest CT w/ oral contrast

Tx:

Primary Repair (left thoracotomy; see above for details of repair)

Esophagectomy if esophagus is too badly damaged or extensive mediastinitis

< 24 hours   *repair* unless esophagus too damaged or mediastinitis

24-48 hours   assess esophagus + mediastinum, if OK, repair, if not resection

> 48 hours   *esophagectomy*

***Boerhaave's have highest mortality for esophageal perforations** – 40%*

<u>Esophageal caustic Injury</u> (Burn Grades)
> **Grade 0**: normal
> **Grade I**: mucosal **hyperemia** and **edema**
> **Grade IIa**: exudates, **superficial ulceration**, sloughing, pseudomembranes
> > **Grade IIb**: above *plus* **circumferential ulcerations**
> **Grade IIIa**: deep ulceration, necrosis, massive hemorrhage, **obliteration of lumen**, charring, **perforation**
> > **Grade IIIb**: above *plus* **extensive necrosis**

<u>Caustic esophageal injury</u>
> **Alkali** – deep liquefaction necrosis, especially liquid (eg Drano, lye)
> > *Worse injury than acid*; also more likely to cause subsequent CA
> **Acid** – coagulation necrosis; mostly causes gastric injury
> **Cx's of caustic ingestion** – esophageal or stomach perforation or necrosis, strictures, CA
> **Initial Tx:**
> > **ABC's, 2 IV's, fluid resuscitation, abx's**
> > *Do not place NG tube; Do not induce vomiting*; NPO
> > Inspect mouth + oropharynx, if injured or hoarseness / stridor → **intubate**
> **Dx** (need all of the following):
> > 1) **CXR** and **AXR** – looking for PTX, effusion, free air, or subcutaneous / mediastinal emphysema
> > 2) **Endoscopy** – need to assess severity of lesion
> > > Do *NOT* go past the point of severe injuries; Figure out injury degree
> > 3) **Gastrograffin swallow** (followed by thin barium) if not intubated
> > > **Chest/abd CT** instead of swallow if intubated
> > 4) **Bronch** – if aspiration suspected
> **Tx:**
> > 1) **Stent** for **mouth burns**
> > 2) **Perforation**
> > > **Signs of perforation** → Free air, pleural effusion, sepsis, subcutaneous or mediastinal emphysema, PTX
> > > **All above indications for going to OR →**
> > > > **Esophagectomy**
> > > > > **Right thoracotomy** – allows removal of entire esophagus
> > > > > *Do not repair caustic perforations*
> > > > **Washout mediastinal area**
> > > > Staple off stomach end
> > > > Chest tubes, decompressing G tube, feeding J tube, cervical esophagostomy
> > > > Gastric pull-up (adults, sub-sternal) or colon replacement (children) in 6-8 weeks (well after recovery)
> > 3) **Peritonitis**
> > > **Exploratory laparotomy** – evaluate stomach, if necrotic, resection of that part; look at esophagus – if that is necrotic also need transhiatal esophagectomy at the same time (do NOT hook-up)
> > 4) **No perforation or peritonitis**
> > > Serial **X-rays and exams**
> > > **Indications for surgery** – sepsis, peritonitis, worsening metabolic acidosis, mediastinitis, free air, mediastinal air, crepitance, contrast extravasation, PTX, pleural effusion, stomach wall air
> > > **Conservative Tx**: IVFs, spitting, abx's
> > > **HD # 3**
> > > > Repeat **gastrograffin/barium swallow**
> > > > Extubate if there is an air-leak
> > > > Start TPN
> > > > NPO until able to swallow their own secretions, then clears
> > > **HD #7**
> > > > Perform careful **EGD in OR** → looking for full thickness injury
> > > > **Grade I-IIa injuries**
> > > > > NPO until they can handle their own saliva (MC 1-3 d)
> > > > > Then start liquids (milk) for 1 week

Then mechanical soft for 3 weeks

Grade IIb or higher injuries

Place gastrostomy (28 Fr Stamm) and feeding J-tube

Pass string from mouth out through Gastrostomy (EGD; future dilatation)

Can dilate stricture from above (mouth) and below (through gastrostomy tube) using the string as a guidewire starting at 3 weeks

Strictures usually take **3 weeks to form**

If esophagectomy needed – alimentary tract *not* restored until after pt recovers from the caustic injury (6-8 weeks)

Strictures usually **cervical** and near **aortic indentation**

Can also get **shortening of esophagus**, requiring PPI or future anti-reflux procedure

Perforation of caustic stricture after attempted dilatation usually requires **esophagectomy** (stricture area too chronically damaged for repair)

Esophageal Foreign Bodies

Sx's: profound saliva, choking, dysphagia, child who won't eat

Dx:

Plain films

Rigid EGD under anesthesia

Path

↑ length of time in esophagus → ↑ perforation risk

MC age groups: children < 10 and adults > 50

Adults

MC overall and **MC edible** – food impaction (meat)

MC non-edible – bones

Children

MC overall and **MC non-edible** – coins

MC edible – meat

MC site overall – UES (just below lip of the cricopharyngeous)

Highest rate of injury – bones and fish bones (10% perforation, 75% injury); Can lead to mediastinitis

Tx:

Rigid EGD in OR (need to intubate 1st)

Pull sharps out w/ tip trailing

Small pressure necrosis or perforations w/ no leakage of contrast – conservative management

Free perforation – surgical repair and drainage

Sentinel bleed w/ esophageal FB – confirm FB, then thoracotomy to remove (aorto-esophageal fistula)

Large and deeply penetrating FB – surgery

Hypopharyngeal FBs – deep inhalation anesthesia and Magill forceps

***NO foreign body should ever be left in the esophagus**

Once in stomach, most FBs pass w/o problem (get serial AXRs)

Dimensions > 2 x 5 cm – unlikely to pass through duodenum (removal indicated)

Disk batteries or coins that do not move after 48 hours – extract

Sharps – watch them pass – 10% need laparotomy

Barium esophagogram and/or **manometry after extraction indicated for:**

1) Anything below cervical esophagus (looking for obstruction/dysfunctional area)

2) Meat or food impaction (looking for obstruction/dysfunctional area)

3) Repeated episode (looking for obstruction/dysfunctional area)

4) Battery removal (looking for perforation)

MC esophageal problem leading to FB – strictures from GERD

In children, food lodging in UES – need to R/O retrobulbar palsies

Gastroesophageal reflux disease (GERD)

Sx's

Heartburn (worse 30-60 minutes after meal), ↑ed lying down or stooping

Heartburn is from **exposure of esophagus to gastric acid**

Choking, regurgitation, aspiration

Precipitants (↓ LES tone) – large meal, fatty food, ETOH, tobacco, caffeine

Many pts just treated **empirically w/ PPI w/o testing**

Make sure pt does not have another cause for pain:

Dysphagia or odynophagia – tumors, strictures, primary motility D/O

Bloating – possible aerophagia and delayed gastric emptying (Dx gastric emptying study)

Epigastric pain – peptic ulcer, tumor

Dx:

Make sure you have following studies before doing a wrap (need to R/O other potential causes of pts pain)

1) **pH test** (*best test* for GERD)

24 hour Ambulatory pH testing

Probe placed **5 cm above LES** as determined by manometry

Most sensitive indicator → > 4.5% of total time w/ pH < 4

Need to be off PPI and H2 blockers for a week before performing this

2) **Manometry** (want 3 readings)

Resting LES is usually < 6 mmHg w/ GERD

MC secondary esophageal motility problem – esophageal deterioration from GERD

Ineffective esophageal motility

Low amplitude contractions (< 30 mmHg) and non-transmitted

Need to R/O primary and secondary esophageal dysmotility D/Os before Nissen fundoplication

For secondary dysmotility D/O, will need **partial wrap** to prevent **dysphagia**

For primary dysmotility D/Os (eg achalasia, DES, nutcracker) → **need different Tx** (see previous sections)

3) **EGD w/ Bx's**

Esophagitis establishes Dx (if not present, can still have GERD)

Barrett's – raised lesions; red

Peptic ulceration – flat, always proximal to squamocolumnar junction

Strictures – need Bx to R/O CA; can also dilate stricture w/ EGD

Also get EGD when worried about GERD Cx's (eg stricture)

4) **Barium Swallow** if unusual sx's or worried about paraesophageal hernia

**Test of choice for suspected para-esophageal hernia

Distinguishes different types of hiatal hernia

Path

Most people w/ GERD have a hiatal hernia

Normal anatomic protection from GERD:

LES competence

Normal esophageal body (ie esophageal motility)

Normal gastric reservoir (eg stomach does not become distended)

GERD caused by **incompetent LES**

Requirements for adequate LES:

Adequate **LES pressure** (MC problem leading to GERD)

Adequate **LES length** (nl 5 cm)

Adequate **abdominal length** (nl 2 cm)

Esophagitis – almost always gets better w/ PPI

MCC of esophageal bleeding – esophagitis secondary to GERD

Peptic Stricture

GERD MCC of benign stricture

Most severe right above the EGJ

Need to **R/O malignancy** w/ strictures (EGD Biopsy)

Tx: medical tx is 95% effective (PPI and periodic EGD dilatation)

All peptic strictures have **shortened esophagus** and will need **Collis gastroplasty** if performing a wrap

Rare non-dilatable strictures may need esophagectomy

Esophageal Shortening

> **RFs for esophageal shortening** – peptic stricture, giant hernia, esophagitis, *previously failed wraps*
>
> Shortening suggested if **EGJ lies 4-5 cm above diaphragmatic hiatus**
>
> Esophagus should lie (freely) 2 cm below hiatus after dissection for wrap (o/w need Collis gastroplasty)

Barrett's

> Present in 10% of pts w/ GERD
>
> **Squamous to columnar metaplasia**
>
> **Specialized intestinal type metaplasia** highest RF for CA
>
> From long standing reflux
>
> *Barrett's NOT reversed w/ PPI or fundoplication*-can stop progression
>
> *CA risk NOT reversed w/ PPI or fundoplication*
>
> Cx's of Barrett's – CA, ulcer, stricture, bleeding, ulcer perforation
>
> **Need Bx's** to R/O CA (adenocarcinoma)
>
> **Surveillance for CA**
>
>> 4 quadrant Bx at 1 cm intervals annually (3-6 month initially)
>>
>> **Risk of adenocarcinoma w/ Barrett's** – 0.5% per year
>>
>> **50 x ↑ed risk of esophageal CA** compared to general population (get adenocarcinoma; relative risk = 50)
>>
>> Make sure the Dx of high grade dysplasia is confirmed by **2 experienced pathologists**
>
> ****Need continual annual surveillance even if you perform a Nissen Fundoplication in setting of Barrett's** - Barrett's never goes away, will always have CA risk
>
> **Indications for esophagectomy w/ Barrett's:**
>
>> **High grade dysplasia** (HGD, or carcinoma in situ)
>>
>>> **→ 20-25% harbor occult CA** at time of Dx
>>
>> **Perforation** – don't want to repair Barrett's area
>>
>> **Refractory bleeding**
>>
>> **Refractory stricture**
>>
>> **CA**
>
> Take **entire Barrett's segment** if performing esophagectomy
>
> *Avoid* intra-thoracic anastomosis w/ esophagectomy for GERD cx's such as HGD Barrett's – can get future reflux w/ intra-thoracic anastomosis (want anastomosis in neck)

Lower esophageal Ring (ie Schatzki's Ring)

> Associated w/ **GERD** (almost all pts have associated hiatal hernia)
>
> Lies at **squamo-columnar junction**; **submucosal fibrosis**
>
> **Sx's:** dysphagia
>
> **Dx:** barium esophagogram (likely not able to see this w/ EGD)
>
> **Tx:**
>
>> **Asymptomatic** – nothing
>>
>> **Symptomatic** – usually food impaction
>>
>>> **Dilatation** and **PPI** (sufficient in majority)
>>>
>>> Surgery for failure of dilatation or intractable reflux (→ wrap and dilatation of ring)
>>
>> *Resection of ring NEVER indicated*

Esophageal webs

> **NOT involved in any motility D/Os**
>
> 1) **Acquired** (MC type; upper esophagus; associated w/ Zenker's, Plummer-Vinson)
>
> 2) **Congenital** (middle to lower esophagus)
>
> **Sx's:** dysphagia
>
> **Dx:** barium esophagogram (may need to evacuate contents 1st)
>
> **Tx:**
>
>> Dilatation 1st
>>
>> Circumferential web excision via longitudinal esophogotomy if dilatation fails
>>
>> ***Esophagectomy NEVER indicated***

Medical Tx:
    GERD

- **PPI** (often empiric Tx, ↑ dose if refractory, 3 months minimum)
- **Elevate head of bed**
- **Weight loss** for obese pts (↓ abd pressure)
- *Avoid* → recumbency for 3 hours after meals, bedtime snacks, fatty foods, chocolate, peppermint, onions, garlic, ETOH, tobacco, NSAID's, drugs that ↓ LES pressure (CCB, anticholinergics)
- **EGD if recurrent, persistent, or worried about cx's of disease**
- **Esophagitis** – re-scope in 6 weeks to makes sure getting better
- **Results of medical Tx**:
  - **Symptom relief in 99%**
  - Improves **esophagitis**
  - Improves **strictures** (grade IV esophagitis)
  - Improves **dysphagia**
  - Decreases need for dilatation
  - Does <u>NOT</u> help Barrett's
  - LES pressure and peristaltic function <u>NOT</u> improved
- **Stricture** – dilatation and PPI (cures 95%)
- **Barrett's** (uncomplicated) – PPI (Barrett's is <u>NOT</u> an indication for wrap)

Absolute indications for surgery
- Perforation
  - Tx: repair perforation + perform reflux operation at same time (do NOT repair Barrett's area perforation – need resection)
- Uncontrolled bleeding (usually Barrett's ulcer or peptic ulcer)
- Unrelieved obstruction
- Gastric necrosis
- Unmanageable aspiration
- CA
- Barrett's w/ High Grade Dysplasia
- High grade squamous cell dysplasia or carcinoma in situ
- Para-esophageal hernia (possibly relative indication)
- Incarceration (possibly relative indication)

Relative Indications for surgery:
- Avoid lifelong medication in young pt
- GERD or cx's (esophagitis, stricture, bleeding) refractory to medical Tx
- Young pt w/ Barrett's (infants, children, adolescents), avoid ↑ in Barrett's
- Chronic Fe^{++} deficient anemia – venous congestion of gastric mucosa
- Resp inhibition from giant hernia
- Chronic gastric ulcer – worried about CA

Surgery
- **Nissen Fundoplication**
  - *Key to hiatal dissection is finding **right crura***
  - *Key to wrap is finding **left crura***
  - Divide short gastric arteries
  - Pull esophagus into abdomen
    - Need to mobilize at least **5 cm of intra-thoracic esophagus**
    - Need at least **2 cm of free esophagus** in abdomen
  - Wrap over **54 Fr Maloney Dilator** (Bougie) to prevent **stenosis**
  - Want fundus wrap **2 cm in length** → make it a **loose wrap but secure** (360-complete)
  - **Approximate crura** – should be able to pass a finger through here (2-0 tevdek sutures)
    - This effectively repairs defect in phrenoesophageal membrane
    - Phrenoesophageal membrane is an extension of **transversalis fascia**
  - **Anchor wrap** to right crura (2-0 tevdek sutures)
  - When dissecting gastro-hepatic ligament and left triangular ligament of liver, watch for **replaced left hepatic** and **right vagus**
- **Partial fundoplication wraps** (Toupet, partial Nissen) – posterior 180 wrap; used if esophagus has motility problem
- **Intra-thoracic fundoplication wraps** (ie Belsey) – approach through chest

Concomitant stricture – balloon dilatation of stricture (or use dilator)
Collis gastroplasty
>   Used when not enough esophagus exists to pull down into abdomen
>   Staple stomach along cardia to lengthen esophagus tube – the wrap
>   will end up going around the neo-esophagus; used for
>   **shortened esophagus**

Difficult delivery of viscera from above diaphragm – incise the hiatus,
>   reduce the contents, and repair hiatus later

Cx's from Nissen
>   **MC intra-op injury** – esophageal perforation (Tx: repair)
>   **MC Cx following Nissen** – dysphagia
>   1) **Dysphagia** (potential causes listed below)
>>   **Dx: Barium esophagogram** (*best initial study*)
>>   a. **Wrap too tight** (dysphagia **early** post-op)
>>>   **MCC of dysphagia following Nissen**
>>>   May be due to **edema**
>>>   > **95% resolve w/ conservative Tx**
>>>   **Tx: clears** for 1 week, can try to **dilate** after 1 week
>>>   **Inability to swallow liquids** or **foamy salvia** → reop
>>   b. **Twisted fundoplication** (MC w/ laparoscopic); Tx: reop
>>   c. **Wrap herniation** above diaphragm (MC w/ laparoscopic)
>>>   **MCC of dysphagia following Redo Nissen**
>>>   From **shortened esophagus** → need to perform **Collis
>>>   gastroplasty** to prevent this
>>>   **Sx's: dysphagia** and **abd/chest pain**
>>>   **Tx:** reop
>>   d. **Slipped fundoplication**
>>>   Wrap slips down around cardia
>>>   **Sx's: dysphagia** and **reflux**
>>>   **Tx:** reop
>>   e. **Two compartment fundoplication** (MC w/ laparoscopic)
>>>   Occurs when body of stomach used for wrap and not
>>>   fundus;
>>>   **Sx's: dysphagia**, **early satiety** and **inability to
>>>   belch/vomit**
>>>   **Tx:** reop
>>   **Late Dysphagia**
>>>   **Dx: Barium esophagogram** *best study* to figure out
>>>   problem; worry about CA and above Cx's
>   2) **Recurrent Reflux**
>>   **Dx: Barium esophagogram**, EGD to look for wrap disruption
>>   a. **Wrap Disruption** – return of reflux Sx's: Tx: reop
>>   b. **Slipped fundoplication** – **Dysphagia + Reflux**
>>>   Wrap is around cardia; Tx: reop
>   3) **PTX** – chest tube
>   4) **Injury to spleen** – possible splenectomy
>   5) **Gas, bloating** or **delayed gastric emptying**
>>   **Simethicone** for bloating or gas
>>   **Reglan** for bloating and delayed emptying
>>   May need **pyloroplasty** if from **injured vagal nerves**
>   6) **Injury to vagus Cx's**
>>   Gallstones (cholecystectomy if symptomatic)
>>   Delayed gastric emptying (Reglan)
>>   Gas bloat syndrome in air swallowers (Tx Reglan + simethicone
>>   usually self-limiting)
>   7) **Both vagus nerves injured** – Tx: pyloroplasty likely needed
>   8) **Late leak** (late) - fevers
>>   Make sure adequately drained (percutaneous drain)
>>   Abx's for at least 1 week, NPO, TPN
>>   Chest/abd CT to R/O abscess
>>   Gastrograffin (then thin barium) swallow to R/O distal stenosis
>>   Wait it out; surgery if still not closed after 6-8 weeks

Hiatal Hernias

Types of hernias

Type I Hernia (99%) – GE junction above diaphragm
- **Fixed** – from esophageal shortening
- **Sliding** – reduces in upright position
- Most pts w/ type I hiatal hernia <u>do not</u> have reflux
- Most pts w/ significant reflux <u>do</u> have type I hiatal hernia

Type II Hernia (para-esophageal hernia)
- GE junction in normal position
- Occurs as a result of **weakness or defect in phrenoesophageal membrane**
- Allows part of the stomach to **migrate** into thorax
- Sx's – chest pain, dysphagia, early satiety
- **Prone to cx's** – incarceration, strangulation, infarction volvulus
- **All of these patients need surgery**

Type III hernia
- Starts out as sliding hernia but then develops a sliding/rolling para-esophageal component
- May also start out as a para-esophageal hernia that gradually expands esophageal hiatus, resulting in concomitant formation of a sliding component
- Either way, all of these pts need surgery

Type IV – Type II or III but also includes another organ besides stomach (spleen, colon)

Incarcerated para-esophageal hernia (Type II, III, or IV hiatal hernias)
- **Sx's:**
  - **Borchardt's triad** – chest pain, inability to vomit, inability to pass NGT
  - **Inability to swallow saliva**
  - **Retching *without* vomiting** (*classic*)

Gastric volvulus (associated w/ Type II, III, or IV hiatal hernias)
- **Sx's**: same as incarceration
- **MC rotation** – organoaxial volvulus

Tx:

Type I – see above GERD section

Type II-IV
- Pre-op Ewol tube to remove esophageal contents (retained food)
- Repair (high risk of incarceration, infarction)
  - If incarcerated – may need to resect necrotic portions of stomach
- Can use Nissen as repair (anchors stomach and closes defect)
- Can also reduce stomach, close phrenoesophageal defect, and place gastrostomy tube to anchor stomach

Leiomyoma
MC benign tumor of esophagus
MC found in **distal 2/3 of esophagus** (where smooth muscle cells are)
Composed of **smooth muscle** (gray-white swirls)
In **muscularis propria** (submucosal)
Sx's: dysphagia, odynophagia (painful swallowing), pressure, lump throat
Dx:
Barium swallow *(best test)* – smooth, convex, semi-lunar filling defect
EGD w/ EUS
Confirms length, location of tumor, R/O CA
Homogenous, hypoechoic
Overlying mucosa intact
Do not biopsy - can form scar and make subsequent resection
difficult w/ ↑ed risk of disrupting the mucosa
Chest CT – confirms hypodense tumor
Indications for surgery
1) **> 5 cm** (worry about malignancy)
2) **Symptomatic** (significant dysphagia or odynophagia)
3) **Diagnosis in doubt**
4) **Intraluminal, pedunculated**, or **mobile** (risk of this flopping back and
acutely blocking airway)
Tx:
Thoracotomy and **enucleation** *(do __not__ resect esophagus)*
Leave the mucosa intact
Leiomyosarcoma → esophagectomy

Fibrovascular polyp (angiofibrolipoma)
2nd MC benign tumor of esophagus
MC found in **cervical esophagus**
Sx's: dysphagia, respiratory symptoms, hematemesis
Dx:
Barium swallow *(best test)* – will show intra-luminal filling defect; can
widen esophagus
__DO NOT EGD these pts unless at time of surgery__ – this thing can flop
out and cause acute airway obstruction
Path
Long, pedunculated intra-luminal mass
Composed of various amounts of fibrovascular and adipose tissue covered
by normal mucosa
Surface is normal mucosa – **can be missed on EGD**
Indications for surgery – all need removal for risk of airway obstruction
> 8 cm - generally requires open surgical removal
< 8 cm - EGD rsxn
Surgery
Need to figure out where the stalk is and remove at that point
Myotomy, take stalk, will create hole in mucosa that you will need to close

Esophageal Cancer

RFs: achalasia, caustic injury (eg lye), ETOH, tobacco, nitrosamines, Barrett's, tylosis (hyperkeratosis hands/feet), long standing GERD, males

Sx's:

    Dysphagia and **weight loss**

    Jaundice worrisome for liver spread

Dx:

    1) **Esophagogram** (*best initial test for dysphagia*) – apple core lesion

    2) **EGD w/ EUS** (best test for T status - depth) and **biopsies**

    3) **Bronch** – needed for tumors in **upper 2/3 of esophagus;** R/O tracheo-bronchial invasion (infiltration or TEF excludes rsxn – take Bx's)

    4) **Chest/abd CT scan**

        Look for mets to **liver, lungs,** and **adrenals** – Bx suspicious lesions (unresectable DZ)

        Look at **celiac, SMA,** and **supra-clavicular nodes** – Bx suspicious lesions (unresectable DZ)

        **Chest CT is the single best test for overall resectability

        EUS – best test for assessing tumor depth

    5) **Labs** – LFTs

    6) **PET scan** – best test for mets; misses lesions < 1 cm; accuracy 85%

    7) **Head MRI** for HA's, **Bone scan** for bone pain or elevated alk phos

    Suspicious Nodes

        Supraclavicular or retrocrural > 0.5 mm – <u>FNA</u>

        Intra-abdominal > 1 cm – <u>EUS</u>, CT guided, or laparoscopic Bx

        Intra-thoracic > 1 cm – <u>bronch w/ Wang needle</u> or mediastinoscopy

    Unresectable Disease

        Mets (MC lung or liver depending on tumor type)

        Positive nodes outside planned area of resection (supraclavicular nodes and celiac nodes are M1, unresectable)

        Hoarseness (RLN involvement)

        Horner's syndrome

        Phrenic nerve involvement

        Malignant pleural effusion

        Malignant fistula (3 month survival, die of **asphyxiation**)

        Airway, vertebral, or other structure invasion

    PFT's if smoker; **EKG** and **cardiac evaluation**

Poor hepatic, pulmonary, or cardiac function big mortality RFs w/ resection

Path

    Most impt prognostic factor – nodal spread

    EGFR (epidermal growth factor receptor) – single worst tumor marker for prognosis

    Spreads quickly along **submucosal lymphatics**

        Mucosal longitudinal lymphatic drainage connected to submucosal

    Adenocarcinoma – **MC esophageal CA** (↑ in caucasians, 50-60s)

        MC in lower 1/3 of esophagus

        MC in background of **Barrett's**

        MC met's – liver

    Squamous cell CA (SCCA, ↑ in African-Americans, 60-70s)

        MC in middle 1/3 of esophagus

        Worry about invasion of **tracheobronchial tree** – need bronch

        MC Met's – lung

    Barrett's confirmed if squamocolumnar junction (SCJ – found on EGD) is 3 cm above the esophagogastric junction (EGJ – found on manometry)

        Pink mucosa; stains blue w/ Toludine blue (nl. esophagus is grey)

            Surveillance - 4 quadrant Bx's 1 cm apart for the length of the Barrett's lesion annually

            0.5% eventually get adenocarcinoma (1 CA in 200 pt years)

            PPI's can lead to pseudoregression – Barrett's covered by squamous

    Esophageal melanoma Tx: resection

Pre-op chemo-XRT (neoadjuvant)

> **Cisplatnin** and **5-FU** (for anything > T1, ie stage II and III, takes 6 weeks)
> T1 - submocosal invasion
>
> May **downstage larger tumors** and make them resectable
>
> Operate within 6 weeks of XRT
>
> **> 20 lbs weight loss** – place laparoscopic J-tube if getting pre-op chemo-XRT

Surgery

1) Need to be able to **tolerate surgery**
2) Need to have **resectable CA** (No obvious distant met's; no celiac or supraclavicular DZ, not invading another structure)

Esophagectomy

> Mortality from surgery – 5%
> Curative in 25%

Ascites, pleural effusions, or nodules (abdomen or chest) suggests mets – thoracoscopic or laparoscopic approach 1st

Previous XRT – ↑ risk for leak, **perform anastomosis outside XRT field**

Poor PFT's (FEV-1 <1 L) – probably not suitable for thoracic approach; consider **transhiatal esophagectomy**

All of Barrett's area needs rsxn if present

Reflux pre-op → **want anastomosis in neck** (less reflux post-op than chest)

Need **10 cm** margins – may need to take part of stomach

MC complication w/ lymphadenectomy – recurrent laryngeal nerve injury

**Right gastroepiploic artery

> ****Primary blood supply to stomach after replacing esophagus** *(is a branch off GDA)*
>
> Have to divide short gastrics and left gastric artery when using stomach as a conduit

Watch for a **replaced left hepatic artery** coming off the left gastric artery in gastro-hepatic ligament

Watch for a **replaced right hepatic artery** coming off the SMA in the hepatico-duodenal ligament; goes behind **neck of pancreas** and will be **lateral to CBD**

Surgical Techniques

> **Transhiatal**
>
> > Abdominal and neck incisions
> > Bluntly dissect intra-thoracic esophagus
> > Will pull stomach up w/ anastomosis in neck
> > ↓ mortality from esophageal leaks w/ cervical anastomosis
>
> **3 hole esophagectomy**
>
> > Abdominal, neck, and right thoracotomy incisions
> > Exposes entire esophagus
> > Anastomosis in neck
>
> **Ivor Lewis** (2 hole)
>
> > Abdominal and right thoracotomy incisions – exposes all of the thoracic esophagus
> > Anastomosis is in the chest
> > Decreased leak rate compared to cervical anastomosis
>
> **Colonic interposition** – good for young pts with benign disease when you want to preserve gastric function; 3 anastomoses required; blood supply depends on **marginal vessels**

Need **pyloromyotomy** if stomach used as conduit (avoids dysphagia)

Incidental liver, peritoneal, lung, or other met's – close and palliate (esophageal stents if obstruction present)

Incidental M1a DZ during resection (eg unexpected positive celiac node for lower tumors or incidental supraclavicular node for upper tumors) – continue w/ resection, resect the nodal area w/ resection

Need contrast study on POD 7 to rule out anastomotic leak

Cx's following esophagectomy

Intra-op

Air Leak

Performing transhiatal, mobilizing intra-thoracic esophagus and anesthesiologist says **air leak**

Likely tear in **distal trachea** or **left mainstem**

Bronch and find tear

Place a long single lumen tube down non-injured bronchus and ventilate (MC will be right bronchus mainstem intubation)

Right thoracotomy to access the distal trachea

Ligate the azygous vein

Primary repair of the tear – 2-0 vicryls, knots on the outside

Bleeding

High and **dark** (w/ transhiatal) – right thoracotomy, look for tear in azygous

Low and **bright** (w/ transhiatal) – left thoracotomy, look for aortic branch tear

Positive or Close Margins w/ Ivor Lewis – drape for 3 hole w/ anastomosis in the neck and resect for additional margin

Chylothorax

May be clear initially because the pt has been NPO

Add fats to TFs or lipids to TPN and will turn white

Wait 1-3 weeks, NPO, TPN, **short to medium chain FA's**

No better or > 2 liters per day - surgery to ligate thoracic duct

Leak (late)

Sx's: fevers, ↑ WBCs, wound infection

Leak on routine gastrograffin study

Dx:

Look at wound

Gastrograffin study

1) **If wound infection** or anastomosis looks **completely apart** on gastrograffin study →

Open wound and assess stomach

May need resection and return of stomach remnant to abdomen if completely necrotic, cervical esophagostomy, followed by later reconstruction w/ colon (wait 3 mos)

If stomach OK, place drains and conservative Tx below

2) **If small leak** and **no wound infection** (contained leak)

Make sure leak adequately drained

Abx's for at least 1 week, NPO, TPN

Chest and **neck CT** to R/O abscess

Gastrograffin (then thin barium) **swallow** to R/O stenosis at anastomosis after 1 week or so

Wait it out

Surgery if still not closed after 6-8 weeks

Repeat chest and neck CT, gastrograffin (then thin barium) studies before operating on leak

Wound infection

Go to OR and open wound → **if necrotic stomach,** see below

Washout, loosely close, leave drains

Gastrograffin (then thin barium) swallow to R/O occult leak

If you find leak, tx as above

Stenosis

Want to start dilating this area early (after 1 week)

Can be a problem if you do not tx early

Necrosis of stomach (can be a highly lethal problem)

Fluid resuscitation and **abx's**

Resect necrotic part – place residual stomach back in abdomen

Place G tube for decompression, feeding J tube

Cervical esophagostomy

Use colon next time (3 months)

Delayed gastric emptying – pyloric obstruction, hiatal obstruction,
redundant intra-thoracic stomach
Reglan may help
Distended intra-thoracic stomach → place NGT carefully

Esophagitis – Tx: PPI
Regurgitation – Tx: Reglan
MC w/ trans-hiatal esophagectomy
Chylothorax
Posterior membranous trachea tears
Blood loss
Right RLN injury
MC w/ trans-thoracic esophagectomy
Respiratory Cx's
Palliation – chemo-XRT, esophageal stents
Palliative esophagectomy may be indicated in rare circumstances
Perforation of unresectable esophageal CA → place stent
Chemo – 5-FU + cisplatin (for node-positive disease, full thickness lesion
or use preop to shrink tumors)
XRT – also used in most pts either pre-op or post-op; ↓s local recurrence
5-YS w/ resection for cure: 25%
Median survival for pts w/ systemic met's – < 6 months
Colonic conduits
Left colon based on **left colic** (MC used)
Right colon based on **middle coli artery**

STOMACH

Normal Anatomy and Physiology
Basic Functions of Stomach
1) kill bacteria ingested
2) break down food to create a larger surface area for digestion
3) holds food and releases it at a constant rate

Blood supply
Celiac trunk – left gastric, common hepatic artery, splenic artery branches
Right gastric artery is a branch off the common hepatic artery
Gastroduodenal artery (GDA) is a branch off common hepatic artery
(comes off after the right gastric artery branch)
Right gastroepiploic is a branch off gastroduodenal artery (GDA)
Left gastroepiploic and **short gastric** are branches of splenic artery
Greater curvature – right and left gastroepiploics and short gastrics
Lesser curvature – right and left gastric arteries
Pylorus – gastroduodenal artery

Innervation – gastroduodenal pain from **afferent sympathetic fibers T5–10**
Mucosa – simple columnar epithelium
Motility
Stomach transit time 3-4 hours
Peristalsis only occurs in the distal stomach
Rapid gastric emptying – previous surgery (MCC), gastrinoma, ulcers
Delayed gastric emptying – opiates, anticholinergics, myxedema
(hypothyroidism), hyperglycemia, diabetes (gastropathy)

Glands
Cardia glands – mucus secreting
Fundus and **body glands**
1) **Chief cells** release **pepsinogen** (1st enzyme in proteolysis)
↑ **release** – acetylcholine (vagus), gastrin, and secretin
2) **Parietal cells** release H$^+$ and **intrinsic factor**
↑ **HCL release** – acetylcholine (vagus), gastrin, and histamine
Inhibitors of parietal cells – **somatostatin**, PGE, secretin, CCK
Intrinsic factor – binds B-12; complex absorbed in **terminal ileum**
Pernicious anemia – lose parietal cells, ↓ed B-12 absorption
Ranitidine blocks histamine receptors (↓s acid production)
Omeprazole Inhibits parietal cell H/K ATPase (proton pump inhibitor)
Antrum and **pylorus glands**
1) **G cells** release **gastrin** – reason antrectomy is helpful w/ ulcer surgery
Inhibited by H$^+$ in duodenum
Stimulated by **protein, acetylcholine**
2) **D cells** secrete **somatostatin** – inhibits gastrin and acid release
3) **Mucus and HCO$_3^-$ secreting glands** – protects stomach
Duodenum glands
1) **Brunner's glands** – secrete pepsinogen and alkaline mucus (protects
duodenum from acid; *jejunum does not have these* (can get **marginal
ulcers** after roux-en-Y gastro-jejunostomy w/ long afferent limb)
2) **Somatostatin, CCK, and secretin** – released w/ antral and duodenal
acidification
Causes of ↑ acid and ↑ gastrin – gastrinoma, antral cell hyperplasia, renal
failure, gastric outlet obstruction, short bowel syndrome
Causes of ↑ gastrin and normal or ↓ acid – pernicious anemia, chronic
gastritis, gastric CA, post-vagotomy, PPI or H2 blocker
Billroth I – antrectomy w/ gastroduodenal anastomosis
Billroth II – antrectomy w/ gastrojejunal anastomosis
Increased diarrhea and **dumping syndrome** w/ Billroth I and II vs. Roux-en-Y
gastrojejunostomy
Trichobezoars (ie hair ball) – hard to pull out w/ EGD
Tx: EGD likely inadequate; *usually need gastrostomy* and removal
Phytobezoars (ie fiber) – MC in diabetics w/ poor gastric emptying
Tx: enzymes to breakdown, EGD, diet changes

Gastric ulcers

RFs: males, tobacco, ETOH, NSAIDs, *H. pylori*, uremia, burns, sepsis, trauma, steroids, chemo, malignancy, XRT

Most (ie type I + type IV) have **normal** acid secretion and ↓ **mucosal defense**

MC location – lesser curve of stomach (85%)

Hemorrhage w/ stomach ulcers has higher mortality than duodenal ulcers

H. pylori – found in 90% of duodenal and 70% of gastric ulcers (↑s acid)

    Best site to Bx for H pylori – antrum

    Best test for Dx of H pylori – <u>histiologic examination</u> of endoscopic Bx's of antrum

Sx's: epigastric pain radiating to back; **relieved w/ eating** but recurs in 30 min; melena or guaiac-positive stools

Cushing's Gastric Ulcer – associated w/ head trauma

Curling's Duodenal Ulcer – associated w/ burns

Type A blood – associated with type I ulcers

Type O blood – associated with type II–IV ulcers

Types

    Type I: lesser curve along <u>body</u> of stomach
        <u>Decreased mucosal protection</u>

    Type II: 2 ulcers (lesser curve and duodenal)
        <u>High acid secretion</u> (similar to duodenal ulcers)

    Type III: pre-pyloric ulcer
        <u>High acid secretion</u> (similar to duodenal ulcers), ↑ risk of bleeding

    Type IV: lesser curve high along <u>cardia</u> of stomach
        <u>Decreased mucosal protection, ; ↑ risk of bleeding

    Type V – ulcer associated with NSAIDs

Surgery for ulcer rarely indicated since introduction of **proton pump inhibitors**

Surgical indications

    Perforation

    Protracted bleeding despite EGD therapy

    Obstruction

    Intractability despite medical Tx (>3 months without relief or 2nd recurrence based on mucosal Bx findings)

    Inability to R/O CA (ulcer remains despite Tx) → requires resection of ulcer

Duodenal ulcers

More common than gastric ulcers

RFs: male, tobacco, ETOH, NSAIDs, *H. pylori*, uremia, burns, sepsis, trauma, steroids, chemo, malignancy, XRT

From ↑ **acid production** and ↓ **defense**

H. pylori – found in 90% of duodenal and 70% of gastric ulcers (↑s acid)

    Best site to Bx for H pylori – antrum

    Best test for Dx of H pylori – <u>histiologic examination</u> of endoscopic biopsies of antrum

Sx's: epigastric pain radiating to back; may **worsen w/ eating** melena or guaiac-positive stools

MC location – 1st portion of duodenum (MC location – <u>anterior</u>)

    Anterior ulcers <u>perforate</u>

    Posterior ulcers <u>bleed</u> from gastroduodenal artery

MC complication of duodenal ulcers – <u>bleeding</u> (usually minor but can be life-threatening)

Surgery for ulcer rarely indicated since introduction of **proton pump inhibitors**

Surgical indications

    Perforation

    Protracted bleeding despite EGD therapy

    Obstruction

    Intractability despite medical Tx (>3 months without relief or 2nd recurrence based on mucosal findings)

    Inability to R/O CA (ulcer remains despite Tx) → requires resection of ulcer
        Although CA incidence is much lower for persistent duodenal ulcers compared to persistent gastric ulcers

Surgical Options for Gastric and Duodenal Ulcer DZ

Roux en-Y gastro-jejunostomy better (compared to Billroth I or Billroth II)
1) Don't get **bile reflux gastritis**
2) ↓**ed of dumping syndrome** w/ Roux limb
Billroth I and Billroth II less commonly performed

Surgical options:
1) Truncal vagotomy and pyloroplasty
2) Truncal vagotomy, antrectomy, and Roux en-Y gastro-jejunostomy
3) Highly selective vagotomy

	Morbidity	Mortality	Recurrence
Highly selective vagotomy	1%	<1%	15%* (? 40%)
Vagotomy and pyloroplasty	5-10%	1-2%	5-10%
Vagotomy and Antrectomy	5-10%	1-2%	<1%

*Best surgeons who have done a lot of these.
Estimated 40% recurrence in surgeons who do not do a lot of these
If highly selective vagotomy out of the scenario due to high recurrence, *best option* is **vagotomy and antrectomy** for most ulcer DZ
Antrectomy does <u>not</u> add to increased morbidity or mortality compared to vagotomy and pyloroplasty
Antrectomy has a much lower incidence of recurrence
Exception to above is in cases of surgery for **duodenal perforation or bleeding**
Because the patient is sick, probably best not to do an antrectomy.
If you decide to perform an ulcer operation in these settings, just go w/ vagotomy and pyloroplasty
For **gastric perforation or bleeding** cases, go w/ antrectomy and vagotomy because you have to resect the ulcer anyway, might as well extend the resection boundaries and remove antrum for most optimal ulcer operation
W/ pyloroplasty, open longitudinally and close transversely
W/ vagotomy, take 1 cm of each vagus nerve so it does not grow back

Intractable Gastric and Duodenal Ulcer DZ

Sx's:
> Persistent ulcer despite 3 months of Tx or recurrence of ulcer < 1 year (all based on EGD mucosal findings, not sx's)
> ***Important to realize that in 10-15% of intractable <u>gastric ulcers</u> it is actually a gastric cancer***
> <u>< 1% of intractable <u>duodenal ulcers</u> are duodenal cancer
> **99% of ulcers** are treated w/ **PPI + H. pylori Tx**

Dx:
> **EGD**
>> Bx of <u>ulcer rim</u> and <u>base</u> x 10 for CA **(gastric ulcers absolutely; some would not do this for duodenal ulcers)**
>> Bx of <u>**antrum**</u> x 10 for **H pylori**
> **Rule Out:**
>> **CA** (10 Bx's), sx - weight loss
>> **Gastrinoma** (serum gastrin), sx - diarrhea
>> **PTH DZ** (check Ca and PTH), sx - kidney stones
>> **Ulcerogenic meds** (NSAID's, ect.)
>> **H. pylori** (10 antral Bx's)
>>> Send for histology to look for H pylori organism *(best test)*
>>> Get rapid **urease assay** (Clo test, not as sensitive as above)

Medical Tx:
> **Proton pump inhibitor <u>*plus*</u> H. Pylori tx:**
>> 1) Clarithromycin + amoxicillin (14 days)
>> 2) **Refractory ulcer –** metronidazole, tetracycline, and bismuth salts

D/C NSAIDS – consider exchanging for **COX-2 selective inhibitor** (eg celecoxib) if no cardiovascular DZ or adding misoprostol (S/Es diarrhea)

D/C smoking and **ETOH**

Re-scope after a month to make sure ulcer is improving (re-biopsy)

Pts who suffered a perforation or bleeding complication →

Should have **H pylori eradication documented** w/ **urea breath test** or **stool antigen** (both are 90% specific and 90% sensitive)

ELISA serology not useful for determining eradication (hangs around for months to years)

If > 3 months w/o relief on escalating doses of **PPI, consider ulcer surgery:**

Increase PPI dose during this time (20, 40, 80mg)

No real max dose, up to 120 mg TID has been safe

Medical failure rate **higher for gastric ulcers** compared to duodenal

Surgical Tx:

Vagotomy, Antrectomy and **Roux-en-Y Gastro-jejunostomy** (for duodenal ulcers include pylorus and duodenal ulcer)

Important that you resect gastric ulcers (High rate of **CA**) send frozen section, may need partial or total gastrectomy

Can perform extended antral rsxn up the lesser curve to get ulcer

Can also just wedge the ulcer out if far from antrum

Bleeding from Duodenal or Gastric Ulcer (Sx's - melena or hematemesis)

MC complication of duodenal ulcers

If massive hematemesis or shock:

ABC's, 2 IV's, fluid resuscitation, place an NGT

T and C for 6 units – transfuse if unstable or significant blood loss

Send coags and correct them

Start PPI (Omeprazole 8 mg/hr IV) if ulcer suspected cause

Intubate for ongoing shock, poor resp status, change in mental status

Medical Tx:

Initial Tx:

NGT – lavage stomach until clear (can help reduce fibrinolysis)

If symptom was melena:

Blood in NGT – UGI source

NO blood and clear fluid w/o bile in NGT - still may be UGI source w/ closed pylorus (eg duodenal ulcer)

NO blood and you see bile in NGT – likely LGI source

Octreotide if unstable and waiting for EGD

Vasopressin if unstable and waiting for EGD

EGD *(best test and best treatment if ulcer)*

Will confirm ulcer (see other causes below)

Tx: Epi injection, cautery

Erythromycin 250 mg IV before EGD will help empty stomach

PPI once ulcer confirmed as cause (Omeprazole IV 8 mg/hr)

RFs for ulcer re-bleeding after EGD is performed

#1 spurting, bleeding blood vessel at time of EGD

(60% chance of re-bleed)

#2 visible blood vessel at time of EGD

(40% chance of re-bleed)

#3 diffuse oozing at time of EGD

(30% chance of re-bleed)

Criteria for surgery following EGD for ulcer (any):

1) **> 4 units of blood** and **still bleeding**

2) In **shock despite multiple blood transfusions**

3) **Recurrent bleed** after maximal EGD Tx

→ *all indications for OR*

Surgery
- **Duodenal Ulcer**
  - **Gastroduodenal artery ligation**
    - **Longitudinal duodenal incision** in 1st **portion of duodenum** (close duodenum transversely)
      - **Superior, inferior,** and **underneath** (U-stitch) stitches for GDA
        - **Pancreaticoduodenal artery** comes off posterior GDA – need to ligate this w/ the U-stitch
        - **Avoid CBD** (don't go too deep) w/ underneath suture
      - **Vagotomy** and **Pyloroplasty** if all of the following criteria met:
        1) Pt has been on **previous PPI Tx**
        2) Pt has been **treated for H. pylori**
        3) Pt is **stable**
  - 99% of ulcer DZ is treatable w/ meds (PPI and tx for H. pylori)
  - Need appropriate ulcer Tx post-op
- **Gastric Ulcer**
  - **Vagotomy, Antrectomy** and **Roux-en-Y Gastro-jejunostomy** (B-I and B-II other options)
    - Important that you **resect gastric ulcers** (High rate of **CA**)
      - Can perform extended antral rsxn up the lesser curve
      - Can just wedge the ulcer out
      - Also a very high rate of **bleeding recurrence** if you just ligate gastric ulcer (40%)
  - **Send ulcer for FS to make sure it's not CA**

DDx Upper GI Bleeding (other than ulcers)
- **Erosive esophagitis** (rarely causes severe bleed) Tx: PPI, EGD w/ cautery + epi
- **Esophageal Varices**
  - Usually see signs of **liver DZ** (jaundice, ascites, abdominal striae)
  - Tx:
    - **Octreotide**
    - **EGD band ligation** (combined w/ octreotide 95% effective)
      - Possible sclerotherapy
    - **Sengstaken-Blakemore tube** if continued bleeding
      - Mainly as a bridge to TIPS procedure
    - **TIPS** if refractory to above (S/E TIPS – encephalopathy)
    - **Open porto-caval shunt** if TIPS not available
- **Gastritis** (usually diffuse bleeding)
  - Tx: PPI, EGD w/ epi and cautery (maybe hard to get because of diffuse bleeding), vasopressin and/or octreotide (95% success rate w/ previous therapies); angio w/ embolization
  - **Massive gastric bleeding diffusely** (rare) → consider gastric devascularization (last resort)
- **Mallory Weiss tear** – usually stop **spontaneously**
  - Tx: EGD w/ epi and cautery if active
  - ****Continued bleeding** → surgery (anterior gastrostomy, oversew vessel); Tend to **re-bleed** w/ angio embolization
- **Dieulafoy's lesion** (ulcer; superficial artery ectasia in **cardia**) or **gastric AVM**
  - Sudden massive GI bleed
  - Tx: EGD w/ epi and cautery (90% success)
  - ****Continued bleeding** → surgery (anterior gastrostomy, oversew vessel) Tend to **re-bleed** w/ angio embolization
- **Gastric antral vascular ectasia** (GAVE; tortuous, numerous, dilated small arterial vessels all throughout antrum; looks like watermelon)
  - Usually causes **chronic bleeding** (not acute or massive)
  - Tx: EGD w/ epi and cautery
  - **Continued bleeding** → angiography and selective vasopressin/embolization (may re-bleed but these large blood vessels make surgery risky)

Aorto-enteric fistula (Hx of previous graft placement)
> Tx: excise graft w/ extra-anatomic bypass usual

CA Tx: resection if possible

GIST tumor Tx: resection

Upper GI but can't find bleeding source (eg too much blood, food) →
Angiography

Having trouble localizing bleeding source despite angiography (eg small
bleed) → Tagged RBC scan

Poor prognostic signs of UGI bleed:
> Age > 60
> Comorbidities
> Variceal bleed
> CA source
> Bright red blood in NGT
> Increased transfusion requirement
> Instability

Obstruction from Duodenal and Gastric Ulcer

Sx's:
> Bloating, fullness, vomiting
> Heaped up area from ulcer, need to make sure not CA
> **Initial Tx** – fluid resuscitation; NGT to decompress, PPI
> Can get **metabolic alkalosis** (hypokalemic, hypochloremic metabolic
> alkalosis)

Dx:
> **UGI** (through NGT)
> **EGD**
>> Bx of <u>ulcer rim</u> and <u>base</u> x 10 for CA
>> Bx of <u>antrum</u> x 10 for H pylori

R/O:
> **CA** (10 Bx's)
> **Gastrinoma** (serum gastrin)
> **PTH DZ** (check Ca and PTH)
> **Ulcerogenic meds** (NSAID's, ect.)
> **H. pylori** (10 antral Bx's)
>> Send for histology to look for H pylori organism (best test)
>> Get rapid **urease assay** (Clo test)

Tx:
> **Normal saline bolus** if dehydrated
>> Maintenance D5 ½ normal saline w/ 20 mEq K
> **1 week** of **NGT decompression, PPI** and **TPN**
> **Repeat UGI** to see if its opening up after 1 week, if not surgery **below**

> **Vagotomy, Antrectomy** and **Roux en-Y gastro-jejunostomy**
>> **Duodenal ulcers**
>>> Almost always have extensive **scarring around duodenum** w/
>>> obstructing ulcers
>>> At risk for **common bile duct** and **ampulla of vater** injury if you
>>> try to resect
>>> If clearly proximal to ampulla, you can resect (unusual case)
>>> **Probably not** going to be able to remove ulcer itself (check
>>> Bx's and make sure not CA)
>>> May need whipple if CA
>> **Gastric ulcers**
>>> Important that you **resect gastric ulcer** (High rate of **CA**)
>>> Can perform extended antral rsxn
>>> Can just wedge the ulcer out
>> **Send resected area for FS** to see if there is CA for both above

Perforation of Duodenal Ulcer or Gastric Ulcer

ABCs, 2 IV, fluid resuscitation, Abx's, PPI

Sx's

Sudden, sharp, severe epigastric pain; generalized peritonitis

Pain can radiate to **pericolic gutters** w/ dependent drainage of gastric content

Higher mortality w/ **gastric ulcer perforations**

Dx:

Upright CXR and **KUB** should show free air (85%)

UGI if Dx still in question

Surgery

Duodenal Ulcer Perforation

Small perforation → omental patch (Graham Patch)

Freshen edges, **try to close hole primarily + omental patch**

Omental onlay patch by taking submucosal bites on either side of hole

NGT, drains (19 Fr JP), **PPI, Abx's** (7 days), **NPO** for 7 days

Gastrograffin and thin barium **UGI** after 7 days to R/O leak, clears after that

Vagotomy and **Pyloroplasty** if <u>all</u> of the following criteria met :

1) Pt has been on **previous PPI Tx**

2) Pt has been **treated for H. pylori**

3) Pt is **stable**

4) Have a **small perforation**

Include ulcer in pyloroplasty

Post op need to treat for ulcer disease

Large perforation (ie omental patch won't work) →**Vagotomy, Antrectomy and Roux en-Y gastro-jejunostomy**

Include ulcer in resection

Can exclude duodenal stump by tacking the anterior to the posterior duodenal wall

Send ulcer for frozen section to make sure its not CA

Gastric Ulcer Perforation

Vagotomy, Antrectomy and **Roux-en-Y Gastro-jejunostomy**

It is important that you **resect gastric ulcer** (High rate of **CA**)

Can perform extended antral rsxn up the lesser curve

Can just wedge the ulcer out

Send ulcer for frozen section to make sure its not CA

For complicated ulcer disease (ie bleeding, perforation, obstruction) – consider post-op intractable ulcer W/U above

Post-gastrectomy complications

Advantages of Roux-en-Y over Billroth I or II for ulcer DZ
1) Do <u>not</u> get bile reflux gastritis
2) ↓ed dumping syndrome

Post-vagotomy diarrhea
MC complication following vagotomy or gastrectomy
Caused by **sustained postprandial organized MMCs** leading to **non-conjugated bile salts in colon**
Tx: cholestyramine, octreotide, anti-motility agents (loperamide)
Surgical option: reversed interposition jejunal graft

Dumping syndrome
Can occur after either gastrectomy or vagotomy and pyloroplasty
From **rapid entrance of carbohydrates into jejunum**
90% resolve w/ medical Tx
2 phases
1. Hyperosmotic load causes fluid shift into bowel (N/V, diarrhea, dizziness, **hypotension**)
2. Reactive increase in insulin and **hypoglycemia** (2nd part rarely occurs); 1-3 hours after 1st part

Dx: Gastric emptying study (*best test,* radionuclide colloid scintography)
Stomach dumps colloid quickly (check glucose 3 hours after)
Tx: small, high protein, low-fat, low-carbohydrate meals
No liquids with meals
No lying down after meals
Octreotide effective (given before meals)
Surgical options (rarely necessary)
Convert Billroth I or Billroth II to Roux-en-Y gastrojejunostomy
Operations that either increase the **gastric reservoir** (jejunal pouch) or **increase the emptying time** (slow emptying, eg reversed jejunal loop or narrowing the G-J anastomosis) can be used

Alkaline reflux gastritis
Sx's: postprandial epigastric pain associated with N/V, **bilious emesis**
Pain <u>not</u> relieved with vomiting
Dx: EGD (*best test*) → evidence of bile reflux in stomach, histologic evidence of gastritis
Tx: PPI, cholestyramine, metoclopramide
Surgical option: conversion of Billroth I or II to Roux-en-Y gastrojejunostomy w/ afferent limb 60 cm distal to gastrojejunostomy

Afferent loop Syndrome (Afferent-loop obstruction, ie biliary limb)
Found w/ Billroth II or Roux-en-Y
Obstruction of afferent limb (RFs – long afferent limb)
Can be caused by stenosis, kinking, volvulus, or adhesions
Sx's: non-bilious vomiting + abd pain → *Pain <u>relieved</u> w/ bilious emesis*
Can cause closed loop obstruction w/ fever, shock, and perforation
Dx:
CT scan (*best test for Dx*) – see a big loop of fluid filled bowel
Does <u>not</u> fill w/ contrast
EGD to look for recurrent tumor, fibrosis, food obstruction, tight or twisted anastomosis – best test to figure out problem
Tx: **Balloon dilation w/ EGD** may be possible
Surgical option: re-anastomosis w/ shorter (40-cm) afferent limb and relieve cause of obstruction (may require conversion of B-II to Roux en-Y gastro-jejunostomy)

Blind Loop Syndrome (biliary limb) - With Billroth II or Roux-en-Y
From **stasis** leading to **bacterial overgrowth** (*E. coli*, GNRs) in afferent limb
Sx's: pain, malabsorption, B-12 deficiency (bacteria use it up, megaloblastic anemia), **steatorrhea** (bacterial deconjugation of bile)
Dx: EGD w/ afferent limb aspirate + culture (*best test*); CT scan may show dilated segment; can check for <u>fecal fat</u> (sudan red)
Tx: Tetracycline and Flagyl; metoclopramide or erythromycin
Surgical option: re-anastomosis with shorter (40-cm) afferent limb

Delayed gastric emptying

> **Chronic gastric atony** following vagotomy
> **Sx's:** N/V, pain, early satiety
> **Dx: gastric emptying study** *(best test),* EGD
> **Tx: metoclopramide, erythromycin**
> **Surgical option:** near-total gastrectomy w/ Roux-en-Y

Small gastric remnant (early satiety)

> Actually want this for roux-en-y gastric bypass pts
> **Dx: upper GI** *(best test);* EGD
> **Tx: small meals**
> **Surgical option:** jejunal pouch construction

Efferent-loop obstruction (gastric limb)

> **Sx's:** distension, N/V, pain
> **Dx: upper GI** *(best test)* can show narrowed area; CT scan may show
> > dilated stomach
> **Tx: balloon dilation possible**
> Surgical option: find site of obstruction on UGI or CT scan and relieve it

Duodenal stump blowout – reop, jejunal patch, lateral duodenostomy tube (or
> can just place in hole and sew around it), drains, feeding J-tube

Lateral duodenostomy tube – placed if the duodenal closure feels unsecure
> after gastrectomy; prevents duodenal stump blow-out; use 14 fr red rubber

PEG complications – insertion into liver or colon can occur

Vagotomies

Vagal denervation

> **Vagal-mediated receptive relaxation of stomach is removed**
> Results in ↑ed gastric pressure and:
> > 1) ↑ **liquid emptying** (all vagotomy forms)
> > 2) ↓ **solid emptying** if just truncal vagotomy is performed w/o
> > > pyloromyotomy (**pylorus constriction** prevents solid emptying)

> **Truncal vagotomy** – divides vagal trunks at level of the esophagus
> **Selective vagotomy** – divides nerves of Latarjet
> **Highly selective vagotomy**- divides individual fibers, preserves crow's
> > foot

> If **complete vagotomy** (truncal or selective) – ↓ed solid emptying
> If **highly selective vagotomy** – normal emptying of solids
> Addition of **pyloroplasty** to either of above results in ↑ed solid emptying

Gastric effects (all vagotomy forms) – ↓ acid output 90%, ↑gastrin, gastrin cell
> hyperplasia

Other non-gastric truncal vagotomy effects (not present w/ HSV)

> **Diarrhea** (40%)
> > **MC problem following vagotomy**
> > Caused by sustained motor-myenteric complexes (MMC's) forcing
> > > bile acids into the colon

> **Cholelithiasis** (gallstones)
> **Other**
> > ↓ Exocrine pancreas function (enzymes, HCO3-)
> > ↓ Postprandial bile flow
> > ↑ Gallbladder volumes
> > ↓ Release of vagally mediated hormones (CCK, secretin)

Summary

> **Truncal or Selective Vagotomy alone** - increases liquid emptying and
> > decreases solid emptying
> **Truncal or Selective Vagotomy and pyloroplasty** - increases liquid
> > emptying and increases solid emptying
> **HSV alone** – increases liquid emptying and normal solid emptying
> **HSV w/ pyloromyotomy** – increases liquid emptying and increases solid
> > emptying

Recurrent or persistent peptic ulcer disease after surgery

Initial Tx: PPI; but also need to w/u the problem

Dx tests you will need:

 UGI – will detect stenosis

 EGD – Bx for CA, Bx for H pylori, suture granuloma, look for stenosis, look for bile gastritis

 Sham feeding study – will detect incomplete vagotomy

 Technetium scan – will detect retained gastric antrum

 Gastrin level – will also need a basal acid output (BAO) level to detect gastrinoma

 Ca level – also will need to check PTH for hyperparathyroidism

Incomplete vagotomy

 **MCC of recurrent peptic ulcer DZ after surgery

 Missed criminal nerve of Grassy; **poorly performed HSV**; misidentification

 Dx – shame feeding (chew but do not swallow) - measure acid output and gastric pH and see if it goes up w/ chewing

Retained gastric antrum - Dx: 1) **technetium scan** will light up retained antrum

 2) **Meal test** (acid level goes up w/ meal) will be positive w/ retained antrum (not w/ gastrinoma)

Stenotic gastric outlet – Dx: UGI *(best)*, EGD; **Tx**: balloon or redo anastomosis

Suture granulomas – Dx: EGD; **Tx**: try to get suture endoscopically if healed

Long afferent loop w/ inadequate neutralization of acid; can present w/ marginal ulcer; **Tx**: PPI; Consider converting to Roux en Y w/ shortened biliary limb or placing it more proximal on the gastric limb

Bile reflux gastritis– Dx: EGD; **Tx**: Reglan, cholestyramine; Consider converting to a Roux en-Y w/ biliary limb 60 cm distal on gastric limb

Gastrinoma – Dx: Serum gastrin + BAO **Tx**: rsxn of the gastrinoma

Hyperparathyroidism – Dx: Ca; **Tx**: surgery for hyperparathyroidism

H. pylori – Dx –EGD and Bx (*histology best*, rapid urease assay);

 Tx: PPI, Bismuth salts, Amoxicillin, Metronidazole

CA – Dx EGD and Bx; **Tx:** possible gastric resection

Ulcerogenic meds - Tx: discontinue the meds

Gastric varices

90% of gastric varices are associated w/ esophageal varices (follow esophageal varices pathway)

10% of gastric varices are isolated

If isolated gastric varices →

 MC from **splenic vein thrombosis** (secondary to **pancreatitis**)

 Unusually from portal HTN or portal vein thrombosis (from cirrhosis or pancreatitis)

 Dx: U/S (look at portal vein and splenic vein)

Splenic vein thrombosis and **gastric varices**

 MCC isolated gastric varices

 Leads **to isolated gastric varices** *without* elevation of pressure in rest of portal system

 These **gastric varices** can bleed

 Splenic vein thrombosis most often caused by **pancreatitis**

 Dx: U/S (look at portal vein and splenic vein and figure out problem

 Tx: splenectomy

Portal HTN and **gastric varices** (*unusual* cause of isolated gastric varices)

 Follow bleeding esophageal varices pathway (see Liver chp)

Mallory-Weiss tear
Sx's: hematemesis after **forceful vomiting episode**; often Hx of ETOH
Bleeding often stops spontaneously
Tear is usually near **lesser curve** of stomach (near GE junction)
NGT – lavage stomach until clear (can help reduce fibrinolysis)
Dx: EGD (can also Tx problem)
Tx:
> **EGD** w/ Epi and Cautery
> If continued bleeding → **anterior gastrostomy** and **oversewing of vessel**

Dieulafoy's ulcer (lesion) - submucosal vascular malformation (1-5 mm)
Sx's: hematemesis
95% in upper stomach and MC on lesser curve
Tx:
> **EGD** w/ Epi and Cautery
> If continued bleeding → **anterior gastrostomy** and **oversewing of vessel**

Stress gastritis
MC 3-10 days after stressful event
MC in fundus 1st
Tx:
> 1) **PPI** (Omeprazole 8 mg/hr)
> 2) **NGT** – lavage stomach until clear (can help reduce fibrinolysis)
> 3) **Vasopressin** and/or **octreotide** (+ above → 95% effective)
> 4) **EGD** w/ cautery (often not effective due to diffuse bleeding)
> 5) **Selective angiography** w/ coil embolization if above fail
> 6) rarely need gastric devascularization

Chronic gastritis
Type A (fundus) – associated w/ pernicious anemia, autoimmune disease
Type B (antral) – associated w/ **H. pylori**

Menetrier's disease – hyperplastic hypersecretory gastropathy
↑ gastric CA risk
Sx's: pain, weight loss, anemia
Path + ulcers + protein loss; mucus cell hyperplasia, ↑ rugal folds
Tx: PPI, protein supplements
Childhood form - from CMV or H pylori; resolves in weeks to months

Acute Gastric Distension
Sx's: severe **abd distension** and **pain** → followed by **bradycardia, hypotension, tachypnea,** and **sweating**
As stomach distends, initiates **vaso-vagal response** (compresses vagus)
RF's – pancreatitis, recent surgery
Can be a life threatening complication
Tx: NGT

Morbid obesity
Central obesity – worse prognosis
NIDDM, HTN, sleep apnea often resolve after surgery
Operative mortality 1%
Pre-op studies (surgical eligibility):
> BMI > 40 or BMI > 35 with co-morbidities (HTN, DM, CAD, pulmonary HTN related to obesity, obstructive sleep apnea)
> **Psychological evaluation –** to r/o overlying psych issue as cause of eating (eg schizophrenia, OCD)
> **Nutrition** assessment R/O metabolic issue causing weight problem
> Have tried at least **2 weight loss programs** and failed over 2 years
> Can't be gaining weight during the evaluation process
> Weight is seriously affecting **quality of life**
> Need to be willing to risk **1% risk of death**
> Need to be done in a center that does a lot of these

Roux-en-Y gastric bypass
Need 75-100 cm of jejunum Roux limb if performing roux-en-Y gastric bypass

Perform **cholecystectomy** during operation if stones present.

UGI on postop day 2

10-15% failure rate due to high carbohydrate snacking

Ischemia – most common cause of leak

Laparoscopic banding
Disadvantage compared to Roux-en-Y – less initial weight (1st 2 years), after 3-4 years weight loss is similar

Benefits over Roux-en-Y

Lower mortality rate: 0.05% vs. 0.5% for Roux-en-Y gastric bypass

Fully reversible

No cutting or stapling of stomach

Shorter hospital stay

Adjustable without additional surgery

No malabsorption issues

Fewer leaks, gastric necrosis, etc

MC Cx - regurgitation of non-acidic food from upper pouch (Productive Burping) Tx: eating less, more slowly, more thoroughly; food can cause obstruction

Jejunoileal bypass
These operations are no longer done

Associated with liver cirrhosis, kidney (stones) problems and osteoporosis ($\downarrow$ Ca)

Need to correct these pts w/ Roux-en-Y gastric bypass if ileojejunal bypasses are encountered

Complications from Roux en-Y gastric bypass
Leak
MCC leak overall – ischemia

MCC early leak – technical error

MCC late leak – ischemia

Sx's:

Pain and **fever**

$\uparrow$ RR, $\uparrow$ HR, elevated WBCs; can be really sick

Initial Tx: ABC's, IV x 2, fluid resuscitation, abx's

Dx:

UGI (*best test*; gastrograffin then barium)

Abd CT – may see necrosis (stomach doesn't light up)

Labs – $\uparrow$WBCs

Tx:

Early Leak (< 7 days) → re-operate

Fix leak

Place a **G-tube** in the distal gastric pouch

Also place a **feeding J-tube** in the distal jejunum if the leak was at the distal anastomosis

NGT in proximal pouch and NPO

Leave Drains

UGI POD # 7

Late leak ($\geq$ 7 days) → Use UGI and an Abd CT scan to assess whether or not leak is contained or if there is stomach necrosis

Contained leak and pt not sick

Percutaneous drainage of fluid collection

Abx's for 1st week, NPO, NGT, TPN, octreotide and PPI

Look for **stenosis** at any of the anastomoses on the UGI

Re-operate in 6-8 weeks if the leak persists

If leak is not contained or pt sick

Re-operate (need to be worried about <u>stomach necrosis</u> as well here)

If the leak is small and tissue looks healthy (unlikely
scenario) can place a stitch to close the leak, place
drains and washout abdomen

If not just a small leak or if tissue looks bad, just leave
drains and washout abdomen

Place a **G-tube** in the <u>distal</u> gastric pouch

If the leak was at the distal anastomosis (J-J), also place
a **feeding J-tube** distal to the anastomosis

NGT in proximal pouch and keep NPO

Abx's for 1st week, octreotide and PPI, feeds through G-
tube or J-tube depending on area of leak

Re-operate in 6-8 weeks if the leak persists

Proximal stomach necrosis

Sx's: pain and **fever**; ↑ RR, ↑ HR, peritoneal signs; can be pretty ill

Initial management – ABCs, IV x 2, fluid resuscitation, abx's

This is usually found at the time of reoperation for a leak

Dx:

UGI (gastrograffin then barium)

Abd CT + IV and oral contrast – proximal stomach won't light up

Labs – ↑ WBCs

Tx:

Re-operate, takedown gastro-jejunostomy, and resect necrotic area
from proximal pouch

Leave the residual healthy proximal pouch in place

Place a **G-tube** in the distal gastric pouch

Place **drains** and washout area

Abx's, feed through G-tube in the distal stomach pouch

Re-do anastomosis if viable stomach left in 6-8 weeks

If too much of the proximal stomach pouch was resected, will likely
need a **jejunal pouch connected to esophagus**

B-12 deficiency (intrinsic factor need acidic environment to bind B-12)

Tx: B-12 shots every month

Fe deficient anemia (bypasses duodenum where Fe absorbed) – Tx: Fe

Gallstones (from rapid weight loss)

Tx: cholecystectomy (try to do this at the time of initial surgery)

Pulmonary Embolism (MCC of death in some series)

Tx: prevent w/ enoxaparin 0.5 mg/kg BID

Aspiration w/ intubation – **Tx:** fiber-optic intubation to avoid this

Marginal ulcers (10%) – occur on the jejunal side of the anastomosis; Tx PPI

Stenosis

Sx's: hiccoughs, large stomach bubble, nausea and vomiting (all sx's of
obstruction)

Tx:

Early – **re-operate** (technical problem)

Late (from ischemia)

For either the proximal gastro-jejunal anastomosis or the distal
jejunal-jejunal anastomosis, may be able to dilate
(pediatric colonoscope is 160 cm and can be used to try
and dilate the distal anastomosis)

Usually responds to **serial dilation**

Gastrointestinal stromal tumors (GIST tumors)

MC benign gastric neoplasm, although can be malignant

Sx: MC asymptomatic; obstruction and bleeding can occur

Dx:

> **EGD w/ Bx** (*best test*) – **95% c-kit positive** (use immunostaining)
>
> **EUS** – hypoechoic, smooth edges

Path

> **Spindle cells**
>> Connective tissue (interstitial cells of Cajal)
>> Autonomic pacemaker cells
>
> ± calcification, ± necrosis
>
> **MC location** – stomach (70%)
>
> **25% malignant** (behave like **sarcomas**)
>> Rare nodal spread (< 10%)
>> **MC mets** – liver
>> **Malignant GIST:**
>>> 1) **> 5-10 mitoses / 50 HPFs** *or;*
>>> 2) **Size > 5 cm**
>
> **c-Kit** – receptor tyrosine kinase (stem cell growth factor receptor)
>
> Now felt to be <u>distinct entities</u> from and far more common than stomach leiomyomas and leiomyosarcomas (c-kit <u>not</u> in leiomyomas or leiomyosarcomas, although these tumors also have spindle cells)

Tx:

> **Wedge resection** (1 cm margins) – <u>no</u> nodal dissection
>
> **Chemo indications** – *all malignant GIST tumors* (defined above)
>> **1st line - Imatinib** (Gleevac); Sunitinib if resistant to Imatinib
>> **Both** receptor tyrosine kinase inhibitors

Mucosal-Associated Lymphoid Tissue Lymphoma (MALT lymphoma)

Low grade B cell NHL from mucosa lymphoid tissue

MC site – stomach (80%)
> Usually confined to stomach (90% of pts, **stage IE**)
> Related to *H. pylori* infection (90%)
> Other sites – other GI tract, lung, Waldeyer's ring (oral tonsils)

Sx's (gastric location)**: Pain** (similar to ulcer) and **weight loss**

Dx: **EUS w/ Bx** (mass or large folds; need to look for **H pylori**)
> **CT chest/abd/pelvis** to stage

Tx:

> **Confined to stomach** (stage IE) or **limited to perigastric nodes** (IIE-1):
>> → *H. pylori eradication* (4 prong - PPI, bismuth salts, amoxicillin, and metronidazole) and **surveillance** → cures 90%
>> → If MALT does not regress after above or if H pylori <u>not</u> present
>>> → *XRT only* (cures 90%), possible resection if that fails
>
> **Advanced DZ** (stage IIE w/ nodes other than peri-gastric, Stage III, and Stage IV) <u>*or*</u> if both above fail → **Chemo** (CHOP-R) ± XRT
>
> **Gastric outlet obstruction** → consider sub-total gastrectomy, then above

Overall 5-YS – 90%

Gastric Lymphoma

MC organ involved in extra-nodal lymphoma (MC type – NHL, B cell)

Higher grade lymphoma than MALT lymphoma

Sx's: similar to ulcer symptoms

Dx:

> **EUS w/ Bx** (mass or large folds)
> **CT chest/abd/pelvic** to stage

Tx:

> **Chemo** (CHOP-R) ± XRT (primary modality, see Spleen chp)
> Surgery usually just for cx's (bleeding, perforation, obstruction)
> **Primary surgery** indicated only for **stage I disease** (tumor confined to **stomach <u>submucosa</u>**) and then only partial resection is indicated
>> (Post-op chemo; <u>No</u> lymph node dissection → just sampling to stage)

Overall 5-YS – 60%

Gastric Cancer

Sx's:

Epigastric pain (unrelieved by eating) and **weight loss**
MC location - Antrum (40%)
Highest risk area – Japan (50% of cancer-related deaths)
RFs – adenomatous polyps, tobacco, previous gastric operations, intestinal metaplasia, atrophic gastritis, pernicious anemia, blood type A, nitrosamines, H pylori (3x ↑ risk), achlorhydria (↓ed acid production – thought to promote bacterial overgrowth)
Prevention – COX-2 inhibitors ↓ incidence of gastric CA

Dx:

EGD w/ Bx (x 10) of lesion *(best test)*
    EUS – Bx of suspicious adenopathy or possible metastatic lesions
Chest/abd/pelvic CT scan
    CT (or U/S) guided Bx of suspicious adenopathy or possible mets
Consider PET scan
UGI – optional

Path

1) **Intestinal gastric cancer** (ie adenocarcinoma)
    Increased in high-risk populations, **older men**; rare in US
    Associated w/ chronic atrophy, dysplasia; has blood vessel invasion;
    Histology – shows <u>glands</u>
    Stage I: 5-year survival w/ surgery – 85%
    Overall 5-year survival – 20%
2) **Diffuse gastric cancer** (ie linitis plastica)
    Diffuse proliferation of **<u>connective tissue</u>**
    In low-risk populations, women
    Histology – lymphatic invasion; <u>no</u> glands
    Less favorable prognosis than intestinal gastric cancer
    Overall 5-year survival – 10%
Adenomatous polyps – 15% CA risk; Tx: endoscopic resection
Krukenberg tumor – gastric CA (or other GI CA) w/ mets to ovaries
Virchow's nodes – gastric CA (or other GI CA) w/ mets to supraclavicular nodes

Tx:

Mets outside area of resection – contraindication to resection unless performing surgery for palliation
Need an R0 resection w/ gastric resection– stomach, omentum, perigastric nodes, celiac nodes
Splenic invasion – resect stomach + splenectomy en bloc
Intestinal gastric cancer
    Need **5 cm margins**
    GE junction tumor → tx like esophageal tumor w/ esophagectomy and 5 cm stomach margin
    Upper 1/3 of stomach → total gastrectomy (not GE junction) and **esophago-jejunal anastomosis** (<u>roux limb</u>)
    Middle or lower 1/3 of stomach → distal gastrectomy and gastro-jejunostomy
Diffuse gastric cancer (linitis plastica)
    Tx: total gastrectomy for all (because of diffuse nature of linitis plastica) and esophago-jejunal anastomosis
Chemo: 5-FU, doxorubicin and mitomycin C (poor response for both types)
Palliation of gastric CA
    Obstruction (can get recurrent aspiration of secretions)
        Proximal lesions – stent
        Distal lesion – bypass w/ gastro-jejunostomy
    Bleeding (low to moderate) – XRT
    Pain (low to moderate) - XRT
    If above fail, consider **palliative gastrectomy** for obstruction, pain, or bleeding

LIVER

Normal Anatomy and Physiology
Blood supply
Arterial blood supply
Right, left and middle hepatic arteries (follows hepatic vein system)

Most **primary and secondary tumors** of liver supplied by hepatic artery (can embolize unresectable tumors)

Hepatic artery variants (replaced arteries)
Right hepatic artery off **superior mesenteric artery** (20%)

MC hepatic artery variant

Behind **neck of pancreas** (travels *posterior* to portal vein)

Posterolateral to CBD

Left hepatic artery off **left gastric artery**

Found in gastrohepatic ligament (lesser omentum) medially

Portal vein
Forms from superior mesenteric vein joining splenic vein (no valves)

Inferior mesenteric vein – enters splenic vein

Portal veins – 2 in liver; 2/3 of hepatic blood flow

Left supplies – II, III, and IV

Right supplies – V, VI, VII, and VIII

Hepatic veins – 3 hepatic veins join the IVC
Left – segments II, III, and superior IV

Middle – segments V and inferior IV

Right – segments VI, VII, and VIII

Middle hepatic vein joins left hepatic vein in 80% before going into IVC; other 20% go directly into IVC

Accessory right hepatic veins – drain medial aspect of right lobe directly into IVC

Inferior phrenic veins – also drain directly into the IVC

Caudate lobe – receives separate right and left portal and arterial blood flow; drains directly into IVC via separate hepatic veins

Hepatoduodenal ligament – where bile duct, portal vein, and hepatic artery meet (portal triad)

Portal triad (ie porta hepatis)
Portal vein posterior

Common bile duct lateral

Proper hepatic artery medial

Pringle maneuver – porta hepatis clamping; will not stop hepatic vein bleeding

Falciform ligament
Separates medial and lateral segments of **the left lobe**

Attaches liver to anterior abdominal wall

Extends to **umbilicus** and carries remnant of umbilical vein

Ligamentum teres
Carries the obliterated umbilical vein to undersurface of liver

Extends from the falciform ligament

Line drawn from the middle of the **gallbladder fossa to IVC** (ie portal fissure or **Cantalies line**) separates right and left lobes

Foramen of Winslow – goes into lesser sac
Anterior – portal triad

Posterior – IVC

Inferior – duodenum

Superior – liver

Glisson's capsule – the peritoneum that covers the liver

Bare area – area on posterior-superior surface not covered by Glisson's capsule

Triangular ligaments – lateral and medial extensions of coronary ligament on posterior surface of liver; made up of peritoneum

Portal triad – enters segments IV and V

Gallbladder – underneath segments IV and V (these areas may need resection w/ Gallbladder CA)

Segments
>   I – caudate
>   II – superior left lateral segment
>   III – inferior left lateral segment
>   IV – left medial segment (quadrate lobe)
>   V – inferior right anteromedial segment
>   VI – inferior right posterolateral segment
>   VII – superior right posterolateral segment
>   VIII – superior right anteromedial segment

Liver Function (carried out by hepatocytes)

>   **Produces** and **excretes bile** required for emulsifying fats
>   **Carbohydrate metabolism**
>>   **Gluconeogenesis** (certain amino acids, lactate or glycerol)
>>   **Glycogenolysis** (breakdown of glycogen into glucose; muscle tissues also do this)
>>   **Glycogenesis** (formation of glycogen from glucose) -stores glycogen
>>   Excess glucose is turned into fat
>   **Protein metabolism**
>>   Produces **albumin**, major osmolar component of blood serum
>   **Cori cycle** – lactic acid made in muscle is transported to liver, converted to glucose, and brought back to muscle
>   **Lipid metabolism:**
>>   **Cholesterol synthesis**
>>   **Lipogenesis** (production of triglycerides)
>   Produces all **coagulation factors** *except* factor VIII,
>>   Also produces protein C, protein S and antithrombin
>   Breaks down **hemoglobin** (→ bilirubin), released in bile
>   Breaks down **toxic substances**
>   Converts **ammonia to urea**
>   Liver stores large amount of **fat-soluble vitamins** (A, D, E, K)
> B_{12} – the only water-soluble vitamin stored in the liver
>   Stores **iron** and **copper**
>   **Immunological effects** – part of reticuloendothelial system
>
>   **Kupffer cells** – liver macrophages
>   **Alkaline phosphatase** – normally located in canalicular membrane
>   **Nutrient uptake** – occurs in sinusoidal membrane
>   **Ketones** – usual energy source for liver
>   *Not* made in the liver → von Willebrand's factor + factor VIII (endothelium)

Bleeding and **bile leak** – MC problems w/ hepatic resection
Hepatocytes most sensitive to ischemia – central lobular (acinar zone III)
75% of normal liver (tri-segmentectomy) can be safely resected w/o liver failure – will regenerate as well

Bilirubin

>   Breakdown product of Hgb (Hgb → heme → biliverdin → bilirubin)
>   Conjugated to **glucoronic acid** (enzyme glucoronyl transferase) in liver → improves water solubility
>   Conjugated bilirubin is then actively secreted into bile
>   **Urobilinogen**
>>   Created from breakdown of bilirubin by bacteria in terminal ileum
>>   Gets reabsorbed in blood, and released in urine
>>   Excess urobilinogen turns urine dark like cola

<u>Bile acids</u> (bile salts)

Bile contains **bile acids** (85%), **phospholipids** (lecithin), **cholesterol**, and **bilirubin, proteins**

Final bile composition determined by active reabsorption of water in the gallbladder (Na/K ATPase dependent; concentrates bile)

Cholesterol is used to make **bile acids**

HMG CoA → (*HMG CoA reductase*) → cholesterol → (*7-alpha-hydroxylase*) → bile acids

HMG CoA reductase – rate-limiting step for cholesterol synthesis

Gallstones in obese pts – overactive HMG CoA reductase

Gallstones in thin pts – underactive 7-alpha-hydroxylase

Bile acids are conjugated to **taurine or glycine** (improves water solubility)

Primary bile acids (C's) – cholic and chenodeoxycholic

Secondary bile acids – deoxycholic and lithocholic

→ are dehydoxylated primary bile acids by bacteria in gut

Lecithin – main biliary phospholipid; solubilizes cholesterol and emulsifies fats in the intestine

Bile salts serve as mechanism for;

1) **excreting cholesterol** *and*
2) **emulsify lipids** and **fat-soluble vitamins** in the intestine

<u>Jaundice</u>

1st **evident under tongue**; occurs when **bilirubin > 2.5**

Maximum bilirubin level is 30 (unless pt has underlying renal disease, hemolysis, or bile duct–hepatic vein fistula)

Unconjugated bilirubin elevation

1) Pre- hepatic causes (eg hemolysis)
2) Hepatic deficiencies of uptake or conjugation (eg cirrhosis)

Conjugated bilirubin elevation

1) Storage deficiency
2) Secretion defects into bile ducts
3) Excretion defects into GI tract (eg stones, strictures, tumor)

Syndromes

Gilbert's disease – abnormal conjugation

MCC of jaundice (5% of the population)

Mild defect in glucoronyl transferase

Mildly high **unconjugated bilirubin**

Crigler-Najjar disease – inability to conjugate

Deficiency of glucoronyl transferase

High **unconjugated bilirubin** → life-threatening (brain damage)

Physiologic jaundice of newborn – immature glucoronyl transferase;

High **unconjugated bilirubin**

Rotor Syndrome – deficiency in storage ability

High **conjugated bilirubin,** good prognosis

Dubin-Johnson syndrome – deficiency in secretion ability

Defect in **anionic transporter cMOAT**

High **conjugated bilirubin;** good prognosis

Acute Liver Failure

Definition - acute hepatic disease + coagulopathy + encephalopathy

Etiology

Viral – HepA, HepB, HepC (rare), HepD + HepB, HepE (esp. w/ pregnancy)

Drugs – acetaminophen, phenytoin

Vascular – ischemic hepatitis, Budd Chiari, hepatic sinusoidal obstructive syndrome (SOS → w/ stem cell TXP, bone marrow TXP)

Auto-immune hepatitis

Misc – acute fatty liver of pregnancy, HELLP, Reye's Syndrome

Acetaminophen toxicity better prognosis than non-acetaminophen cause

Sx's:

N/V, malaise, jaundice; **progressive change in mental status**

Outcome determined by course of encephalopathy

Encephalopathy

Stage I – change in mental status

Stage II – lethargy, confusion

Stage III – stupor

Stage IV – coma (80% mortality – *acute fulminate hepatic failure*)

Liver failure leads to inability metabolize **ammonia, mercaptanes, and false neurotransmitters** → get encephalopathy

Tx:

Lactulose

Cathartic – gets rid of ammonia producing bacteria

Also prevents NH_3 uptake by converting it to ammonium (NH_4)

Titrate to 2–3 stools/day

Limit protein intake (< 70 g/day); give **branched chain amino acids** – metabolized by skeletal muscle (impt energy source for body)

Neomycin – gets rid of ammonia producing bacteria

↑ed ICP can occur from cerebral edema, consider monitoring

Tx: Normal ICP is 10; > **20 needs treatment**

Want cerebral perfusion pressure > **60**

Raise head of bed

Relative hyperventilation for modest cerebral vasoconstriction (pCO_2 30–35); ↓s brain edema and ↓s ICP; Don't over-hyperventilate and cause cerebral ischemia from too much vasoconstriction

Mannitol – load 1 g/kg x 1 dose, can give 0.25 mg/kg q4h after that (draws fluid out of brain and ↓s ICP)

Barbiturate coma – if above not working

CV – hypotension from decreased SVR (similar to sepsis)

Tx: volume replacement, norepinephrine

Pulmonary – MC resp alkalosis; impaired peripheral O2 uptake (shunting); ARDS; hepatopulmonary syndrome Tx: may need intubation

GI – GI bleeding

Renal – hepatorenal syndrome, ATN, Tx: CVVH may be necessary

Heme - coagulopathy;Tx: correct for procedures or bleeding (Vit K ± FFP)

Infection – ↑ed risk; low threshold for **abx's**

Endocrine – hypoglycemia common; Tx: D-10

Criteria for likely requiring Liver TXP for survival:

Acetaminophen Toxicity

1) pH < 7.3 (regardless of other values) *or;*

2) PT > 50, Cr > 3.4, and stage III or IV coma

All other causes

1) PT > 50 (regardless of other values) *or;*

2) Any 3 of the following:

Age < 10 or > 40

Halothane, drug, or idiopathic hepatitis

Jaundice > 7 days before encephalopathy

PT > 25

Bilirubin > 17.5

Cirrhosis

Fibrosis and nodular regeneration from hepatocellular injury

**Best indicator of synthetic function w/ cirrhosis – prothrombin time (PT)

Mechanism

> **Hepatocyte destruction** → fibrosis and scarring of liver → ↑ hepatic
> pressure → portal venous congestion → lymphatic overload →
> leakage of splanchnic and hepatic lymph into peritoneum → **ascites**
>
> Normal portal vein pressure < 12 mmHg
>
> **Coronary veins** act as collaterals between portal vein and systemic
> venous system of lower esophagus
>
> **Shunts** can decompress portal system

Sx's: jaundice, ascites, spider angiomata, palmar erythema

Dx:

> Identify **specific cause of cirrhosis** (Bx + serologies as needed)

1) **R/O liver CA** (w/ recent weight loss) - Abd CT and AFP
2) Assess patency of **portal venous system, hepatic veins** and **artery** –
   duplex U/S
3) Assess **electrolytes** (often ↓ Na$^+$, ↓ albumin, ↑ PT)
4) Figure out **Child-Pugh Score** - this correlates w/ mortality elective shunt

	1 point	2 points	3 points
Albumin	>3.5	3– 3.5	<3.0
Bilirubin	<2.5	2.5–4	>4
Encephalopathy	None	Minimal	Severe
Ascites	None	Treatable w/ meds	Refractory
INR	< 1.7	1.7-2.3	> 2.3

Child's A (5-6 pts)	2% mortality w/ shunt
Child's B (7-9 pts)	10% mortality w/ shunt
Child's C (10 or greater)	50% mortality w/ shunt

5) Figure out **MELD score** (model for end stage liver disease, **bilirubin, INR, Cr**)

> **MELD** = 3.78[natural log serum **bilirubin** (mg/dL)] + 11.2[natural log **INR**] +
> 9.57[natural log serum **creatinine** (mg/dL)] + 6.43
>
> **Max score – 40** (all values > 40 are given score of 40)
>
> **MELD score > 15** likely to get benefit from liver TXP
>
> **MELD score < 15** more likely to die from liver TXP itself than their
> underlying liver disease
>
> MELD does not take into account **hepato–pulmonary syndrome**
>
> **Aminopyrine breath test** – felt to be *the most prognostic test* of liver
> function reserve; not used very much clinically

6) **Child class C or MELD ≥ 15** – consider placement on TXP list

> **Indications for TXP**
>
> > Recurrent or severe encephalopathy
> > Refractory ascites
> > Recurrent variceal bleeding
> > Hepatorenal or hepatopulmonary syndrome
> > Hepatocellular CA (no single lesion > 5 cm or ≤ 3 lesions w/ largest
> > ≤ 3 cm)
> > Fulminant hepatic failure
>
> **Contraindications to TXP**
>
> > Advanced HIV
> > Active substance abuse
> > Sepsis
> > Extra-hepatic malignancy
> > Severe comorbidity (cardiopulmonary especially)
> > Persistent non-compliance
>
> **Liver TXP 1 year survival** - 90% (80% 5-year)

General Tx of cirrhosis:

    ↓ **salt intake** (1 gm/d) and ↓ **fluid intake** (1-1.5 L/d)

    Diuretics:

        Spironolactone (max dose 400 mg/d) counter acts ↑aldosterone seen w/ liver failure (impaired hepatic metabolism)

        Lasix (max dose 350 mg/d); correct electrolytes w/ fluid diuresis

    Norfloxacin 400 mg QD for SBP prophylaxis (use in pts w/ previous SBP or who are admitted for UGI bleeding)

    Propanolol for prophylaxis against UGI bleed (only pts w/ **varices** or **previous UGI bleed**)

    Isosorbide dinitrate in addition to propanolol may further ↓ UGIB bleed

Pre-op preparation:

    Nutritional supplementation if severely malnourished for 2 weeks before elective surgery (eg tube feeds)

    Pre-op removal of ascites – replace w/ albumin I.V. (1 g for every 100 cc removed); Use salt-poor albumin (25% albumin in 50 cc bottle)

    Correct coagulopathy – all have abnormal PT; **Tx** – Vit K ± FFP

    Umbilical Hernia

        Resect necrotic skin area, primary closure if infected

        Place **prolene mesh** if not infected

    ***No** hemorrhoidectomies or elective cholecystectomy in cirrhotic pts*

    ***No** epidural or spinal anesthesia → risk of bleeding*

    Post-op – medical tx for ascites as above

Hepatic encephalopathy

    Stage I – change in mental status

    Stage II – lethargy, confusion

    Stage III – stupor

    Stage IV – coma

    Stage I, II, and III – asterixis

    Stage III and IV – encephalopathy, hyper-reflexia, clonus, rigidity

    Development of **asterixis** is a sign that liver failure is progressing

    Liver failure leads to **inability metabolize** → ↑ammonia, mercaptanes, false neurotransmitters

    Need to R/O other causes of encephalopathy:

        CXR – PNA, effusion

        ABG – O2 sat

        Labs

            Hct, guaiac stools, and place **NGT** – R/O GI bleed

            Blood, urine, sputum, and **ascites** for culture (infection)

            Electrolytes – check for hepato-renal syndrome or electrolyte disorders; glucose, ammonia

        Drugs – sedatives, MSO4

        Head CT – for stroke

        Paracentesis if ascites – SBP

    Tx:

        Lactulose

            Cathartic that gets rid of ammonia producing bacteria in gut and acidifies colon

            Prevents NH_3 uptake by converting it to ammonium (NH_4)

            Titrate to 2–3 stools/day

        Neomycin – gets rid of ammonia producing bacteria

        Limit protein intake (<70 g/day)

            Give **branched chain amino acids** – metabolized by skeletal muscle

        Possibly embolize previous therapeutic shunts or embolize other major collaterals

        Lactulose and spironolactone can cause a **non-ion gap metabolic acidosis**

Ascites

Medical tx of cirrhosis outlined above controls ascites in 90%
> Spironolactone and lasix to diurese 1 L/d, steady weight loss

Paracentesis

> **PRN for symptomatic ascites** (Tx of choice for large volume ascites; remove 4-6 liters); Replace w/ salt-poor **albumin** (25% albumin in 50 cc), 1 gm for each 100cc taken off
>
> Also used for either 1) new onset ascites *or* 2) possible infection (ie possible SBP → abd pain, fever, change in mental status, ↑ WBC, acidosis); *coagulopathy <u>not</u> a contraindication*

TIPS

> 90% of shunts are open at 1 year
>
> Improves TXP-free **survival**, improves **creatinine clearance** and **decreases ascites**
>
> **Makes encephalopathy <u>worse</u>** (shunted blood does not undergo liver metabolism)
>
> Consider for **refractory ascites**, Child's A or B, and minimal encephalopathy

Peritoneo-venous shunt (Denver, Leveen Shunt)

> **Denver Shunt** – peritoneal to R IJ connection (need to pump Q4 hrs)
>
> *Contraindications* – coma, organic renal failure, severe hepatic failure (total bilirubin > 6), large pleural effusion
>
> **Cx's:** clot, sepsis, CHF, DIC; *Hardly ever used anymore* – no improvement in survival; only 50% open at 1 year
>
> **Pleural effusions associated w/ ascites** (usually unilateral, R > L)
>> **Tx:** <u>NO</u> chest tube (↑ Cx's), Tx aimed at controlling the ascites (which controls pleural effusion); respiratory distress → thoracentesis

Umbilical hernia w/ ascites

> Conservative tx (non-surgical) has only a 25% success rate (emergency surgery for incarcerations in 50%)
>
> **Risks** – rupture and evisceration; incarceration and strangulation
>
> **Emergency surgery** for umbilical hernia and ascites has ↑ed mortality
>
> *Do not wait* until hernia sac has ruptured to fix umbilical hernias in pts w/ ascites – should fix these electively
>
> (Follow pre-op preparation above before surgery)

Bleeding Esophageal Varices

Tx:

> Place an **NGT,** T and C for 6 units of blood (keep **Hct > 30**)
>
> **Send coagulation studies** and **correct them** (Vit K and FFP)
>
> **EGD w/ sclerotherapy** (cautery) and **banding** (effective in 90%)
>
> **Vasopressin** (splanchnic artery constriction) - pts w/ a history of CAD should receive **NTG** while on vasopressin
>
> **Octreotide** (↓'s portal pressure by ↓ing blood flow),
>
> **Blakemore tube** (not as effective for gastric varices; Need to intubate the pt w/ this; let down after 24 hours to re-assess); Risk of rupture of esophagus (*hardly used anymore*)
>
> **TIPS** – needed for refractory emergent variceal bleeding
>> **If TIPS is not available** → need to place **porta-caval shunt** (<u>not</u> a spleno-renal shunt in this situation – would <u>not</u> completely decompress the portal system)
>
> **SBP Abx prophylaxis** (variceal bleed high risk for SBP, norfloxacin)
>
> **Child's A w/ non-emergent bleeding as only problem**, can perform elective **spleno-renal shunt** (Spleno-renal shunts will **worsen ascites**)
>
> **Propanolol** – may help prevent re-bleed, no good role acutely
>> **Isosorbide Dinitrate** in addition may further ↓ risk of bleed
>
> Can get late **strictures** from sclerotherapy, usually easily managed w/ dilatation
>
> Bleeding varices have 33% mortality with 1st episode
>> 50% re-bleed w/ 50% mortality

Hepatorenal syndrome

Progressive **renal failure** and **oliguria** despite normal filling pressures in pts w/ cirrhosis (not responsive to fluid challenge)

Type I – rapidly progressive

Type II – more indolent course (median survival 6 months)

Sign of end stage liver disease that ultimately is only treated w/ transplantation → All other therapies are temporizing measures

Often has a precipitating event (GI bleed, over-diuresis, infection, drugs)

Impt to R/O other causes of renal failure [renal toxic drugs, pre-renal and post-renal failure, intrinsic renal failure, infection (SBP)]

Dx:

1st **Volume challenge** (will <u>not</u> work w/ hepatorenal syndrome, will work w/ pre-renal azotemia→ **main difference** between the two)

U/S to R/O post-renal obstruction (eg kidney stone)

Paracentesis to R/O infection

Urinalysis – no protein or RBCs (electrolytes from hepatorenal syndrome are the same as pre-renal, see Critical Care chp)

Central line – shows normal CVP and filling pressures

R/O drug causes

Renal Bx – shows normal renal tissue

Tx (all bridges to TXP):

Midodrine and **octreotide** combined (*best therapy*)

Albumin and vasoconstrictors may be helpful

TIPS

Liver TXP eventually needed

Hepatopulmonary syndrome

Hypoxia from **intra-pulmonary vascular shunting**, CXR normal

Dx: contrast ECHO shows right to left shunt

Tx: oxygen, *liver TXP only definitive Tx*

Spontaneous bacterial peritonitis (SBP)

Fever and abd pain (peritonitis)

RFs – ascites fluid total protein < 1, previous SBP, current GI bleed

Dx: Fluid - WBCs > 500, PMNs > 250, positive cultures

Gram stain (less sensitive, more helpful for free perforation)

MC organism – E. coli, others - pneumococci, streptococci

Most commonly **one organism**; if not mono-organismal, need to worry about bowel perforation or abscess

Tx:

3rd **generation cephalosporins** (usually respond in 48 hrs, if not, reconfirm you dx)

IV albumin 1.5 gm/kg at time of Dx + 1 gm/kg on HD #3 ↑s survival

Pts usually respond within 48 hours → if not, repeat paracentesis (worry about bowel perforation or abscess)

Portal vein embolization for liver regeneration

Portal vein embolization for liver regeneration can ↑ volume and density of contra-lateral liver lobe.

Useful pre-op in pts undergoing liver resection who have limited hepatic reserve

Results in a "nodular " regeneration

Postpartum liver failure w/ ascites (hepatic vein thrombosis)

Ovarian vein thrombosis (often infected → thrombophlebitis) → leads to IVC thrombus formation → leads to **hepatic vein thrombosis**

Related to relative **hypercoaguable state** following pregnancy

Pts w/ **hypercoaguable syndromes** more susceptible

Can also get portal vein thrombosis (ie ascites w/o liver failure)

Infectious pelvic thrombophlebitis also involved (fever)

Dx: SMA arteriogram with venous phase contrast

Tx: heparin + abx's (usually have **thrombophlebitis** of ovarian vein)

<u>TIPS</u> (trans-jugular, intra-hepatic, portosystemic shunt)
- Decompresses portal system
- **Used for:**
    - Protracted **bleeding**
    - Refractory **ascites**
    - **Progressive coagulopathy**
    - **Visceral hypoperfusion**
- Allows antegrade flow from portal vein to IVC
- **S/Es**: development of **encephalopathy**; clotting of the shunt; bleeding
- **Porta-caval shunt** – same improvements as above but ↑ encephalopathy and ↑ mortality related to procedure (rarely used anymore unless TIPS unavailable)

<u>Splenorenal shunt</u>
- Low rate of encephalopathy; can leave the spleen
- **Need to ligate:**
    - **Left adrenal vein**
    - **Left gonadal vein**
    - **Inferior mesenteric vein**
    - **Coronary vein**
    - **Pancreatic branches** of splenic vein
- Careful dissection of the splenic vein off pancreas – leave the spleen intact
- Used <u>only</u> for **Child's A** who present just w/ **bleeding only** (unusually used anymore)
- *These are **contraindicated** w/ refractory ascites as spleno-renal shunts **can worsen ascites***
- Also, you do <u>not</u> decompress the portal system w/ this shunt – you <u>do</u> decompress esophageal and gastric varices
- **Child's B or C w/ indication for shunt → TIPS**
- **Child's A** that just has **bleeding as symptom** → consider splenorenal shunt (more durable); otherwise TIPS

<u>Portal hypertension</u>
- **Pre-hepatic causes** – portal vein thrombosis (50% of portal HTN in children) schistosomiasis, congenital hepatic fibrosis
- **Hepatic causes** – cirrhosis
- **Post-hepatic causes** (or sinusoidal) – Budd-Chiari (hepatic vein occlusion), constrictive pericarditis, CHF, SOS (sinusoidal obstructive syndrome)
- Normal portal vein pressure < 12 mmHg
- **Coronary veins** – act as collaterals between portal vein and systemic venous system at lower esophagus (azygous system)
- **Portal HTN** – can lead to esophageal variceal hemorrhage, ascites, splenomegaly, and hepatic encephalopathy
- **Shunts** (eg TIPS) can decompress portal system

<u>Portal hypertension from portal vein thrombosis</u>
- Usually caused by **extra-hepatic thrombosis of portal vein**
- *MCC of massive hematemesis in children*
- **Etiologies** – cirrhosis, CA, hypercoaguable state, surgery, trauma
- **Dx:** U/S or abd CT
- **Tx:**
    - Control UGIB from esophageal varices if present (no anticoagulation)
    - If not bleeding → anticoagulation for acute thrombosis to prevent clot propagation
    - Consider **trans-hepatic direct thrombolysis of portal vein clot** (avoids systemic tPA) for refractory or recurrent bleeding (place sheath from hepatic vein to portal vein, remove portal vein clot, then place shunt)
    - Surgical shunt for refractory bleeding if above fail (porto-caval to decompress portal system, want portal pressure < 12 mmHg)

Unusual causes of cirrhosis
Hemochromatosis (too much iron, dark skin):
> **Tx: phlebotomy** (#1), deferoxamine

Wilson's Disease (too much copper, Kayser-Fleischer rings);
> **Tx: penicillamine** and pyridoxine

Alpha-1 antitrypsin (also get emphysema) – **Tx:** TXP
Sinusoidal obstructive syndrome (occlusion of hepatic venules and sinusoids)
> Associated w/ **liver stem cell TXP**
>> **Tx: supportive**, **UDCA** (urodeoxycholic acid) prophylaxis in pts undergoing stem cell TXP

Budd-Chiari Syndrome
Occlusion of hepatic veins and IVC
Etiologies – hypercoaguable state (esp polycythemia vera), CA, webs, trauma, OCPs, idiopathic (50%)
> **Primary** (75%) – thrombosis of hepatic veins
> **Secondary** (25%) – compression from outside
> **MC identifiable cause** – polycythemia vera

Sx's: RUQ abd pain, ascites (MC sx) and **hepatomegaly** *(classic triad)*
Dx:
> **Retrograde hepatic vein angiogram** *(best test*, may also be able to tx)
>> Catheter is in the IVC and you retrograde inject
>
> Duplex U/S (often initial test)
> CT scan w/ triple phase contrast
> **Liver Bx → sinusoidal dilatation** and **centrilobular congestion**

Tx:
> **Anticoagulation** (heparin, then warfarin), **thrombolysis if acute**
> **TIPS** if refractory (needs to connect to IVC <u>above</u> obstruction)
> **Porta-caval shunt** if TIPS not available (needs to connect to IVC <u>above</u> obstruction)
> **TXP** if refractory to above (10% have <u>recurrence of Budd-Chiari</u> after TXP)

Splenic vein thrombosis
Can lead to **isolated gastric varices** w/o portal HTN (<u>no esophageal varices</u>)
Gastric varices can bleed
MCC isolated splenic vein thrombosis – pancreatitis
Tx: splenectomy

Primary sclerosing cholangitis (PSC)

Usually in **men** (50-60's)

RFs – ulcerative colitis (70% of pts w/ PSC have UC), retroperitoneal fibrosis, Riedel's thyroiditis, pancreatitis, and diabetes

Sx's: fatigue, fluctuating jaundice, pruritis (from **bile acids**), weight loss, malabsorption, steatorrhea

Dx: ERCP *(best test)* – multiple **strictures** and **dilatations** (beaded appearance) in biliary system (MRCP another option)

Path

Autoimmune disease (**p-ANCA** in 70%)

Progressive fibrosis of **intrahepatic** and **extrahepatic ducts** leads to **portal HTN** and **hepatic failure**

Unusually can have **isolated** intrahepatic or extrahepatic duct inflammation and fibrosis

Bacterial cholangitis <u>unusual</u> unless biliary tract manipulation

Does <u>not</u> get better after colon resection for ulcerative colitis

Risk for cholangiocarcinoma

Tx:

Liver TXP is usually the only definitive tx

At risk for **recurrent PSC after Liver TXP** (20% at 5 years)

Although unlikely, this DZ can be only on **one side of the liver** → may be able perform **lobectomy**

Although unlikely, this DZ can be only **extra-hepatic** → **Choledochojejunostomy** may be effective

PTC tube drainage to palliate may be an option

Balloon dilatation of dominant strictures may provide some symptomatic relief

UDCA (urodeoxycholic acid) – ↓ pruritis and sx's (↓ bile acids), ↓ LFTs

Cholestyramine – ↓ pruritis and sx's (↓ bile acids)

Fat soluble vitamins

Primary biliary cirrhosis

Usually in **women**

Sx's: fatigue, pruritus, jaundice, xanthomas

Dx:

Anti-mitochondrial Ab's + ↑ **LFTs** → **diagnostic**

Cholestatic pattern – ↑ alk phos, AST, and ALT

M2-IgG – anti-mitochondrial Ab that is the *most specific test*

**Do <u>not</u> have to get liver Bx, can diagnose based on above

Path

Autoimmune DZ (associated w/ Hashimoto's thyroiditis)

Progressive fibrosis of **small-sized** intra-hepatic ducts

Leads to cholestasis → cirrhosis → portal hypertension

**No increased risk of CA

Tx:

Better survival than PSC, many pts can have normal lifespan and survival w/o liver TXP

TXP often needed

Can **recur after liver TXP** (20% at 5 years)

UDCA (urodeoxycholic acid) – ↓ pruritis and sx's (↓ bile acids), ↓ LFTs

Cholestyramine – ↓ pruritis and sx's (↓ bile acids)

Immunosuppression (MTX, cyclosporine) → may have some benefit

Fat soluble vitamins

Liver Cysts

DDx:

> **Simple cysts** (or polycystic liver DZ)
> **Echinococcus**
> **Hepatic cystadenoma or cystadenocarcinoma**
> **Biliary cystadenoma or cystadenocarcinoma**

Sx's: pain, bowel obstruction, weight loss, fevers or chills; foreign **travel** (Mediterranean)

Dx:

> **Send serology**: hemagglutinin + ELISA for echinococcus
> **Abd and Pelvic CT** (and U/S)
>> The following suggest **hepatic or biliary cystadenoma/-carcinoma:**
>>> **Complex or septated** cyst
>>> Underlying **mass**
>>> **Frond like projections**
>>> Really **thick wall**
> **ERCP** w/ Echinococcus to r/o biliary connection
> After you have ruled out echinococcus, perform **percutaneous aspiration** if **symptomatic** or **suspicious** on CT or U/S →
>> **Bile** → get **ERCP** to look for leak area
>>> Send fluid for **cultures and cytology**
>>> **Likely simple cyst w/ erosion into bile duct** → wedge cyst out (or just simple un-roofing laparoscopically), cautery to the remaining epithelium
>>> Also need to worry about **CA** (biliary or hepatic)
>>> Send cyst wall for FS (and fluid for cytology) to make sure this is not a CA
>>> Perform IOC (w/ methylene blue) if having trouble locating the leaking duct
>> **Pus** (Infection) → leave **percutaneous drain**
>>> Send fluid for **cultures and cytology**
>>> **Abx's**
>>> **Repeat CT** after medical tx to see if there is an underlying mass (make sure not necrotic CA)
>>> Surgery if recurs
>> **Blood** → **resect cyst** (make sure resectable if you think its CA)
>>> Most likely bleeding into **simple cyst** from an exposed vessel
>>> Also need to worry about **CA** (biliary or hepatic)
>>> Send fluid for **cytology**
>>> **Simple cyst w/ bleeding** → wedge cyst out (or just simple un-roofing laparoscopically), cautery to the remaining epithelium
>>>> Send cyst wall for FS (and fluid for cytology) to make sure this is not a CA
>>> **CA** (biliary or hepatic) – formal resection
>> **Mucin** → **formal hepatic resection** for hepatic or biliary cystadenoma/-carcinoma (possible wedge if just adenoma; lean towards formal resection)
>> **Clear fluid** (and nothing else) → simple cyst
>>> **> 95% recur** after **simple aspiration**
>>> **Laparoscopic un-roofing** (*best Tx*) if symptomatic

Echinococcus Cyst (hydatid cyst)

> ↑ed in **right lobe** of liver
> **Sheep** – carriers; **dogs** – human exposure
> **Dx:**
>> **ELISA** for **IgG Ab's** (*best test*)
>> **Abd CT** – ectocyst (**calcified**) + endocyst (**double cyst wall,** *classic*)
>> May have daughter cysts
>> **Preop ERCP** – check for communication w/ biliary system in pts w/ jaundice, ↑ LFTs, or cholangitis
>> ****Do not aspirate** → *can leak out and cause <u>anaphylactic shock</u>*

Tx:

>> **Preop albendazole** (2 weeks)
>> Pack bowel w/ **hypertonic saline** soaked towels and aspirate cyst
>>> **Inject ETOH** if no connection w/ the biliary system
>>>> ***Avoid* rupture of cyst and spillage of contents** *(anaphylaxis)*
>> **Need to remove all of the cyst wall** (ectocyst) off liver
>> Can use **IOC** (w/ **methylene blue** in biliary tract) if can't find biliary connection (need to ligate the connection to prevent biloma)
>> **Albendazole** post-op

Solitary simple cysts

Congenital; cx's from these cysts are <u>very rare</u> (pain, infection, biliary or bowel compression, bleeding) – **vast majority left alone**

↑ed in **right lobe,** women

Walls have **blue hue** (do <u>not</u> contain bile)

Percutaneous drain if infected

Laparoscopic un-roofing for pain or compressive sx's (*best Tx*)

Percutaneous drainage has almost **100% recurrence**

Polycystic liver Disease

Associated w/ polycystic kidney DZ

Sx's: compressive (portal HTN, bowel, resp difficulty)

Tx: may need excision of larger cysts if causing sx's (liver TXP last resort)

Hepatic cyst-adenoma/-adenocarcinoma

U/S will show **papillary-like fronds** within the cyst itself; often **complex**

Mucin production

Usually **intra-hepatic**

Adenoma considered **pre-malignant**

Tx: formal resection unless adenoma (wedge)

Biliary cyst-adenoma/-adenocarcinoma

U/S will show characteristic **very thick cyst wall** and **septated**

Mucin production

Usually **intra-hepatic**

Usually have **calcifications**

Adenoma considered **pre-malignant**

Tx: formal resection usual (if adenoma possibly wedge)

Liver Abscess

Pyogenic abscess (need to make sure this is not CA)

MC type of hepatic abscess (80%)

MC organism – E. coli (GNR's MC class)

MCC overall – biliary tract disease w/ ascending infection (related to CBD stones, stricture, and CA), **multiple** abscesses usual w/ biliary source

Other causes

Biliary tract manipulation or **stents**

**Distant infection

(appendicitis or diverticulitis → bacteremia → Liver abscess)

Sx's: fever, chills, weight loss, RUQ pain, sepsis

15% mortality w/ sepsis

Dx:

Abd CT – ↑ in **right lobe**

↑ **LFTs** and ↑ **WBCs**

Blood cultures positive in 60%

Tx:

Percutaneous drainage + abx's (cover GPCs, GNRs, anaerobes)

Surgical drainage if unstable, continued signs of sepsis, or multiple abscess not amenable to percutaneous drainage

Need to make sure **biliary system is unobstructed**

Always send aspirated fluid for **cultures** and **cytology** (R/O CA)

Re-CT after drainage stops and abscess gone to look for CA

If no history of infection or biliary tract manipulation, need to worry about CA

Amoebic abscess (entoamoeba histolytica)

Travel to Mexico or Latin America (fecal-oral transmission)

Primary infection in **colon** → amoebic colitis

Reaches liver via **portal vein**

↑ed in **right lobe** of liver, usually single

Sx's: fever, chills, RUQ pain, jaundice, hepatomegaly

Dx:

Agglutinin + immuno-electrophoresis Ab tests (positive in 90%)

↑**LFTs** and ↑**WBCs**

Abd CT - can be helpful

If extra-intestinal infection only → stool cx's usually negative

Cultures of abscess often **sterile** → protozoa only in **peripheral rim**

Tx:

Flagyl 1st line *(not drainage)*

Sx's should get better in few days, if not think **super-infection**

Percutaneous drainage if refractory or contaminated

Most do *not* require aspiration (anchovy paste)

Surgery only for free rupture

Schistosomiasis abscess

Travel to middle east (Egypt); in water (penetrates skin)

↑ed in **right lobe** of liver

Sx's: maculopapular **rash**, RUQ pain, can cause **variceal bleeding**

Dx:

Agglutinin + immuno-electrophoresis Ab tests

↑ eosinophils

Stool and **urine O and P**

Diffuse **petechiae** in rectum (lives in **mesenteric venules**)

Tx:

Praziquantel 1st line *(not drainage)* + control of variceal bleeding

Percutaneous drainage if refractory or contaminated

Most do *not* require aspiration

Necrotic tumor – see hepatocellular carcinoma below

Echinococcal Cyst – (see cyst section above)

Hepatic adenomas

80% symptomatic (MC RUQ pain)

50% risk of **significant bleeding** (rupture) – main reason for resection

5% risk of **malignancy**

MC in **right lobe** of liver

RFs – women on OCPs, autoimmune disease, steroids

Sx's: pain or discomfort, palpable mass, hypotension (from hemorrhage – up to 25% present w/ rupture)

Dx:

Abd CT / MRI – hypervascular, homogenous tumor

Sulfur colloid scan – negative (cold)

No uptake; *No Kupffer cells in adenoma*

Tagged RBC scan – negative

AFP – normal

**No FNA – bleeding risk

Tx:

Asymptomatic (or very mildly symptomatic) *and* on **OCPs / steroids** *and* ≤ **4 cm** →

1) **D/C OCPs / steroids** *and;*

2) **Serial CT scans** (every 4-6 weeks)

Make sure mass ↓s in size and eventually completely goes away (takes 6-12 months) → if not, **resection**

> **4 cm** → **resection**

↑ **in size or worsening CT findings** (eg hemorrhage areas) while following → resection

Worsening sx's → resection

Not on OCP's or steroids → resection

Significantly symptomatic → resection

Consider **embolization** if multiple and unresectable

Focal nodular hyperplasia (FNH)

No malignancy risk, very rare rupture

Dx:

Abd CT / MRI

Hypervascular; homogenous (completely fills in arterial phase)

Characteristic '**central stellate scar**' (70%) → *Not* seen w/ adenoma or HCC

Sulfur colloid scan – positive in 70% (hot scan)

Kupffer cells uptake colloid

Not seen w/ HCC or adenoma (No Kupffer cells in adenoma or HCC)

Tagged RBC scan – negative

AFP – normal

FNA – not sensitive enough to DDx FNH vs. adenoma (shows hepatocytes)

Tx:

No resection → **conservative Tx** unless enlarging, worsening sx's, or if unsure of Dx: if surgery needed, wedge resection 1st

D/C OCP's or **steroids** and follow **serial CT scan**

If unsure of Dx (50% cases) → need to follow hepatic adenoma pathway

Hemangiomas

MC benign liver tumor

Rupture rare, women

Sx's: most asymptomatic

NO FNA → risk of **hemorrhage

Dx:

Abd CT / MRI shows **peripheral to central enhancement** (diagnostic)

Tagged RBC scan – positive (*best test*, can be used as confirmatory test if diagnosis still in doubt)

Tx:

No resection – conservative Tx unless very symptomatic, then **surgery ± pre-op embolization** (if child → steroids, see Pediatric Surgery chp)

XRT + steroids for unresectable disease

Hepatocellular CA (HCC, hepatoma)

MC cancer worldwide (MCC – Hep B)

Liver mets to **primary hepatocellular CA ratio = 20:1**

RFs – viral hepatitis (HepB, HepC, and HepD), ETOH, primary sclerosing cholangitis, hemochromatosis, alpha-1-antitrypsin deficiency, alfatoxins, hepatic adenoma, steroids

NOT RFs – primary biliary cirrhosis, Wilson's Disease

In US, 80% occur in setting of **cirrhosis**

Sx's: abd pain, weight loss, ascites, jaundice

Dx
- **CT scan** (triple phase scanning) or **MRI**
  - Often have **mosaic pattern** (non-homogenous, necrotic areas)
  - **Vascular** in arterial phase, **relatively avascular** in venous phase
  - Can have **single** or **multiple** tumors
  - Can be **nodular** or **diffuse**
  - Look for **mets, vessels,** or **nodal involvement**
- **Labs** – **AFP-L3** and **DCP** (Des-gamma carboxyprothrombin, not elevated in liver diseases except HCC, in which 90% have elevation)

Path
- **Best prognosis types** – clear cell, lymphocytic, fibrolamellar (young pts)
- **Worst prognosis** – diffuse nodular
- **AFP level** correlates w/ tumor size
- **Other tumor types:**
  - **Hepatic sarcoma**
    - **RFs** – PVC, Thorotrast, arsenic → rapidly fatal
  - **Cholangiosarcoma**
    - **RFs** – clonorchiasis infection, ulcerative colitis, hemochromatosis, primary sclerosing cholangitis, choledochal cysts
    - Intrahepatic worse survival than extrahepatic
    - Tumor size and satellite nodules correlate w/ outcome

Staging
- **Stage I** - Single tumor (any size) not invading blood vessels.
- **Stage II**
  - 1) Single tumor (any size) w/ invasion of blood vessels *or*
  - 2) Multiple tumors < 5 cm
- **Stage IIIA**
  - 1) Multiple tumors $\geq$ 5 cm *or:*
  - 2) Tumor involving a major branch of portal or hepatic vein(s)
- **Stage IIIb**
  - 1) Tumor invading other organ (other than gallbladder) *or;*
  - 2) Tumor invading visceral peritoneum
- **Stage IIIc** - positive regional nodes
- **Stage IV** - mets or distant lymph nodes

Tx:
- Only **15% can be resected** (eg cirrhosis, porta hepatic lymph node involvement, mets, or not enough liver would be left for survival)
- **For resection, need:**
  - 1) **En bloc resection** – can resect multiple tumors in same lobe or some tumors w/ direct invasion of another organ or peritoneum
  - 2) **Retain enough liver for survival** (child's A or some child's B cirrhosis)
  - *Contraindications to resection:*
    - **Nodal disease** (most likely portal nodes, stage IIIc)
    - **Mets** (most likely peritoneal studding; stage IV)
    - **Child's C cirrhosis**
  - **Diagnostic laparoscopy** before laparotomy
  - Formal resection requires a **1-cm margin**
- Consider **liver TXP** if <u>no</u> systemic DZ (see Cirrhosis section for criteria)
- **5-YS w/ resection** – 30%; **Tumor recurrence** → most likely in liver
- **Sorafenib** (multireceptor tyrosine kinase inhibitor) – if unresectable or mets
- **Palliative Tx** – cryotherapy, radiofrequency ablation, intra-arterial chemo

Liver nodule found at laparotomy for other reasons
Incidental colorectal CA mets
If previous CT showed no other nodules, intra-op U/S shows no other nodules, and lesion is amenable to simple wedge → resection

If difficult to take → just Bx it, finish your procedure, re-stage at 8 wks (chest/abd/pelvic CT, LFTs, CEA) if no other mets → resection

If not having surgery for colon CA → just wedge or core needle Bx, send for frozen section (may contraindicate resection, eg - pancreatic, gastric CA)

Intra-op U/S – *best Dx study for liver mets* (gives number, location, relationship to blood vessels)

Metastatic and primary tumors of liver are supplied by **hepatic arteries:**
Malignancies are generally vascular in arterial phase and avascular in venous phase

Primary liver tumors – generally <u>hypervascular</u>

Metastatic liver tumors – generally <u>hypovascular</u>

Normal Anatomy and Physiology

Gallbladder lies underneath **segments IV** and **V**

Cystic artery is a branch off the right hepatic artery, located in triangle of Calot

Triangle of Calot - cystic duct (lateral), common bile duct (medial), liver (superior)

1) **Right hepatic artery** branches (lateral) and 2) **gastroduodenal artery**
  retroduodenal branches (medial) supply **hepatic and common bile duct**
  The 9- and 3-o'clock positions when performing ERCP sphincterotomy
  Considered longitudinal blood supply

Aberrant posterior right hepatic artery (segments VI and VII)
  1% of the population
  At risk of injury w/ cholecystectomy (found in Triangle of Calot)
  Injury can result in **ischemia to segments VI** and **VII**
    (Sx's – fevers, pain, ↑LFT's, liver abscess)

Cystic veins – drain into **right branch of portal vein** and into liver

Lymphatics – found on **right side** of common bile duct

Innervation

  Parasympathetic fibers – left vagus (anterior trunk)
  Sympathetic fiber – splanchnic and celiac ganglions (T7-T10)

Gallbladder

  Mucosa is **columnar epithelium**
  No submucosa
  Common bile duct and hepatic duct do **not** have **peristalsis**
  Fills by **contraction of sphincter of Oddi** at ampulla of Vater
    Morphine – contracts sphincter of Oddi
    Glucagon – relaxes sphincter of Oddi
  After cholecystectomy, total bile acid pools ↓

Normal sizes

  CBD < 8 mm, (< 10 mm after cholecystectomy)
  Gallbladder wall < 4 mm
  Pancreatic duct < 4 mm

Highest concentration of CCK and **secretin cells** – duodenum

Rokitansky-Aschoff sinuses – invagination of epithelium into muscle layer of gallbladder wall; formed from ↑ gallbladder pressure; harmless

Ducts of Luschka

  Small accessory bile ducts that course along the gallbladder fossa
    Don't actually drain into the gallbladder
  MC originate in the right lobe of the liver
  MC drain into the extra-hepatic bile ducts
  Can be injured w/ cholecystectomy
  Dx of leaking Duct of Luschka – HIDA (*best test*)

Aberrant posterior right hepatic duct (from **segments VI** or **VII**)
  1% of the population
  Enters common bile duct **separately** from right hepatic
  Lies in gallbladder bed fossa and at risk of injury w/ cholecystectomy

Bile excretion

  ↑ed bile excretion – CCK, secretin, vagal input
  ↓ed bile excretion – VIP, somatostatin, sympathetic input
  Gallbladder contraction – CCK (constant, tonic contraction)

Composition and Essential Functions of bile

  1) Fat-soluble vitamin absorption + essential fatty acids
  2) Bilirubin excretion
  3) Cholesterol excretion

  Gallbladder concentrates bile by **active resorption of Na and water**

	Hepatic Bile	Gallbladder Bile
Na (mEq/L)	140-180	225-375
CL (mEq/L)	50-100	1-10
Bile Salts (mEq/L)	1-50	250-350
Cholesterol (mEq/dl)	50-150	300-700

Final bile composition determined by active (Na/K ATPase) **reabsorption** of water in the gallbladder (concentrates bile)

Bile Salts (see Liver chp for synthesis)

Bile salt pool (6 gm) cycles 6 x/day

Small amount (10%) of bile salts lost in stool

90% of excreted bile salts are reabsorbed (**enterohepatic circulation**):

1) **Active resorption** of <u>conjugated</u> bile acids in **terminal ileum** (45%, Na/K ATPase)

Conjugated bile salts absorbed <u>only</u> in terminal ileum

2) **Passive resorption** of <u>non-conjugated</u> bile acids in **small intestine (40%) and colon (5%)**

Postprandial emptying of gallbladder bile maximum at 2 hours (80% emptied)

Bile is secreted by **bile canalicular cells** (20%) and <u>**hepatocytes**</u> (80%)

Color of bile from **conjugated bilirubin**

Stercobilin – breakdown product of conjugated bilirubin in gut; is what gives stool brown color

Urobilin – breakdown product of conjugated bilirubin in gut; some gets reabsorbed and released in urine which gives it yellow color

Gallstones can form after terminal ileum resection from malabsorption of bile acids

Gallstones

10% of the US population has gallstones

MC asymptomatic

Only 10% of gallstones are radiopaque on X-ray

Cholesterol stones (non-pigmented stones)

MC stone type in US (80%)

This type formed almost *exclusively* in the gallbladder (secondary stone)

Yellow to green

From **cholesterol insolubilization:**

1) **Too much cholesterol** or **too little bile salts**

2) **Stasis** or **incomplete emptying** contributes → makes bile too concentrated from increased water absorption

3) **Mucin glycoproteins** in bile also affect cholesterol crystallization – promote **calcium nucleation** and nidus for stone formation

Cholesterol stones in obese pts – overactive HMG CoA reductase

Cholesterol stones in thin pts – underactive 7-alpha-hydroxylase

Cholesterol stone RFs – age > 40, female, obesity, pregnancy, rapid weight loss, vagotomy

Pigmented stones (calcium bilirubinate stones)

MC stones worldwide (25% of stones in US)

Solubilization of **unconjugated bilirubin** and precipitation of **calcium bilirubinate**

Dissolution agents do not work for pigmented stones (mono-octanoin)

Black stones

Almost always form in gallbladder (secondary stone)

From **hemolytic disorders** (eg hemolytic anemia, sickle cell anemia, spherocytosis → all ↑ bilirubin) or **cirrhosis** (↓ conjugation)

Also in pts on **chronic TPN** (liver disease, ↓ conjugation) or w/ **terminal ileum resection** (↑unconjugated bilirubin absorption)

Important development factors for black stones

1) **Increased bilirubin load** (esp unconjugated bilirubin)

2) **Decreased hepatic function**

3) **Bile stasis**

Tx: cholecystectomy if symptomatic

Brown stones (primary CBD stones, formed in ducts)

- **MC type of primary stone** (ie forming in the bile ducts)
- Can form in gallbladder but mostly forms in **bile ducts**
- **From infection** causing deconjugation of bilirubin
- **MC infection causing brown stones - E. coli** (produces beta-glucoronidase, which deconjugates bilirubin, leading to formation of **calcium bilirubinate**)
- Increased in Asians
- Need to check for ampullary stenosis, duodenal diverticuli, and abnormal sphincter of Oddi in these pts
- Almost all pts w/ primary stones need **biliary drainage procedure** – ERCP w/ sphincteroplasty (90% successful)

Cholesterol stones and **black stones** found in CBD considered **secondary common bile duct stones**

Cholecystitis

Obstruction of cystic duct (MC by a gallstone) results in gallbladder wall distention and inflammation

Sx's:

- **RUQ pain** worse 1-2 hours after meal (esp fatty meals), N/V, appetite loss
- **Referred pain** to shoulder or scapula
- **Persistent pain** (unlike biliary colic, which has transient pain + obstruction)
- **Murphy's Sign** – pt resists deep inspiration w/ deep palpation to RUQ secondary to pain
- **MC organism w/ cholecystitis** – E. Coli; others - klebsiella, enterococcus

Dx:

Labs

- **LFT's** (↑**Alk phos**); If other LFT's elevated, need to worry about **CBD stone** → pt needs **ERCP**
- ↑ **WBC** usual
- Amylase and lipase (can get mild elevations w/ cholecystitis; if significantly ↑ed need to worry about **CBD stone** →**ERCP**)

U/S

- *Best initial test for either jaundice or RUQ pain*
- **95% sensitive** for picking up stones
- **Acute cholecystitis findings** – gallstones, GB wall thickening (> 4 mm), pericholecystic fluid, sonographic Murphy's
- **Stones** – hyper-echoic focus, posterior shadowing, movement of focus w/ change in position
- **Dilated CBD** (> 8 mm if gallbladder present) suggests CBD stone (also potentially benign or malignant stricture if not associated w/ stones)
- **Dilated pancreatic duct** (> 4 mm) suggests CBD stone (also potentially benign or malignant stricture if not associated w/ stones)

HIDA scan (Hepatobiliary Imino-Diacetic Acid Scan)

- Also called **cholecystokinin cholescintigraphy** (CCK-CS)
- ***Most sensitive test for cholecystitis***
- Used if U/S is non-diagnostic; checks for **chronic cholecystitis** and **biliary dyskinesia**
- **Technetium** (Tc) is given, taken up by liver, and then excreted in biliary tract (99mTc-*HIDA* cholescintigraphy)
- **Cholecystokinin** (CCK) is given
- **Results**
    1) If **gallbladder cannot be seen** →cystic duct obstruction by **stone**; **Tx:** cholecystectomy
    2) If **>60 minutes to empty** after meal→ **chronic cholecystitis Tx:** cholecystectomy
    3) If **gallbladder ejection fraction < 40%** after 1 hour → **biliary dyskinesia**
       Tx: cholecystectomy (95% get relief)

ERCP pre-op indications (signs that a CBD stone is present):
  Jaundice
  Cholangitis (RUQ pain, fever, jaundice)
  Elevated **amylase** (> 1000) **or lipase** (possible gallstone pancreatitis)
  Elevated **bilirubin** (> 4; CBD stone, possible cholangitis)
  Elevated **AST or ALT** (> 500; CBD stone, possible cholangitis)
  U/S showing stone in CBD or dilated CBD

Tx

Cholecystectomy (semi-urgent, usually within 72 hours; give broad
  spectrum abx's) – vast majority of pts
  Dissect out **cystic duct** and find **cystic artery**
      Be careful of **accessory right hepatic artery** and
          accessory right hepatic duct and that you do not
          mistakenly have **CBD** - need to see the **cystic duct
          enter the GB**
      Also need to see the **cystic artery go onto the GB**
  2 clips on the proximal cystic duct and 1 distal
  2 clips on the proximal cystic artery and 1 distal
Cholecystostomy tube
  CT or U/S guided percutaneous cholecystostomy tube
  For pts who are **very ill and cannot tolerate surgery**
  When pt stable, perform cholecystectomy
Suspected CBD stone intra-op
  1-2% of pts undergoing cholecystectomy will have a retained CBD
      stone and 99% of pts w/ retained CBD stones can have them
      cleared w/ ERCP
  Stones ≤ 2 mm – leave them, will pass on their own
  Stones > 2 mm
      One option w/ CBD stone intra-op is to close w/ post-op ERCP
          (unless skilled in laparoscopic CBD exploration, avoids
          open procedure; *best option for vast majority*)
      If large stone which you feel can't be cleared w/ ERCP –
          consider CBD exploration (small stones leave alone,
          almost always pass)
  CBD exploration
      Intra-op cholangiogram (1:1 Omnipaque: normal saline
          solution) to identify stones (usually inject through cystic
          duct remnant)
      Can give **glucagon** to dilate ampulla and force stone through
          w/ injection (saline)
      Fogarty balloon catheters can be used to remove stone
      Choledochoscope w/ attachments - pull stone out or push it
          through
      Stone forceps can be used
      Duodenostomy + open sphincterotomy an option if above
          fail
ERCP
  Best Tx for **late common bile duct stone**
  Sphincterotomy + grasper and other tools used to remove stone
  Risk's – bleeding, pancreatitis, perforation of bile duct or duodenum
Bleeding intra-op
  Press neck of GB against bleeding site to get control
  See if you can safely clip it; if not, go w/ right subcostal incision and
      ligate bleeder
Place drain if worried about **bleeding or biliary injury**
Bile duct injury intra-op – open and repair
  Partial transection – primary repair over stent
  Complete transection – hepatico-jejunostomy or
      choledochojejunostomy over stent
Diarrhea after cholecystectomy – excess **bile salts in gut** (not stored in
  gallbladder anymore)

Acalculous cholecystitis

MC after severe burns, prolonged TPN, trauma, major surgery, cardiac surgery

Primary pathology – **bile stasis** leading to distention and ischemia

RFs – narcotics, fasting, increased viscosity (eg dehydration, ileus, transfusions)

Sx's: RUQ pain, N/V

Dx:

> **U/S** – dilated GB, sludge, gallbladder wall thickening, pericholecystic fluid, **NO stones**
>
> **Labs** – ↑ WBCs, ↑alkaline phosphatase
>
> **HIDA scan** – is positive

Tx: cholecystectomy; **percutaneous cholecystostomy tube** if pt is too unstable (tube stays in for 6-8 weeks to form tract)

Other Disorders

Gallbladder empyema (ie suppurative cholecystitis)

> Pus fills the gallbladder
>
> More frequent in **diabetics** and **immunosuppressed**
>
> **MC organism** – E. coli
>
> **Sx's**: severe, rapid-onset abdominal pain, N/V, **septic shock**
>
> **Tx: emergent cholecystectomy** or drainage w/ PTC tube, broad spectrum abx's
>
> **If hypotensive** – stabilize pt before OR (volume resuscitation, start abx's)

Gangrenous cholecystitis

> Gallbladder wall becomes **necrotic** – **can perforate**
>
> More frequent in diabetics
>
> **Sx's**: severe, rapid-onset abdominal pain, N/V, **septic shock**
>
> **Tx: emergent cholecystectomy**
>
> **If hypotensive** – stabilize pt before OR (volume resuscitation, start abx's)

Emphysematous cholecystitis

> High **perforation rate** and **mortality rate** (5-10%)
>
> More frequent in **diabetics** and immunocompromised
>
> From **gas forming organism** in gallbladder wall (MC- **clostridium perfringens**; E. coli + Klebsiella also usually present)
>
> **Dx: U/S** or **X-ray** shows **gas in gallbladder wall** ± air in **lumen**
>
> **Sx's**: severe, rapid-onset abd pain, N/V, **septic shock**
>
> **Tx: emergent cholecystectomy**
>
> > **If hypotensive** – stabilize before OR (volume resuscitation, abx's)

Biliary Colic

> Transient cystic duct obstruction caused by passage of a gallstone
>
> Resolves in 4-6 hrs

Air in biliary system

> MC occurs w/ previous ERCP and sphincterotomy
>
> Can also occur w/ **cholangitis** or **erosion of biliary system into duodenum** (eg gallstone ileus)

Bacterial infection of bile

> **MC route** (w/o previous biliary tract manipulation) – dissemination from **portal system**
>
> Can also get retrograde infection from bacteria in duodenum (usually prevented by **sphincter of Oddi**)

Highest incidence of positive bile cultures

> MC w/ **post-op strictures** (**MC** – E. coli, often polymicrobial)

Choledocholithiasis Cx's – cholangitis, pancreatitis, stricture

Mirizzi Syndrome

> **Sx's:** jaundice, RUQ pain, possible cholangitis
>
> Compression of common hepatic duct by stone in infundibulum or chronic inflammation
>
> Sometimes a **fistula** can form between the gallbladder and CBD
>
> The CBD can also become **scarred** w/ time
>
> **Tx:** cholecystectomy, possible CBD reconstruction (choledocho-jejunostomy)

Porcelain gallbladder – diffuse calcification of gallbladder wall; ↑ed risk for CA

Gallbladder polyps
>5% of asymptomatic pts
>**70% are cholesterol polyps** (cholesterolosis)
>>**Benign, epithelial covered, yellow spots**
>>From buildup of **lipid laden macrophages** in the lamina propria
>>Almost always **multiple** when they occur
>
>**Other types**
>>**Inflammatory polyps** – chronic inflammation, narrow stalk, benign
>>**Adenomas** (considered <u>pre-malignant</u>) – can be tubular or papillary; pedunculated or sessile
>>**Adenomyomatosis** – thickened nodule of mucosa that grows through Rokitansky-Aschoff sinuses into muscular layer and often beyond (once thought to be benign but CA reported)
>>**Heterotopic tissue** – pancreas, stomach
>>**Other benign lesion** (eg lipoma, etc)
>>**Adenocarcinoma**
>
>**RFs for malignancy** – size >1 cm, pts > 60 years old, sessile polyps, primary sclerosing cholangitis (PSC)
>**Cholecystectomy indications:**
>>1) **Stones are also present**
>>2) **> 1 cm**
>>3) **Sessile**
>>4) **Malignant looking on U/S**
>>5) **Associated w/ PSC**

Granular cell tumor – benign neuroectoderm tumor of gallbladder
>Sx's of cholecystitis
>Tx: cholecystectomy

Shock following laparoscopic cholecystectomy
>**Early** (1st 24 hours) – hemorrhagic shock, clip fell off cystic artery
>**Late** (after 24 hours) – septic shock from accidental clip on CBD w/ subsequent cholangitis (usually this occurs at **median 7 days**)

Ceftriaxone – can cause gallbladder sludging and cholestatic jaundice

Indications for asymptomatic cholecystectomy – pts undergoing liver TXP or gastric bypass procedure (w/ stones)

Delta bilirubin – bilirubin bound to albumin, half-life of 18 days; takes awhile to clear after long-standing jaundice

T-tube – can be placed for complex biliary issues
>Is a **percutaneous tube** to the **CBD**
>Takes **3 weeks for a tract to form**
>Can work through this tract after 3 weeks by removing the T-tube and using choledochoscopy tools (eg to remove retained stones) – **avoids potential reoperative laparotomy**
>The tract will eventually close after removing the T-tube

Ursodiol (Actigall) – dissolves gallstones < 2cm; indicated for either:
>1) pts w/ cholecystectomy indications who are too high risk for surgery <u>or</u>
>2) prevention of gallstone formation in pts w/ rapid weight loss

Cirrhosis w/ gallstones – <u>no</u> elective cholecystectomy (high mortality)

Cholangitis

If in shock → fluid resuscitation 1st, start abx's, and stabilize pt before ERCP
Next most impt issue here is to get the biliary system decompressed
Sx's

> **Charcot's triad** – RUQ pain, fever, and jaundice (classic)
> **Reynolds' pentad** – Charcot's triad plus **mental status changes** and **shock** (ie sepsis)
> **MCC** – gallstones
> **MC organism** – E. coli; others - Klebsiella, GNR's, enterococcus

DDx: Stones (MC problem), **Stricture** (benign or malignant), **Choledochal cysts** (rare), **Duodenal diverticuli** (rare), **biliary stent w/ obstruction**

Dx:

> **U/S** (usual initial test) – CBD will be dilated (**> 8 mm**, > 10 mm after cholecystectomy) if due to obstruction of biliary system
> **ERCP** (best test)
> **Labs** – ↑ LFTs, ↑ WBCs, positive blood cultures

Path

> **Cholo-venous reflux** occurs at ≥ 20 mmHg, get **systemic bacteremia**
> **Late cx's of cholangitis** - stricture and hepatic abscess
> **MC serious cx** - Renal failure (related to **sepsis)**
> **Mortality** – 5%

Tx:

> **Reynolds' pentad** → **fluid resuscitation + start abx's**
> > Optimize hemodynamics for **septic shock**
> > *Do this before ERCP* (stabilize pt before ERCP)
> **ERCP**
> > Decompression of biliary system - try to remove stone or place temporary stent past stricture
> > If that fails, place a **PTC tube** to decompress
> > If that fails, take to OR and place an intra-op **T-tube** to decompress
> > Work up cause of blockage (gallstones, malignant or benign stricture) after pt recovers
> If due to **gallstones**, should have **cholecystectomy** in near future (likely **before discharge)**
> **Cholangitis due to infected PTC tube** → change PTC tube

Recurrent pyogenic cholangitis (oriental cholangiohepatitis)

MC in East Asia
Recurrent cholangitis from **primary CBD stones** and subsequent **strictures**
Calcium bilirubinate stones
MC organism – E. coli; others - C. sinensis, A. lumbricoides, T. trichiura
Initial Tx:

> ERCP, sphincterotomy, dilatation of strictures; No stents
> PTC if that fails
> Abx's or anti-parasitic meds

Long term Tx – often need hepatico-jejunostomy for long tern relief (best option)

Bile duct injuries intra-op

MC after laparoscopic cholecystectomy (vs. open)
2/3 of bile duct injuries are discovered **intra-op**

> 1/3 post-op at median time of **7 days** (Sx's – N/V, RUQ pain, low fever)

MCC CBD Injury

> ***Excess cephalad retraction of gallbladder fundus** (70% of injuries)
> > You think it's the cystic duct but really is the CBD brought up from excess traction (considered a **Class III injury)**
> > Minimize risk of injury by visualizing the triangle of Calot (want to see the cystic duct going into the gallbladder)

Intraoperative cholangiography (IOC) does not prevent injuries

> May limit severity; ↑ early diagnosis of injury

Aberrant right posterior hepatic duct (MC from segments VI and VII)

> Enters common bile duct **separately**
> Risk of injury with cholecystectomy

Sx's: Bile staining at time of cholecystectomy

Dx:

> Make sure **cystic duct clip** has not fallen off
>
> **Look for location** of bile drainage
>
> Consider an **IOC to help find leak** (can inject methylene blue to see leak or contrast agent + x-ray; laparoscopic or open) – usually given through the **cystic duct remnant**

Tx:

> **CBD injury**
>
>> **If injury < 50% circumference** of common bile duct, perform **primary repair** (over stent to prevent stenosis)
>>
>> In all other cases **hepatico-jejunostomy** or **choledocho-jejunostomy** (mucosa to mucosa apposition, place stent)
>>
>> *You do not attach to duodenum (won't reach)*
>
> **Duct of Luschka** (< 2 mm) → can just ligate
>
> **Aberrant right posterior duct** (segment VI and VII)
>
>> **MC aberrant hepatic duct** (MC aberrant duct injured w/ cholecystectomy)
>>
>> Enters CBD separately (need to look for these in triangle of Calot)
>>
>> **If ≤ 2 mm**, just ligate; may need **IOC** to look for attachment to CBD (would need to ligate that as well)
>>
>> **If > 2 mm**, will need to open and perform hepatico-jejunostomy or choledocho-jejunostomy; may need **IOC** to look for attachment to CBD (would need to ligate that)

Sepsis, jaundice, or persistent nausea and vomiting early following cholecystectomy (days)

DDx:

> **Leak** (from CBD, cystic duct remnant, Duct of Luschka) w/ <u>bile peritonitis</u>
>
> **Blockage** (retained stone, stricture from clip)
>
> **Seroma**

Sx's for the above arise at a median of **7 days** after cholecystectomy

Septic Patient

> **Initial Tx** – fluid resuscitation and abx's 1st if in shock
>
> Next is **drainage of biliary system or fluid collection** → likely **infected**
>
> W/U cause of blockage or leak after pt recovers

Dx and Tx

> **U/S** *(best test)* → find **fluid collection** (leak) or **dilated ducts** (blockage):
>
>> 1) **If fluid collection on U/S**, likely a **bile leak**→
>>
>>> **Place percutaneous drain into collection**
>>>
>>>> Send for cultures and cytology
>>>>
>>>> If just a seroma, just drain it
>>>>
>>>> If fluid is **bilious** → proceed below
>>>
>>> **Need to define leak** (size and location) →
>>>
>>>> Get **ERCP** (PTC if that fails, MRCP if that fails, HIDA if that fails, IOC if that fails)
>>>
>>> **Small Leaks:**
>>>
>>>> a. **Duct of Luschka** (< 2 mm, likely need **HIDA** to find)
>>>>
>>>> b. **Small accessory duct** (< 2 mm)
>>>>
>>>> c. **Cystic duct remnant** (clips fell off the cystic duct)
>>>>
>>>> d. **Small laceration in CBD** (< 2 mm)
>>>>
>>>> → all above treated w/ **ERCP, sphincterotomy, temporary stent** (across leak if possible), and percutaneous **drainage of fluid collection**
>>>>
>>>>> Back-up option if you can't get ERCP is to place a **PTC tube** which will likely take care of problem by decompressing system (small leaks will seal)
>>>>
>>>> Leave drain and stent for 6 weeks, then re-ERCP (or possibly HIDA for Duct of Luschka):
>>>>
>>>>> → pull stent and check for leak in drain for a week, if no leak pull drain

> → **persistent leak after 6 weeks** (rare w/ small leaks)→ OR for hepatico- or choledocho-jejunostomy

Large Leaks

> **Large or complete duct transection** → hepatico- or choledocho-jejunostomy (need Roux limb)
>
> For leaks that cause **early symptoms** (< 7 days) → OR
>
> For leaks that cause **later symptoms** (≥ 7 days) →
>
> > **Wait 6-8 weeks** before OR (just keep drain in until then; consider ERCP stent)
> >
> > Operation too difficult after 1 week secondary to dense adhesions and friable tissue

2) **If dilated ducts on U/S** (and no fluid collection) represents **obstruction** → get **ERCP** (PTC if that fails, MRCP if that fails, HIDA if that fails, IOC if that fails)

> **Need to define:**
>
> > **Cause** of the blockage → **retained stone** or **clip** (stricture from ischemia unlikely this early post-op)
> >
> > **Location** of the blockage

a. **Retained stone** →

> Get **ERCP + sphincterotomy**, remove stone
>
> If that fails, **PTC tube** (may be able to remove stones through PTC tube w/ stone grasper)
>
> If that fails, follow operative procedures for stones below

b. **Clip** across duct or a **stone** that can't be removed → Eventually need OR

> **Try to get biliary system decompressed** (ERCP w/ stent, PTC if that fails) unless its < 7 days and you are just going to operate
>
> > For problem that causes early sx's (< 7 days) → OR
> >
> > For problem that causes late sx's (> 7 days) → **wait 6-8 weeks** before OR
>
> If **you cannot get the pt decompressed** (can't get stent w/ ERCP or PTC) → OR for definitive surgery (no matter what the time period)

Operative Procedures for obstruction:

1) **Retained Stones** (not amenable to above)

> **IOC** if you do not know where the stone is from ERCP
>
> **CBD exploration w/ Choledochoscopy** (stone forceps to remove stones); **IOC** to make sure you got all the stones
>
> **If you still can't get stones out w/ above** → duodenostomy and open sphincterotomy; Remove stones w/ stone forceps or Fogarty catheters
>
> **If you still can't get stones out w/ the above** *(rare)* → choledocho-jejunostomy; Ligate the distal end of the duct
>
> **Retained stones vs. primary stones** (< 2 years vs. > 2 years)
>
> > **If > 2 years** (primary stone) → you have to do a biliary drainage procedure at some point (ERCP w/ sphincterotomy or open sphincteroplasty)
> >
> > **If < 2 years** → just have to get stone out (retained stone)

2) **Clip across duct**

> Can't just remove clip because **duct is too damaged** by clip
>
> Choledocho-jejunostomy or hepatico-jejunostomy (make sure mucosa to mucosa)
>
> **Place a stent across the anastomosis** to prevent stricture (T tube stent brought out through jejunum)
>
> Leave **drains**

Anastomotic leaks following TXP or hepaticojejunostomy → usually handled with ERCP and stents

Jaundice Evaluation

w/o previous surgery or late after cholecystectomy/biliary surgery (mos to years)

MCC of late post-op stricture after cholecystectomy – ischemia

DDx:

    1) **CBD stones**

        Previous cholecystectomy → need to check for ampullary stenosis, duodenal diverticuli, abnormal sphincter of Oddi (considered primary stones if > 2 years)

        No previous cholecystectomy → will need cholecystectomy this admission (ERCP 1st to remove stones)

    2) **Stricture** (benign or malignant)

        Benign stricture – chronic pancreatitis, previous cholangitis, ischemia related to previous cholecystectomy or other biliary surgery, pancreatic pseudocyst

            Usually long and **tapering**

            Benign strictures are very rare w/o antecedent biliary tract manipulation, pancreatitis, cholangitis, or trauma → *would most likely represent a <u>malignancy</u>*

        Malignant stricture – Bile duct, ampullary, duodenal, pancreatic, GB, or liver CA

            Usually **abrupt cut-off**

    3) **Primary liver disease** (eg cirrhosis)

    4) **Hemolysis**

Dx

    1st U/S (*best initial test for jaundice or RUQ pain*) – looking for dilated ducts

        GB may be distended along w/ biliary system

        May or may not see stone

        If ducts not dilated, need to think **primary liver disease** or **hemolysis**

    2nd ERCP (if ducts are dilated)

        Need to define blockage (stone or stricture) and **at what level**

        PTC if ERCP fails to define blockage

        MRCP if that fails

        HIDA if that fails

    3rd Abd CT (3 mm cuts) if there appears to be **a stricture** or if you **do not see stones on ERCP**; look for causes of malignant strictures (eg pancreatic or other CA)

Tx

    1) <u>**Stones**</u> – try to remove w/:

        ERCP (removes 99%)

        PTC if that fails (possibly remove through PTC tube w/ stone forceps)

        Open choledocotomy if that fails

        Transduodenal incision and **open sphincterotomy** if that fails

        Choledocho-jejunostomy or hepatico-jejunostomy as a last resort if that fails (very rare, oversew distal CBD)

        In OR, you get stone out, and pt stable, need **cholecystectomy** if GB still present

        If previous cholecystectomy and **> 2 years out** (ie primary CBD stone) and ERCP failed to remove stone initially (not able to cannulate duct or perform sphincterotomy, ect.) → need duodenostomy and open sphincterotomy while you are in there; If you have primary stones, likely have problem w/ sphincter of Oddi and need this drainage procedure

        If previous cholecystectomy and **< 2 years out** (ie secondary retained CBD stone) → no additional procedures after stone out

    2) <u>**Stricture**</u> (malignant or benign)

        R/O malignancy if stricture (or if you cannot clearly see stones)

            Get Bx's – duodenum, ampullary region, bile duct (brush Bx), either w/ **ERCP** or through **PTC**

            Abd CT (3 mm cuts) - look for pancreatic, bile duct, GB, liver, duodenal, and ampulla CA (consider MRI)

Very unlikely to get benign stricture without a Hx of biliary tract surgery, pancreatitis, cholangitis, or trauma → **this is CA until proven otherwise**

Malignant stricture

Start w/ mets w/u → chest/abd/pelvic CT, LFT's

Depending on CA, may need bile duct resection, whipple, or hepatic resection

Benign stricture

ERCP – 75% of late benign biliary strictures successfully treated w/ ERCP, sphincterotomy, balloon dilatation, and temporary stents (*has improved over the years*)

RFs for failure – pancreatitis induced strictures, occult CA causing stricture

Technique of placing **numerous stents** past stricture has improved outcome

**Note – Early post-op strictures (*eg bile duct injury from clips) not usually amenable to ERCP intervention (see previous section)*

Surgery

Even if you think it's a benign stricture, keep looking for CA

Kocher maneuver to find the portal triad if pt has had **previous biliary surgery**

Palpate duodenum, pancreas, and portal triad to confirm no CA

Send resected bile duct for frozen section to confirm no CA (also send suspicious nodes)

Hepatico-jejunostomy or **choledocho-jejunostomy** (Roux-en-Y) if just bile duct is dilated

Need **whipple** if you have a **dilated pancreatic duct as well**

T-Tube to stent anastomosis is brought out through jejunum and attached to abdominal wall

Hemobilia

MCC – <u>iatrogenic</u> (eg PTC tubes); others – trauma, infection, aneurysms, CA
MC arrangement – fistula between bile duct and hepatic arterial system
Sx's: UGI bleed, RUQ pain and **jaundice** *(classic)* ± **melena**
See **blood in PTC tube** if present
Dx: EGD - shows blood coming out of ampulla of vater
Tx: Angio embolization (cures 95%); operation if that fails

Gallstone ileus

Fistula between **gallbladder** and **2nd portion of duodenum**
Gallbladder releases stone, causing **small bowel obstruction** (SBO)
Usually occurs **in elderly**
MC site of obstruction – terminal ileum
Sx's: N/V, distension, abdominal pain (SBO sx's)
Dx: AXR and **CXR** → **air in biliary tree** (pneumobilia) + **SBO** *(Classic)*
Tx:
> **Initial Tx** – fluid resuscitation, NPO, NGT to decompress
> Remove stone w/ **longitudinal enterotomy** proximal to obstruction (milk it out)
> Can leave gallbladder and fistula if pt too sick
> If not to sick → **cholecystectomy, resect fistula,** and **close duodenum**

Bile Duct CA (cholangiocarcinoma)

Elderly, males
RFs – ulcerative colitis, choledochal cysts, sclerosing cholangitis, chronic bile duct infection, *C. sinesis* (liver fluke), typhoid, congenital hepatic fibrosis, cirrhosis
Sx's: painless jaundice (early), then **weight loss** (late, *classic*); cholangitis
Dx:
> **U/S** *(best initial test for RUQ pain or jaundice)* – dilated ducts
> **ERCP** w/ brush Bx
> **MRCP** – may help define lesion (these tumors can be hard to find)
> **Chest/abd/pelvic CT scan** – looking for invasion, mets
> Consider CT angio for assessment of vascular structures
> **Labs** – ↑ in bilirubin and ↑ alkaline phosphatase
> *Discovery of a **focal bile duct stenosis** in pts w/o a history of biliary surgery, cholangitis, or pancreatitis is **bile duct or gallbladder CA** until proven otherwise (press for Dx here)*

Path
> Invades contiguous structures early – only <u>10% resectable</u>
> **Overall 5-YS** – 5% (after resection for cure 25%)

Tx:
> **Staging laparoscopy**
> Often resectability can only be determined at **time of surgery**
> **Non-resectable tumors** →
>> **Lymph node** spread beyond hepatoduodenal ligament (eg celiac, SMA, para-aortic, IVC nodes)
>> **Main portal vein or proper hepatic artery** invasion or encasement
>> **Direct invasion of adjacent organs** (eg stomach, colon, duodenum, abdominal wall)
>> **Mets** (including liver)
>> Above criteria for <u>Klatskin tumors</u>
> **Upper ⅓** (Klatskin tumors)
>> **MC type** (75%), worst prognosis, usually unresectable
>> **Tx: hepatic lobectomy** (often w/ extended resection) and **stenting** of contralateral bile duct if mostly localized to a lobe (and you feel you can reconstruct any vascular or bile duct issues)
> **Middle ⅓** – **Tx: hepatico-jejunostomy**
> **Lower ⅓** – **Tx: whipple**
> Palliative stenting for unresectable DZ

Gallbladder adenocarcinoma

MC cancer of biliary tract (although still rare)

4 x more common the bile duct CA

Usually have associated **gallstones**

RFs

> **Porcelain gallbladder** (or calcifications of GB wall, 5-10% risk) → these
> pts need cholecystectomy
>
> **Primary sclerosing cholangitis** (PSC)
>
> **Gallbladder adenomas** (esp. in setting of PSC)
>
> Others – obesity, chronic cholecystitis, native Americans

Sx's: jaundice initially, followed by **RUQ pain**

Dx:

> **U/S** *(best initial test for RUQ pain or jaundice)*
>
> **Chest/abd/pelvic CT scan** (majority have mets at time of Dx)
>
> **ERCP** (or MRCP) to define biliary anatomy if jaundiced (get brush Bx's)
>
> > **Mid-bile duct obstruction** not caused by stones is gallbladder CA
> > (or bile duct CA) until proven o/w
>
> **Labs** – LFT's often elevated

Path

> 1st spreads to **segments IV** and **V**
>
> 1st nodes are **cystic duct nodes** (right side of portal triad)
>
> **MC site of mets** – liver
>
> High incidence of **tumor implants** in **trocar sites** when discovered after
> laparoscopic cholecystectomy
>
> Laparoscopic approach *contraindicated* for gallbladder CA
>
> 80% present w/ **stage IV disease** – <u>only 20% resectable</u>
>
> **Best prognosis** – papillary sub-type

Tx:

> 1) **Confined to mucosa + lamina propria** (T1, stage I-a, <u>*no muscle*
>   *invasion*</u>) – cholecystectomy sufficient
>
> 2) **Muscle invasion only** (T2, Stage I-b, muscularis propria invasion)
>   a) Wedge resection of **segments IV and V** w/ 2-3 cm margin <u>*and*</u>;
>   b) Stripping **portal triad lymph nodes** (regional lymphadenectomy)
>
> 3) **Beyond muscle** and **resectable** (Stage IIa or greater, T3 or T4 tumors)
>   a) Formal **resection of segments IVb and V** (possible right
>   hepatectomy) w/ 2-3 cm margins <u>*and;*</u>
>   b) Stripping **portal triad lymph nodes**
>   Depending on invasion, may need **CBD resection w/ hepatico-
>   jejunostomy** (also consider if cystic duct involved)
>
> **Non-resectable tumors→**
>
> > **Lymph node** spread **beyond hepatoduodenal ligament** (eg
> > involvement of celiac, SMA, para-aortic, IVC nodes)
> >
> > **Main portal vein or proper hepatic artery** invasion or encasement
> >
> > **Direct invasion of $\geq$ 2 extrahepatic organs or structures** (eg
> > stomach, colon, duodenum, abdominal wall)
> >
> > **Mets** (including liver)
>
> **Chemo-XRT post-op** – 5-FU and mitomycin based (some benefit)

Overall 5-YS: 5% (after resection for cure 30%)

PANCREAS

Normal Anatomy and Physiology
- **Head** (including uncinate), **neck, body,** and **tail**
- **Uncinate process** – rests on aorta, behind SMV and SMA

Blood supply
- **Head**
  - **Superior** (off GDA) and **Inferior** (off SMA) pancreaticoduodenal arteries
  - Each has **anterior** and **posterior** branches
    - ***Inferior pancreaticoduodenal artery is the 1st branch* off SMA**
      - **Middle colic is first branch going to bowel
  - **Body** - great, inferior, and caudal pancreatic arteries (all splenic artery branches)
  - **Tail** – splenic, gastroepiploic, and dorsal pancreatic arteries
  - **Venous drainage into the portal system**
  - **SMA** and **SMV** – behind neck of pancreas (SMV to the right of the SMA)
  - **SMA** and **SMV** – lie anterior to the 3rd and 4th portions of duodenum
  - **Portal vein** – forms behind neck of pancreas (SMV and splenic vein)

Lymphatics – celiac and SMA nodes

Exocrine function of pancreas
- **Ductal cells** – secrete HCO3⁻
  - Have **carbonic anhydrase**
  - ↑ flow leads to ↑HCO$_3^-$ and ↓ Cl⁻
- **Acinar cells** – secrete pancreatic **digestive enzymes** and Cl⁻
  - **Enzymes** – amylase, lipase, trypsinogen, chymotrypsinogen, carboxypeptidase
    - ***Amylase and lipase* –** only pancreatic enzymes secreted in **active form;**
      - **Amylase** - hydrolyzes alpha 1-4 linkages of glucose chains
      - **Lipase** – converts TAGs to FFAs and mono-acylglycerides
  - **Enterokinase** – released by duodenum, converts trypsinogen to trypsin
  - **Trypsin** then activates other pancreatic enzymes including trypsinogen
    - ***Trypsin can also autoactivate in acidic environments* (pH < 6)**

Endocrine function of pancreas
- **Alpha cells** – glucagon
- **Beta cells** (center of islets) – insulin
- **Delta cells** – somatostatin
- **PP cells** – pancreatic polypeptide
- **Islet cells** – also have VIP, serotonin, neuropeptide Y, GRP
- Islet cells receive **majority of blood supply** compared to size
- Blood travels to islet cells first, then travels to acinar cells

Hormonal control of pancreatic exocrine function
- **Secretin** – ↑s HCO$_3^-$ release mostly (ductal cells)
- **CCK** – ↑s enzyme release mostly (most potent pancreatic acinar cell stimulant)
- **Acetylcholine** (vagus) – ↑s HCO⁻ and enzymes
- **Somatostatin** – ↓s exocrine and endocrine function
- **Glucagon** – ↓s exocrine function
- **CCK and secretin release** – mostly by cells in **duodenum**

Development
- **Ventral pancreatic bud**
  - Contains duct of Wirsung
  - Migrates **posteriorly**, to the right, and clockwise to fuse with dorsal bud
  - Forms **uncinate** and **inferior portion of pancreas head**
- **Dorsal pancreatic bud** - tail, body, and superior aspect of pancreatic head
  - Contains duct of Santorini
- **Duct of Santorini** – small accessory pancreatic duct that drains directly into duodenum
- **Duct of Wirsung** – major pancreatic duct, merges w/ CBD before duodenum
- **Ampulla of Vater** – fusion of pancreatic duct and CBD
- **Sphincter of Oddi**
  - Controls introduction of bile and pancreatic secretions into duodenum
  - Marks transition from **foregut to midgut** (where celiac stops supplying gut and SMA takes over)
  - ERCP w/ sphincterotomy open this

Annular pancreas

From **failure of clockwise rotation** of the **ventral pancreatic bud**
2nd portion of duodenum trapped in pancreatic band
Sx's: feeding intolerance (vomiting; duodenal obstruction); pancreatitis (adults)
RFs - Down's syndrome
Dx:

> **AXR** – double bubble sign (duodenum and stomach distension)
> **UGI** – will show stenosis

Tx: duodeno-jejunostomy (MC; or duodenoduodenostomy)
> ***Pancreas is not resected***
> **If pancreatitis is the problem → ERCP w/ sphincteroplasty**

Pancreas divisum

Failed fusion of pancreatic ducts
Most asymptomatic
Can result in **pancreatitis** from Duct of Santorini (Accessory Duct) stenosis
Dx: ERCP

> **Minor papilla** will show long and large duct of Santorini
> **Major papilla** will show short duct of Wirsung

Tx:

> **ERCP w/ sphincteroplasty** if symptomatic
> May need open sphincteroplasty if that fails
> If long standing, may cause chronic pancreatitis

Heterotopic pancreas

MC location – duodenum
Usually asymptomatic; surgical resection if symptomatic

Acute pancreatitis

MCC – Stones (35%) and **ETOH** (30%)
> **Other causes** – ERCP, trauma, hyperlipidemia, hypercalcemia, viral
> infection, meds (eg Imuran, lasix, steroids, CSA, HIV drugs)
> **RF for necrotizing pancreatitis** – obesity

Mortality rate – 10% (Hemorrhagic pancreatitis mortality up to 50%)
Pancreatitis w/o obvious cause (eg no stones, ETOH, ect.) → need to worry
about **malignancy**
Sx's:

> Abd pain radiating to back; N/V, fever, anorexia, jaundice
> > **Fox's** sign(inguinal ligament ecchymosis)
> > **Cullen's** sign (peri-umbilical ecchymosis)
> > **Grey Turner** sign (flank ecchymosis)
> > → all signs of **retroperitoneal hemorrhage**

Dx:

> ****U/S of RUQ**
> > *All pts need this*
> > Check for **stones** and biliary **obstruction**
> > **Proceed w/ ERCP if obstructed** (sphincterotomy, stone extraction)
> **Abd CT** – if really sick to check for signs of **infected necrotic pancreatitis**
> or **abscess** (necrotic pancreas will not light up w/ contrast)
> **Sentinel loop** – dilated small bowel near pancreas as a result of
> inflammation (can be confused w/ SBO)
> **Pleural effusions** – can occur w/ pancreatitis
> **Labs** – ↑WBCs, ↑amylase, ↑lipase

Ranson's Criteria:

On Admission	*After 48 hours*
Age > 55	Hct decrease of 10
WBC > 16	BUN increase of 5
Glucose > 200	Ca < 8
AST > 250	PaO2 < 60
LDH > 350	Base deficit > 4
	Fluid sequestration > 6 L

8 Ranson criteria met → mortality rate near 100%

Path

From impaired extrusion of zymogen granules and activation of
degradation enzymes in the pancreas → leads to **autodigestion**

MCC death – infection, usually GNRs

Hemorrhagic pancreatitis

> Usually results in **retroperitoneal bleeding** (Fox's, Cullen's, and
> Gray-Turner's Signs)
>
> *Rarely* results in massive bleeding and hypotension →
>
> > Usually from **arterial pseudoaneurysm** formation and rupture
> >
> > **Tx: angio + embolization**, *not open surgery*
> >
> > Tissue **too friable** for surgery and embolization is Tx of choice.

ARDS – from release of phospholipases

Coagulopathy and **DIC** – from release of proteases

Pancreatic fat necrosis – from release of phospholipases

Other cx's – shock, renal failure, GI bleeding (coagulopathy, portal vein
thrombosis)

Tx:

NPO, aggressive **fluid resuscitation** (up to 10 L/d) and **ICU care**

Correct coagulopathy (eg PT) w/ hemorrhagic pancreatitis (eg FFP)

Abx's for stones, severe pancreatitis, severe necrosis, failure to improve,
fever, or infection

Enteral feeds (naso-jejunal if possible, use fluoroscopy; can be naso-
duodenal) ↓ **infectious cx's** and ↑ **survival** compared to TPN
(given after acute period)

ERCP w/ sphincterotomy and stone extraction if **gallstone pancreatitis**
(immediately after Dx if pt stable)

Pts w/ gallstone pancreatitis should undergo **cholecystectomy** when
recovered from pancreatitis (at **same admission**, need **pre-op ERCP**
to check for stones)

Morphine should be avoided → can contract the sphincter of Oddi and
could worsen attack

Surgery only indicated for **infected necrosis** or **abscess:**

> 1) **Necrosis** (20%; infected necrosis 5%)
>
> > ***Leave sterile necrosis alone**
> >
> > Want to try and *avoid* **operating on these pts** (70% mortality
> > in 1st few days of acute pancreatitis if operated on)
> >
> > **Sx's of infected necrosis** – really high WBCs, persistent fever,
> > multi-organ failure, positive blood cultures
> >
> > If pt worsening and worried about infected necrosis →
> >
> > > Consider CT guided sample of fluid to see if it is infected
> > > (**gas bubbles** on CT scan suggests infection)
> > >
> > > CT guided drainage of infected necrosis is ***not effective***
> >
> > If infected and pt not doing well, proceed w/ OR and scoop out
> > dead pancreas, leave **drains**
> >
> > Usually **GNRs**
> >
> > May need **multiple debridements**
>
> 2) **Abscess**
>
> > **Tx:** Need **open debridement**
> >
> > CT guided drainage of pancreatic abscesses is ***not effective***

Mildly increased amylase and lipase found w/ cholecystitis, perforated
ulcer, sialoadenitis, SBO, intestinal infarction

Chronic pancreatitis

Corresponds to irreversible parenchymal fibrosis

Islet cells usually preserved, **exocrine function** decreased

MCC – ETOH (80 %); **2nd** – idiopathic

Sx's: pain (MC), **weight loss**, **steatorrhea**, malabsorption (fat soluble vitamins)

Dx

 Abd CT – shrunken fibrotic pancreas w/ **calcifications**

 Chain of lakes (advanced DZ) → alternating segments of dilation
 and stenosis in pancreatic duct

 U/S – shows pancreatic duct > 4 mm, cysts, and atrophy

 ERCP – *very sensitive* at diagnosis of chronic pancreatitis

Tx:

 Analgesics + pancreatic enzyme replacement (pancrealipase) 1st line Tx

 TPN for acute exacerbations

 Celiac block (splanchnicectomy) effective in 30%

 Surgical indications:

 1) **Pain** that interferes w/ quality of life or addiction to narcotics
 2) Failure to rule out **malignancy**
 3) **Biliary obstruction**
 4) **Abscess**

 Surgical options:

 Puestow procedure – pancreatico-jejunostomy

 For **ducts ≥ 8 mm** (most pts improve)
 Open main pancreatic duct and anastomosis to jejunum

 Distal pancreatic resection – for normal duct size and only distal
 portion of gland is affected or for failed Puestow surgery

 Whipple – may be needed to pts w/ **isolated pancreatic head** DZ
 and normal duct size

 80% get pain relief w/ surgery

 Common bile duct stricture

 Proximal dilation can occur w/ chronic pancreatitis

 Tx:

 ERCP w/ dilatation and stent as a 1st step (75% successful)
 Hepatico-jejunostomy or choledocho-jejunostomy if that fails for
 pain, jaundice, cholangitis

 Need whipple if both CBD and pancreatic duct are dilated

 Splenic vein thrombosis

 Chronic pancreatitis is MCC of **isolated splenic vein thrombosis**

 Can get **bleeding** from **gastric varices** that form as collaterals

 Tx: EGD to control acute gastric variceal bleeding; **splenectomy**

Pancreatic ascites (or pancreatic pleural effusion)

MC due to leaking **pancreatic pseudocyst** or leak from **pancreatic duct**

 (can leak retroperitoneal to get above diaphragm → pleural effusion)

MC found with **chronic pancreatitis**

**Majority close spontaneously

Try to wait it out

Tx:

 Almost exactly like pancreatic fistula

 Tap ascites or pleural effusion – Send fluid for culture and cytology

 Repeated taps of ascites or pleural fluid may be needed initially
 Fluid will be high in **amylase** (> 1000)

 Consider abx's 1st week

 Octreotide (to ↓ pancreatic output)

 Follow electrolytes

 Abd CT to R/O abscess or fluid collection

 If moderate to high output (> 200 cc/d) → NPO and TPN

If failure to resolve w/ medical Tx after 6-8 weeks →

 ERCP, sphincterotomy, temp stent to try and get it to close

If that fails after 6-8 weeks, for distal lesions perform **distal pancreatectomy**

 Possibly **whipple** for proximal lesions

Do not be in a hurry to operate on these pts

Pancreatic pseudocysts

DDx:

Pseudocyst
Serous cystadenoma
Mucinous cystadenoma or cystadenocarcinoma
Mixed cystadenoma or cystadenocarcinoma
Papillary cystadenoma or cystadenocarcinoma

Sx's:

Pain (MC sx), **weight loss**, and **bowel obstruction** (compression)
MCC – pancreatitis (acute or chronic)
Very unusual to have a pancreatic pseudocyst without a history of
   pancreatitis, pancreatic trauma (MC children), or pancreatic surgery
   → *need to worry about CA in these pts*

Dx:

Abd CT (*best test*): need to look for:
   Signs of **acute** (edema, fluid) or **chronic pancreatitis** (shrunken
      pancreas, calcifications, dilated ducts)
   Masses (worry about **CA**)
   Complex cyst (septations, frond-like projections – more likely **CA**)
U/S to help evaluate the cyst

Path

Pseudocysts MC in **head of pancreas**
Small cysts (< 5 cm) usually resolve spontaneously
High in **amylase**
Nonepithelialized sac (true pancreatic cysts have epithelial sac)
(see below for pseudocyst cx's)

Pseudocyst Criteria:

1) Need Hx of **pancreatitis, pancreatic surgery,** or **trauma** *and:*
2) **Not** a complex cyst (no fronds or septae; no associated mass) *and:*
3) **Not** growing on serial CT scan
If above not met, need to worry about CA

Tx:

*Only need to tx pseudocysts that are either: 1) continually symptomatic
   or 2) are growing → asymptomatic pseudocysts leave alone*
1) **Continued sx's:**
   Expectant management up to **3 months** (± **TPN** if unable to eat)
   After 6 weeks of sx's → get **ERCP** to check for duct involvement:
      If **duct involved:**
         Perform sphincterotomy + stent (across leak possible)
         Drain pseudocyst percutaneously
         Remove stent after 6 weeks
         If you still have a leak, will need **cysto-gastrostomy**
            (endoscopic or open) after 3 months
      If **duct not involved:**
         Try to **drain pseudocyst percutaneously**
         If recurs or not able to drain → **cysto-gastrostomy**
            (endoscopic or open) after 3 months
   Need **3 months** of conservative Tx before cysto-gastrostomy to
      allow **pseudocyst to mature →**
      Cyst wall needs to thick and **mature** to be able to sew to it
      Also, for endoscopic cysto-gastrostomy to work, pancreatic
         pseudocyst needs to be **attached** (scarred) **to posterior
         stomach wall**
   Send Bx of cyst wall + fluid to make sure its **not CA**
   Open cystogastrostomy – posterior stomach sewn to cyst wall
2) **Pseudocysts that continue to grow** (inability to R/O malignancy)
   Tap cyst fluid (try to drain completely)
   Send fluid for **cultures** and **cytology**
   No glycogen, no mucin, and **high amylase** (> 5,000) →
      Likely a pseudocyst (make sure it meets other criteria above)
      Tx: Expectant management up to 3 months (see above)
      Continues to grow → resection (CA risk)

Glycogen → likely a **serous cystadenoma or a mixed mucinous/serous cystadenoma**

> **Tx: resection** if pt can tolerate surgery
>
> Although **serous cystadenomas** are generally considered to be benign, CA has been reported
>
> Also, if it's **mixed serous/mucinous** (can't tell this from just the tap) there is a definite CA risk

Mucin → **mucinous cystadenoma/cystadenocarcinoma** (pre-malignant)

> **Tx: resection**

Pancreatic mucinous or mixed cystadenocarcinoma

> **5-YS after resection** – 40% (compared to 20% for pancreatic ductal adenocarcinoma)

Cx's of pancreatic pseudocyst

> **SBO** – conservative Tx 1st, drain pseudocyst if possible, may need cysto-gastrostomy
>
> **Intra-abdominal bleeding from erosion into vessels**
>> **MCC bleeding from pancreatic pseudocyst**
>> Usually associated w/ a **pseudoaneurysm**
>> **Tx: angio embolization** *(best,* very difficult to operate in pts w/ pancreatic pseudocyst and bleeding)
>
> **Infection** – external drainage and abx's *(best Tx)*
>
> **Portal vein thrombosis**
>> EGD control of variceal bleeding if present
>> If not bleeding → heparin, transhepatic or systemic thrombolytics
>>> TIPS or possible porto-caval shunt for severe sx's if above fail
>> Drain pseudocyst to decrease compression
>
> **Splenic vein thrombosis** – initial EGD control of gastric variceal bleeding; **splenectomy**
>
> **Bowel erosion** – resection and placement of cysto-gastrostomy

Pancreatic insufficiency

> MC after long standing pancreatitis or after total pancreatectomy (> 90% of function must be lost)
>
> Generally refers to **exocrine function**
>
> **Sx's**: malabsorption and steatorrhea
>
> **Dx:** fecal fat testing (sudan red)
>
> **Tx:** High-carbohydrate, high-protein, low-fat diet with **pancreatic enzyme replacement** (pancrealipase)

Pancreatic Etiologies for Biliary Stenosis

> Includes pseudocysts, fibrosis, CA
>
> **Cx's:** biliary cirrhosis, cholangitis
>
> Should be treated if symptomatic or causing cirrhosis
>
> **Tx:**
>> **Benign** – ERCP w/ stent (treats 75%) ; choledocho-jejunostomy if that fails
>> **Malignant** – whipple if resectable; stents if not

Pancreatic adenocarcinoma (ductal)

Epidemiology

4th leading cause of CA death in US

RFs – **smoking (#1),** obesity, chronic pancreatitis

Not a RF - ETOH

Genetic RFs – HNPCC, Peutz-Jeghers, ataxia-teleangiectasias

Males (50-60's)

Sx's:

Painless jaundice (tumor in head), then **weight loss**

New onset **atypical DM,** unexplained **malabsorption,** unexplained
pancreatitis, pain (growth into nerves or retroperitoneum)

Migratory thrombophlebitis (Trousseau's sign)

Supra-clavicular adenopathy (Virchow's node)

Path

> 95% of pancreatic tumors arise from **exocrine pancreas**

Lymphatic spread 1st

Majority in **head** (70%)

Most cures w/ pancreatic head disease

90% **ductal** adenocarcinoma

Other tumors of exocrine pancreas (have more favorable prognosis):

Papillary cystadenocarcinoma

Serous cystadenomas (vast majority benign)

Mucinous cyst-adenomas/-adenocarcinomas
(adenomas considered pre-malignant)

Mixed cyst-adenomas/-adenocarcinomas
(adenomas considered pre-malignant)

CA 19-9 – serum marker for pancreatic CA

k-*ras* oncogene (GTPase) – present in 90%

15% resectable

5-YS survival with resection – 25%

Dx:

If jaundice – start w/ U/S

If mid-epigastric pain or other sx – start w/ CT scan

U/S → dilated ducts, ERCP after that

ERCP – find cause of obstruction

ERCP good at differentiating dilated ducts secondary to chronic
pancreatitis vs. CA

Signs of CA on ERCP – duct w/ irregular narrowing, displacement,
destruction

Try to get **brush Bx** of ducts; look for ampullary adenoma or CA

Try to place **decompressing stent**

When no stones causing problem, need **abd CT**

Abd/pelvic CT (3 mm cuts; triple phase imaging)

Pancreatic head CA – **double duct sign** (pancreatic duct + bile duct
dilatation)

Check for **gross invasion** or **loss of patency** of **portal vein, SMV,**
and IVC (*unresectable* DZ) → often can't tell for sure until
laparotomy (limited involvement resectable→ place **vein patch**)

Check for **retroperitoneal invasion** (*unresectable*)

Check for **encasement of SMA** (*unresectable*)

Check for **celiac, portal triad** near liver, and **SMA nodal** (nodal
systems outside area of resection) and **liver mets** →
unresectable, get EUS or percutaneous Bx of area)

Distal peri-portal, peri-pancreatic, and peri-duodenal nodes you can
take w/ specimen (can still resect)

Pain as sx → still possibly resectable

MR angiogram or contrast angiogram if worried about vessel involvement

No mass on CT scan – EUS, ERCP or MRI / MRCP may reveal mass or
malignant ductal strictures

EUS-guided Bx (avoids seeding) or **CT guided Bx** (risk of seeding) for
suspicious nodes

Can also use above for primary Dx – although can avoid Bx altogether if you are going to take mass out anyway (ie no mets or nodes outside area of resection)

Labs – possible ↑ LFTs (esp alk phos and bilirubin), amylase, lipase

Tx:

Resection if resectable (whipple or distal pancreatectomy)

Diagnostic laparoscopy before whipple – if mets to peritoneum, omentum, or liver → close and palliate

Whipple (pancreaticoduodenectomy) removes pancreatic head, duodenum, CBD, and gallbladder, ± gastrectomy →
1) pancreatico-jejunostomy, 2) choledocho-jejunostomy, and 3) gastrojejunostomy then performed to Roux limb of jejunum

Distal pancreatectomy – does <u>not</u> require roux limb (just oversew it)

Prognosis based on vascular + nodal invasion; ability to get clear margin

Bleeding behind neck of pancreas after blunt dissection – SMV Divide pancreas to control bleeding

Post-op chemo-XRT → 5-FU + gemcitabine

↑s survival w/ R0 or R1 resection

Gemcitabine – nucleoside analogue anti-metabolite

Erlotinib – multi-receptor tyrosine kinase inhibitor (EGFR group)
Used for locally advanced, <u>unresectable, or metastatic pancreatic CA</u> (erlotinib + gemcitabine)

Palliation

Stents (or PTC tube) or **gastrojejunostomy** (or stent) **as palliation** (for jaundice or obstruction, respectively)

Celiac plexus block – for painful unresectable DZ (50% effective)

Chemo-XRT (5-FU and gemcitabine) to palliate (↑s mean survival)

XRT for pain

Pancrealipase for fat malabsorption

Cx's from Whipple:

MC Cx – delayed gastric emptying; Tx – metoclopramide

Pancreatic duct or bile duct leak

Both **Early** (< 7 days; eg anastomotic breakdown) and **Late** (> 7 days; eg fistula) – tx like pancreatic fistula (see pancreatic fistula below)

The tissue planes are very friable early after surgery → will end up doing more damage w/ reop

Usually presents as ↑ed drainage from pancreatic drains

Can present w/ N/V and **large fluid collection** on U/S (Tx: percutaneous drainage, leave drain, send for amylase, lipase, and cytology; rest same as pancreatic fistula)

Vast majority of fistulas resolve on their own

Nausea and vomiting after Whipple

DDx – delayed gastric emptying, potential biliary, pancreatic duct leak

Dx: U/S *(best test)* or CT scan

Marginal ulceration – from acid; on **jejunal side; Sx's** - pain
Tx: PPI

Abscess → open drainage (hard to drain pancreatic abscess w/ percutaneous drainage), abx's

Pancreatitis → Abx's if severe or complicated, TPN (or J tube feeds), NPO

Bleeding after whipple or other pancreatic surgery – go to **angio for embolization as 1ˢᵗ move** *(Not re-operation)*

Try and coil embolize the bleeding vessel

Try to avoid surgery as 1ˢᵗ move; if you have to go, pack everything off 1ˢᵗ, then ligate bleeders

The tissue planes are very friable early after surgery and bleeding is extremely hard to control operatively

High volume centers (> 12/year) have ↓ed perioperative mortality

5-year survival after resection – 25%

30% if node negative

10% if node positive

Pancreatic fistulas

Sx's:
1) Leakage of fluid from wound after pancreatic surgery
2) Pancreatic drain w/ ↑ed fluid after pancreatic surgery
3) Fluid collection around pancreas from **injured pancreatic duct** (surgery, trauma or pancreatitis → place drain)

Majority are **asymptomatic**

Majority **close spontaneously** (especially if low output < 200 cc/d)

Try to wait it out w/ **conservative Tx**

Dx: fluid can be clear or murky; **amylase in fluid** (in 1000s)

Tx:
1) **Control drainage** (ostomy or percutaneous drain)
2) **Consider abx's** for 1st week if you think there is an infection in tract
3) **If high output** (> 200 cc/day) → NPO and TPN (distal feedings if J tube)
4) **If low output** (< 200 cc/day) → let pt eat and avoid cx's of TPN
5) **Octreotide** (↓s pancreatic output, ± results)
6) Follow **electrolytes**

Abd CT – look for **abscess,** undrained **fluid collection, pseudocyst**

If failure to resolve w/ medical Tx after 6-8 weeks → **ERCP and stent** (try to get stent across duct leak if possible)

Rare to have to operate (or re-operate) for pancreatic fistula → Do <u>not</u> rush to re-operate

Ampullary villous adenoma (carcinoma)

Villous tumor in ampulla of Vater

Sx's: obstructive jaundice and **heme positive stools** *(classic)*

Can cause pancreatitis

Dx:

Get ERCP w/ Bx's to truly define this lesion

High false negative rate w/ Bx (ie biopsy misses CA harboring in adenoma) – 70% of adenomas have CA in them at pathology

Tx:

Need to resect locally

Incision in 2nd portion of the duodenum

Send for FS to confirm benign (whipple if malignant cells detected)

Likely will end up w/ open **sphincteroplasty** and/or **ductoplasty** after rsxn of benign tumor

Do <u>not</u> perform whipple if benign

Nonfunctional endocrine tumors

30% of pancreatic endocrine neoplasms

90% of nonfunctional endocrine tumors are **malignant**

Sx's: pain, weight loss, jaundice

More **indolent and protracted** course compared w/ pancreatic adenocarcinoma

MC met's – liver

Dx: W/U same as adenocarcinoma

Resect if resectable

5-FU and **streptozosin** may be effective

5-YS after resection – 50%

Functional endocrine pancreatic tumors

70% of pancreatic endocrine neoplasms
Octreotide for treating mets – effective for all _except_ somatostatinoma
Octreotide scan for locating – effective for all _except_ insulinoma
Tumors MC located in pancreatic head → gastrinoma and somatostatinoma
All of these tumors can respond to **debulking**
Liver mets – 1st for all
Streptozosin – toxic to islet cells of pancreas

Insulinoma

MC islet cell tumor of pancreas
90% benign
Evenly distributed throughout pancreas
DDx hypoglycemia:
    Insulinoma
    Congenital hyper-insulinemia or functional islet cell hypertrophy
    Liver DZ (poor glycogen stores)
    Tumors
        Hepatoma (diffuse hepatoma replaces liver, no glycogen stores)
        Mesothelioma (Insulin-like growth factor-1 expressed)
    Munchausen's Syndrome

Sx's:

    Whipple's triad
        1) **Fasting hypoglycemia** (< 50)
        2) **Sx's of hypoglycemia**, (palpitations, ↑ed HR, and diaphoresis)
        3) **Relief w/ glucose**

Dx:

    Labs
        1) **Insulin to glucose ratio > 0 .4 after fasting (72 hours)**
        2) Fasting glucose **< 50**
        3) Fasting insulin **> 24**
        4) **↑ C peptide** and **pro-insulin** → if _not_ elevated suspect
            Munchausen's syndrome (self-injection of insulin)
        The above are **diagnostic**
    Localization:
        Abd CT (or MRI) – check for liver tumors or mesothelioma
        EUS (endoscopic U/S) – finds 80% of these
        Selective arterial calcium stimulation w/ **hepatic venous insulin**
            sampling (localizes tumor – Ca^{++} causes release of insulin)
            Used if trouble localizing w/ above
        Notably, many of these tumors will <u>NOT</u> light up on octreotide scan

Tx:

    Enucleate if < 2 cm (has pseudocapsule)
        Can have multiple lesions (enucleate each if < 2 cm)
    Formal rsxn if >2 cm (whipple or distal pancreatectomy)
    Look around for node DZ
    Check serum glucose level after removal
        To make sure you got the insulinoma
        The 1/2 life of insulin is **4 minutes**
    Trouble finding tumor:
        Intra-op U/S to help localize (hyper-echoic densities, posterior
            shadowing)
        Still can't find tumor – _avoid blind pancreatic resection_ and
            perform post-op **selective arterial calcium stimulation** w/
            hepatic venous insulin sampling to localize the tumor
    Mets:
        Streptozosin and **5-FU**
        Octreotide
        Diazoxide (inhibits release of insulin)

<u>Gastrinoma</u> (Zollinger-Ellison syndrome; ZES)

MC pancreatic islet cell tumor in **MEN-1 pts**

75% sporadic and **25%** related to **MEN-1**

50% malignant

> **Pancreatic** more commonly malignant than duodenal
>
> **Sporadic** more commonly malignant than MEN associated

50% multiple (esp w/ MEN)

Majority (75%) **in gastrinoma triangle**

1. Common bile duct
2. Neck of pancreas
3. Third portion of the duodenum

Sx's:

1) **Refractory or complicated ulcer disease** (many ulcers, abd pain)
2) **Diarrhea** (improved w/ PPI)

Dx:

Always need **1)** fasting **serum gastrin level** *and:* **2) stomach basal acid output** to make Dx:

1) **Serum gastrin**
   > **>200 pg/ml** (c/w gastrinoma but <u>not</u> diagnostic; nl 0-115;)
   > > 1000 pg/ml → virtually diagnostic

2) **Basal Acid Output (BAO):**
   > **> 15 mEq/hr** (no previous vagotomy, nl 3-5) → c/w gastrinoma
   > > 5 mEq/hr (previous vagotomy) → c/w gastrinoma

3) **Gastrin > 200** <u>and</u> **BAO > 15** → diagnostic of gastrinoma

Secretin stimulation test
> Pts w/ gastrinoma will have an ↑ in gastrin (> 200 increase)
> Normal pts have ↓ gastrin w/ secretin

Abd CT (or MRI) to localize; look for multiple tumors

Octreotide scan (*best test for localizing tumor*) – if can't localize on CT
> May be good to get in all pts as 50% have multiple tumors; all the tumors may <u>not</u> show up on Abd CT

EUS – also good at localizing tumors

Screen for hyperparathyroidism before operating (PTH and Ca^{++}) – needs to be treated before gastrinoma

Tx:

Duodenum
> **< 2 cm** – duodentomy w/ resection, dissection of regional nodes
> **> 2 cm** – formal resection (ie whipple), dissection of regional nodes
> Be sure to check pancreas for separate primary (50% multiple)

Pancreas
> **< 2 cm** – enucleation, dissection of regional nodes
> **> 2 cm** - formal resection (ie whipple), dissection of regional nodes
> Look around for multiple tumors (gastrinoma triangle)

Can't find tumor →
> Perform duodenostomy and look inside duodenum for tumor (20% of microgastrinomas there)

> ***Blind pancreatic resections are generally <u>not</u> indicated***

Unresectable tumor w/ symptomatic ulcers:

1) **Maximal PPI –** see if it controls sx's
2) **Debulking + mets ablation** – ↓s sx's
3) **Streptozosin** and **5-FU**
4) **Octreotide**

> If above fail, total gastrectomy often best Tx for sx's (*vagotomy and antrectomy <u>won't work</u>* – HCl secreting cells in body of stomach)

> Can get 20-30% 5-YS in pts w/ liver mets so palliation impt here

.**Antral G cell hyperplasia** – can ↑ BAO and gastrin levels, but not to same degree as gastrinoma; Tx: PPI usual

Somatostatinoma

Majority **malignant**
> ****Worst prognosis** of pancreatic endocrine tumors (85% have mets at Dx)

Most in **head of pancreas**
Sx's: diabetes, gallstones, and **steatorrhea** (classic triad)
Dx: fasting somatostatin level
Tx: resection of tumor, cholecystectomy with resection
Mets – streptozosin and **5-FU**

Glucagonoma

Majority **malignant**
Most in **distal pancreas**
Sx's: diabetes and **dermatitis** (70%, **necrolytic migratory erythema**), wt loss,
stomatitis
Dx: fasting glucagon level ≥ 500-1000 pg/mL
Tx: resection
Skin rash tx – Zinc, amino acids, or fatty acids
Mets – streptozosin and **5-FU, octreotide**

VIPoma (Verner-Morrison Syndrome)

Majority **malignant**
Most in **distal pancreas** (10% extra-pancreatic – retroperitoneal, thorax)
Sx's: watery diarrhea, hypokalemia, achlorhydria (WDHA syndrome)
Hypokalemia from diarrhea
Diarrhea associated with VIPoma will <u>not</u> get better w/ PPI
Dx: exclude other causes of diarrhea; **fasting VIP levels**
Tx: resection
Mets – interferon and **5-FU** (work very well); debulking may also help

SPLEEN

Normal Anatomy and Physiology
Vascular supply
- **Short gastrics** and **splenic artery** (off celiac trunk) considered end arteries
- Short gastrics come off splenic artery
- Splenic vein is posterior and inferior to splenic artery (both behind spleen)

Red pulp (85%)
- Acts as a **filter for aged** or **damaged RBCs**
- **Pitting** – the removal of abnormalities in RBC membrane
  - **Howell-Jolly bodies** – nuclear remnants
  - **Heinz bodies** – hemoglobin (siderocytes)
  - **Pappenheimer bodies** - iron
- **Culling** – removal of less deformable and old RBCs

White pulp (15%)
- **Immunologic function**
- Contains **lymphocytes + macrophages**
- The major site of **bacterial clearance that lacks preexisting Ab's**
  - Site of removal for **poorly opsonized bacteria, particles,** and **other cellular debris**
- Serves as antigen-processing center for **dendritic cells + macrophages**
  - Antigen processing involves **helper T cells** (adaptive immunity)
- **Largest producer of IgM**
- **MC immunoglobulin in spleen** – IgM

Tuftsin
- An **opsonin**; produced in spleen
- Binds PMN's and macrophages; **stimulates phagocytosis** + chemotaxis

Properdin
- An **opsonin**; produced in spleen
- Activates **alternate complement pathway** (fixes complement) →
  complement products facilitate destruction of target organism

Hematopoiesis
- Occurs in spleen before birth and in conditions like myeloid dysplasia

Accessory spleen – most commonly found at splenic hilum (20% of pts)

MC non-traumatic condition requiring splenectomy – ITP
- **Indication for splenectomy** – ITP far greater than for TTP

Postsplenectomy changes
- ↑RBCs, ↑WBCs, ↑platelets
- Will see **Howell-Jolly, Heinz,** and **Pappenheimer bodies**
- ↑ **spur cells** and **target cells**
- If platelets >1-1.5 x 10^6, need ASA (most of these changes transient)
- Liver picks up some splenic functions

MC splenic tumor (and MC benign splenic tumor) - Hemangioma
- Tx: splenectomy if symptomatic

MC malignant splenic tumor – Non-Hodgkin's lymphoma

MCC splenomegaly – Non-Hodgkin's lymphoma

Splenic cysts – surgery if **sx's** or **> 10 cm** (CA risk)

Reticuloendothelial system – monocytes and macrophages;
- **Locations –** spleen, liver, lymph nodes, (Kupffer cells), lung (alveolar macrophages)

Immune thrombocytopenic purpura (ITP)

Etiologies – many (drugs, viruses, etc)

Sx's:

Most pts asymptomatic

Purpura, petechiae, gingival bleeding, bruising, soft tissue ecchymosis

In children < 10 years → usually resolves **spontaneously** (90%)

Often after **viral infection**

Path

Low platelets (< 100,000)

Spleen is normal

Caused by **anti-platelet Ab's** (IgG, useful in Dx) bind platelets (at plasma membrane glycoproteins); platelets then get chewed up by **macrophages** in spleen, leading to bleeding diatheses

Tx:

Initial

Steroids *(#1 primary therapy)*

Gammaglobulin for steroid-resistant DZ

Anti-Rh Ab's (RhoGAM) **in Rh positive pts**

Overwhelms macrophage Fc receptors, can't bind Ab's bound to platelets

Tx directed at keeping platelets > 20,000 to avoid spontaneous bleeding (eg intra-cerebral hemorrhage)

Avoid giving platelets if possible

Romiplostim (Nplate) – ↑s platelet formation; for chronic ITP

Acute Bleeding

Steroids (methyprednisilone 1 gm/d)

Gammaglobulin (IV-IG)

Platelets may be needed in this situation to stop profuse bleeding

Refractory ITP

Rituximab (anti-CD20, destroys B cells)

Can try Azathioprine, Cyclophosphamide

Splenectomy → **80% respond after splenectomy

Splenectomy indicated for those who **fail steroids** and **medical tx**

1) Removes the source of IgG production (B cells in the spleen)

2) Removes the source of phagocytosis

Pre-splenectomy issues:

Gammaglobulin 1 week pre-op (prolongs life of platelets)

Platelets given after splenic artery is ligated (*classic*, usually given if plts < 50, not required)

Hydrocortisone 100 mg Q 8 hours (adult), wean over a week post-op (start at beginning of case)

Give immunizations – strep pneumoniae, H. influenza, and N. meningitides (2 weeks before operation best)

Post-splenectomy issues:

Immunizations if not already given

ASA for plt > 1-1.5 x 10^6

Prophylactic Daily Augmentin for 6 months in children < 10

Helps prevent IPSI (PSSS)

Explain to parents need to bring child to ER w/ any fever

Early Abx's in these pts w/ any infection

MC organisms w/ IPSI – strep pneumoniae

Persistent thrombocytopenia post-op

Look at smear for **asplenic changes** in RBC (should see Howell-Jolly, Heinz and Pappenheimer bodies if no spleen is present)

If asplenic changes not present, consider **accessory spleen** (MC located at the hilum; Dx – CT scan)

Tx: steroids, IVIG, reoperation if accessory spleen

Thrombotic thrombocytopenic purpura (TTP)

Loss of platelet inhibition – leads to thrombosis and infarction, profound thrombocytopenia (not Ab mediated)

Sx's (*classic pentad*)

> **Low platelets** (profound)
> **Mental status changes**
> **Kidney failure**
> **Fever**
> **Microangiopathic hemolytic anemia** (anemia, jaundice, and a characteristic blood film)

Path

> **Primary TTP** (60% of cases)
>> Majority (80%) arise from deficiency or inhibition of **enzyme ADAMTS13** (responsible for **cleaving large vWF molecules**)
>> These large vWF molecules go uncleaved and cause thrombosis
>> Red blood cells passing microscopic clots subject to shear stress which leads to **hemolysis**
>
> **Secondary TTP** (40% of cases) – CA, bone marrow TXP, pregnancy, platelet inhibitors, immunosuppressants, HIV, autoimmune DZ
> Deaths usually from **intracerebral hemorrhage** or **acute renal failure**

Tx:

> **Plasmapheresis** *(#1 primary therapy)* – gets rid of vWF molecules
> **Immunosuppression** – steroids, vincristine, cyclophosphamide
> *Splenectomy rarely indicated*
> If splenectomy performed, pre-op and post-op issues same as ITP
> Survival rate for primary TTP – 90%
> Survival for secondary TTP – 30%

Overwhelming post-splenectomy infection (OPSI)

(Post-splenectomy sepsis syndrome, PSSS)

Lifetime risk after splenectomy: 2-3%

Increased Risk OPSI:

> MC in **children aged ≤ 5** *(the younger the pt, the higher the risk)*
> MC **< 2 years after splenectomy** (80% of all cases)
> MC w/ **non-traumatic causes for splenectomy** (eg malignancy, hemolytic D/Os such as **thalassemia**)
>> Thalassemia specifically considered higher risk
>
> Usually in pts w/ **immunocompromise, CA**, or **hematologic disorders**
> *Highest risk for OPSI* – Wiskott-Aldrich syndrome (immune deficiency resulting in ↓ed antibody production); also other indications associated w/ ↓ed immunity

Path

> Condition is due to a **specific lack of immunity to capsulated organisms** (lack of **IgM** immunoglobulin)
> **MC organism w/ OPSI** – strep pneumoniae (pneumococcus)
>> others - H influenza, N, meningitides, S. aureus, group A strep

Mortality rate 50% (highest in **children**)

Prevention

> One should try and delay splenectomy until **after 5 years of age**
>> Allows antibody formation; child can get **fully immunized**
>
> Pts should be immunized against **Pneumococcus, Meningococcus, H. influenzae** at least **2 weeks before elective splenectomy** or 2 weeks after a traumatic splenectomy
> Booster immunization every 3 years **for pneumococcal vaccine**
> They also need an **annual influenza virus immunization**
> Prophylactic Augmentin given to children < 10 for 6 months (every day)
> Explain to parents they need to bring child to ED for any **fever**.
> **Early broad-spectrum I.V. abx's** for suspected infection
> These pts need **abx prophylaxis** for **dental procedures**

Lymphoma

1) **Hodgkins**
   MC symptom – painless swollen lymph node in neck
   Superficial adenopathy ± mediastinal adenopathy
   Nodal DZ w/ orderly anatomic spread to adjacent nodes
   Reed Sternberg cells
   MC sub-type – nodular sclerosing
   Lymphocyte predominant – better prognosis
   Lymphocyte depleted – worst prognosis

2) **Non-Hodgkins lymphoma** (includes 40+ types of lymphoma)
   Diffuse; nodal and extra-nodal DZ usual; non-contiguous spread
   Sx's reflect involved sites (eg abdominal fullness, bone pain)
   MC type – B cell (90%)
   Worse prognosis than Hodgkin's
   Generally **systemic disease** by the time the diagnosis is made

B symptoms (constitutional) – fever, night sweats, weight loss (worse prognosis)

Dx:
   Excisional lymph node biopsy (need **architecture**, not just cells)
   FNA and core needle are <u>not adequate</u> for initial diagnosis
   Generally need **1 cm³ of tissue** for architecture
   Bone marrow Bx
   Chest/abd/pelvic CT
   Does NOT reliably detect spleen or liver involvement; thus may need
   2nd imaging modality (→ **gallium MRI** or **PET**)
   Lumbar puncture if CNS involvement suspected
   Head CT if CNS clinically suspected
   Bone scan for bone pain or elevated alkaline phosphatase

Staging
   A – Asymptomatic
   B – Symptomatic (eg night sweats, fever, weight loss) – unfavorable
   I – 1 LN region
   II – ≥ 2 LN regions (non-contiguous) same side of the diaphragm
   III – LN regions on both sides of the diaphragm
   IV – disseminated involvement of one or more extra-lymphatic organs (eg
   liver, bone, lung, or any other nonlymphoid tissue except spleen)

Tx:
1) **Hodgkins**
   ABVD (MC) – doxorubicin (Adriamycin), bleomycin, vinblastine,
   dacarbazine
   Involved field XRT for **bulky DZ**
   These pts are at high risk for **2nd malignancies** related to **therapy**
   From XRT and **chemo** – leukemia, lung CA
   From XRT only – breast CA
   Also at risk for earlier onset **coronary atherosclerosis**

2) **NHL**
   CHOP-R (MC) – **C**yclophosphamide, doxorubicin (**H**ydroxy-),
   vincristine (**O**ncovin), **P**rednisone, and **R**ituximab (anti-DC20,
   kills B cells)
   Involved field XRT for **bulky DZ**
   Add methotrexate for CNS prophylaxis if high risk (para-nasal sinus,
   testicular, bone, breast, peri-orbital, para-vertebral involvement)

Staging laparotomy rarely performed anymore as it does not impact Tx
Surgery today involves:
   Getting lymph node tissue for Dx (eg, axillary dissection, groin
   dissection, mediastinoscopy, cervical dissection)
   Tx of Chylous effusion (see Thoracic chp)
   Rarely need more open Bx (eg laparoscopic Bx of retroperitoneal
   lymphoma) if you can't find easily accessible lymph node
   Splenectomy for isolated splenic lymphoma (rare)
MCC of chylous ascites – lymphoma

Overall 5-YS
   Hodgkins Lymphoma – 85%; **Non-Hodgkins Lymphoma** – 65%

Hypersplenism definition (4 cardinal signs)
    1) **Cytopenia** (↓**platelets** and/or ↓**RBCs** and/or **WBCs)** *and;*
    2) **Compensatory response** in bone marrow *and;*
    3) **Splenomegaly** *and;*
    4) **Correction of cytopenia following splenectomy**

W/ splenomegaly:
    If hypersplenism overlies problem, splenectomy helps
    If hypersplenism does **not** overlie problem (eg portal HTN) – no
      splenectomy
Hemolytic anemias (membrane protein defects)
    Hereditary Spherocytosis
      **MC congenital hemolytic anemia requiring splenectomy
      Spectrin deficit (membrane protein) deforms RBCs, get **splenic**
        sequestration → splenomegaly
      Sx's: pigmented stones, anemia, jaundice
      Splenectomy after age 5 (**immunizations**)
      Tx: splenectomy and **cholecystectomy**
      Splenectomy is **curative**
    Hereditary Elliptocytosis
      Sx's: mechanism and tx as above; less common
      Spectrin and **protein 4.1 deficit** (membrane protein)
Hemolytic anemias (non–membrane protein defects)
    Pyruvate kinase deficiency
      **MC congenital hemolytic anemia <u>not</u> involving a membrane
        protein requiring splenectomy
      Congenital hemolytic anemia
      Altered glucose metabolism
      RBC survival increased w/ splenectomy (may be required in minority)
    Warm antibody autoimmune hemolytic anemia
      MC autoimmune hemolytic DZ (usually IgG against RBCs)
      Indication for splenectomy – if refractory to steroids and IVIG
    Beta thalassemia
      Most common thalassemia
      Major – both chains affected; **Minor** – 1 chain, asymptomatic
      Sx's: pallor, poor body growth, head enlargement
      Persistent Hgb F
      Most die in teens secondary to hemosiderosis
      Splenectomy may ↓ hemolysis and sx's
    Sickle cell anemia – Hgb A replaced w/ Hgb S
      Spleen usually autoinfarcts and *splenectomy <u>rarely</u> required*
    G6PD deficiency
      Precipitated by infection, certain drugs, fava beans
      Splenectomy <u>rarely</u> required
Platelet Problems – ITP (see above) and **TTP** (see above)
Myelofibrosis w/ myeloid metaplasia of the spleen – causes splenomegaly
    and consumption of blood products (anemia, thrombocytopenia)
Felty's Syndrome
    Rheumatoid arthritis, neutropenia, splenomegaly, infections
    Tx: occasional splenectomy for symptomatic splenomegaly w/ neutropenia
Always need splenectomy:
    1) **Hereditary spherocytosis**
    2) **Hereditary elliptocytosis**
    3) **Splenic vein thrombosis** (w/ gastric variceal bleeding)
    4) **Echinococcal Cyst** (MC splenic cyst)
Usually need splenectomy
    1) *Refractory* **Warm antibody type autoimmune hemolytic anemia**
    2) *Refractory* **ITP in adult**
    3) **Splenic Abscess (MC organism** – streptococcus; followed by staph)
    4) **Isolated splenic lymphoma** (rare)
    5) **Myelofibrosis w/ myeloid metaplasia (MMM)** if transfusion dependent,
      is causing pain, or causing severe thrombocytopenia

Other spleen problems

Spontaneous splenic rupture – mononucleosis (MC), malaria, sepsis, sarcoid, leukemia, polycythemia vera)

Splenosis – splenic implants; MC after trauma

Hyposplenism – see Howell-Jolly bodies, Heinz bodies, Pappenheimer bodies, Target cells and Spur cells

Pancreatitis – MCC of splenic artery or splenic vein thrombosis

Splenic artery aneurysms – females; can be secondary to fibromuscular dysplasia, atherosclerosis (see Vascular chp)

Myeloid metaplasia – spleen acts as bone marrow

Special Isolated Lymphoma areas

1) **Duodenum** - chemo ± XRT *(No whipple)*
   If 3rd or 4th portion of duodenum consider resection
2) **Ileum and Jejunum** – wide en bloc resection (include nodes), then chemo ± XRT
3) **Colon lymphoma** (MC cecum) – wide en bloc resection (include nodes), then chemo ± XRT
4) **Anal lymphoma** (↑ w/ AIDS) – chemo ± XRT
5) **Pancreatic lymphoma** – chemo ± XRT
6) **Gastric lymphoma** – surgery only if stage I DZ, o/w chemo ± XRT
7) **Splenic lymphoma** (marginal zone lymphoma) – either splenectomy, chemo, or watchful waiting
8) **Thyroid lymphoma** – chemo ± XRT

SMALL BOWEL

Normal Anatomy and Physiology
Small intestine – nutrient and water absorption
Large intestine – water absorption
Duodenum
   Bulb (1st portion) – 90% of ulcers here; ulcers more distal think about
      gastrinoma
   Descending (2nd) – contains ampulla of Vater
   Transverse (3rd) – overlies the SMA and SMV
   Ascending (4th) – distal portion held in place by ligament of Treitz
   Vascular supply
      Superior pancreaticoduodenal artery (anterior and posterior
         branches) – off gastroduodenal artery
      Inferior pancreaticoduodenal artery (anterior and posterior
         branches) - off SMA (*1st branch of the SMA*)
      Many communications between these artery systems
   Anatomical features
      Descending (2nd) and transverse (3rd) portions are **retroperitoneal**
      3rd and 4th portions – transition point at acute angle between the
         aorta (posterior) and SMA (anterior)
Jejunum
   Apx 100 cm long
   Has long vasa recta coming off **SMA**
   Circular muscle folds
   Maximum site of all absorption except:
      Iron (duodenum) - Both **heme** and **Fe transporters**
      Bile acids (ileum – non-conjugated; **terminal ileum** – conjugated)
      B$_{12}$ (terminal ileum)
      Folate (terminal ileum)
   95% of all **NaCl** and **water** absorbed in **jejunum** (maximum site water
      absorption)
Ileum
   Apx 50 cm long
   Has short vasa recta coming off **SMA**
   Flat appearance
SMA eventually branches off the **ileocolic artery**
Normal bowel sizes
   Small bowel   3 cm
   Transverse colon   6 cm
   Cecum   9 cm
Migrating motor complex (MMC, gut motility)
   Phase I – rest
   Phase II – acceleration and gallbladder contraction
   Phase III – peristalsis
   Phase IV – deceleration
   Motilin is most important hormone in migrating motor complex (*initiates
      phase III peristalsis*)
Intestinal brush border
   Microvilli covered w/ simple columnar cells
   Intra-membrane enzymes here break down **carbohydrates** (eg maltase,
      sucrase, limit dextrinase, lactase) and allow absorption
Crypts of Lieberkuhn
   Secrete **carbohydrate processing enzymes** (eg maltase and sucrase)
   Basal portion contains **multipotent stem cells**; with mitosis one daughter
      remains a stem cell while the other differentiates and moves up crypt
      and eventually to microvilli

Cell types
    Absorptive cells
    Goblet cells – secrete **mucus** (Mucin)
    Enterochromaffin cells (APUD, serotonin release, carcinoid precursor)
        Serotonin (5-HT) impt for **gut secretion, peristalsis,** and **nausea**
        Ondansetron blocks serotonin receptors in brain to <u>prevent nausea</u>
    Brunner's glands (in duodenum) – secrete **alkaline solution**
        1) **protects duodenum from acid**
        2) **lubricates**
        3) creates **alkaline environment** for activation of enzymes
    Paneth cells – **host defense** against microbes
        When exposed to **bacteria antigen** (GPCs, GNRs, LPS, Lipid A, etc)
            they release intra-luminal anti-microbials
        1) **Anti-defensins** – create pores in bacterial → cell lysis
        2) **Lysozyme** – destroy bacterial cell wall
        3) **Phospholipase A2** – destroys bacterial cell wall
    Peyer's patches (GALT; gut associated lymphoid tissue)
        Highest concentration in ileum, many cell types:
            B cells (germinal centers)
            T cells (between follicles)
            Macrophages
            Dendritic cells (APCs – antigen presenting cells)
    M cells – specialized endothelium overlying Peyer's Patches
        Sample intraluminal antigens and present them to APCs in Peyer's
            Patch
        APC cells activate lymphocytes, which then pass to mesenteric lymph
            nodes for regional response, and finally to the thoracic duct
    IgA – produced from mucosal linings and released intra-luminally
        Can also come from mother's milk
        Released from **plasma cells**

Carbohydrate, fat and protein digestion (see Nutrition section)
Bile salt metabolism (see Biliary System section)

<u>Assessment of bowel viability intra-op</u> (options)
    (eg incarcerated hernia, mesenteric ischemia)
    1) **Wrap bowel** in warm moist towel, see if it pinks, up
    2) **Doppler** mesenteric border
    3) **Fluorescein dye injection** (1 gm of fluorescein dye) and Wood's lamp to see
        if bowel glows

<u>Bowel prep</u>
    Noon – 1 gallon of Go-lytely
    1 pm – neomycin and erythromycin
    3 pm – neomycin and erythromycin
    5 pm – neomycin and erythromycin
    8 pm – Fleet's enema
    Morning of surgery – Fleet's enema
    Cefoxitin within 30 minutes – 2 hours before incision

<u>Celiac sprue</u>
    Autoimmune DZ (inflammatory reaction interferes w/ absorption)
    Gluten (gliadin) sensitivity
    Sx's: FTT, diarrhea
    Dx:
        Endoscopy w/ tissue Bx (*Best Test*) – ↑ed lymphoid elements, villous
            atrophy, enlarged crypts of Lieberkuhn, loss of small bowel
            architecture
        Serology – **anti-transglutamase Ab's** (99% specific, 90% sensitive)
    Tx: avoid wheat, barley, and rye

Crohn's disease (CD)

Transmural inflammation of GI tract and **skip lesions**

DDx:

- **Crohn's DZ**
- **Ulcerative colitis**
- **Infectious** (salmonella, shigella, campylobacter, giardia, entamoeba histolytica, C. difficile)
- **Celiac sprue**
- **Irritable bowel syndrome**

Bimodal age distribution – 20's and 60's

RFs – Ashkenazi Jews, smokers

Sx's:

Intermittent **abdominal pain, diarrhea,** and **weight loss**

Mucus containing, non-grossly bloody diarrhea usual

Toxic megacolon or toxic colitis

Fever, tachycardia, ↑WBCs, bloating

Extra-intestinal manifestations

Arthritis, pyoderma gangrenosum, erythema nodosum, ocular disease, growth failure, megaloblastic anemia (folate + B-12 malabsorption), gallstones, kidney stones

Anal disease MC sx of **Crohn's Disease** (large skin tags)

Can occur anywhere from **mouth to anus** (**MC site** - terminal ileum):

Small bowel only	30%
Small bowel and **large bowel**	50%
Large bowel only	20%
Isolated upper tract	rare

90% pts w/ CD eventually need an operation

Dx:

1) **Trying to make Dx:**

Colonoscopy w/ Bx's *(best test* for making Dx)

Try to get to terminal ileum, intubate it, and take terminal ileum Bx's (**MC location of Crohn's DZ**)

Avoid colonoscopy if toxic megacolon or toxic colitis suspected

Findings – non-friable mucosa, cobble-stoning, aphthous ulcers, long deep fissures

UGI w/ SBFT and **enteroclysis**

Enteroclysis uses real time fluoroscopy of small intestine while contrast is flowing through; picks up strictures, etc

If fairly symptomatic and has chronic strictures, take to OR

Barium enema – look for obstruction or strictures

Abd and Pelvic CT scan

Try to identify **abscess** or **lead point**

All pts w/ suspected or confirmed Crohn's need an **abd/pelvic CT scan** before operating on them

EGD – consider if UGI disease is suspected

R/O infectious cause at initial w/u – stool cx's, O and P (giardia and entamoeba histolytica), C. difficile toxin

2) **Acute exacerbation:**

Obstruction →

Abd/Pelvic CT scan

Serial abdominal series

Toxic megacolon or toxic colitis →

Abd/Pelvic CT – look for abscess or perforation

Serial abdominal series – looking for perforation or progressive colon dilatation

↑ **WBCs**

No colonoscopy

Medical Tx
1) **Stable CD**
   a) **5-ASA compounds**
      Can be given in enema form for left sided DZ
   b) **Azathioprine or 6-mercaptopurine** (need frequent WBC, LFT, and drug metabolite checks)
   c) **Loperamide** (ie anti-diarrheals) only for mild disease
   d) **Low residue diet** (avoid fiber such as cereal, bread, nuts or vegetables)

   Steroids
   > ***Avoid chronic prednisone if possible***, can be used for flares
   Try to **cut back** steroid dose once sx's under control
   Failure to wean high steroid dose down after 3-6 months is an indication for surgery
   Steroids can be give in enema form for isolated left sided CD

   Fistulas
   > **Enterocutaneous fistulas** – *add* Infliximab + flagyl
   > **Colovesicle fistula** – *add* Infliximab + flagyl (UTI prevention)
   > **Perianal** or **anorectal-vaginal fistulas**
   >> *Add* Infliximab + flagyl + ciprofloxacin

2) **Acute exacerbation**
   Defined as acute flare (mild, moderate, or severe), abd pain, diarrhea, obstruction, toxic megacolon, or toxic colitis
   a) Continue **medical tx** as above (5-ASA and 6-MP drugs)
   b) **If moderate to severe** → **IVF's, NPO, NGT** and **TPN**
   c) *Add* **Flagyl** (→ mild DZ, unknown mechanism):
      Good for **active**, **fistulizing**, or **perianal CD**
      Causes **irreversible peripheral neuropathy** if used long term in 50%
      > *Add* **Ciprofloxacin** to flagyl for:
      >> i) Fever, ↑WBCs, or possible toxic megacolon / colitis
      >> ii) Perianal or anorectal-vaginal fistula
   d) *Add* **Steroids** (→ moderate DZ, *best tx for acute exacerbations*)
      Hydrocortisone 100 mg Q 8 hours
      Consider **budesonide** (Entocort) as substitute for other steroids
      > Only for **isolated ilio-cecal CD**
      > ↓ed systemic absorption, ↓ed S/Es
      > <u>Not</u> effective for UC
   e) *Add* **Infliximab** (→ severe DZ)
   f) **TPN** – may induce remission and fistula closure w/ small bowel CD
   <u>NO</u> loperamide w/ acute exacerbation
   <u>NO</u> NSAID's
   Serial abdominal series and exam

   Indications for surgery w/ acute exacerbation:
   > **↑ing WBCs**
   > **Persistent tachycardia** despite resuscitation
   > **Worsening clinical exam**
   > **Sepsis**
   > **Bloody BM's > 6-12/d** (unusual w/ CD)

   5-ASA compounds
   > **Pentasa** – small intestine and colon
   > **Mesalazine** (Asacol) – terminal ileum and colon
   > **Sulfasalazine** – colon only

Surgical indications – unlike UC, surgery for CD is <u>not</u> curative; **segmental resection** usual *except* toxic megacolon, toxic colitis, or colon perforation (need subtotal colectomy)
Failed medical TX or **chronic high does steroid** requirement
Obstruction
> Usually just partial from inflammation → initially medical Tx
> **If that fails** (give it 3-5 days) → OR
> If due to **fibrotic stricture** (chronic partial obstruction getting worse despite medical tx) → OR

Abscess
> Tx: **percutaneous drainage** (CT guided; R/O distal obstruction)
> **Localized abscess** is <u>not</u> a contraindication to primary anastomosis
>> (place some omentum in area)

Toxic megacolon or toxic colitis (less common w/ CD than w/ UC)
> Medical tx initially
> **Colonic perforation** (10%) → OR (**subtotal colectomy**, <u>not</u>
>> segmental)
> Not improving w/ medical Tx: (give 3-5 days) or worsening clinical
>> picture → OR (**subtotal colectomy**, <u>not</u> segmental)

Hemorrhage – unusual w/ CD but can occur
> **Tx:** OR for significant hemorrhage, resection of area

Blind loop obstruction – can get dilated, isolated bowel loop
> **Tx:** need to go to OR for resection

CA or dysplasia – CD pt's ↑ risk for **small bowel** and **colon CA**;
> **Tx:** resection

Fissures
> <u>*NO* lateral internal sphincteroplasty in pts w/ CD</u>
> Tx: sitz baths, bulk, lidocaine jelly, stool softeners, NTG cream for
>> chronic ones

Hemorrhoids or perianal skin tags w/ CD → <u>*NO*</u> resection

Enterocutaneous fistula (MC small bowel)
> Can usually be treated conservatively
> **Dx:**
>> **UGI w/ SBFT + barium enema** to R/O **distal stenosis**
>>> Will need resection or stricturoplasty if obstruction present
>> **Abd CT** to R/O **abscess** (percutaneous drain if present)
> **Tx:**
>> **High output fistulas – NPO**, TPN, ostomy and medical tx (see
>>> section for enterocutaneous fistula Tx below)
>> **Low output fistulas** (< 200 cc/d – let pt take PO and avoid
>>> TPN cx's, o/w same as above; if that fails, NPO)
>> Continue **maintenance Tx**
>> *Add* **Infliximab**
>> *Add* **Flagyl**
>> Conservative Tx for 6-8 weeks (need to be patient w/ these)
>> OR if that fails for resection of involved segment, primary re-
>>> anastomosis, and coverage w/ omentum

Anorectal-vaginal fistulas
> **Dx:**
>> **MRI** – define **fistula** and R/O **abscess**
>> **Endoscopy w/ EUS** – define **fistula** and R/O **abscess**
>> **Cystoscopy** to R/O entero-cystic fistulas if suspected
> **Tx:**
>> Continue **maintenance Tx**
>> ***Add* Infliximab**
>> ***Add* Cipro** and **Flagyl**
>> Can try medical tx for 6-8 weeks
> **Surgery:**
>> **Low fistula → rectal advancement flap** (see Rectum and
>>> Anus chp)
>> **High fistula → resection of involved bowel** w/ primary re-
>>> anastomosis if possible, close defect in vagina, omentum
>>> interposition, temporary ileostomy
>> If severe peri-anal and peri-rectal DZ, APR w/ colostomy may
>>> be only viable option

Perianal fistula (fistula-in-ano)

Often **initial area** for Crohn's presentation

Dx:

> **MRI** – define **fistula** and R/O **abscess**
> **Endoscopy w/ EUS** – **define fistula** and R/O **abscess**
> EUS and MRI *best Dx studies*

Initial Tx for all perianal fistulas:

> 1) **Unroof fistula** (eg fistulotomy), open entire tract
> 2) **Drain** any **internal abscess**
> 3) Continue **maintenance Tx**
> 4) ****Infliximab** *(best medical Tx for perianal fistulas)*
> 5) **Cipro + Flagyl** (3 weeks)

> ***Most** perianal fistulas will heal w/ medical Tx (esp simple fistulas)*

Refractory *simple* perianal fistula

> Defined as fistulas w/ **internal opening below dentate
> line** (in lower 1/3 external sphincter)
>
> **Tx:**
>
> > Place **Seton stitch** (goes through fistula) for 6-8
> > weeks to allow drainage, remove Seton,
> > closure of internal opening, curettage out
> > tract
> >
> > Note - Setons used to be tightened over time to cut
> > through the tract but no longer done due to
> > high rate of **incontinence**

Refractory *complex* perianal fistula

> Defined as fistulas w/ **internal opening above dentate
> line** (in upper 2/3 external sphincter or higher)
>
> **Tx:**
>
> > 1) **Rectal advancement flap** (see Perianal Disease
> > section) – contraindicated if rectal/anal
> > mucosa has inflamed active CD *or*:
> > 2) APR w/ colostomy – reserved for severe perianal
> > and peri-rectal DZ that won't heal w/ medical
> > Tx or tolerate rectal advancement flap

Entero-vesicle Fistula

Can often be treated conservatively

Dx:

> **Cystoscopy** *(best test for Dx)* if suspected
> **UGI w/ SBFT** and **barium enema** to R/O **distal stenosis**
> Will need resection or stricturoplasty if obstruction present
> **Abd CT** to R/O **abscess** (percutaneous drain if present)

Tx:

> Continue **maintenance Tx**
> *Add* **Infliximab**
> *Add* **Flagyl (**prevent UTI's)
> Try conservative tx for 6-8 weeks (need to be patient w/ these);
> OR after that for resection of involved segment, primary
> re-anastomosis, closure of bladder, and omentum
> interposition
> Consider earlier surgery of pt is suffering from **repeated UTI's**

Surgery Issues

Peri-operative steroids and **bowel prep** (if not obstructed)
Operative findings of CD

> Creeping fat
> Skip lesions (segmental DZ)
> Transmural involvement
> Cobble-stoning
> Fistulas

CD usually **spares rectum** (unlike UC)

If **peri-rectal DZ present,** may respond to resection of small bowel

W/ resection, do not need clear margins, just **2 cm from gross disease**

Diffuse disease of colon and **rectum** – proctocolectomy + ileostomy procedure of choice (**_NO_ _ileoanal anastomosis)_**

**No** J pouches (or Kock pouch) w/ CD

Incidental finding of inflammatory bowel disease in pt w/ presumed appendicitis who has normal appendix (eg terminal ileitis) **– remove appendix** if cecum not involved (avoids future confounding diagnosis)

Duodenal CD (get strictures, ulceration, or edema)

Medical management as above, surgical management below

Tx: for 1st + 2nd portions of duodenum

1) **Gastro-jejunostomy + vagotomy** usual

Vagotomy to avoid **marginal ulceration**

Should also perform pyloroplasty

2) **Stricturoplasty** if just a short stricture (unusual)

Tx: for 3rd + 4th portions of duodenum

1) **Duodeno-jejunostomy** usual

2) **Stricturoplasty** if just a short stricture (unusual)

**Do not perform whipple for duodenal Crohn's**

Stricturoplasties

Consider if pt has multiple strictures to save small bowel length

Stricturoplasties probably not good for a pt's 1st operation as it leaves disease behind

Longitudinal incision on anti-mesenteric border; close transversely; resection if stricture is long

10% leakage, abscess or fistula rate w/ stricturoplasty

50% recurrence rate requiring surgery for CD after resection

Cx's after terminal ileum resection (or from **severe terminal ileum disease** which has become non-functional for absorption)

1) ↓ed **B-12** and **folate uptake** can result in **megaloblastic anemia**

2) ↓ed **bile salt uptake** causes osmotic **diarrhea** (bile salts) and **steatorrhea** (↓ fat uptake) in colon

3) ↓ed **bile salt uptake** can result in the formation of **gallstones**

4) ↓ed **oxalate binding to Ca** secondary to increased intra-luminal fat → oxalate then gets absorbed in colon → released in urine → **Ca-oxalate kidney stones** (hyperoxaluria)

CA surveillance

Pts w/ Crohn's pan-colitis are at same CA risk as UC

Surveillance for Crohn's pan-colitis same as for UC

Duodenal diverticula

R/O gallbladder disease (chronic cholecystitis) origin

Gallbladder to duodenal fistula (which is how a gallstone ileus occurs)
should be R/O w/ U/S and abd CT

Frequency of diverticula – duodenal > jejunal > ileal

70% of duodenal diverticula are in **2nd portion of duodenum**, often within **2 cm of ampulla**

Tx:

Observe unless **perforated, bleeding, obstruction,** or highly **symptomatic** (pancreatitis or biliary obstruction)

Can be difficult cases – underlying concept is to figure out something *other than a whipple* to tx symptomatic duodenal diverticula

1) **Outside 2nd portion of duodenum**

Usually just **resection w/ primary closure**

Consider **jejunal serosal patch** over defect if primary closure not an option or **duodeno-jejunostomy** (if 3rd or 4th portions of duodenum)

If 1st portion of duodenum may need temporary gastrojejunostomy

2) **2nd portion of duodenum**

Juxta-ampullary diverticula

Intra-luminal resection w/ primary closure – if enough tissue is present between diverticula and ampulla (external resection or perform duodenostomy and resect diverticula from inside lumen)

If you don't think you can get primary closure (ie diverticula is immediately adjacent to or in the ampulla)

→ **w/ biliary obstruction** – hepatico-jejunostomy

→ **w/ pancreatic obstruction** – ERCP w/ stent

Enterocutaneous fistulas

Sx's: drainage from wound

< 7 days → operate (it's not a fistula, it's a leak)

Assess anastomosis

Run small bowel

Assess fascia

Send cultures of fluid

Primary repair ± ostomy or resection w/ primary anastomosis ± ostomy

≥ 7 days – conservative Tx (fascia intact; no fascitis, peritoneal signs, or sepsis)

If > 200 cc/day → NPO + TPN; if < 200 cc/d – allow pt to eat w/o TPN

Abx's (usually just for the 1st week)

H2 blockers (↓'s gastric secretion)

Octreotide (↓'s pancreatic secretion)

Stoma appliance (make sure replacing at least cc for cc w/ TPN or TFs)

Abd/pelvic CT to r/o abscess or fluid collection

High output drainage – place on loperamide; get it down to 500-700 cc/d

R/O FRIENDS (RFs for fistula; abd/pelvic CT, barium enema, UGI +SBFT):

Foreign body – look into fistula tract for stitch or other foreign body

Radiation

Inflammatory bowel DZ – find on UGI w/ SBFT, barium enema, colonoscopy

Epithelialization – scrape the epithelial cells off tract

Neoplasia – send Bx of area to cytology

Distal obstruction – get barium enema and UGI w/ SBFT

Sepsis or infection – Abx's; R/O **abscess** on abd/pelvic CT

Likely will close on its own w/ time → give it 6 weeks

After 6 weeks if still open →

Get **fistulogram** – look for **abscess**

Repeat **UGI w/ SBFT** – to look for leak and distal obstruction

Repeat **Barium enema** to assess for distal obstruction

Repeat **abd CT** scan to look for abscess

Re-operate after 6 weeks of conservative Tx → resection of fistula segment, primary re-anastomosis; diversion if left sided colon

Bowel Obstruction

Initial Tx: fluid resuscitation, NPO, NGT to decompress

Sx's:

N/V, crampy abd pain, previous surgery or XRT

If still **passing gas** – partial bowel obstruction

Fever – need to worry about perforation

Look for **hernias** and **rectal masse;**, guaiac stools

Dx:

1st **Abdominal series**: air-fluid levels, distended loops of small bowel, distal decompression

2nd **CT scan** for all pts unless you think its from a **hernia** (inguinal or ventral) or **adhesions**

Previous CA → need a CT scan (possible recurrence)

Path

Get **bacterial overgrowth**

3rd **spacing of fluid** into bowel lumen (all need volume resuscitation)

Air w/ bowel obstruction from **swallowed nitrogen**

MC w/o previous surgery

Small bowel – hernia

Large bowel – cancer

MC w/ previous surgery

Small bowel – adhesions

Large bowel – cancer

SBO etiologies – adhesions by far MC, hernia, internal volvulus, tumor

SBO w/ no previous surgery and no hernia – likely CA source

LBO etiologies – colorectal CA, volvulus (cecal or sigmoid), diverticulitis, Ogilvie's (see Large Bowel chp)

Tx:

SBO

NG tube, IV fluids, bowel rest, correct electrolytes (esp K and Mg)

Serial exams and labs → cures 80% of partial, 20% of complete SBO

Surgical indications:

Non-reducible hernia (inguinal or ventral)

Persistent tachycardia (despite resuscitation)

Progressing pain

Peritoneal signs

Fever

↑ed WBCs

Failure to resolve (3-5 days)

OR

Run bowel and look for **sites of obstruction** (may be more than one)

Surgical options:

Lysis of adhesions (LOA; best option and by far the MC procedure)

If you have been trying to work on area for **over 1 hour** and not making much progress, consider another option below:

1) Resection of associated bowel

2) Bypass

3) Just bring up ostomy

Perform LOA unless to hazardous, then just **bypass, resection, or ostomy** (avoid closed loops)

XRT w/ matted bowel → likely too difficult to resect, just **bypass** (jejuno-jejunostomy); make sure this isn't recurrent CA

Ovarian CA carcinomatosis causing obstruction

Can you resect for possible cure? Safely and leaving enough bowel behind? Bypass or ostomy if you cannot resect it

Debulking for ovarian CA helps chemo-XRT

Other CA carcinomatosis – usually just bypass, bring up ostomy, or just close

Special Bowel Obstruction Issues
    Large incarcerated Ventral hernia
        Usually place permanent mesh unless:
            Bowel looks viable but battered
            You have performed bowel resection
            You have made enterotomies
            → any of the above, then just primary closure of abdominal wall
                If you can't get abdominal wall closed primarily, just place
                    omentum over the bowel and use vicryl mesh (will
                    dissolve w/ time); let granulate in; then skin graft
    Previous CA surgery + XRT → now w/ matted area + obstruction
        Figure out what is causing the obstruction (CA recurrence,
            adhesions, or radiation fibrosis)
        Biopsy to confirm problem
            Don't perform lysis of adhesions when its actually a local
                recurrence
            CA recurrence – resect if resectable (while leaving enough
                bowel behind for survival)
            Adhesions – LOA
            Radiation fibrosis – likely need to just bypass
    Wilkie disease (superior mesenteric artery syndrome)
        Partial obstruction of the 3rd portion of the duodenum by the SMA
        Sx's: Young pts; weight loss and bilious emesis
            sx's better in prone position
        RFs – total body cast, prolonged recumbency, spinal rods
        Dx: UGI series
        Tx: duodeno-jejunostomy

Carcinoid Tumors

Sx's:
- Abd pain (mistaken for appendicitis), possible **SBO**
  - Pain from **mass** effect or **vasoconstriction** + **fibrosis** (desmoplastic reaction)
- **Carcinoid syndrome** (10% of pts) – intermittent **facial flushing** + **diarrhea** (*hallmark;* **liver mets** bypass metabolism) ± hypotension

Dx:
- **Abd CT**
- **Octreotide scan** (*best test* for detection and localization)
  - **Highest sensitivity** for **localizing tumor** not seen on CT scan
- **Urine 5-HIAA** (> 25 mg/d; not all have this, serotonin breakdown product)
  - **False positive 5-HIAA** – fruits
- **Chromogranin A** serum level (glycoprotein, <u>100%</u> of tumors have this)
  - *Highest sensitivity for detecting tumor*

Path
- **Kulchitsky cells** (neural crest cells, neuroendocrine)
  - Part of amine precursor uptake decarboxylase system (APUD)
  - Produce serotonin, bradykinin, kallikrein, chromogranin, ect.
  - **Serotonin → diarrhea**
    - **Tryptophan** is precursor to **serotonin**
      - ↑ serotonin production leads to tryptophan deficiency + **niacin deficiency → pellagra** (diarrhea, dermatitis, dementia)
  - **Kallikrein → facial flushing**
  - **Bradykinin → hypotension** (from kallikrein; powerful vasodilator)
- **Carcinoid Syndrome** (10% of all carcinoids)
  - Intermittent **facial flushing** (MC sx) + **diarrhea** (*hallmark sx's*)
  - Can also get **bronchoconstriction** and **right heart valve lesions** (tricuspid valve insufficiency)
  - Caused by **bulky liver mets** – liver usually metabolizes compounds released form carcinoid but liver mets bypass liver
  - **Gastrin** – can ↑ sx's
  - **Rectal carcinoids** <u>rarely</u> cause Carcinoid Syndrome (can bypass liver w/ Batson's Venous Plexus → IVC, 1% incidence)
  - **Bronchial carcinoids** <u>rarely</u> cause Carcinoid Syndrome (not metabolized by liver before systemic circulation, 1% incidence)
- **MC site** – <u>appendix</u> (50% of all carcinoids, only 2% malignant)
  - **MC tumor of appendix**
  - Ileum and rectum next most common
- Site w/ **highest mets** and **highest Carcinoid Syndrome** rate – <u>ileum</u> (35% malignant, 20% Carcinoid Syndrome)
- **Small bowel carcinoid** (other than appendix)
  - At risk for **multiple primaries** (10%) + **2nd unrelated GI CA** (20%)
  - Look around for other tumors (small bowel, colon) at time of resection

Tx:
- **Carcinoid in appendix**
  - < 2 cm, not involving base, and <u>no</u> mets → **appendectomy**
  - ≥ 2 cm, involving base, or mets → **right hemicolectomy**
- **Carcinoid anywhere else in GI tract** (*except* rectal)
  - → treat like CA (segmental resection w/ lymphadenectomy)
  - **Rectal carcinoids** (see Colon and Rectum chp)
- **Debulking** – good for palliation if suffering form carcinoid syndrome
- If resection of liver met is performed, perform **cholecystectomy** in case of future **hepatic arterial embolization** or **intra-arterial chemo**
- **Chemo**
  - **Octreotide** – useful for carcinoid syndrome or mets
    - **Interferon** if octreotide fails to control sx's
  - **Streptozocin + 5-FU** – used for mets
  - **Flushing Tx** – alpha-blockers (eg phenothiazine, cyproheptadine)
- **5 -YS w/ mets** – 30%

Benign small bowel tumors
Rare
Benign are more common than malignant
MC benign SB tumor – leiomyomas (usually extra-luminal)
Adenomas
> **MC in ileum**
> **Sx's:** bleeding, obstruction
> Need resection when identified

Malignant small bowel tumors
Adenocarcinoma (rare)
> **MC malignant small bowel tumor**
> High proportion in **duodenum** (40%)
>> 70% of duodenal adenocarcinomas are in 2nd portion of duodenum
>>> Mostly originate in ampulla (**ampullary adenocarcinomas**)
>>> Often from **ampullary villous adenoma** (see Pancreas chp)
>> **RFs for Duodenal CA** – FAP, Gardner's, polyps, adenomas
> **Sx's:** obstruction, jaundice
> **Tx:**
>> Resection and adenectomy if resectable
>> **Duodenal adenocarcinoma**
>>> If in 1st or 2nd **portions of duodenum** – need **whipple** (high likelihood **ampulla** is involved)
>>> If in 3rd or 4th **portions of duodenum** – resection w/ **duodeno-jejunal anastomosis** (do <u>not</u> have to resect pancreas)

Leiomyosarcoma
> **MC sites** – jejunum and ileum
> Most **extra-luminal**
> DDx leiomyoma vs. leiomyosarcoma (>5 mitoses/HPF, atypia, necrosis)
> **Tx:** resection; <u>no</u> adenectomy required (sarcoma)

Lymphoma
> **MC small bowel site** – <u>ileum</u> (↑ed lymphoid tissue - Peyer's Patches)
> **MC type** – <u>B cell</u>
> **Sx's:** SBO
>> **Post-TXP** – ↑ risk of bleeding and perforation
>> **Mediterranean variant** – young males, **clubbing**
> **RFs** - Wegener's disease, SLE, AIDS, Crohn's, celiac sprue, post-TXP
> **Dx::** abd CT, UGI w/ SBFT, node sampling
> **Tx** (for lymphoma isolated to specific area below):
>> 1) **Duodenum** - chemo ± XRT *(No whipple)*
>>> If 3rd or 4th portion of duodenum consider resection
>> 2) **Ileum and Jejunum** – wide en bloc resection (include nodes), then chemo ± XRT
>> 3) **Colon lymphoma** (MC cecum) – wide en bloc resection (include nodes), then chemo ± XRT
>> 4) **Anal lymphoma** (↑ w/ AIDS) – chemo ± XRT
>> 5) **Pancreatic lymphoma** – chemo ± XRT
>> 6) **Gastric lymphoma** – surgery only if stage I DZ, o/w chemo ± XRT
>> 7) **Splenic lymphoma** (marginal zone lymphoma) – either splenectomy, chemo, or watchful waiting
>> 8) **Thyroid lymphoma** – chemo ± XRT
> **Surgery for bowel lymphoma** – wide en bloc resection w/ negative margins (same as for other CA), mesenteric + para-aortic lymph node sampling outside zone of resection, and liver biopsy
> (see Spleen chp for lymphoma chemo)

Peutz-Jeghers syndrome (AD)
Sx's:
Mucocutaneous (ie oral) melanotic **skin pigmentation** (patches); freckles
Gastrointestinal hamartomatous polyps (entire GI tract) – can cause
obstruction → 1st presentation often **intussusception**

Path
Have ↑ **extra-intestinal malignancies** (eg pancreas, liver, lungs, breast,
ovaries, uterus, small bowel and testicles)

MC CA w/ Peutz-Jeghers – breast CA

Some ↑ed risk of **intestinal malignancies**, but not significant enough to
warrant prophylactic resection (related to adenomatous changes in
hamartomatous polyp)

No significant increased risk of colon CA →
NO prophylactic colectomy

Mean survival – 57 years of age

Screening
GI

EGD + colonoscopy every 1-2 years (earlier if blood loss anemia)
When to start depends on family Hx

Remove polyps > 5 cm, if **hemorrhagic,** or thought to have
malignant changes; use push endoscopy (will reduce
surgery for bowel obstructions); some remove all polyps if
not too many

UGI w/ SBFT every 2 years

RUQ U/S yearly

Push endoscopy – upper endoscopy using a rigid overtube to
prevent coiling in the stomach → gets further down small bowel;
uses 200 cm scope

Uterus, ovary and cervix – annual Pap smear, pelvic exam and
transvaginal U/S beginning in teens

Breast – breast exams at age of 20
Mammograms at age 25 and yearly (consider breast MRI)

Testicles – yearly U/S and exam

Intussusception in adults
Can occur from small bowel or cecal tumors

MCC in adults – cecal adenocarcinoma

Worrisome for **CA in adults** (70% have **tumor lead point**, eg cecal CA)

*Do **not** try to reduce w/ barium enema in adults → go to OR for resection*

Tx: operative reduction, resection of lead point

Causes of steatorrhea (Excess fat in feces)
Gastric hypersecretion of acid → ↓ pH → ↑ intestinal motility; interferes with
fat absorption (eg gastrinoma)

Interruption of bile salt resorption interferes with micelle formation (eg terminal
ileum resection)

Lack of pancreatic enzyme secretion (eg chronic pancreatitis)

Defective mucosal cells (eg inflammatory bowel disease)

Short bowel syndrome

Tx: control diarrhea (loperamide); ↓ oral intake (esp fats); pancrealipase, PPI

Short Bowel Syndrome (short gut syndrome)

Inability to absorb enough water and nutritional elements to be off TPN
Dx is made on sx's, not length of bowel.
Sx's: diarrhea, steatorrhea, weight loss, nutritional deficiency (lose fat, B-12, electrolytes, water), abd pain

Dx:

Sudan red stain – checks for **fecal fat**
Schilling test – checks for B-12 absorption (**radiolabeled B-12 in urine**)
Probably need at least 75 cm to survive off TPN; 50 cm with competent iliocecal valve

Tx:

H2 blockers to reduce acid
Octreotide
Loperamide
Pancrealipase
Restrict fat with diet resumption
Vitamins
Lactase
TPN for flares (chronic TPN leads to chronic liver DZ)
Small bowel TXP
Growth Hormone

Hypersecretion of acid → ↓ pH → ↑intestinal motility; interferes w/ fat absorption → steatorrhea
Interruption of bile salt resorption interferes with micelle formation and causes steatorrhea (if terminal ileum gone)

Non-healing fistula

"FRIENDS"

Foreign body
Radiation
Inflammatory bowel disease
Epithelialization
Neoplasm
Distal obstruction
Sepsis or infection of tract

High output fistulas

Usually w/ **proximal bowel** (duodenum or proximal portion of jejunum)
Less likely to close w/ conservative tx

Colonic fistulas are more likely to close than those in small bowel
Persistent fever – need to check for abscesses (fistulogram, abdominal CT, UGI w/ SBFT)
Most fistulas **iatrogenic** and treated conservatively 1st (see enterocutaneous fistulas above)
50% close w/ medical Tx
Surgical options: bowel resection (containing fistula) and primary re-anastomosis

Stomas

Loop ileostomies – 1% obstruction rate
Parastomal hernias – highest rate w/ loop colostomies
MC stomal infection – Candida
Diversion colitis (eg Hartmann's pouch)
Secondary to ↓ short-chain fatty acids
Tx: short-chain fatty acid enemas
MCC stoma stenosis – ischemia; Tx: dilation if mild
MCC fistula near stoma – Crohn's disease
Abscesses – usually underneath stoma site often caused by irrigation device
Ileostomy – increased risk of **gallstones** and **uric acid kidney stones**
Post-op ostomy (eg colostomy or ileostomy) **that appears dark below the level of the fascia** – re-op and revise (too compressed by fascia, has twist, or too devascularized); If bowel looks OK at level of **fascia – leave alone**

Appendix
Appendicitis
Sx's:
1st anorexia

2nd abd pain (peri-umbilical)

3rd vomiting

Pain gradually migrates to **RLQ** as peritonitis sets in.

MC in pts 20-30's

Dx:
Can have normal WBC count

CT scan – diameter **> 7 mm** or wall thickness **> 2 mm** (looks like a bull's eye), fat stranding, no contrast in appendiceal lumen; try to give rectal contrast

All women < 50 get → B-HCG, pelvic exam, and pelvic U/S (or Abd CT)

MC area to perforate – midpoint of anti-mesenteric border

MCC in children – lymph node hyperplasia (can follow a viral illness)

MCC in adults – fecalith

Luminal obstruction followed by:
1) distention of appendix

2) venous congestion and thrombosis

3) ischemia

4) gangrene necrosis

5) rupture

Non-operative situation
CT scan shows walled-off perforated appendix

Tx:
Percutaneous drainage and interval appendectomy at later date as long as sx's are improving

F/U barium enema or colonoscopy to R/O perforated colon CA

Children and elderly
Have higher propensity to **rupture** secondary to delayed diagnosis

Children often have **higher fever** and more **vomiting and diarrhea**

Elderly – sx's can be minimal; may need right hemicolectomy if cancer suspected

Appendicitis is unusual to rare in infants

Perforation – pt generally more ill; can have evidence of sepsis

Necrotic base after appendectomy
Just inflamed or minimal necrosis → staple across cecum and place some omentum there

Extensive necrosis of the cecum→ cecectomy

Late fever or abd pain after appendectomy →
Abd CT – look for abscess

If **contained** → percutaneous drainage

If **not contained** → OR, clean out area (lower midline to mobilizing omentum)

At reoperation, If you find a **hole in the cecum**→ options:

Very small hole → repair (if easy to repair), omental flap, clean out abdomen, leave drains, Abx's

Moderate size hole → partial cecal resection, omental flap, leave drains, Abx's

All of cecum necrotic → cecectomy or right hemi-colectomy + primary anastomosis, omental flap, Abx's

Appendicitis during pregnancy
1) *MCC of acute abd pain in 1st trimester*

2) *Most likely to occur in 2nd trimester* (but is not most common cause of abd pain)

3) *Most likely to perforate in 3rd trimester* (confused w/ contractions)

If open procedure → need to make incision where pt is having pain – *underline appendix is displaced superiorly by uterus*

Usually have **RUQ pain** in 3rd trimester
Pain may be exacerbated w/ pt lying on **right side**
35% fetal mortality w/ rupture
Women w/ suspected appendicitis need beta-HCG drawn ± abd U/S
to R/O OB/GYN causes of abd pain
No prophylactic tocolytics (start w/ sx's of **pre-term labor** or
uterine contractions; see Trauma chp)

Appendix Mucocele (mucinous cyst-adenoma or cyst–adenocarcinoma)
Mucin buildup leading to **dilated appendix**
Can rupture causing **abdominal mucin accumulation** or **peritoneal mets**
Pseudomyxoma peritonei (malignant rupture) – **peritoneal implants** that
secrete mucin, cause **bowel obstruction**
Can be caused by other **mucin secreting tumors** (eg Ovarian)
MCC of death w/ pseudomyxoma peritonei – **SBO** from CA spread
Needs resection if not metastatic
Benign – appendectomy
Malignant – right hemicolectomy

Terminal regional ileitis – mimics appendicitis (RLQ pain)
1) enlarged mesenteric LN's
2) symmetric inflammation and thickening of terminal ileum and cecum
Use above to DDx regional ileitis *vs.* appendicitis
Infectious organisms causing ileitis – yersinia, campylobacter,
salmonella
5% is actually early Crohn's

Gastroenteritis – N/V, diarrhea

Presumed appendicitis but find ruptured ovarian cyst, thrombosed ovarian vein,
or regional enteritis <u>not</u> involving cecum → **still perform appendectomy**
(as long as cecum at base of appendix is not involved)

Ileus

Etiologies – surgery (MC), electrolyte abnormalities (**↓K** and **↓Mg**), peritonitis,
ischemia, trauma, drugs, pancreatitis
Ileus – dilatation is uniform throughout stomach, small bowel, colon, and rectum
w/o decompression
Obstruction – there is bowel decompression distal to obstruction

Typhoid enteritis (salmonella) – rare bleeding / perforation; fever, headaches,
maculopapular rash, leukopenia, abd pain, constipation ; Tx: Bactrim

COLON and RECTUM

Anatomy and Physiology

Colon secretes K^+ and reabsorbs Na^+ and **water** (mostly right colon and cecum)

Layers
> Mucosa (columnar epithelium)
> Submucosa
> Muscularis propria
> Serosa

Retroperitoneal portions – ascending, descending, sigmoid colon, and rectum
Peritoneum – covers anterior portions of upper and middle ⅓ of rectum

Muscle layers
> **Muscularis mucosa** – circular/longitudinal interwoven inner layer
> **Muscularis propria** – circular layer of muscle
> **Taenia coli** – three bands that run longitudinally along colon. At rectosigmoid junction, the taenia broaden and completely encircle bowel as 2 discrete muscle bands

Plicae semilunaris – transverse bands across colon that form haustra

Vascular supply
> **Ascending** and **2/3 of transverse colon** supplied by **SMA**
> > (eg ileocolic, right colic and middle colic arteries)
> **1/3 transverse, descending colon, sigmoid colon,** and **upper portion of rectum** supplied by **IMA** (left colic, sigmoid branches, superior rectal artery)
> **Marginal artery** – travels along colon margin, connecting SMA to IMA (provides collateral flow)
> **Arc of Riolan** – a short direct connection between IMA and SMA
> 80% of blood flow goes to mucosa and submucosa
> **Superior rectal artery** – branch of **IMA**
> **Middle rectal artery** – branch of **internal iliac** (the **lateral stalks** during LAR or APR contain the middle rectal arteries)
> **Inferior rectal artery** – branch of **internal pudendal** (a branch of internal iliac)
> Rectal arteries = hemorrhoidal arteries

Watershed areas
> **Splenic flexure** (Griffith's point) – SMA and IMA junction
> **Rectum** (Sudeck's point) – superior rectal and middle rectal junction
> Colon more sensitive to ischemia than small bowel due to ↓ed **collaterals**

Venous drainage
> Generally follows arterial except IMV, which goes to the splenic vein
> Splenic vein joins SMV to form portal vein behind neck of pancreas
> **Superior** and **middle rectal veins** drain into **IMV** and eventually the portal vein
> **Inferior rectal veins** drain into internal iliac veins and eventually caval system (can get isolated lung mets w/ low rectal tumors)

Nodal supply
> **Ascending, transverse, descending,** and **sigmoid areas** follow arterial supply
> **Superior and middle rectum** – drain to IMA nodes
> **Lower rectum** – primarily to IMA nodes, also to internal iliac nodes
> Bowel wall contains submucosal and mucosal lymphatics

External anal sphincter – under voluntary (CNS) control
> The continuation of **puborectalis muscle**
> **Inferior rectal** (anal) branch of **internal pudendal nerve** (sympathetic) and **perineal branch of S4**
> The puborectalis is part of the **levator ani muscle group** (striated muscle)

Internal anal sphincter – involuntary control
> The continuation of **muscularis propria** (colon circular layer, smooth muscle)
> Innervation by **pelvic splanchnics** (S2-S4, parasympathetic, <u>No</u> voluntary control)
> ***No*** *pudendal innervation*; Normally contracted

Meissner's plexus – inner nerve plexus to bowel
Auerbach's plexus – outer nerve plexus to bowel
Distances from anal verge

Anal canal	0–5 cm
Rectum	5–15 cm
Rectosigmoid junction	15–18 cm

Levator ani – marks transition between anal canal and rectum
Short-chain fatty acids – main nutrient of colonocytes
Denonvillier's fascia (anterior) – recto-vesicular fascia in men; recto-vaginal
    fascia in women
Waldeyer's fascia (posterior) – recto-sacral fascia
Colonic inertia – slow transit time; pts may need subtotal colectomy
    R/O mechanical obstruction (eg malignancy, stricture, volvulus)
    R/O systemic DZ (eg diabetes, hypothyroidism, scleroderma, diffuse
        dysmotility D/Os)
    Tx:
        ↑ **fiber** (30 gm/d) and ↑**water** (cures 95%)
        If that fails:
            Measure **colonic transit time** (radiopaque markers given w/
                plain films on days 3 and 5 – 80% of markers should be
                gone by day 5)
            Assess **pelvic floor function**
                Defography
                Anorectal manometry – sphincter muscles should relax
                    when trying to have a bowel movement
            Can try **biofeedback** if pelvic floor dysfunction
            Consider **subtotal colectomy** and **ilio-rectal anastomosis** for slow
                colonic transit time (should have failed multiple other Tx's)

Rectocele
    Anterior wall of rectum bulges into vagina; weakness in recto-vaginal fascia
    RFs – multiparous women
    Tx: kegel exercise, pessary; surgery to **re-appose** and **re-inforce fascia**
        between vagina and rectum

Pouchitis
    Diversion or disuse proctitis (eg Hartman's Pouch after sigmoid
        resection)
        Sx's: mucus drainage from pouch (from sloughing of dead mucosa)
        Tx: short-chain fatty acid enema
    Infectious pouchitis (eg J-pouch or Kock pouch)
        Sx's: purulent material, fever, can be bloody
        Tx: cipro + flagyl; if refractory to abx's, may need pouch take-down

Lymphocytic colitis
    Sx's: watery diarrhea and inflammatory bowel sx's
    Dx: colonoscopy looks normal but Bx shows lymphocytes in epithelium
    Tx: diet modifications (↓ fat, caffeine, lactose), steroids sulfasalazine
Steroids S/Es - Cushing's syndrome, mania, insomnia, hypertension,
    hyperglycemia, osteoporosis, and avascular necrosis

Ulcerative Colitis
    Inflammation of the **colonic mucosa**
    DDx:
        Ulcerative Colitis
        Crohn's Disease
        Infectious colitis (C. difficile, campylobacter, salmonella, shigella, E. Coli
            O157:H7, amebic, CMV, giardia)
        Ischemic colitis
        Mesenteric ischemia
        Celiac sprue
    Age of onset – 20-25 years
    Ashkenazi Jewish
    Acute Disease → fluid resuscitation, NPO, NGT

Sx's:
>
> **Bloody diarrhea, abd pain, fever,** and **weight loss** *(classic)*
> **Toxic megacolon** or **toxic colitis** → fever, tachycardia, ↑ed WBCs,
>> bloating, > 6 bloody BM's/day, hypotension
>
> Strictures and fistula unusual (unlike Crohn's disease)
> **Spares anus** (unlike Crohn's disease)
> Rectal exam → **bleeding is universal**
> **No skip lesions**

Dx:
>
> **Trying to make Dx:**
>> **Colonoscopy w/ multiple Bx's** *(best test)*
>>> *Not if toxic megacolon suspected*
>>> Starts distally in **rectum**, is **contiguous**
>>>> (No skip areas like Crohn's disease)
>>>
>>> Mucosal friability w/ pseudopolyps, collar button ulcers
>>> **Full colonoscopy** when disease 1st discovered to R/O CA
>>>> (esp if pt has had long-standing problems)
>>
>> **R/O infectious cause at initial w/u:**
>>> Stool cultures, O and P (giardia, entamoeba histolytica), C.
>>> difficile toxin
>>
>> **Barium enema** – w/ chronic disease see loss of haustra, narrow
>>> caliber, short colon, loss of redundancy
>
> **Acute exacerbation:**
>> T and C for 6 units of blood; check coagulation studies (correct them)
>> Labs – WBCs may be elevated; check Hct
>> **Abd/pelvic CT scan** – to look for perforation or abscess
>> **Serial abdominal series** – to look for progressive dilatation w/ toxic
>>> megacolon or perforation
>>
>> *No colonoscopy*

Medical Tx:
>
> 1) **Stable Ulcerative Colitis**
>> a) **5-ASA** compounds (sulfasalazine)
>>> For isolated left sided CD, can give in enema form
>>
>> b) **Azathioprine or 6-mercaptopurine** (frequent wbc, LFT, and
>>> metabolite checks)
>>
>> c) **Loperamide** and anti-diarrheals only for mild disease
>> d) **Low residue diet** (avoid fiber such as cereal, bread, nuts or
>>> vegetables)
>>
>> Steroids
>>> Avoid chronic prednisone if possible; use for flares
>>> Try to **cut back steroid dose** once sx's under control
>>> **Failure to wean high steroid dose** down after 3-6 months is
>>>> an indication for surgery
>>>
>>> Can be give in enema form for isolated left sided colitis
>
> 2) **Acute exacerbation** (mild, moderate, or severe bloody diarrhea and abd
>> pain; obstruction, toxic megacolon, toxic colitis, hemorrhage)
>> a) **Medical Tx as above** (5-ASA and 6-MP compounds)
>> b) **Moderate to severe DZ** → **IVF's, NPO, NGT,** and **TPN**
>>> **T and C for 6 units** – transfuse if bleeding
>>
>> c) *Add* **Antibiotics** (cipro + flagyl) – for fever, ↑ed WBC, or if worried
>>> about toxic megacolon or toxic colitis
>>> Abx's are not as effective for UC exacerbations compared to
>>>> CD exacerbations
>>
>> d) *Add* **Steroids** (moderate DZ; *best Tx for acute exacerbation*)
>> e) *Add* **Infliximab** (severe DZ) ± **cyclosporin** (severe DZ)
>> **Serial abdominal series and exams**
>>> Transverse colon > 6 cm on KUB (→ toxic megacolon)
>>> *No loperamide w/ acute exacerbation*

Indications for surgery w/ acute exacerbation:
↑ing WBCs
Persistent tachycardia despite resuscitation
Worsening clinical exam
Sepsis
Bloody BM's > 10-12/d
Perforation
50% w/ toxic megacolon or toxic colitis will require surgery
MC Perforation w/ UC – transverse colon
MC Perforation w/ CD – distal ileum

Surgery:
Surgery is **curative** for UC
5% get colectomy w/ 1st attack (severe acute fulminant ulcerative colitis)
Surgical indications:
Significant hemorrhage
Refractory toxic megacolon or **toxic colitis** (fails to improve after 72 hrs)
Persistent obstruction or stricture
Dysplasia (*any dysplasia* → *including low grade*)
Cancer
Intractability or failed medical Tx (> 10-12 bloody stools / day)
Systemic Cx's (MC is failure to thrive)
Long standing DZ (> 10-20 years; as prophylaxis against colon CA)
Failure to wean high dose steroids
Perforation
Emergent or urgent surgery
Usually perform **total procto-colectomy and ileostomy**
Can perform ileoanal anastomosis w/ J pouch at a later date when stable
Do not hook up in acute setting (eg toxic colitis, toxic megacolon, hemorrhage, perforation, significant obstruction)
Elective surgery
Usually total procto-colectomy, rectal mucosectomy, J-pouch (from ileum), and w/ ilio-anal anastomosis; need temporary loop ileostomy
Can also just perform **APR and place ileostomy** (want **ileostomy output < 500-1000 cc/d;** use loperamide)
If performing elective surgery in pt w/ **long-standing DZ**, need **total colonoscopy** pre-operatively to R/O CA
Also need **peri-operative steroids** and **bowel prep** before surgery
Ileoanal anastomosis
Total proctocolectomy, rectal mucosectomy (4 cm of cuff), J-pouch (from ileum) and ileal-anal anastomosis
Need temporary diverting loop ileostomy (6–8 wks) while pouch heals
May **protect bladder** and **sexual function** better than APR
Need lifetime **surveillance** of residual rectal area
15% of ileoanal anastomoses eventually **need resection** (APR +ileostomy) secondary to 1) **CA** or **dysplasia,** 2) refractory **proctitis / sepsis** *or* 3) **incontinence** (MC reason for takedown)
Try to get BM's down to 6-8/day
Cx's
Leak – MC major morbidity after surgery → can lead to sepsis
Infectious pouchitis – Tx: Flagyl
Disuse pouchitis (occurs w/ diversion) – Tx: short chain fatty acid enemas
Bladder dysfunction
Sexual dysfunction
Anastomotic stenosis – dilate
Dysplasia or CA in the residual rectal mucosa – Tx: APR
Contraindications to J pouch and ileoanal anastomosis:
1) **Not** used with Crohn's disease
2) **Don't hook-up w/ acute fulminant colitis, hemorrhage, or perforation** → just do total proctocolectomy w/ residual rectal stump (to hook up to later) + ileostomy; hook-up 6-8 weeks later
3) **Can't perform this w/ severe rectal DZ and incontinence**

CA risk
> **1-2% per year starting 10 years after initial diagnosis**
> CA more evenly distributed throughout colon
> *Pan-colitis at highest risk for developing colon CA*
> **Left sided colitis** and co-existent **primary sclerosing cholangitis** pts are high risk
> ****Cancer risk is _not_ elevated in pts w/ isolated ulcerative proctitis**
> *Any dysplasia is an indication for total colectomy (technique as above)*

Prophylactic Colectomy
> Some experts recommend **prophylactic colectomy at 10 years** *(safest answer)* however there has been some shift to surveillance
> At 20 years, especially in pts w/ **family Hx** of colon cancer, pts diagnosed at a **young age**, and pts w/ **primary sclerosing cholangitis**, the case is strong for prophylactic colectomy

Surveillance
> Should start at 8 years for pts w/ pan-colitis and 15 years for pts w/ isolated left sided colitis to look for dysplasia
> **Low grade dysplasia** – 20% actually have colon CA
> **High grade dysplasia** – 40% actually have colon CA

Extra-intestinal manifestations:
> **MC extra-intestinal manifestation requiring total colectomy** – failure to thrive in children
> **Does _not_ get better w/ colectomy** → primary sclerosing cholangitis, ankylosing spondylitis
> **Gets better with colectomy** → ocular problems, arthritis, anemia
> **50% get better** → pyoderma gangrenosum (deep necrotic ulcers)
> > Tx: steroids
> Can get thromboembolic cx's w/ UC
> **HLA B27** – sacroiliitis and ankylosing spondylitis

	Crohn's	Ulcerative Colitis
Clinical Features		
Location	Small and large bowel	Colon only backwash ileitis 10%
Anatomic distribution	Skip lesions (often rectal sparing)	Contiguous involvement (rectum 1st)
Gross bleeding	50%	Universal
Perianal disease	70%	Rare
Fistula	Yes	No
Endoscopy		
Mucosal involvement	Skip lesions	Contiguous
Discrete aphthous ulcers	Common	Rare
Surrounding mucosa	Normal	Abnormal
Longitudinal ulcer	Common	Rare
Cobble-stoning	Yes, if severe	No
Rectal involvement	Sparing common	Involved in 90%
Mucosal friability	Uncommon	Common
Vascular pattern	Normal	Distorted
Path		
Transmural inflammation	Yes	No
Granulomas	Common	No
Fissures	Common	Rare
Submucosal fibrosis	Common	No
Submucosal inflammation	Common	Uncommon

Amoebiasis (amoebic dysentery, amoebic colitis)

Contaminated food and water with feces that contain cysts

10% become carriers for *Entamoeba histolytica*

Primary infection – colon; **secondary infection** – liver

RFs – travel to Mexico, ETOH; fecal-oral transmission

Sx's: similar to UC (dysentery, can be bloody); chronic more common form (3–4 bowel movements/day, cramping and fever)' 90% asymptomatic

Dx:

Stool O and P

Serology – 90% have anti-amoebic antibodies

Endoscopy – patchy red areas

Tx: Flagyl and **diiodohydroxyquin** (Iodoquinol)

Actinomyces (<u>not</u> a fungus)

Present as a mass, abscess, chronic draining fistula, or induration – can be confused w/ perforated CA or diverticulitis; can also occur in oral cavity

Crosses tissue planes easily

Most commonly misdiagnosed disease

Suppurative and granulomatous

Gram positive rods (GPRs) and **yellow sulfur granules**

Cecum most common location

Tx: High dose PCN G (or amoxicillin + drainage of any abscess)

Lymphogranuloma venereum

Chlamydia infection; homosexuals

Causes ulcers, proctitis, tenesmus, bleeding, and adenopathy; ± fistulas

Tx: doxycycline, hydrocortisone; drainage of any abscesses

Large bowel obstruction
Initial Tx – fluid resuscitation, NPO, NGT
DDx: Colon CA (MC)
Diverticulitis (#2)
Sigmoid volvulus
Cecal volvulus
Pseudo-obstruction (Ogilvie's syndrome)
Sx's:
Abd pain + distension, failure to pass gas or stool, $\pm$ N/V
Small caliber stools, weight loss → suspect **colon CA**
Fever, chills, tenderness, local peritoneal signs → suspect **diverticulitis**
Old person, nursing home, laxatives→suspect **sigmoid volvulus** (or cecal)
Narcotics, very sick, and in the hospital → suspect **pseudo-obstruction**
Dx:
AXR and **CXR** (or CT scan) – look for distension
Proctoscopy – look for rectal mass
1) If likely **diverticulitis** → Abd/Pelvic CT scan
2) If likely **CA, sigmoid volvulus,** or **pseudo-obstruction**→ Colonoscopy
Go all the way to cecum even if a mass is already found – need to make sure there is not a **concomitant colon CA** more proximal
Can get **Bx** and get Dx if **colon CA**
Can **de-torse** if **sigmoid volvulus**
Can **decompress** if **pseudo-obstruction**
3) If likely **cecal volvulus**– operate (very hard to de-torse + will likely recur)
Colon perforation w/ obstruction
Most likely in **cecum** (Law of LaPlace tension = pressure x diameter)
Closed-loop obstructions – worrisome; can have rapid progression and perforation w/ minimal distention; a competent **iliocecal valve** can lead to closed-loop obstruction.
Surgical management of colon obstruction w/ colon CA:
Perforation
Right – resection, ostomy, and MF or HP (**2 stage**, unlike trauma)
Left – resection, colostomy, MF or HP (**3 stage**)
No perforation, un-prepped bowel (total obstruction):
Right sided lesions – primary anastomosis (**1 stage**)
Left sided lesions – resection, colostomy, MF or HP (**3 stage**)
No perforation, prepped bowel (partial obstruction, could clean out)
Right sided lesions – primary anastomosis (**1 stage**)
Left sided lesions – can perform 1°anastomosis but also place temp ileostomy (**2 stage**)

Ogilvie's Syndrome (colonic pseudo-obstruction)
RFs – opiates, bed-ridden pts, infection, major surgery, and trauma
Sx's: **abd distension** and **pain**, ± N/V, rectal exam reveals *air-filled rectum*
Dx: AXR – massive, diffusely dilated colon; **if free air** → perforation
Tx:
1) Make sure pt does **not** have: 1) **true large bowel obstruction** (should have air filled rectum w/ Ogilvie's, not with large bowel obstruction) *or;* 2) **perforation** (peritoneal signs)
2) **IVF's** to replace volume deficit
3) **Replace electrolytes** (K, PO4, Mg)
4) **Stop drugs** that slow the gut (eg narcotics)
5) **Place NGT** (± rectal tube)
6) **Neostigmine** 2.5 mg IV should be given if the above fails
7) **Colonoscopy** to decompress the colon if **cecum is $\geq$ 12** or failure of medical Tx over 24-48 hours
Recurrence rate after colonoscopy is 30% (may be ↓ed w/ Neostigmine)
Neostigmine can cause **bradycardia – have atropine immediately available**.
Acetylcholinesterase inhibitor
Others S/Es - ↑ secretions, salivation, diarrhea
If colonoscopy fails to decompress, proceed with **cecostomy**
Need right hemi-colectomy w/ colostomy and MF if bowel not viable

Sigmoid volvulus

Initial Tx: fluid resuscitation, NPO, NGT

Sigmoid colon folds over on itself, causing closed loop obstruction

Sx's:

>Pain, distention, obstipation – causes closed loop obstruction
>Debilitated; psychiatric pts; laxative abuse
>Usually with high-fiber diets (Iran, Iraq)

Dx:

>**Abd/pelvic CT** (best test) – shows closed loop obstruction
>**AXR** – Bent inner tube sign or Ace of Spades appearance; point (or line) goes to RUQ
>**Gastrograffin enema** – may show bird's beak sign (tapered colon)

Tx:

>**Peritoneal signs**
>>→ *Do **not** attempt decompression*; just go to OR for detorsion
>>**Non-gangrenous bowel** → just de-torse, pexy, close, rectal tube, bowel prep, back in 2-3 days for resection
>>**Gangrenous bowel** → do not un-torse the bowel (releases IL-1, TNF, etc); just resection, colostomy and MF or HP
>
>**No peritoneal signs**
>>→ **decompress w/ colonoscopy** (80% reduce, 50% will recur)
>>Then place a rectal tube, give bowel prep
>>Perform sigmoid colectomy during same admission
>>**If necrotic bowel** found w/ colonoscopy (eg black) – don't de-torse w/ colonoscopy, go to OR for resection
>>**If you can't de-torse w/ colonoscope, go to OR:**
>>>**If bowel viable→** de-torse, pexy, close, rectal tube, bowel prep, back in 2-3 days for resection
>>>**If bowel not viable** → rsxn, colostomy and MF or HP

Cecal volvulus

Initial Tx: fluid resuscitation, NPO, NGT

Less common than sigmoid volvulus

Dx

>**Abd/pelvic CT** – shows closed loop obstruction
>>Can appear as a **SBO**, w/ dilated cecum in the RLQ
>
>**AXR** – has an Ace of Spades appearance; the point (or line) goes to LUQ

Tx: right hemicolectomy best Tx (gangrene or no gangrene) w/ 1° anastomosis

If frail pt and **incontinent** → consider just colectomy and MF or HP

Diverticulitis

Diverticula - MC location is sigmoid colon (90%), **mucosal out-pouching** from increased intra-luminal pressure (straining due to low fiber diet; is a **false diverticulum**)

Result of **perforations in mucosa** in diverticulum w/ adjacent fecal contamination

Denotes infection + inflammation of colonic wall + surrounding tissue

Initial tx: Fluid resuscitation, NPO, abx's

DDx: diverticulitis, perforated colon CA (pencil stools or weight loss), appendicitis (right sided pain), TOA or other ovarian problem, volvulus (nursing home patient; laxatives), ischemic colitis, inflammatory bowel DZ

Sx's

>LLQ pain, fever, tenderness, constipation
>Signs of **complicated diverticulitis** requiring CT scan include:
>>1) Obstructive sx's
>>2) Fluctuant mass on exam
>>3) Localized peritoneal signs
>>4) Temp > 39
>>5) WBC > 20,000
>>6) Failure to resolve w/ medical tx

Labs – ↑ WBCs

Dx:

Abd and Pelvic CT *(best test)* – bowel wall thickening, fat stranding
Get if worried about complicated diverticulitis (see above)
May see free perforation or abscess
Make sure you see diverticuli on the CT scan, if not, most likely CA
Need F/U barium enema on all pts w/ diverticulitis to R/O cancer
Colonoscopy <u>*contraindicated*</u> *in acute phase (perforation risk)*
Barium enema also <u>*contraindicated*</u> *in the acute phase*

Tx:

Uncomplicated diverticulitis
14 days of Abx's (cipro + flagyl)
Bowel rest for 5-7 days – clears when sx's improving and pt is
passing gas
IV abx's for severe episode
Surgery if fails to improve or if gets **worse**
25% will have a Cx (MC - abscess formation, Tx: percutaneous drain)
If resection required, **pre-op ureteral stent** can help avoid ureteral
injury; rsxn, colostomy and MF if acute

Complicated Diverticulitis
Abscess
If contained → percutaneous drainage
Not contained → OR, rsxn, colostomy and MF
Free perforation – w/ perforation, can suddenly feel better (relief of
obstruction) then worse (peritonitis) → OR, rsxn, colostomy and
MF
Obstruction – try conservative management and see if pt opens up
If pt fails to improve (3-5 days) → OR, rsxn, colostomy and MF
Fistula
Colo-vesical fistula MC in men
Colo-vaginal fistula MC in women
Colo-vesical fistula
Sx's: fecaluria, pneumaturia → get **Cystoscopy** *(best
test)* to confirm problem
Can also get **UA** to look for enteric contents
Tx: bowel prep, Abx's; resection of involved bowel; repair
defect in bladder or vagina (chromics); interpose
omentum; re-connect bowel; diverting ileostomy
Colo-vaginal fistula (see Rectum and Anus chp)
Inability to exclude CA → elective resection
Late sigmoid strictures can form → resection of stricture if severe
Recurrent Diverticulitis
2nd attacks associated w/ 50% recurrence rate
Cool down inflammatory process w/ abx's
Elective rsxn in 6 weeks (barium enema to R/O CA, bowel prep,
ureteral stents) – temporary ileostomy (2 stage procedure)
Indications for elective resection
1) **recurrent** diverticulitis
2) diverticulitis requiring **hospitalization in pt aged < 40**
3) diverticulitis **complicated** by **abscess or obstruction** (treat w/
percutaneous drain for abscess and conservative Tx: bring
back in 6 weeks for elective resection)
Right-sided diverticulitis – 80% discovered at the time of incision for
appendectomy; Tx: right hemicolectomy, primary anastomosis
Ureteral stents – place pre-op for elective or semi-elective sigmoid
resection for **diverticulitis**
Getting ready to take down colostomy after previous colon rsxn:
Barium enema to R/O distal stenosis or leaks
CT scan to look for any abscesses
Ureteral stents and bowel prep
W/ resection, need to take **all of the sigmoid colon to the upper rectum**
(*where **taenia coli disappear***); proximal margin extended beyond
sigmoid colon if thickened colon w/ chronic inflammation present

Colorectal cancer

Epidemiology
- 3rd **MC CA in US**
- 2nd **MCC CA death in US**
- Rare before 40, 90% occur > age 50
- 25% of pts have positive Fam Hx
- **MC location** – sigmoid colon
- **ASA** and **NSAID's** ↓ risk of adenomas but ↑ bleeding risk
    - **Adenomas** – villous, sessile, and large (> 2 cm) → ↑ed CA risk
- **RFs** – diet high in red meat
- ? Association w/ **strep bovis** and **clostridium septicum** species

Major RFs
- **FAP** (100% lifetime risk; tumor suppressor gene)
- **HNPCC** (80% lifetime risk; mismatch DNA repair genes)
- **Inflammatory Bowel Disease** (UC and CD involving colon)

Sx's: change in bowel habits, constipation, small caliber stools, bleeding; iron deficient microcytic anemia, pain

Dx:

- **Total colonoscopy**
    - Barium enema if not able to get to cecum – r/o **synchronous lesions**
    - *You need to evaluate the entire colon*
- **TRUS** (trans-rectal U/S) for **rectal lesions** *(best test for T and N status)*
    - T3 or T4 rectal lesions get neoadjuvant chemo-XRT
    - Good at assessing depth of invasion and sphincter involvement
    - Good for assessing recurrence or presence of enlarged nodes
- **Abd/pelvic CT** – look for liver mets; *best for M status (distant disease)*
- **CXR** – look for lung mets
- **LFT's**
- **CEA** (useful for prognosis, to detect recurrence, and follow response to therapy; *NOT useful as a screen*)

Path

- **MC site for colorectal CA** – sigmoid colon
    - Although 50% of colon CA is proximal to splenic flexure
- **Most impt prognostic indicator** – node status (spreads to nodes 1st)
- **MC site for mets** – liver; others – lung (#2)
    - Portal vein → **liver mets**
    - Iliac vein → **lung mets**
    - **Isolated liver or lung mets sh**ould be resected
    - 5% get drop metastases to **ovaries**
    - **Rectal CA** – can metastasize to **spine directly via Batson's plexus** (venous)
    - **Colon CA** typically does not go to bone
- **Better prognosis** – lymphocytic penetration
- **Worse prognosis** – mucinous (Signet Ring Cell), mucoepidermoid, pts w/ obstruction or perforation, ↑ CEA, vascular / nerve / lymphatic invasion, rectal tumors, ulcerative tumors
- **Main gene mutations:**
    - **APC gene** (adenomatous polyposis coli gene; tumor suppressor)
        - APC protein binds **glycogensynthasekinase** [GSK] and is involved **in cell cycle regulation** and **cell movement**
    - **p53** – tumor suppressor
        - p53 protein - **transcription factor** for RNA polymerase involved in **cell cycle regulation**
    - **k-ras** – oncogene
        - ras protein - **GTPase** (G protein) involved in **transmembrane signal transduction** and **cell cycle regulation**
    - **DCC gene** (deleted in colorectal cancer) – oncogene, ? mechanism

Staging

T

Tis: involves only the mucosa; has not grown beyond muscularis mucosa (inner muscle layer).

T1: through muscularis mucosa and into submucosa

T2: through submucosa and into muscularis propria (outer muscle layer).

T3: through muscularis propria and into subserosa (or non-peritonealized peri-colic or peri-rectal tissue)

T4: through the wall of the colon or rectum and into nearby tissues or organs (or perforates visceral peritoneum)

Tis, N0, M0: *carcinoma in situ* or *intra-mucosal carcinoma*

N

N0: No lymph nodes

N1: 1 to 3 nearby lymph nodes.

N2: 4 or more nearby lymph nodes.

M M0: No mets., **M1:** mets

Stage

Stage I:	**T1, N0, M0 or T2, N0, M0**
Stage IIA:	**T3, N0, M0**
Stage IIB:	**T4, N0, M0**
Stage IIIA:	**T1, N1, M0 or T2, N1, M0**
Stage IIIB:	**T3, N1, M0 or T4, N1, M0**
Stage IIIC:	**Any T, N2, M0**
Stage IV:	**Any T, Any N, M1**

Tx:

Ultimately resection for all unless stage IV

(Although some stage IV DZ should be resected, see below)

En bloc resection includes:

Associated **mesocolon**

Regional **adenectomy**

Adequate **margins** ($\geq$ 2 cm)

Take Waldeyer's and Denonvillier's **fascia** for rectal tumors

Rectal tumors

T3, T4 or positive nodes get neoadjuvant chemo-XRT

T1 or T2 w/ negative nodes – just resection

Need 2-cm margins

Exceptions:

T1 rectal lesion and going for trans-anal excision →

Can accept 2-3 mm margins (other criteria must also be fulfilled – see T1 rectal CA below)

Pedunculated adenoma or rectal sessile adenoma w/ small focus of T1 CA →

Can accept 2-3 mm margins (other criteria must also be fulfilled – see polyp section below)

Standard resection techniques:

Right hemi-colectomy – take right colic and ilio-colic arteries and all associated nodes

Transverse colectomy – take the middle colic artery and all associated nodes

Extended right hemicolectomy – for tumors at the hepatic flexure

Takes the right colic, the ilio-colic and the middle colic arteries

Will need to resect most of the transverse colon

Left hemi-colectomy – take left colic artery and all associated nodes

Extended left hemicolectomy – for tumors at the splenic flexure

Take left colic and middle colic arteries

Most **right-sided** and **transverse colon CA** can be treated w/ **primary anastomosis w/o ostomy**

Left sided colon CA – leave temporary loop ileostomy

Low anterior resection (place temporary ileostomy)

Sigmoid colon ± rectum

Take sigmoidal ± rectal arteries and associated nodes

Leave main inferior mesenteric artery (and left colic) intact to supply left colon

**Need at least 2 cm margin

2 cm from levator ani muscles or **6 cm from anal verge** → *If not, perform APR*

Apx 2 cm from the anal verge is the dentate line

Apx 2 cm from dentate line is levator ani muscles

You need a 2 cm rectal cuff for EEA stapler (1 cm is donut, 1cm is the staple line)

These distances vary

Easier to perform LAR in women compared to men because their pelvic bones are wider

The EEA stapler takes **1 cm of tissue** w/ staple line

Preoperative chemo-XRT

Produces complete response in some w/ rectal CA; preserves sphincter function in some

Still need resection w/ complete response (25% have occult CA)

Uncontrolled bleeding from sacral veins

Suture ligation, bone wax, thrombin can all be tried

If unsuccessful, pack and damage control, bring back next day

Local recurrence after LAR → Tx: APR (re-stage pt 1st)

Abscess following LAR – percutaneous drain unless severely septic (then reop + washout)

Leaks and **Fistulas** (see Wound Healing chp)

Getting ready to takedown temporary ileostomy after LAR –

Barium enema to R/O stricture at LAR anastomosis

Abd/pelvic CT to R/O occult abscess

Abdominoperineal resection

Removes rectum and anus w/ permanent colostomy

Rectal pain w/ rectal CA → APR

Can have post-op **impotence + bladder dysfunction** (nerves)

Indicated for malignant lesions not amenable to LAR (*not for benign tumors*)

Risk of local recurrence higher w/ rectal CA than w/ colon CA in general

Watch for the **ureters** (travel over iliacs) and **iliac vessels**

Watch for **pudendal nerves** (in pelvic sidewall, risk of incontinence) when taking down the lateral stalks

Lateral stalks contain **middle rectal arteries**

Low rectal T1 lesion (limited to submucosa) – assess w/ **TRUS**

Can be excised trans-anally if:

1) **< 4 cm** in size

2) **< 1/3 circumference**

3) **Negative margins** (need at least **2 mm margin**)

4) **Well differentiated**

5) **No neuro / vascular / lymphatic invasion**

6) **< 8 cm away** (LAR if > 8cm)

Otherwise pt needs APR or LAR

Low rectal T2 or higher – assess w/ **TRUS**

Tx: pre-op chemo-XRT if T3, T4 or positive nodes, **then APR or LAR**

If tumor disappears after pre-op chemo-XRT → **LAR or APR still standard of care**

Trans-anal excision of T2 lesions has ↑ed recurrence (25% vs 15%) and ↓ **survival** (75% vs 65%) compared to T1

Post-op (chemo-XRT)

> **Stage III and IV colon CA** – adjuvant chemo (<u>no</u> XRT)*
> > *consider adjuvant chemo for **high risk stage II** colon CA
> > > (obstruction/perforation, adherence to adjacent structures, lymphatic / vascular/ neuro invasion, poor differentiation)
>
> **Stage II and III rectal CA** – neoadjuvant chemo-XRT, surgery, then adjuvant chemo
>
> **Stage IV rectal CA** – chemo-XRT ± surgery (possibly just colostomy)
>
> **Chemo**
> > **5-FU, Leucovorin,** and **oxaliplatin** (FOLFOX, 6 cycles)
> > **If mets**, *add* **Bevacizumab** (monoclonal Ab to vascular endothelial growth factor-A, VEGF)
>
> **XRT** (5000 rads)
> > ↓'s **local recurrence** and ↑s **survival** when combined w/ chemo
> > **XRT damage** – rectum MC site of injury → vasculitis, thrombosis, ulcers, strictures, bleeding
> > Pre-op chemo-XRT may downstage (can have complete response) allowing LAR vs. APR
> > **Really high risk surgical pts** → possibly chemo-XRT only tx
> > **Repeat proctoscopy w/ TRUS** if giving pre-op chemo-XRT for rectal CA (should basically re-stage pt after neoadjuvant chemo-XRT)

5-YS for Colorectal CA (based on stage)

Stage	
Stage I	95%
Stage II	80%
Stage III	65%
Stage IV	10%

Follow-up

> 1) **H and P + CEA** (T2 or greater) every 6 months for 5 years
> > **CEA** (1/2 life 18 days) – if persistently elevated after colectomy but can't find source despite extensive w/u → 2nd look laparotomy
>
> 2) **Chest/abd/pelvic CT** every year for 3 years (only high risk pts)
>
> 3) **Colonoscopy**
> > Mainly to check for new colon CA's; metachronous lesion
> > **Perform after 1 year**, unless not performed initially due to obstructing mass, in which case it should be performed after 3 months
>
> **20% of pts have a recurrence, of those w/ recurrence:**
> > 50% occur within 6 months
> > 100% occur within 3 years
> > 5% have another primary – *main reason for surveillance*

Special Issues

> **Mets to liver** are fed primarily by **hepatic artery** (which would be route of intra-arterial chemotherapy or embolization).
>
> **Intra-op U/S**
> > Best method of picking up liver mets
> > Conventional ultrasound: 10 mm
> > Abd CT: 5–10 mm
> > Abd MRI: 5–10 mm (better resolution than CT)
> > Intraop U/S: 3–5 mm
>
> **Liver met discovered at time of colon resection**
> > If really easy to remove, just wedge it out w/ 1 cm margin (use **intra-op U/S**)
> > If not really easy to remove, just take a wedge or needle Bx and send it to path
> > > Finish the operation you were there to do
> > > Re-stage after 6-8 weeks (Abd/ Pelvic CT, CXR, CEA, LFT's)
> > > If no other mets detected, resect colon met
> > > Metastases usually do <u>not</u> create more metastases

Obstructing CA

1) **Partial Obstruction** → try to **decompress**

NGT, IVF's, NPO

Metastatic, resectability and **synchronous tumor work-up**
(carefully try to get the colonoscope past the lesion)
Bowel prep (slow, over 2 days); rectal tube if low lesion
Resection

2) **Total Obstruction** (not passing gas, significant sx's) → **need resection** (also for **partial obstruction** if **not able to decompress, peritoneal signs** or **free air**)

Left sided colon → colectomy, colostomy, MF or Hartman's pouch (3 stage procedure)
Total colonoscopy prior to takedown to search for other tumors

Right Sided or transverse colon → colectomy, primary anastomosis (1 stage) unless perforation (then 2 stage)

Rectal → is likely to be a deep lesion

Best Option

Try to core out or place stent so you can give **bowel prep**
Can place rectal tube for bowel prep
Perform **colonoscopy** and w/u for **metastatic DZ**

If too high to core out trans-anally, just resect and place colostomy and MF or HP

Low but can't core out – likely a very deep lesion → APR usual (colostomy and MF or HP)

3) **Perforation** → resection and colostomy or ileostomy w/ either right (2 stage procedure) or left (3 stage procedure) lesions

4) **Obstructing left sided lesions w/ cecal perforation** → sub-total colectomy, ileostomy

Unresectable mets at time of APR (eg peritoneal mets, bulky mets throughout liver)

→ *May __not__ need APR* (avoids morbidity associated w/ APR)

If **obstructed or near obstructed** → place colostomy and mucus fistula; avoids morbidity of APR in pt w/ terminal dz

If **bleeding** was a significant sx, best to proceed w/ APR

If **rectal pain** was a significant sx, best to proceed w/ APR

If not rectal CA (ie colon CA) – still resect lesion

Unresectable liver mets – consider cryoablation, RF, or chemo-embolization

Unresectable mets during pre-op work-up for colon or rectal CA

→ no rsxn unless **obstructed** (or near obstruction), or if **bleeding or pain** is a significant sx

Unresectable disease w/ ascites – peritoneal dialysis cath to drain PRN

Resectable liver mets pre-op

Liver mets

Resect if completely resectable and leaves adequate liver function (need 1 cm margin)

Number of tumors, size, and location are not factors for resection as long as you can resect all of the tumor(s) and leave enough liver behind for survival

5-year survival after resection of isolated liver mets – 35%

Poor prognostic indicators after resection of liver mets:

Disease free interval < 12 months
> 3 tumors
CEA > 200 (ug/L)
Size > 5 cm
Positive nodes
Synchronous primary and liver met

Intra-op U/S – *best method* of picking up intra-hepatic mets
>Also use palpation

Wedge or **formal liver resection** depending on location, number, and liver reserve

Formal hepatectomy has improved loco-regional control over wedge resection (eg mets to segments 1 and 2 → left hepatic lobectomy + caudate resection if sufficient liver reserve)

Lung mets (isolated) – 25% 5-year survival rate in selected pts

Colorectal CA invasion of adjacent organs (T4) is **resected en bloc** (eg partial bladder resection, pancreas, liver, any other organ) → this is still stage II disease if pt has negative nodes and no mets

Colon Cancer Screening
Normal risk
1) **FOBT** (x3) and **digital rectal exam** every year and **Flexible sigmoidoscopy** (goes to 60 cm) every **5 years** each starting at **age 50**

or;

2) **Colonoscopy** every **10 years** starting at age **50**

Positive FOBT requires colonoscopy

Positive polyp on sigmoidoscopy requires colonoscopy

If worried about getting all of polyp, **repeat colonoscopy in 3 mos**

Colonoscopy surveillance after successful polypectomy →
>**High risk** (≥ 3 adenomas, high grade dysplasia, villous, or size ≥1 cm) → **3 years**
>**Low risk** → **5 years**

High-risk
FOBT (x3) and **digital rectal exam** every year starting at **age 40** (or 10 years before 1st relative got colorectal CA)

Colonoscopy every 2–3 years starting at **age 40** (or 10 years before 1st relative got colorectal CA)

No colonoscopy w/ recent MI, splenomegaly, or pregnancy (if fluoroscopy planned)

FOBT (fecal occult blood test; **globin detection** most sensitive) –
>↓s mortality by 1/3 due to earlier Dx

Familial adenomatous polyposis (FAP)
All have cancer by age 40 (100% lifetime risk); autosomal dominant

Mutation in **APC tumor suppressor** (20% spontaneous → no Fam Hx)
>Involved in **cell cycle regulation** and **cell adhesion**

Polyps not present at birth

Polyps are present in **puberty** (**1000's**, carpeted)

Do not need colonoscopy for surveillance with suspected FAP → just need flexible sigmoidoscopy to check for polyps (teens)

Need **total colectomy** prophylactically at **age 20**

Also get **duodenal** and **periampullary polyps** and **adenocarcinoma** → need to check duodenum for polyps and CA w/ EGD every 1-2 years (remove polyps if found)

Newly discovered FAP (hundreds of polyps on sigmoidoscopy)
1) Perform **complete colonoscopy** and **metastatic w/u**
>Abd/pelvic CT, CXR, LFT's, and CEA before surgery
>Will also detect any associated **desmoid tumors** (eg Gardner's syndrome)
2) Need **EGD** to look for duodenal tumors
3) Offer genetic counseling to rest of the family

Surgery
Total proctocolectomy, **rectal mucosectomy,** and **ileoanal pouch** (Kock or J-pouch)

Need lifetime **surveillance of residual rectal area**

Total proctocolectomy w/ end ileostomy also an option

*Following colectomy, MCC of death w/ FAP is **periampullary CA of duodenum** (would need whipple)*

Cx's after J-pouch

MC Cx after J-pouch – incontinence (may need APR)

Ileal pouchitis

Sx's: bloody diarrhea, urgency

Dx: colonoscopy – erythematous, friable pouch w/ RBCs or WBCs in the lamina propria

Tx: cipro and **flagyl**

Refractory pouchitis or sepsis may require APR w/ ileostomy

Dysplasia (any) or **CA** of residual rectal area → APR

Gardner's syndrome (FAP variant)

1) **Colon CA** (APC gene)

2) **Osteomas** (odd **bumps on forehead** or other **bony protuberances**)

Benign – leave alone

3) **Desmoid tumors:**

Benign but locally invasive; increased recurrences

Tx:

Wide local excision if localized

If involving significant small bowel, excision <u>not</u> indicated → often not completely resectable and can cause worsening fibrosis w/ attempted excision

NSAIDs, anti-estrogens, chemo-XRT may help

These may prevent you from being able to perform a J-pouch if involving the base of the mesentery → try to resect if you can, o/w just go w/ end ileostomy

Turcot's syndrome (FAP variant) – **colon CA** and **brain tumors**

<u>Lynch syndromes</u> (hereditary non-polyposis colon cancer, HNPCC)

Autosomal dominant, fewer polyps than APC (< 100)

Defects in **DNA mismatch repair genes** (hMSH2, hMLH1, hPMS1, hPMS2)

Predilection for **right-sided** (eg cecal CA) and **multiple colon CAs**

80% lifetime risk of developing colorectal CA

Lynch I – just colon CA risk

Lynch II – also ↑ed risk of ovarian, endometrial, bladder, stomach, pancreas, others

**Amsterdam criteria ("3, 2, 1")

3 relatives (1 first degree relative to the other 2)

over **2** generations

1 relative w/ cancer before age 50

Amsterdam II criteria same as I except includes any combination of CA (endometrial, gastric, small bowel, ovarian, renal, brain, ect.)

Need **surveillance colonoscopy**:

1) Starting at age 21 or 10 years before primary relative got CA

2) Every 2 years until age 40, then every year

If a specific CA runs in family, develop a screening regimen for that CA (ie urine cytology at 30 years, then every 1-2 years for bladder CA)

Total colectomy should be performed with the 1st colon CA operation

↑ed risk of future colon CA → 50% get metachronous CA within 10 years

Often have multiple primaries

Women

Annual pelvic exam, trans-vaginal U/S, and CA-125 starting at age 25

Endometrial Bx's as sx's arise

Mammograms starting at age 30

Self breast exams starting at age 20

Consider **TAH and BSO** after child-bearing years

Polyps

Hyperplastic polyps – MC polyp; no CA risk

Tubular adenoma – MC intestinal neoplastic polyp (75%)

Usually pedunculated

Villous adenoma – most likely to be symptomatic

Usually sessile and larger than tubular adenomas

50% of villous adenomas have **cancer**

Increased CA risk – > 2 cm, sessile, and villous lesions

Most **pedunculated polyps** removed endoscopically

Sessile polyps may need segmental resection (stain area w/ methylene blue so you can find it at time of resection)

If not able to get all of the polyp, need segmental resection (MC w/ sessile)

False-positive FOBT – beef, vitamin C, iron, antacids, cimetidine

High-grade dysplasia – basement membrane is intact (carcinoma in situ)

Intra-mucosal cancer – into muscularis mucosa (carcinoma in situ → still not through basement membrane)

Invasive cancer – into submucosa (T1)

Polypectomy shows T1 lesion – polypectomy adequate if:

Margins clear (2-3 mm)

Well differentiated

No vascular / lymphatic / neuro invasion

O/W need a formal colon resection

Extensive _low_ rectal villous adenomas with atypia

Trans-anal excision (can try mucosectomy) as much of polyp as possible

***No APR unless CA is present** (if T1 CA is present, trans-anal excision may still be adequate, see below)*

Pathology shows T1 lesion after trans-anal excision of _low_ villous adenoma → trans-anal excision adequate if:

Clear margins (2-3 mm)

Is **well differentiated**

No vascular / lymphatic / neuro invasion

→ O/W need formal rectum resection

Pathology shows T2 lesion or greater after trans-anal excision of **rectal polyp** → pt needs APR or LAR (pre-op chemo-XRT if T3 or T4)

Juvenile Polyposis

Sx's: usually painless rectal bleeding; anemia, failure to thrive, anergy

Even though they are **hamartomatous colonic polyps,** there is a chance for adenomatous changes, which in turn leads to risk of adenocarcinoma

10% lifetime risk of colorectal CA (↑ed number of polyps ↑s risk)

Colonic surveillance every 2 years; _NO_ prophylactic colectomy

Current recommendation is that these polyps be **removed**

Cronkite-Canada syndrome

Older pts (50-60's)

Often associated w/ **chronic diarrhea** and **protein-losing enteropathy**

Hamartomatous polyps; atrophy of nails + hair, patchy hypopigmentation (eg vitiligo)

Polyps most frequent in **stomach** and **colon**

10% lifetime risk CA, related to adenomatous changes in the hamartomatous polyps and subsequent malignant changes

Peutz-Jeghers Syndrome (see Small Bowel chp)

Carcinoid of colon and rectum

Represents 15% of all carcinoids; infrequent carcinoid syndrome

Usually small at time of Dx

Mets related to tumor size: < 1 cm → rare, 1-2 cm → 10%, > 2 cm → 70%

Low rectal carcinoids:

< 2 cm → wide local excision with negative margins

> 2 cm _or_ invasion of muscularis propria → APR

Colon or high rectal carcinoids – formal resection w/ adenectomy

Neutropenic Typhlitis

Inflammation of cecum; can also get neutropenic enterocolitis

Follows chemotherapy when WBCs are low (nadir, **neutropenia**); also HIV pts

Sx's: abd pain

Can mimic surgical DZ (eg appendicitis)

Often see **pneumotosis** on plane film or abd CT scan (*not an operative indication in this circumstance)*

Avoid endoscopy for risk of perforation

Tx:

> **Abx's**
>
> **GCSF** to ↑ WBCs → pts will improve when WBCs recover
>
> Only operate w/ **perforation**

Radiation Proctitis (radiation colitis)

1) **Acute radiation Proctitis** (1st few weeks) - present w/ diarrhea and tenesmus

   Tx: conservative Tx (steroid enemas) unless perforation (rare)

2) **Late radiation Proctitis** (months to years)

   Can present as **bleeding** (MC Cx), **obstruction**, **fistula** or **ulcer** (get Bx)

   R/O **CA recurrence** w/ late problem

   a) **Bleeding** from **rectum** – *Formalin fixation of rectum* (*best Tx*); argon beam, cautery, epinephrine injection, rectal rsxn (last resort)

   b) **Obstruction** from **strictures**

   > **Dx:**
   >
   > > **Abd CT**
   > >
   > > **Barium Enema**
   > >
   > > **Sigmoidoscopy w/ Bx's**
   > >
   > > > Not w/ acute radiation proctitis to prevent perforation
   > > >
   > > > Chronic see pale edematous mucosa w/ ulcerations
   > > >
   > > > **Need to R/O original CA**
   >
   > **Tx:**
   >
   > > Low residue diet, possible steroids
   > >
   > > **Conservative tx for 6-8 weeks;** consider stricture **dilatation**, local trans-anal **excision** of strictured area (some use laser to ↓ bleeding), or just **divert** w/ ostomy

   c) **Fistulas**

   > **Abd CT** to R/O abscess, recurrent CA
   >
   > **Barium enema** to R/O distal obstruction, recurrent CA
   >
   > **Biopsy** area to R/O recurrence
   >
   > (see Rectum and Anus chp for tx)

   Try to avoid APR for radiation proctitis

3) **Late radiation Colitis** (eg XRT for previous ovarian CA)

   If you need surgery (eg obstruction), **rsxn of bowel only when safe, o/w bypass**

   > Leave extended length on ileostomies and colostomies expecting contraction
   >
   > Be cautious and perform **bypasses** when needed here
   >
   > Need to take **Bx's to R/O CA recurrence**

Lower GI Bleeding
Initial Tx:
2 IV, fluid resuscitation, NPO, <u>NGT</u> (R/O UGI source)
T and C for 6 units, transfuse to keep Hct > 30
Correct coags w/ FFP, cryo, and plts

DDx:
Diverticulosis
Angiodysplasia (colonic or small bowel)
UGI bleed
CA
Ulcerative colitis (bloody diarrhea)
Ischemic colitis (bloody diarrhea, will have abd pain)
Hemorrhoid
Fissure
Anal ulcer

Sx's
Melena or hematochezia (both can occur w/ UGI bleed)
    Stool guaiac can stay positive up to 3 weeks after bleed
Hematemesis – bleeding from pharynx to ligament of Treitz
Melena – tarry stools (need as little as 50 cc of blood)
Azotemia after GI bleed – from production of urea from bacterial
    metabolism of intraluminal blood (↑ BUN)

Dx (initial steps for all LGIB):
1) **NGT to R/O UGI source**
    Need to see bile and no blood
    If you see just clear fluid w/ NGT, you have <u>NOT</u> ruled out an UGI
        source (pylorus was closed, could have potential bleeding
        duodenal ulcer)
    Perform EGD if you have not ruled this out
2) **Proctoscopy** (in ER) to R/O rectal and anal source (hemorrhoids,
    fissure, anal ulcer)
    Low Rectal CA – try local tx (epi, cautery, packing)
    Hemorrhoids or ulcer → ligate in OR
Hard to find bleeds (eg intermittent):
    Arteriography – bleeding must be ≥ 0.5 cc/min
    Tagged RBC scan *(most sensitive test)* – bleeding must be ≥ 0.1
        cc/min

Tx:
Stages of LGIB (guidelines):
1) **In shock** (SBP 60 despite blood transfusions)
        → **OR for total abdominal colectomy** (R/O UGIB +
            proctoscopy 1st, as above)
    Include terminal ileum w/ resection
    Ileostomy; leave portion of rectum (enough to get make an
        anastomosis to later)
    Consider scoping though **mouth** (pediatric colonoscope – 160
        cm; telescope the bowel along the scope), **anus**, and
        make an **enterotomy** for **intra-op enteroscopy** if pt
        stabilizes to try and find the source (looking in small
        bowel as well as large bowel) – trying to avoid total
        colectomy for a pt w/ a small bowel bleeding source
2) **Massive LGIB** (SBP 90 despite multiple blood transfusions)
        → **Angio then OR**
    Figure out which side of the colon bleeding is coming from or if
        small bowel
    Vasopressin and **octreotide** to slow bleeding
    Then take pt to the OR for appropriate resection
3) **Moderate LGIB** (BP 120) → **colonoscopy**
    Can cauterize bleeder if **angiodysplasia**
    If **diverticulosis**, careful w/ cautery (usually thin walled)
    Intubate terminal ileum to look for small bowel source
    Find problem but can't control w/ scope → resection

4) **Mild LGIB** (or moderate LGIB and can't find source) →
    Upper and **lower endoscopy**
    Angiography
    Tagged RBC scan – bleeding must be ≥ 0.1 cc/min *(most sensitive test)*
    Video capsule study
    Meckel scan (technetium-99 pertechnate scintography)
    Colectomy for bleeding (have un-prepped bowel)
        Left hemi-colectomy – colostomy and MF or HP
        Right hemi-colectomy – primary anastomosis (if not in shock)
    Recurrent diverticular or angiodysplasia bleeds → Tx: resection
    If stops bleeding while in hospital w/o surgery and you have not found source, repeat above studies + Meckel scan in hopes of localizing (try for 1 week, then discharge)
    Small bowel source for LGIB is rare

Diverticulosis bleeding
    MCC of lower GI bleed
    MC on **left side** (although higher proportion of right sided ones bleed)
    Arterial bleeding – disrupted vasa rectum
    Usually causes **significant bleeding**
    75% stop spontaneously; recurs in 25%
    Tx:
        Endoscopic tx (epi, careful cautery, band, clip), surgery if that fails
        Diverticula thin walled so careful w/ cautery
        Recurrent bleeding → resection

Angiodysplasia bleeding
    MC on **right side** of colon
    Venous bleeding
    Bleeds are usually less severe than diverticular bleeds but are more likely to recur (80%)
    Soft signs of angiodysplasia on angiogram – tufts, slow emptying
    20% of pts w/ angiodysplasia have **aortic stenosis**
    Tx:
        Endoscopic tx (epi, cautery, band, clip), surgery if that fails
        Aminocaproic acid for diffuse disease (eg small + large bowel)
        Recurrent bleeding → resection (unless diffuse disease)

Small bowel bleeding
    Rare; can be hard to Dx
    DDx – angiodysplasia, tumor, Meckel's, Crohn's, vasculitis
    Dx: video capsule study, Meckel scan, tagged RBC scan, angiography
Hemoglobin absorption from GI tract can result in **jaundice**

Diverticuli

Herniation of mucosa through colon wall at sites where arteries enter muscular wall

Is a false diverticula

Thickening of circular muscle adjacent to diverticulum with **luminal narrowing**

Caused by **straining (↑ intraluminal pressure)**

Most diverticuli occur on **left side** (80%) in the sigmoid colon.

Bleeding from diverticulosis is more common on the **left side** but a higher proportion of right sided diverticula bleed

Diverticulitis is more likely to present on **left side**

Present in 35% of the population

Ischemic colitis

Initial Tx: fluid resuscitation, NPO, abx's

DDx: Ischemic Colitis, Mesenteric ischemia, Infectious DZ (eg campylobacter, salmonella, shigella; C. difficile; entamoeba histolytica), Diverticulitis, Sigmoid volvulus

Sx's

LLQ abdominal pain

Bloody diarrhea (possible non-bloody diarrhea)

RFs

Ligation of IMA at surgery (eg AAA repair) or **IMA thrombosis**

Recent low flow state (eg CHF, MI, sepsis, cardiopulmonary bypass)

Results in **left colon ischemia**

Dx:

Colonoscopy *(best test)*

Splenic flexure and **lower sigmoid / upper rectum** most vulnerable with low flow states (watershed areas)

Griffith's Point (splenic flexure) – SMA (middle colic) and IMA (left colic) junction

Sudeck's Point – superior rectal (off IMA) and middle rectal (off internal iliacs) artery junction

Middle and Lower Rectum are <u>spared</u>

Supplied by middle (off internal iliac) and inferior (off internal pudendal) rectal arteries

This is important, as you will need to go all the way past splenic flexure to make sure pt does not have ischemic colitis

Will see cyanotic edematous mucosa covered with exudates →

Dusky (ischemic, not trans-mural) → optimize C.O. (swan, a-line, Keep Hct > 30); Abx's; Re-scope next day; ICU care

Black (necrotic, trans-mural) → rsxn

If **gangrenous colitis** suspected (eg peritonitis) or worsening clinical status → <u>NO</u> colonoscopy and go to OR (left hemicolectomy including sigmoid colon usual)

Tx:

Stabilize pt as outlined above (fluid resuscitation, abx's)

Optimize C.O. (swan, a-line, foley; dopamine, dobutamine)

Serial exams

Go to OR for **peritoneal signs** or **full thickness ischemia** on colonoscopy (ie black bowel)

Other surgery indications – refractory colitis, hemorrhage, stricture, or refractory sepsis

Resection of necrotic bowel, ostomy and MF

Medical Tx effective in 50% of cases

Mesenteric ischemia

Initial Tx: fluid resuscitation, optimize hemodynamics, NPO, abx's, ICU

DDx: emboli, thrombosis, NOMI, venous thrombosis, bowel perforation, diverticulitis, appendicitis, ischemic colitis

Sx's:

Pain out of proportion to physical exam – hallmark for <u>SMA embolism</u>

Previous food fear or weight loss – hallmark for <u>SMA thrombosis</u> or <u>visceral angina</u>

Pt may have had multiple other studies in an attempt to diagnose the problem without success 'the great mimic'

GI bleed due to **mucosal sloughing**

RFs

Recent angiography, CABG, atrial fibrillation, endocarditis, or MI (all more likely <u>arterial embolus</u>)

Vasculopathy (more likely <u>arterial thrombosis</u> or visceral angina)

Low flow state (eg sepsis, ARDS, cardiogenic shock → <u>NOMI</u>)

Hyper-coaguable state (<u>venous thrombosis</u>)

Exam

 Atrial fibrillation (more likely <u>embolus</u>)
 Weak femoral pulses (**vasculopathy;** more likely <u>thrombosis</u> or <u>visceral angina</u>)
 Peritoneal signs – late finding
 Celiac or SMA bruit (from occlusive DZ)

Dx:

 1st Angiogram *(best test)* – gives road map
  The 1st study to get in most instances
  Need to look at the **lateral view**
 CT angiogram – can identify compromised bowel (bowel wall thickening, intramural gas, portal venous gas, vascular occlusion)
 Labs – ↑ WBCs, metabolic acidosis and ↑ed lactate (late)

Etiology (acute mesenteric ischemia)

Arterial Embolism	50% *(MCC mesenteric ischemia)*
Arterial Thrombosis	25%
NOMI	15%
Venous thrombosis	5%

Overall mortality 60%

Superior Mesenteric Artery Embolism (50%)

 MC occurs near **origin of SMA** (**MC source** – <u>Heart</u>, A-fib)
 Pain out of proportion to exam *(hallmark)*
 Usually sudden onset
 Hematochezia and peritoneal signs occur late
 Often history of **recent angiography, atrial fibrillation**, endocarditis, or recent MI

 Dx:

  Angiogram → MC the proximal jejunum is spared
   Need <u>lateral view</u>
   Usually see a **meniscus** on angio about **5 cm down the SMA**

 Tx:

  a. **Stabilize pt** as outlined above (fluid resuscitation, abx's)
  b. May be able to try **selective intra-arterial infusion of thrombolytic** at site of embolus
   Criteria – <u>No</u> peritoneal signs and **< 8 hours** since onset of pain
   If peritoneal sx's develop or sx's don't improve in 4 hours → OR
   Need to get **guidewire** and **infusion catheter** past occlusion 1st

  c. **OR if above fails →**
   Finding the SMA:
    Pull transverse meso-colon superiorly
    Look for **Ligament of Treitz** and cut through this going medially → you eventually get to SMA
    Other landmark is the **middle colic artery** in the transverse meso-colon → goes directly to SMA
    Fogarty balloon embolectomy, **heparin flush** proximally + distally until good backflow x 2
    Send embolus to path and make sure its not an **atrial myxoma** (ECHO to look for myxoma)
   Resect compromised bowel
    Dusky → leave and wait for 2nd look
    Black → rsxn
    Perform ostomies or leave bowel stapled in the abdomen until 2nd look
    No anastomoses (safest move; take down in 6-8 weeks; risk of breakdown due to previous poor flow)
   Post-op: ICU care, 2nd look next day

Superior Mesenteric Artery Thrombosis
  MCC – atherosclerosis
  Usually have history of **chronic problems:**
    Food fear from mesenteric angina (see below)
      Visceral angina occurs 30 minutes after meals
    Weight loss
    Other **peripheral vascular disease present** (weak distal pulses)
    Possible **hypercoaguable state**
  Angio → MC the proximal jejunum is involved (need lateral view)
    See thrombus right at origin of SMA
    Usually have **2 vessel DZ** w/ mesenteric thrombosis
    If **no peritoneal signs** and **< 8 hours** – **PTA w/ stent** *(best initial Tx)*
    Use angio to determine how far along the SMA to plug into for bypass
      if you can't PTA
    Look at celiac and IMA as well (made need to bypass one of these as
      well; MC the celiac)
  Tx:
    a. **Stabilize pt** as outlined above (fluid resuscitation, abx's, ect.)
    b. **PTA ± stent** w/ selective intra-arterial **thrombolytic infusion** (tPA)
      Criteria – No peritoneal signs and < 8 hours since pain onset
      If peritoneal sx' develop or sx's don't improve in 4 hours → OR
      Need to get **guidewire** and **infusion catheter** through clot 1st
    c. **OR if above fails →**
      Finding the SMA (same as SMA embolism)
      Usually need to bypass the obstruction
        Many options for this
        Could also perform endarterectomy
        Basic principle is to hook into **non-diseased arterial
          system** (aorta normally, can also used the iliac
          vessels) and **bypass the stenotic area** w/ either
          PTFE or saphenous vein graft
      Resect compromised bowel
      Dusky → leave and wait for 2nd look
      Black → rsxn
        Perform ostomies or leave bowel stapled in abdomen until
          2nd look
        No anastomoses (safest move; take down in 6-8 weeks;
          risk of breakdown due to previous poor flow)
      Post-op: ICU care and **2nd look next day**
Non-Occlusive Mesenteric Ischemia (NOMI)
  Etiologies – spasm, low flow states, hypovolemia, hemoconcentration,
    Digoxin, high dose pressors, cocaine, sepsis → final common
    pathway is **low cardiac output state** to visceral vessels
  RFs – prolonged shock, CHF, prolonged cardiopulmonary bypass
  Sx's: abd pain
  Tx:
    Stabilize pt as outlined above (fluid resuscitation, abx's, ect.)
    Glucagon, papavarine, nitrates can increase visceral blood flow
      (can give these directly through the angio catheter used to
      make diagnosis)
    Optimize C.O. (Swan, a-line, foley; Fluid, Dopamine, Dobutamine)
    ICU care
    Go to OR for peritoneal signs with resection of necrotic bowel
Mesenteric Vein Thrombosis
  Usually **short segments** of intestine involved
  Bloody diarrhea, crampy abdominal pain
  RFs – vasculitis, hypercoaguable state, portal HTN, inflammation
    (pancreatitis, peritonitis), pregnancy, or trauma history
  Dx: Angio – need venous phase
  Tx:
    Stabilize pt as outlined above (fluid resuscitation, abx's, ect.)
    Heparin, possibly systemic thrombolytics

Optimize C.O. Fluid, Dopamine, Dobutamine)

Can try mesenteric vein thrombectomy if diagnosed early

Go to OR for peritoneal signs, resection of necrotic bowel and 2nd look next day

Chronic mesenteric angina

Sx's: abd pain and **weight loss** (secondary to **food fear**)

Pain occurs 15-30 minutes after meals

Dx: angio (almost always have **2 vessel DZ**; eg celiac and SMA)

Need **lateral visceral vessel aortography** to see origins of celiac and SMA

Arc of Riolan - important direct collateral between SMA and celiac

Tx: PTA + stent *(best Tx);* may need bypass graft

Median Arcuate Ligament syndrome

Results in **celiac** compression

Hear a bruit near epigastrium; have chronic pain, weight loss, diarrhea

Tx: transect median arcuate ligament, possible need for arterial reconstruction

Other colon diseases

Colitis – *Salmonella, Shigella, Campylobacter,* CMV, other viral infections, *Giardia*

TB enteritis – presents like Crohn's (stenoses)

Tx: 5 drug therapy; surgery with obstruction

Yersinia infection – mimics appendicitis; fever, RLQ abd pain, N/V

Causes **mesenteric lymphadenitis** (MC organism)

Usually have **diarrhea, no peritoneal signs**

Comes from contaminated food (feces/urine)

Usually in **children**

CT scan shows **enlarged lymph nodes**

Tx: tetracycline or Bactrim

Megacolon

Risk for volvulus; enlargement proximal to non-peristalsing bowel

Hirschsprung's disease – rectosigmoid most common. Dx: rectal biopsy

Trypanosome cruzi (Chagas Disease) – MC acquired cause, secondary to destruction of nerves in Auerbach's plexus

Chilaiditi's Syndrome – loop of colon goes above liver and can be confused w/ free air; will see haustra

RECTUM and ANUS

Anus arterial supply – inferior rectal artery
Venous drainage
> Above dentate – internal hemorrhoid plexus
> Below dentate – external hemorrhoid plexus

Nodal Drainage
> Superior and middle rectum – IMA nodes
> Lower rectum – primarily IMA nodes, also to internal iliac nodes
> **Upper 2/3 anal canal** (above dentate) – internal iliac, pelvic nodes
> **Lower 1/3 anal canal** (below dentate) – inguinal nodes

Dentate line – transition from columnar to stratified squamous epithelium

Hemorrhoids

> Left lateral, right anterior, and right posterior hemorrhoidal plexuses
> **External hemorrhoids** can cause pain when they thrombose
>> Are distal to dentate line
>> Covered by sensate squamous epithelium; cause pain, swelling, itching
>> Do not band external hemorrhoids (painful)
> **Internal hemorrhoids** cause bleeding or prolapse
>> **Primary** – slides below dentate w/ strain
>> **Secondary** – prolapse reduces spontaneously
>> **Tertiary** – prolapse must be manually reduced
>> **Quaternary** – can't reduce

Tx:
> High fiber diet, stool softeners, sitz baths, lidocaine jelly
> **Surgical indications:**
>> **Thrombosed external hemorrhoid** → lance open to relieve pain
>> **Recurrent bleeding**
>> **Large external component**
>> **Moderate to severe pain**
> 1) Can **band** primary and secondary internal hemorrhoids
> 2) **Hemorrhoidectomy** for **tertiary + quaternary internal hemorrhoids**
>> Resect down to **internal sphincter** in all 3 areas (taking the mucosa and submucosa)
>> If anal canal getting tight, consider only doing 2 quadrants: make sure you can insert 3 fingers after resecting hemorrhoids

Post-op – stool softeners, bulk fiber, sitz baths, lidocaine jelly

Cx's
> **Urinary retention** (MC Cx following hemorrhoidectomy, 20%)
>> **Pelvic musculature spasm** after local anesthesia wears off
>> **RFs** – DM, females, large extent of resection, pre-op urinary issues
>> **Post op pain control** and **limiting fluids** intra-op helps reduce this
>> **Tx:** place urinary catheter
> **Eschar can slough post-op** causing **light bleeding late** (5-10 days)
>> **Tx:** stool softeners to avoid local trauma; avoid ASA and NSAIDs
>> **Significant bleeding** needs an exam under anesthesia

Anal fissure

> Caused by a **split in the anoderm** from large, hard stools
> **90% in posterior midline**
> **Sx's:**
>> Occurs w/ **straining bowel movements** (eg **constipation** due to heavy narcotic use after back surgery, perineal surgery, etc)
>> **Pain** and **bleeding** after defecation
>> **Chronic ones** usually have a **sentinel pile**
>> **Anoscopy + rectal exam** to confirm Dx (**pain** reproduced w/ **rectal exam**)
> **Medical Tx** (90% heal)
>> **Sitz baths**
>> **Bulk** and **water hydration**
>> **Lidocaine jelly**
>> **Stool softeners** (colace)

NTG cream (for chronic ones)

Avoid suppositories (cause irritation, pain)

Surgical Tx: lateral subcutaneous internal sphincterotomy

Do _NOT_ go past the dentate line

Do _NOT_ go through the mucosa

Do _NOT_ cut external sphincter

Feel for groove between internal and external sphincter

Use 11 blade to make a transverse cut

Fecal incontinence is most serious cx of surgery; bleeding, infection

Lateral or recurrent fissures → Worry about inflammatory bowel DZ, STD's, or infection (rule these out)

Do _not_ perform sphincterotomy if secondary to Crohn's disease

Anal cancer

Association with **HPV** and previous **XRT**

The **dentate line** is an important landmark for how SCCA is treated

1) **Anal Canal Lesions** (above dentate line)

Squamous Cell CA (eg Epidermal CA, Mucoepidermoid, Basaloid, Cloacogenic)

Sx's: pruritis, bleeding, palpable mass

Dx: get Bx of lesion, Abd CT, CXR, and LFT's

Tx:

Chemo-XRT 1st line _(NOT surgery)_

a) **Nigro protocol**: **Chemo** (5-FU and mitomycin) + **XRT**

This cures 80%.

Need to get FNA of clinically positive **inguinal nodes** and **spread the XRT field** to include the inguinal area if CA is present

b) **Re-Bx anal area** 1 month after chemo-XRT as well as inguinal FNA if pt had previous positive nodes

→ give another cycle of chemo-XRT if either is positive

c) **Re-Bx the anal area** again 1 month after 2nd cycle of chemo-XRT as well as inguinal FNA if patient had previous positive nodes

If **anal area** still positive → APR

If **inguinal nodes** still positive → **inguinal LN dissection** (see Skin and Soft tissue chp for technique)

If **Cloquet's node** (in the femoral sheath) is positive or abd CT shows **bulky iliac and obturator nodes** →iliac and obturator node dissection

Adenocarcinoma

Dx: get Bx of lesion, Abd CT, CXR, and LFT's

Tx: APR usual

WLE if :

< 4 cm

less then 1/3 circumference

Limited to **submucosa** (T1 lesions only)

Well-differentiated

No vascular/lymphatic invasion

Need apx **2-3 mm margin**

Post-op chemo-XRT same as rectal CA

Melanoma

3rd MC site for melanoma (skin and eyes #1 and #2)

30% have spread to **mesenteric lymph nodes**

Hematogenous spread to **liver + lungs** early (most deaths)

MC sx – rectal bleeding

Most tumors lightly **pigmented or no pigment at all**

Perform mets w/u before resection (eg abd/chest CT)

Tx: **Thick melanoma** (> 4 mm) **– APR**

Thin (superficial) **melanoma** (< 1 mm) – local resection

Intermediate melanoma (1-4 mm) – case by case; APR safest

2) **Anal Margin Lesions** (<u>below</u> dentate line)
Better prognosis than anal canal lesions
Squamous cell and **Basal cell** CA treated similar to other skin CA
Paget's often a marker for a **separate internal malignancy**

Squamous cell CA
Sx's: ulcerating, slow growing; **better prognosis** than anal canal CA
MC Met's – inguinal nodes
Dx: Biopsy
Tx:
Lesions < 5 cm (T1 and T2) and **negative nodes** →
WLE w/ **1-2 cm margin** *(No APR → follow below)*
Lesions > 5 cm (T3), **involving sphincter** (T4; fixed lesion,
would require APR), **positive nodes,** *or* **recurrence** →
1) **Induction chemo-XRT** (5-FU + cisplatin)
2) **XRT to inguinal nodes** if positive (get inguinal lymph
node Bx if clinically suspicious nodes)
3) **APR** if above fails
5-YS for node positive DZ – 80%
Sphincter preservation in 80%

Bowen's Disease
Intra-epidermal squamous cell CA (eg Erythroplasia of Queyrat)
Does <u>NOT</u> invade dermis
Almost always associated w/ **HPV**
HPV **6** and **11** can cause high grade anal intra-epithelial neoplasia
(can eventually degenerate into SCCA – see above for tx)
Dx Biopsy
Tx:
High grade Bowen's
Imiquimod
Topical 5-FU
Cautery ablation
Avoid wide excision (high recurrence rate due to HPV
infection even w/ wide margins)
Follow these lesions w/ regular Bx's (monitor for CA)
WLE w/ clear margins reserved for:
Malignant transformation (SCCA)
Intractable sx's (intractable itching, crusting, burning)
NO APR for just Bowen's DZ

Paget's Disease (extra-mammary Paget's Disease)
Intra-epidermal adenocarcinoma (has positive PAS stain)
Origin is underlying **apocrine glands** or **separate internal CA**
Does <u>NOT</u> invade dermis although is **slowly progressive** and can
encompass whole anal area
Often a marker for a **separate internal malignancy** (eg rectal
adenocarcinoma)
Sx's: can have intractable itching; slow growing; can often be
confused w/ **chronic dermatitis**
Dx: Biopsy
Tx:
WLE w/ clear margins
If too extensive, **cautery ablation** (or CO2 laser)
NO APR just for Paget's (although if a separate internal
malignancy is found, APR may be necessary)
Many of these pts have or will develop a separate colorectal CA
Check for and follow for other internal and external CA (eg
associated low rectal adenocarcinoma)
Extra-mammary Paget's Disease
MC sites – genital (eg vulva, penis), perianal, axilla
Often patchy looking
If left untreated, is a slowly progressive DZ

Condylomata acuminata (genital wart)

> Cauliflower mass; papillomavirus (95% → **HPV type 6 or 11**)
> **Dx:** Biopsy
> **Tx:** laser surgery, Imiquimod, Gardasil vaccination to prevent
> ***No APR for just condylomata acuminata***
> **Giant type** (felt to be low grade verrucous carcinoma, seen in HIV
> pts, does <u>not</u> have mets) – need WLE

Basal Cell CA – central ulcer, raised edges, rare mets

> Tx: WLE usually sufficient w/ 3-5 mm margins
>   Rare need for APR unless sphincter involved

Anal incontinence

Neurogenic (gaping hole w/ laxity of levators, eg spinal cord injury)

> No good treatment (possible colostomy)

Abdominoperineal descent

> Trauma to levator ani, puborectalis, and external anal sphincter muscles +
> pudendal nerves

Anus falls below levators

MCC – vaginal childbirth

Tx:

> **High fiber diet, Bulk** (limit to 1 BM/d)
> This type can be surgically repaired w/ anterior sphincteroplasty

Anterior Sphincteroplasty

> Place in lithotomy
> Begin dissection in **anterior 1/2 of anus** between internal and
> external sphincters
> Need to watch for the internal pudendal nerves bilaterally (lateral)
> Dissect out **external sphincter, puborectalis mm**, and **distal
> levator ani muscles**
>> Overlap these muscles w/ silk sutures to tighten the sphincter
>> These muscles were displaced laterally from the trauma
>> Wrap over a Hegar dilator to avoid stenosis
>> **Tightening of external sphincter** biggest component

Stenosis post-op

> **Tx:** sitz baths, bulk, lidocaine jelly, stool softeners
> **Anal dilatation under anesthesia** over several weeks
> Can be mucosal or muscle stenosis; if mucosal, can resect and
> take flap from surrounding skin to cover if not improving
> w/ dilatation

Abscesses (peri-rectal and peri-anal)

Can be very painful on exam

Abscess **superior** to **levator ani muscles**

> → drain through the **rectum** (send for cultures and cytology if appropriate)

Abscess **inferior** to **levator ani muscles**

> → drain through the **skin** (send for cultures and cytology if appropriate)
> **Infra-levator abscesses**
>> **Perianal**
>> **Intersphincteric** – can form horseshoe abscess
>> **Ischiorectal abscesses** – can form horseshoe abscess
>> **Horseshoe abscess** – abscess has horseshoe appearance
>> (between internal and external sphincters)

Need to R/O fistulo in ano

> Drain the abscess as above
> Probe w/ a coronary probe to find possible hole
> Inject saline into abscess and look inside anus to see if there is a
> connection

Abx's for cellulitis, DM, pt's w/ hardware (eg prosthetic valve)

WTD dressings and try to heal from the bottom up

Horseshoe abscess do <u>not</u> need an extensive incision, they will drain through the
opening you make

Perianal Fistulas and Perirectal Fistulas (fistulo in ano)

Sx's:

Can present as a **perianal or perirectal abscess** or as **fistula w/ soiling**
Need to look for a fistula in pts w/ abscess

Goodsall's Rule

Posterior fistulas (90% of fistulas) connect to anus at posterior midline
Anterior fistulas connect to the anus in a straight line
Fistulas that are <u>not</u> posterior and in midline → need to r/o
inflammatory bowel DZ (colonoscopy, UGI w/ SBFT, possible
enteroclysis)

Dx:

Probe previous abscess (if present) w/ coronary probe to find possible hole
Inject saline into abscess and look inside anus to see if there is a
connection

Trouble finding it or recurrent:

MRI *(best test)* to R/O **abscess** and define fistula (percutaneous
drain abscess if present)
Endoscopy w/ EUS to fully **define fistula** and look for **abscess**

Tx:

Superficial fistulas (simple fistulas, most cases)
Fistulas in **lower 1/3 of external anal sphincter** (internal opening
below dentate line)
Make sure any associated **abscess is drained**
Opening up the tract will <u>not</u> have an impact on incontinence
→ **Unroof fistula** – can just place a probe through the fistula and un-
roof it using the probe as a guide
Curettage out the fistula tissue and let it close by 2° intention
This method is safe as long as you are not cutting through the
external sphincter too much

Deep fistulas (complex fistulas)
Fistulas in **upper 2/3 of external anal sphincter** (internal opening
above dentate line)
Make sure any associated **abscess is drained**
Do <u>NOT</u> just unroof or cut through fistula – causes <u>incontinence</u>
→**Rectal mucosa advancement flap** *(best surgical Tx)* to cover
internal opening (mucosa over opening is excised and rectal
mucosa advancement flap covers area), curettage out
remaining fistula tract
Another option is placing a vessel loop **Seton stitch** (goes through
fistula) for 6-8 weeks to allow drainage, remove Seton, closure
of internal opening, curettage out tract
Note - Setons used to be tightened over time to cut through the tract
but no longer done due to high rate of **incontinence**

Levator ani muscle forms the pelvic floor and turns into the **puborectalis** then
the **external sphincter**
Internal sphincter is continuation of the **circular band** of muscle in the colon
Central tendon separates vagina and external sphincter

Anorecto-vaginal fistulas

Causes:

Obstetrical trauma (MCC), others - infection, IBD, XRT, CA
You need to figure out the cause before you start treating this
(Crohn's Disease → see Small Bowel chp for Tx)

Dx:

Find source of problem if not due to trauma:
Abd CT – looking for CA or IBD
Barium enema
Pelvic U/S
Bx both ends of fistula; looking for CA, IBD, infection
Cystoscopy to R/O entero-cystic fistulas if suspected
Consider **MRI** to define fistula and R/O **abscess** (drain if present)
Consider **Endoscopy w/ EUS** to fully **define fistula** and look for **abscess**

Simple:
>**Low to mid vagina**
>Secondary to obstetrical **trauma or infection**
>**Tx:**
>>Many obstetrical ones heal spontaneously (allow 6-8 weeks of conservative Tx)
>>If due to **inflammatory bowel DZ,** can try 6-8 weeks of aggressive Tx before surgery – may heal
>>**Rectal advancement flap** (trans-anal approach)
>>>Used if medical tx fails
>>>Lift a flap of mucosa and internal sphincter
>>>Cut out fistula hole
>>>Approximate internal sphincter that remains in rectal wall to cover remaining fistula hole
>>>Suture flap (containing internal sphincter + mucosa) into place (will end up w/ a double layer of internal sphincter muscle)

Complex:
>**High** in **vagina**
>Pts w/ **previous XRT or CA**
>**Tx:**
>>Abdominal or combined perineal approach usual
>>**Resection and re-anastomosis of bowel** w/ placement of temporary loop ileostomy
>>**Close vagina primarily**
>>Need good tissue for anastomosis
>>Interpose omentum between the rectum and vagina if possible

Rectal prolapse
>Secondary to **pudendal neuropathy** and **laxity of anal sphincter + pelvic floor**
>**RFs** – laxative abuse, multiparous, straining, females, long standing diarrhea, age, COPD (coughing)
>Prolapse starts 6–7 cm from anal verge
>**Types**
>>**Full-thickness rectal prolapse** – entire rectum protruding through anus
>>**Mucosal prolapse** – just rectal mucosa (not entire wall)
>>**Internal intussusception** – rectum collapses but does not exit anus
>**Tx:**
>>**High fiber diet** and **stool softeners** (prevent straining)
>>**For full thickness prolapse** (all layers of bowel wall) _and_ have to manually reduce or can't manually reduce →
>>>1) **Old frail lady** → **Altemeier procedure** (pull rectum out anus, resect it, then primary anastomosis)
>>>2) **Good condition pt – Low anterior resection** and **pexy of residual colon** (possible **just pexy** if little redundant sigmoid)
>>**Incarcerated rectal prolapse not manually reducible** – **sugar (sucrose)** used as osmotic agent to reduce edema and size, can then reduce, bowel prep, and go for elective procedure
>>If above fails or if viability of bowel in question → **LAR or Altemeier**

Pilonidal cysts
>Sinus or abscess formation over sacrococcygeal junction
>MC in men; often get infected; contain **hair**
>**Tx:** abx's, drainage, and packing; follow-up surgical resection of cyst

AIDS anorectal problems
>**Kaposi's sarcoma** – see purple nodule with ulceration
>>**MC CA in pts w/ AIDS** (see Skin and Soft Tissue chp)
>**CMV** – see shallow ulcers. Tx: ganciclovir
>**HSV** – MC rectal ulcer
>**B cell lymphoma** – can look like an abscess or ulcer
>Need biopsies of these ulcers to figure out the problem

HERNIAS

Inguinal Anatomy
External abdominal oblique fascia
- Forms the **inguinal ligament** (inferior portion of inguinal canal → shelving edge)
- Forms roof (anterior portion) of inguinal canal
- You cut through this to get to the inguinal canal

Internal abdominal oblique
- **Muscle portion** forms cremasteric muscles
- **Fascia** combines w/ **transversalis fascia** to form the **conjoined tendon**, which serves as the **floor** of the inguinal canal

Transversalis fascia
- Along w/ **conjoined tendon** forms inguinal canal floor
- Beneath this are the femoral vessels

Inguinal ligament (ie Poupart's ligament)
- Arises from external abdominal oblique fascia
- Runs from anterior superior iliac spine to the pubis
- This is anterior to where the femoral vessels exit the pelvis
- Forms inferior portion of inguinal canal

Lacunar ligament – where inguinal ligament splays and insert into pubis
- Connects the inguinal and pectineal ligaments (forms an arc)
- Femoral vessels and nerve go through the arc (between inguinal and pectineal ligaments

Pectineal ligament (ie. Cooper's ligament)
- Posterior to inguinal ligament
- Posterior to the femoral vessels (lies right against the bone)

Conjoined tendon
- Composed of the aponeurosis of the internal abdominal oblique and transversus abdominus muscles
- Along w/ the transversalis muscle, forms the inguinal canal floor

Internal ring – entrance to canal from peritoneum

External ring – exit from canal into scrotum

Hesselbach's triangle
- Rectus muscle, inferior inguinal ligament, and inferior epigastrics
- **Direct hernias** – inferior and medial to epigastric vessels
  - From weakness in abdominal wall; Rare in females
  - Higher **recurrence** than indirect
- **Indirect hernias** - superior and lateral to epigastric vessels
  - **MC type**
  - From persistently patent processus vaginalis
  - Higher risk of **incarceration** than direct
- **Pantaloon hernia** – direct and indirect components
- **Incarcerated hernia** – can lead to bowel strangulation; should be repaired emergently if it can't be reduced
- **Sliding hernias**
  - Visceral peritoneum coming from a retroperitoneal structure makes up part of the sac
  - The retroperitoneal organ is included in the herniated tissue
  - **Males** (MC gender for sliding hernia) – cecum or sigmoid usual
  - **Females** – ovaries (MC) or fallopian tubes usual
  - Bladder can also be found
- **Females w/ ovary in canal**
  - Ligate **round ligament** (lets ovary fall back into pelvis)
  - Return ovary to peritoneum
  - Perform biopsy of ovary if looks abnormal

Vas deferens – runs medial to cord structures

RFs for adult inguinal hernias – age, obesity, heavy lifting, COPD (coughing), constipation, straining (BPH), ascites, pregnancy, peritoneal dialysis

Inguinal Hernia Repair

Bassini – conjoined tendon and transversalis (superior) approximated to inguinal ligament (inferior); reconstructs floor of the inguinal canal

McVay (Cooper's ligament repair) – conjoined tendon and transversalis fascia (superior) approximate to Cooper's ligament (inferior)

Need relaxing incision in external abdominal oblique fascia

Lichtenstein repair – mesh reforms inguinal canal floor; sewn between conjoined tendon and inguinal ligament; **recurrence ↓ed** (↓tension)

Laparoscopic inguinal hernia repair

Dissect peritoneum off abdominal wall

Starting at pubic tubercle, horizontal staples in abdominal wall going over to anterior, superior iliac spine (you are outside peritoneum)

Avoid the epigastric vessels

Inferiorly, staple mesh to **inguinal ligament** – avoid area where the spermatic cord and vessels enter inguinal canal (although due need staples medial to this to avoid recurrence)

Close the peritoneum over the mesh

No staples in pubic bone→ can cause post-op pain or ostitis (Tx NSAIDs)

No mesh w/ bowel compromise → can just suture the conjoined tendon to the inguinal ligament

Recurrence rate after laparoscopic repair – 4%

MCC of recurrence after laparoscopic hernia repair →

Medial separation of mesh from fascia at inguinal ligament

Usually because mesh is ***too small***, also failure to attach mesh medially

Want tension free repair

Hernias in infants and children

Just perform high ligation (nearly always indirect)

Open sac prior to ligation to make sure nothing important is in there

Inguinal hernia in elderly (why are they straining?)

Rectal exam and colonoscopy to R/O **colon CA**

BPH – from rectal exam and PSA; **Tx**: prazosin

Severe COPD w/ incarcerated inguinal hernia

Can repair under **local** w/ anesthetic injection into the **ilioinguinal nerve** (medial to anterior superior iliac spine) and direct injection into groin

Trouble reducing inguinal hernia contents at time of repair **→** options

1) **Divide inguinal ligament at internal ring** (*best option*; repair it later, best for incarcerated indirect hernias) *or*:

2) **Incise into abdominal wall musculature** (external abdominal oblique, internal abdominal oblique, and transversus) staying extra-peritoneal

Help reduce at level of abdominal wall w/ gentle traction

May be useful for direct hernias *or*:

3) Can also perform laparotomy

Find knuckle of incarcerated bowel and inspect (possible laparotomy)

You find a **Femoral hernia** when exploring for inguinal hernia and can't reduce contents **→ Cut through inguinal ligament** and floor of inguinal canal to free up bowel; end up doing a **McVay repair**

Cx's:

Urinary retention – MC early Cx following hernia repair

RF's – males, ↑ed narcotic usage, age

Tx: foley, leg bag if persistent

Constipation – very frequent, give colace w/ pain meds

Wound infection – 1%

Recurrence rate – 1%, lower w/ mesh

Testicular atrophy – MC from dissection of distal component of hernia sac causing vessel disruption; **thrombosis of spermatic cord veins**

MC after indirect hernia repair

Pain after hernia – MC compression of **ilioinguinal nerve**

Tx: local infiltration can be diagnostic and therapeutic

If that doesn't work go in and **resect nerve**

Cord lipomas – remove

Ilioinguinal nerve injury

MC nerve injury after **inguinal hernia repair**

Loss of cremasteric reflex; numbness on ipsilateral penis, scrotum and inner thigh

Nerve usually injured at **external ring**

Nerve is **anterior to cord structures**

Genitofemoral nerve injury

MC nerve injury w/ **laparoscopic hernia repair**

Genital branch

Gives branches to **cremaster** (motor) and **scrotum** (sensory)

Genital branch runs **posterior and inferior to the cord**

Femoral branch

Goes to upper **lateral thigh** (sensory)

Runs **lateral to iliac vessels**

Femoral hernia

Sx's: mass just below inguinal ligament

Femoral canal boundaries:

Superior – inguinal ligament

Inferior – pectineal ligament

Medial – lacunar ligament (attaches to the pubis; connect the inguinal and pectineal ligaments)

Lateral – femoral vein

Femoral canal structures

NAVEL (lateral to medial) – femoral nerve, femoral artery, femoral vein, empty space, lymphatics

High risk of incarceration → may need to **divide inguinal ligament** to reduce bowel

Hernia passes under the inguinal ligament

Have characteristic **bulge** on anterior-medial thigh **below ligament**

Can repair w/ **McVay** or **low inguinal approach**

Ventral hernias

Ventral hernia repairs can be major operations

Can present as a **large abdominal mass** after operation

CT scan to confirm ventral hernia

RFs – obesity, smoking, COPD, previous hernia repair (esp large defects)

Laparoscopic repair *(best Tx option)*

Avoids big incision, helps w/ post-op recovery

Open Hassan in LUQ for 1st port, insufflate; find optimal place for ports

Take down adhesions and bowel

Find fascia, cut and place mesh in the abdomen

Dual mesh – smooth PTFE on inside so bowel doesn't stick; marlex interstices on outside for fibroblast in-growth

Prolene sutures to hold the mesh up, then place **screw tacks**

No mesh w/ bowel compromise – just repair enterotomy and close (abx's, back in 6 weeks)

0.1% incidence of placing veress needle or trocar into bowel / blood vessel

If overlying skin is necrotic from pressure →

Place on Abx's and remove this area w/ hernia repair

Need **compartment repair** *(best option*, separates the abdominal wall muscle compartments to cover the defect)

Primary repair also an option (20% recurrence)

*Do **not** place mesh w/ necrotic area* (infected)

Skin graft placed over bowel after necrotizing fasciitis and now has hernia → leave it alone

MCC ventral hernia recurrence after repair (5%) – separation of mesh from posterior fascia

MC Cx after ventral hernia repair – seroma (can cause bulge) – leave unless very symptomatic (Tx: aspiration)

Other hernias
Umbilical hernia
RFs – African-Americans; males; Obesity or ascites in adults
Tend to **close spontaneously in children** (esp if < 2.5 cm)
Delay repair until **age 5**
Risk of incarceration is in adults, <u>not</u> children

Spigelian hernia (ie lateral ventral hernia)
Lateral border of rectus muscle (hernia through **linea semi-lunaris**)
Almost always **inferior to semi-circularis band** (ie below umbilicus, lacks of posterior sheath)
Occurs in **internal abdominal oblique aponeurosis** w/ the rectus muscle
Usually **no bulge**, high risk of **incarceration**, MC on **right**

Sciatic hernia (posterior pelvis)
Herniation through **greater sciatic foramen**
Sx's: uncomfortable **mass in gluteal area**
Bowel obstruction may also occur, high rate of strangulation

Obturator hernia (anterior pelvis)
Herniation through **obturator canal**
Sx's: elderly **women**, multiparous, bowel gas below superior pubic ramus
Howship-Romberg sign – inner thigh pain w/ internal rotation *(classic)*
Tx:
> Operative reduction, may need mesh
> Check other side for similar defect
> Dx usually made at time of surgery for small bowel obstruction

Richter's hernia - non-circumferential incarceration of nonmesenteric bowel wall
Can cause **bowel strangulation** and **perforation <u>w/o</u> obstruction**

Petit's hernia – inferior lumbar triangle hernia, borders:
External abdominal oblique
Latissimus dorsi (or lumbodorsal aponeurosis)
Iliac crest

Grynfelt-Lesshaft hernia – superior lumbar triangle hernia
Internal abdominal oblique
Lumbodorsal aponeurosis
12th rib (or posterior lumbocostal ligament)

Littre's hernia – incarcerated Meckel's Diverticulum

Incisional hernia – MC type to recur; inadequate closure most common cause

Parastomal hernia
↑ed w/ **colostomies** compared to ileostomies
> ****50% five-year incidence for colostomies**
> **RFs** – fascial opening too large; stoma lateral to rectus sheath, obesity, COPD, Age

Do <u>not</u> need to fix these unless symptomatic – generally well tolerated
Absolute repair indications – obstruction; incarceration w/ strangulation
Relative repair indications – incarceration, severe prolapse, stenosis, intractable dermatitis, pain, cosmesis, difficulty w/ stoma appliance
Tx:
> Generally, **relocating the ostomy** is the preferred tx
> **True hernias** – remove and place in rectus muscle
> **Pseudohernia** – secondary to being in the oblique muscle; need to move to rectus
> **Prolapse** – keep stoma at same site, fix mesentery (ostomy is in rectus and the fascia is intact but bowel is prolapsing through)

Rectus sheath
Anterior – complete sheath from costal cartilages to pubis
Posterior – absent below semicircularis (below umbilicus)
Anterior portion – external abdominal + internal abdominal oblique aponeurosis
Posterior portion – internal abdominal oblique + transversalis aponeurosis

Rectus sheath hematomas
Usually after trauma; epigastric vessel injury
Painful abdominal wall mass, may have overlying discoloration
Mass more prominent + painful w/ **rectus muscle flexion** (Fothergill's sx)
Tx: non-operative usual, surgery if expanding (ligate epigastric vessels)

UROLOGY

Gerota's fascia – fascia that encloses the kidney
Anterior to posterior structures – renal vein, renal artery, renal pelvis
    Right renal artery crosses posterior to the IVC
    Left renal vein crosses anterior to the aorta (MC)
Ureters cross **over iliac vessels**
Left renal vein – can be ligated from IVC
    Has collaterals (left adrenal vein, left gonadal vein, left ascending lumbar vein)
    Right renal vein does not have these collaterals and cannot be safely ligated
Epididymis – connect the efferent ducts at the rear of each testicle to vas deferens
Seminal vesicles – are connected to the vas deferens
MCC renal insufficiency following surgery – hypotension intra-op

Kidney Stones
    Sx's: severe colicky pain, restlessness
    Dx:
        UA – blood or stones
        Abd CT – stones and associated hydronephrosis
            90% opaque
    Types of stones
        1) **Calcium oxalate stones** (radio-opaque)
            MC kidney stone (75%)
            ↑ed after **terminal ileum resection** due to **oxalate reabsorption** in
                colon
            Prevention
                ↑ **fluids, urine alkalinization** (potassium citrate) and **oxalate**
                    restriction after terminal ileum resection
        2) **Magnesium ammonium phosphate stones** (15%; radio-opaque)
            Struvite stones
            Associated w/ **kidney infections** and **urea splitting organisms** such
                as *Proteus mirabilis*
            Can cause **staghorn calculi** that fill the renal pelvis
            Prevention – ↑ **fluids** and **abx's**
        3) **Uric acid stones** (7%; radio-lucent)
            RFs – gout, ileostomies, short gut, thiazide diuretics,
                myeloproliferative D/Os
            W/ ileostomy, loss of alkaline fluid from ileostomy lowers urinary pH
                and volume, leading to uric acid stone formation.(short gut
                similar mechanism)
            Prevention: ↑ **fluids, urine alkalinization** (potassium citrate) and
                allopurinol
        4) **Cysteine stones** (2%; radio-dense to radiolucent)
            Are associated w/ **congenital disorders** of cysteine metabolism
            Prevention –
                ↑ **fluids**
                Urine alkalinization (potassium citrate)
                Penicillamine
                Tiopronin (↓s rate of cysteine solidification and excretion)
    Surgery for kidney stones:
        Intractable pain or infection
        Progressive obstruction
        Progressive renal damage
        Solitary kidney
        > 6 mm not likely to pass
        Tx:
            ESWL *(best therapy*; extracorporeal shock wave lithotripsy)
            Ureteroscopy w/ stone extraction or placement of stent past stone
                obstruction
            Percutaneous nephrostomy tube (temporary)
            Open nephrolithotomy or urethrotomy (last resort)

Testicular cancer

MCC cancer death in men 25-35

Vast majority of solid tumors of testicles are malignant

90% of tumors are **germ cell** – seminoma or non-seminoma

Undescended testicles (crypto-orchidism) – ↑s risk of testicular CA

> MC get seminoma

Sx's: painless hard mass *(classic)* ± gynecomastia

Dx:

> Cardinal finding is **mass in substance of testis**
>
> > 95% of solid testicular tumors are **malignant**
>
> **U/S** *(1st test)* – make sure not a hydrocoele (will transluminate if so)
>
> **Labs** *(get before orchiectomy so you have levels)* – **AFP, B-HCG,** and
> > **LDH** (correlates w/ tumor bulk)
>
> **Orchiectomy**
>
> > Through an **inguinal incision** (*not trans-scrotal* → do not want to
> > > disrupt lymphatics)
> >
> > *****The testicle and attached mass are the biopsy specimen***
> > Do not stick a needle through scrotum to get Dx
>
> Once Dx of CA made, need **CT chest/abd/pelvis** to check for
> > retroperitoneal and mediastinal tumor burden + mets

**Overall 5-YS survival – 90% (100% if no mets, 85% w/ mets)

> Seminoma better survival than non-seminomatous

Seminoma

> **MC testicular tumor**
>
> 10% have beta-HCG elevation
>
> ***No AFP elevation*** (if elevated, tx like non-seminomatous)
>
> Spreads to retroperitoneum
>
> ****Seminoma is extremely sensitive to XRT**
>
> **Tx:**
>
> > **All stages get:**
> >
> > > 1) **Orchiectomy** *and;*
> > > 2) **Retroperitoneal XRT** (para-aortic and ipsilateral pelvic)
> > > > Gets occult **retroperitoneal mets**
> > > > If **para-aortic nodes** in abdomen enlarged, extend XRT
> > > > > to **mediastinum**
> >
> > **Chemo** (cisplatin, bleomycin, etoposide) reserved for either:
> > > **Systemic mets** *or*
> > > **Bulky retroperitoneal or mediastinal nodes**
> > **Surgical resection** of **residual mets** after chemo-XRT

Non-seminomatous testicular CA

> Types – teratoma, choriocarcinoma, yolk sac, embryonal
>
> **AFP** and **beta-HCG** – elevated in 90%
>
> Spreads hematogenously to **lungs**
>
> Spreads to **retroperitoneum**
>
> Tumors w/ increased **teratoma components** more likely to metastasize to
> > **retroperitoneum**
>
> XRT never used as primary tx for non-seminomatous
>
> **Tx:**
>
> > **Stage I**
> >
> > > 1) **Orchiectomy** *and;*
> > > 2) **Retroperitoneal lymph node dissection** (prophylactic; this
> > > > is Stage II or greater if tumor is present)
> >
> > **Stage II or greater:**
> >
> > > 1) **Orchiectomy**
> > > 2) **Retroperitoneal lymph node dissection** (para-aortic +
> > > > ipsilateral pelvic)
> > > 3) **Chemo** (cisplatin, bleomycin, etoposide)
> > > 4) Surgical resection of residual mets after chemo

Other testicular tumors – Non-Hodgkins lymphoma (older pt)

MC location for primary extra-gonadal germ cell tumor – mediastinum (see
> Thoracic chp)

Prostate Cancer

MC CA in US for men
2nd MCC CA death in men (#1 - lung CA)
Lifetime risk – 15%
Lifetime risk of dying from prostate CA – 3%
RFs – age, Fam Hx, African-Americans
Sx's:
> Asymptomatic (MC)
> Obstructive
> Irritative (frequency, dysuria, urgency)
> Hematuria, erectile dysfunction

Screening – mortality benefit from screening <u>not</u> established (DRE or PSA)
> **PSA**
>> Not very specific or sensitive
>> 15% of Stage I prostate CA have PSA < 4 and normal DRE
>> Offer to men $\geq$ 50 (or high risk $\geq$ 45) and life expectancy > 10 years
>> **PSA** can be ↑ed w/ prostatitis, BPH, and chronic catheterization

Dx
> **TRUS w/ Bx** (6-12 Bx's) – histology correlates w/ prognosis
> **Imaging** to look for spread:
>> **Bone scan** – for PSA > 10, high Gleason grade, clinically advanced tumor, or elevated alk phos
>> **CT abd/pelvis** – poor accuracy in detecting extra-capsular spread and nodes
>> **Endorectal coil MRI** – best for assessment of extra-capsular spread
> **Labs** – alk phos, PSA; ↑ alk phos → ↑ mets or extracapsular DZ
> **Gleason grade** (0 - 10)

Path
> **MC site** – posterior lobe
> **MC mets** – bone (**Osteoblastic** - x-ray demonstrates **hyperdense** area)
> Many pts **impotent** after resection; can get incontinence
> Can also get urethral **strictures**

Tx:
> **Stage I** (Tia – nonpalpable, not on imaging) + **Stage II** (T1 or T2 – both confined to capsule of prostate) *either*:
>> 1) **Watchful waiting** (likely if age >75 or limited life expectancy) <u>or</u>:
>> 2) **XRT** <u>or</u>;
>> 3) **Radical prostatectomy** w/ **pelvic LN dissection** (if lifespan >10 yrs)
> **Stage III** (extends thru capsule)
>> → **XRT + androgen ablation**
> **Stage IV** (invades adjacent structures or mets)
>> → **XRT + androgen ablation**

Androgen deprivation options:
> 1) **Bilateral orchiectomy** *(best therapy)*
> 2) **GnRH analogues** (leuprolide, goserelin) – cause ↓ FSH and ↓LH
> 3) **Anti-androgens** (flutamide, bicalutamide) – block androgen receptor

XRT can help w/ **bone pain** or **local recurrence**
Chemo if hormone refractory
W/ prostatectomy, PSA should go to 0 after **3 weeks** (1/2 life 3 days) → if not, get bone scan to check for mets

Prognosis
> High **PSA level,** high **Gleason grade,** and ↑ **age** are predictors of mets
> 5-year survival (disease-free)
>> | | |
>> |---|---|
>> | Confined to organ | 95% |
>> | Extension through capsule | 75% |
>> | Seminal vesicle invasion | 45% |
> Compared to watchful waiting, surgery ↓s prostate CA mortality and ↓s overall mortality in **pts aged < 75**
> **Mean survival w/ met's** – 2-3 years (all become androgen independent)
Prophylaxis – **Finasteride** ↓'s total number of prostate CA but ↑'s number of high Gleason grade tumors

Renal cell carcinoma (RCCA; hypernephroma)

MC primary tumor of kidney
> **MC kidney tumor** – mets from breast CA

RF – smoking

Sx's: abd pain, mass, and **hematuria** *(classic triad)*; often incidental finding
> other - new onset **left sided varicocele** (L. testicular vein→ L. renal vein)

Dx:
> **CT chest/abd/pelvis**
>> **Disrupts renal contour**
>>> **Can often be fairly certain about RCCA based on CT scan but can <u>not</u> exclude RCCA w/ CT scan
>>
>> *Biopsy <u>not</u> useful* – hard to DDx from oncocytoma; also high risk of bleed (unfavorable risk-benefit ratio)
>> Essentially all masses need some sort of resection (<u>cysts</u> are observed unless complex)

Path
> **Solid tumor** – 90-95% solid renal masses are RCCA
>> **± necrosis**, ± **calcification**
>> **MC subtype** – clear cell (75%)
>> Others – papillary, chromophillc, chromophobic, oncocytic, collecting duct
>
> **MC mets** – lung (30% have **mets** at time of dx)
> **Paraneoplastic syndromes:**
>> **Erythrocytosis** from **erythropoietin** secreting tumors
>> **HTN** from **renin** secreting tumors
>> **Stauffer syndrome** – ↑ed LFTs; improves after successful resection
>> **Others** – PTHrp (hypercalcemia), ACTH (Cushing's), insulin (hypoglycemia)
>
> **Von Hippel–Lindau syndrome** – multifocal and recurrent RCCA (clear cell type), renal cysts, CNS tumors, pheochromocytomas
> **Wide range of 5-year survival** – related to tumor size + degree of spread:
>> **Stage I** (< 4 cm)   > 95%
>> **Stage IV** (eg mets to lungs)   5%
>
> **Oncocytomas** – benign tumors
> **Angiomyolipomas** – benign hamartomas; can occur w/ tuberous sclerosis

Tx:
> **Radical nephrectomy** – Tx of choice for majority
>> Takes kidney, adrenal gland, fat, Gerota's Fascia, and regional nodes
>
> **Consider partial nephrectomy if:**
>> 1) RCCA on **limited area of kidney** (eg < 4 cm) *and;*
>> 2) If total nephrectomy would result in **dialysis** (eg pt creatinine 2.5)
>> **Bilateral small tumors** – partial nephrectomies (avoid dialysis)
>
> **Limited to small part of kidney and not sure if its RCCA**
>> → partial nephrectomy (or enucleation) initially
>> **Path shows RCCA < 4 cm** (stage I) w/ **good margin** → partial nephrectomy only can be performed (esp if elevated creatnine)
>> **Path shows RCCA > stage I** → total nephrectomy
>
> **Chemo-XRT** (doxorubicin based), **interferon** and IL-2 (all marginal benefit)
> **Sunitinib** (for mets or unresectable RCCA)
>> Multi-targeted receptor tyrosine kinase (MRTK) inhibitor
>> Inhibits angiogenesis and proliferation

Special situations
> **Isolated lung mets** – resection
> **RCCA has predilection for growth into IVC** (even right atrium)
>> Can still resect even if going up IVC
>> Pull tumor thrombus out of IVC (± cardiopulmonary bypass)
>
> **Partial nephrectomies**
>> Consider for pts who would require dialysis after nephrectomy
>
> **Embolization** to palliate large tumors or as pre-op for large tumors

Transitional cell CA of renal pelvis – Tx: radical nephroureterectomy

Bladder cancer

Males (4:1); prognosis based on stage and grade
RFs – smoking, aniline dyes, cyclophosphamide, occupational exposure
MC type – transitional cell CA (90%)
Sx's: painless hematuria (*classic*)
Dx:

    UA cytology
    Cystoscopy
    Possible IVP

Tx:

    T1 (muscle <u>not</u> involved)
        Intravesical BCG (or valrubicin) or t**ransurethral resection**
    T2 or greater (muscle involved):
        1) **Cystectomy** (w/ ileal conduit) + **bilateral pelvic lymph node dissection** <u>and</u>;
        2) **Chemo-XRT** (MVAC: methotrexate, vinblastine, Adriamycin cisplatin)
        Men – include **prostatectomy** in resection
        Women – include **TAH + BSO**, and **anterior vaginal wall**
    Mets – chemo-XRT only

Overall 5-YS after <u>cystectomy</u> – 60%
    5-YS for T1 tumors – 95%
Ileal conduit
    Avoid stasis as this predisposes to infection, stones (calcium resorption), ureteral reflux
    Can get **hyperchloremic metabolic acidosis** (NH_4^+ reabsorption)
    ↑s serum – K^+, Ca^{++}, NH_4^+ and Cl^-
    ↓s serum - Na^+
Squamous cell CA of bladder – schistosomiasis

Testicular torsion

Peaks in 15-year-olds
Involved testis often not viable at exploration
    Usually just intravaginal torsion of spermatic cord if viable
Torsion MC is towards midline
Dx:

    U/S – can be used to aid in dx (shows no blood flow to testis)
    If suspicion high → **skip U/S and immediate detorsion**

Tx:

    Trans-scrotal incision
    De-torse testis
    Bilateral **orchiopexy** if testicle viable
    If not, resection and orchiopexy of contralateral testis
    100% viable if within 6 hours

Ureteral trauma

If going to repair end to end:
    Spatulate ends.
    Use **absorbable suture** to avoid stone formation.
    Stent ureter to avoid stenosis
    Place drains
Avoid stripping soft tissue on ureter - compromises blood supply.

Urethral and bladder trauma (see Trauma chp)

Benign prostatic hyperplasia (BPH)

Arises in **transitional zone**
Sx's: nocturia, frequency, dysuria, weak stream, urinary retention
Dx: DRE – enlarged prostate; TRUS
Initial Tx

    Alpha blocker – terazosin (Hytrin), doxazosin (Cardura), relax smooth muscle

5-alpha-reductase inhibitors – finasteride (Proscar), dutasteride (Avodart)
→ inhibits the conversion of testosterone to dihydrotestosterone (inhibits prostate hypertrophy)

Surgery (TURP – trans-urethral resection of prostate)

Indications – recurrent UTIs, gross hematuria, stones, renal insufficiency, failure of medical Tx

Post-TURP syndrome (ie **seizures**)

Hyponatremia secondary to irrigation w/ water (as opposed to normal saline); can precipitate **seizures** from cerebral edema

Tx: careful correction of Na with diuresis (see Fluid / Electrolytes chp)

Most pts w/ TURP have **retrograde ejaculation**

Neurogenic bladder (spastic bladder)

MC secondary to spinal injury
Accidental voiding, often of large amounts of urine
Injury above T-12
Tx: surgery to improve bladder resistance

Neurogenic obstructive uropathy (flaccid bladder)

Incomplete emptying of the bladder, can have frequency
Injury below T-12; can occur with APR
Tx: intermittent catheterization

Urinary Incontinence

Stress incontinence (often w/ cough, sneeze)

MC type of incontinence; MC in women

Pelvic floor weakness leading to hypermobile urethra or **loss of sphincter mechanism**

RFs – multiparous women, age, obesity, prostatectomy

Tx:

Kegel exercises to strengthen pelvic floor

Alpha-adrenergic agents

Surgery for **urethral suspension or pubovaginal sling** (best)

Urge incontinence (urgency or frequency)

Involuntary **detrusor contraction** *without* neurologic disorder

Tx: anticholinergics, behavior modification (timed voiding, bladder training), cystoplasty (rarely needed), urinary diversion (last resort)

Neuropathic incontinence (urgency or frequency)

Detrusor contraction associated w/ **neuro condition** (eg spinal cord dysfunction, stroke, multiple sclerosis)

Leads to **decreased bladder capacity**

Tx: underlying neurologic disorder, behavior modification, anti-cholinergics, intermittent catheterizations, surgical cystoplasty or urinary diversion

Overflow incontinence

Incomplete emptying and enlarged bladder

Obstruction (eg BPH) leads to distention and leakage

Tx: medical tx of BPH, possible TURP

Congenital incontinence – continuous leakage and nocturnal enuresis

Sphincter mechanism is bypassed

Tx: surgical correction (bladder exstrophy, ureteral diversion, etc)

Other urologic diseases

Varicocele – abnormal enlargement of veins draining testis

New onset left sided varicocele – worrisome for **renal cell CA** (left gonadal vein inserts into left renal vein, obstruction by renal tumor causes varicocele)

Can also be from other **intra-abdominal, pelvic, or retroperitoneal malignancy** placing pressure on **gonadal veins**

Is found in scrotum on **posterior portion** of testicle (different from testicular tumor)

↑ **infertility risk** due to thrombosis/compression → **improved fertility w/ high spermatic vein ligation**

Hydrocoele in adult – accumulation of clear fluid in tunica vaginalis
>**New onset adult** (ie secondary hydrocoele) – suspect **testicular tumor**
>Can also occur w/ trauma, infection (eg epididymitis)
>U/S – translucent – look for associated tumor
>MC found on **anterior portion testis**
>No therapy needed for adults if asymptomatic and no significant underlying
>>causes (eg tumor)

Spermatocele
>**MC cystic structure of scrotum**
>Fluid filled cystic structure superior and separate to testis along epididymis
>Tx: surgical removal if symptomatic
>These do <u>not</u> impair fertility

Ureteropelvic obstruction – Tx: pyeloplasty (relieves obstruction)

Vesicoureteral reflux – Tx: re-implantation into bladder w/ long bladder muscle
>portion (prevents reflux)

Ureteral duplication
>**MC urinary tract abnormality**
>Tx: re-implantation in bladder if obstructed
>Not a contra-indication to kidney donation for TXP

Ureterocele
>MC at junction of ureter and bladder
>MC in females
>MC associated w/ **ureteral duplication**
>**Sx's**: UTI's, retention; **Tx:** resect and reimplant ureter in bladder if sx's

Hypospadias – ventral urethral opening
>Tx: repair at 6 months with penile skin

Epispadias – dorsal urethral opening Tx: surgery

Horseshoe kidney – usually joined at lower poles
>**Cx's**: UTI, urolithiasis, hydronephrosis
>**Tx:** may need pyeloplasty for obstruction

Polycystic kidney disease – resection of cysts only if symptomatic
>(decompression of large cysts)

Persistent urachus – connection between umbilicus and bladder
>10% have bladder outlet obstruction (eg wet umbilicus)
>**Dx: voiding cystourethrogram** (will also show any obstruction)
>Tx: resection of sinus and cyst w/ closure of bladder; relieve obstruction

Epididymitis – inflammation or infection of epididymis
>**MCC sudden scrotal pain**
>**U/S –** increased blood flow to epididymis
>**MC infection –** Chlamydia; others – gonorrhea, E coli (Tx: abx's)
>Sterile epididymitis can occur w/ abdominal straining (Tx: NSAIDs)
>Children should be screened for urinary tract abnormality

Pneumaturia
>**MCC –** diverticulitis and subsequent formation of colo-vesical fistula

WBC casts – seen w/ pyelonephritis and glomerulonephritis

RBC casts – just w/ glomerulonephritis

Interstitial nephritis – fever, rash, arthralgias, eosinophils (caused by a variety
>of drugs, viruses, etc)

Vasectomy – 50% pregnancy rate after repair of previous vasectomy

Priapism
>**Tx:** aspiration of corpus cavernosum w/ dilute epinephrine
>May need to create a communication through glans w/ scalpel to relieve
>RFs – sickle cell anemia, hypercoaguable states, trauma, intracorporeal
>>injections for impotence, sildenafil

SCCA of penis – standard care is penectomy w/ 2-cm margin

IV Indigo carmine or methylene blue – can be used to check for urine leak

Phimosis found at time of laparotomy – Tx: need dorsal slit

Erythropoietin – ↓ production in pts w/ chronic renal failure **(low Hct)**

Peyronie's Disease – thick plaques in tunica albuginea cause penile curvature
>**Tx: conservative Tx** for up to 1 year (colchicines, Vit E)
>If that fails to relieve sx's, need **Nesbit operation** (tissue on opposite side
>>of plaque is shortened to straighten curve – *plaque is <u>not</u> excised*)

Normal Anatomy

Fallopian tubes carry ovum from ovaries to uterus

Ampullary portion of fallopian tube → MC site of ectopic pregnancy

Ligaments

Round ligament – maintains **anteversion** of the uterus

Starts at uterus, goes through inguinal canal, eventually attaches to labia majora

Broad ligament – contains uterine vessels

Connects the sides of the uterus to the floor and walls of pelvis

Infundibulopelvic ligament – contains ovarian artery, nerve, and vein

Fold of peritoneum that extends out from ovary to pelvic wall

Cardinal ligament – holds cervix and vagina in place at base of broad ligament; Contains uterine artery and vein

U/S – often study of choice for Dx of disorders of female genital tract

Pregnancy

Can see pregnancy on U/S at **6 weeks**

Gestational sac seen at beta-HCG of **1500**

Fetal pole seen at beta-HCG of **6000**

Mittelschmirtz

Rupture of graffian follicle or follicular swelling

Pain can be confused w/ appendicitis

Occurs 14 days after 1st day of menses

Negative pelvic exam and negative U/S

Tx: Nothing

If already in OR for RLQ pain and you find this, perform appendectomy and close

Not sure if Graffian Follicle:

4 quadrant wash, send for cytology

Bx cyst wall (or mass)

Bx omentum

Look at all visceral surfaces for met's, biopsy these areas, send to cytology

F/U w/ OB

Abortions

Missed

Dx: 1st trimester bleeding, closed os, U/S – positive sac, no heartbeat

Embryo or fetus has died but no miscarriage yet

Threatened – 1st trimester bleeding, positive heartbeat

Possibly due to **subchorionic hematoma** – Tx: bedrest

Incomplete – abortion tissue protrudes through os

Ectopic (see below for management)

Acute abd pain, positive beta-HCG, and negative U/S for sac

Other sx's – missed period, vaginal bleeding, hypotension

RFs – previous tubal manipulation, PID, previous ectopic, smoking

MC location – ampullary portion of fallopian tubes

Life-threatening – hemorrhage and shock can occur

Ectopic Pregnancy

1) **Abdominal/pelvic pain**

2) **Positive B-HCG**

3) **U/S cannot find conception**

4) **Hypotension**

The above = **ruptured ectopic pregnancy → go to the OR**

May be able to see ectopic pregnancy on U/S

Laparoscopy to confirm Dx is an option if pt is stable

Un-ruptured ectopic pregnancy

Salpingotomy, evacuate hematoma, hemostasis, repair tube w/ vicryls

Can also try medical Tx (eg methotrexate) to try and terminate pregnancy

Ruptured ectopic pregnancy – salpingectomy if unstable; o/w salpingotomy as above

Pregnancy and need for surgery

Call OB/GYN to help w/ the problem

If you go to OR, start **tocolytics** only w/ **initiation of pre-term labor** or w/ uterine irritability

Mg drip – need serum levels of **Mg 4-6** (9-13 causes resp depression)

S/Es – pulm edema, resp depression, cardiac arrest

Terbutaline (S/Es – pulm edema, resp depression, cardiac arrest)

Indomethacin enemas (S/Es – GIB)

Nifedipine (PO) – used when off Mg drip (maintenance); S/E - hypotension

Try to stall surgery (if possible, depends on cause) until **2nd trimester**

Too early risk **spontaneous abortion** (1st trimester, 10-15%)

Too late risk **preterm labor** (3rd trimester, 10-15%)

1% risk of fetal demise in 2nd trimester w/ surgery

Place surface fetal heart rate monitor and **a tocodynometer** to monitor strength of contractions

Can also use **trans-vaginal HR monitor** and **tocodynometer**

Normal fetal HR 120-160

Late decelerations – signify a significant **deficit in fetus oxygen supply**

Need to correct this (roll pt to the left and off IVC)

Give volume

Potential C-section

Cefotetan OK w/ pregnancy

Keep pCO_2 low w/ surgery (monitor ET-CO2)

If you have to do fluoro, shield uterus w/ lead (**fluoro sent from below** so shield below pt)

Laparoscopy

Can usually perform w/ pregnancy (although probably not in 3rd trimester)

Keep inflation CO_2 pressure < 15 mmHg

Roll to pt to left and off IVC

Hassan technique for entry – high entry above fundus (above umbilicus)

Avoid touching uterus

Monitor ABG to keep CO_2 low (30-40; *avoids* fetal acidosis)

Need trans-vaginal **fetal HR monitor** and **tocodynometer** (as above)

MC CA during pregnancy – lymphoma

Pregnancy w/ acute cholecystitis

Initial Tx - → abx's and NPO (95% treated w/o intervention)

1st or 3rd trimester – consider percutaneous cholecystostomy tube if refractory to abx's (avoids general anesthesia and surgery risks while relieving problem); cholecystectomy in 2nd trimester or after delivery

2nd trimester – laparoscopic cholecystectomy

If you need **ERCP** – use **uterine shielding**; can perform sphincterotomy and stone retrieval

Pregnancy w/ appendicitis

MC problem requiring surgery with pregnancy

May have **RUQ pain** in 3rd trimester - appendix moves **towards RUQ** w/ pregnancy

Pain may be exacerbated w/ pt lying on **right side**

Dx

Get an U/S 1st (diameter > 7, thickness > 2)

CT scan if that doesn't demonstrate appendicitis

Can perform laparoscopically if in 1st or 2nd trimester; open probably best for 3rd trimester

If open appendectomy, **mark site of incision over the site of maximal pain** before you put pt to sleep - *appendix is displaced superiorly by uterus*

↑**rupture risk** from **misdiagnosis** (esp 3rd trimester, confused w/ contractions)

Appendicitis w/ pregnancy – ↑ risk of premature labor (10-15%) and fetal loss (5-10%); 20-25% fetal mortality w/ ruptured appendix

Pregnancy w/ small bowel obstruction

Sx's: not passing gas, crampy abd pain
Plain films – AFL's, dilated loops (may need serial studies)
Fluid resuscitation (important for the fetus)
NGT decompression
Surgery has more prominent and **earlier role** (90% eventually require
    operation)
    Conservative Tx for 24 hours then go to OR
    Necrotic bowel often found w/ delay in pregnant pts
    Generous laparotomy; avoid manipulation of uterus
    If **volvulus** in present, just pexy unless necrotic, definitive Tx after delivery

Pelvic inflammatory disease

Increased risk of **infertility** and **ectopic pregnancy**
Sx's: pain, N/V, fever, vaginal discharge
MC in first 1/2 of menstrual cycle
RFs – multiple sexual partners
Dx: cervical motion tenderness *(best),* cervical cultures, Gram stain
    Gonococcus – diplococci
    Chlamydia – MC STD; granuloma lymphadenopathy
        Obligate intracellular pathogen
        Can be asymptomatic
Tx: ceftriaxone + doxycycline

HPV – condylomata, vesicles
Syphilis – positive dark-field microscopy, chancre

Tubo-ovarian abscess

Sx's: fevers and chills; **RFs** - previous PID, IUD use
Dx:
    Cervical motion tenderness and **adnexal mass** on pelvic exam
    Get B-HCG to r/o ectopic pregnancy
    U/S for diagnosis
Tx: percutaneous drain + abx's (doxycycline and ceftriaxone)
    If you have to operate (radiology not available or can't get drain) →
        laparotomy, evacuate abscess, place drain, abx's

Ovarian torsion – Dx: U/S Tx: relieve torsion, check for viability; rsxn if necrotic

Incidental ovarian tumor when performing another procedure

Stop
4 quadrant wash, send for cytology
Biopsy mass
Bx omentum
Look at all visceral surfaces for met's, biopsy these areas, Send to cytology
F/U w/ OB or appropriate physician
If original procedure elective (eg laparoscopic gastric bypass) – likely abort
    procedure
If non-elective – finish procedure
Do __NOT__ perform oophrectomy

Endometriosis

Sx's:
    Dysmenorrhea, dyspareunia, and **infertility** *(classic)*
    Rectal involvement can cause bleeding during menses → rectal
        endoscopy shows **blue mass**
    Catamenial PTX – endometriosis in lung that can cause recurrent PTX
MC site – ovaries
Many women w/ infertility have endometriosis
Tx: progesterone, OCP's, Danazol, NSAID's

Ovarian cancer

MCC of gynecologic CA death (non breast CA)
2nd **MC gynecologic CA** (#1 - endometrial CA)
↓ed risk – OCPs, bilateral tubal ligation, multiparous
↑ed risk – nulliparity, late menopause, early menarche, unopposed post-
menopausal estrogen replacement. BRCA,HNPCC, Ashkenazi Jews
Often a **delay in Dx** (60% stage III or IV at Dx)
80% occur in **post-menopausal women**
Sx's: pelvic or abd pain, bloating, feeling full, painful sex, urinary sx's
Dx: U/S and **CA-125;** diagnostic laparoscopy
Types

1) **Epithelial** tumor
MC ovarian CA type
MC ovarian tumor type in post-menopausal women
**Serous tumors (60% benign, 30% malignant, 10% borderline)
MC ovarian tumor overall (50% of all tumors)
MC malignant ovarian tumor overall (40% of all tumors)
Papillary elements → malignant
Mucin tumors (cystadenocarcinoma, often has papillary elements)
Clear cell – very aggressive, *worst prognosis*
Brenner – transitional cells like bladder (can be benign or malignant)
Endometroid

2) **Sex cord** tumors
Granulosa cell (estrogen secreting, precocious puberty)
Sertoli-Leydig (androgens, masculinization)
Choriocarcinoma (beta-HCG)

3) **Germ cell** tumor(dysgerminoma, choriocarcinoma, embryonal, teratoma)
Teratoma → **MC benign ovarian tumor (30% of all tumors)
Adults- 95% benign teratomas, 5% malignant (children ↑ malignant)
Germ cell MC ovarian tumor in female children (60% malignant,
MC - dysgerminoma)
Struma ovarii (thyroid tissue, hyperthyroidism)

Worst prognosis CA – clear cell type
Best prognosis CA – malignant germ cell tumors
MC mets to ovary (ie Krukenberg tumor) – GI cancer (**colon CA** MC; if
from stomach CA, path will show **signet ring cells**) and breast
Meige's syndrome – pelvic ovarian tumor (classically fibroma) that causes
ascites + hydrothorax (↑ on right); **tumor excision cures syndrome**

Stage

I	Confined to **one or both ovaries**
II	Disease **confined to pelvis**
III	Spread **throughout abdominal cavity** or **positive nodes**
IV	Distant **mets**

Bilateral ovary involvement still **stage I**
MC initial regional spread – contralateral ovary

Tx:

All stages get
1) **Total abd hysterectomy + bilateral salpingo-oophrectomy**
2) **Pelvic** and **para-aortic LN dissection**
3) **Omentectomy**
4) **4 quadrant washes + Bx's** (under right diaphragm, pericolic
recess, pelvic sidewall)
Pelvic exenteration (above + bladder, rectum and vagina) **+ stripping of
essential organs** may be indicated for advanced tumors
Chemo – cisplatin + paclitaxel for residual DZ; often given **intra-peritoneal**
XRT – of some benefit (for residual DZ after surgery)
****Special case – confined to single ovary, stage I, low grade and low
risk tumor** (eg malignant teratoma), **in young female who wants
pregnancy** – consider unilateral salpingo-oophrectomy
Debulking tumor – can be effective and improves prognosis for advanced
CA (helps chemo-XRT); tumor nodules left behind should be ≤ 1 cm
Overall 5-YS – 35% (late stage at Dx)

Endometrial cancer

MC gynecologic CA in US

3rd MCC gynecologic CA death (1st ovarian CA, 2nd cervical CA)

Sx's: vaginal bleeding

> **Vaginal bleeding in postpartum pt** is endometrial CA until proved otherwise (need endometrial Bx)

RFs – nulliparity, obesity, unopposed estrogen, Tamoxifen, polycystic ovaries, early menarche, late menopause, polyps, breast or ovarian CA, XRT

Often occurs in setting of **endometrial glandular hyperplasia**

Most endometrial cancers are found **early** (as opposed to ovarian CA)

Types

> **MC type** – endometrioid adenocarcinoma
> **Worst prognosis** – serous, papillary, and clear cell
> Rare endometrial stromal sarcomas (**MC** - leiomyosarcomas)
> **Endometrial polyps** have 0.1% chance of malignancy
>> Polyps can present w/ increasing **menstrual flow**

Dx: endometrial curettage or brush Bx; D&C (**routine screening** w/ RF)

Stage

> I – limited to endometrium
> II – invades cervix only
> III – invades the vagina, peritoneum, or ovary; positive nodes
> IV – invades bladder or rectum (IVA) or distant mets (IVB)

Tx:

> **Stage I** – TAH + BSO (abdominal approach, _not vaginal_)
> **Stage II, III,** and **IV** or **high grade tumors →**
>> 1) TAH + BSO + para-aortic / pelvic LN dissection
>> 2) post-op XRT

Overall 5-YS – 75% (early stage at Dx)

Cervical cancer

Sx's: vaginal bleeding, painful sex, discharge

PAP smear has greatly ↓ed incidence of cervical CA

All associated w/ **HPV** (MC HPV 16 and 18)

MC type – SCCA; Goes to **obturator nodes 1st**

Dx:

> **PAP smear** – looks for cervical intraepithelial neoplasia (CIN) or cervical dysplasia; if present, need a Bx (called colposcopy Bx)
> **Colposcopy Bx** – if severe CIN (microscopic DZ w/o basement membrane invasion) or more invasive lesion found, need conization Bx
> **Conization Bx** – inner lining of cervix is removed
>> If no basement membrane invasion (eg carcinoma is situ or high grade intra-epithelial neoplasia) → all that is necessary

Stage

> **CIS** full-thickness epithelium; no stromal or basement membrane invasion
> **I** cervix only
> **II** upper 2/3 of vagina
>> **A** – no parametrial invasion, **B** – parametrial invasion **(impt for tx)***
>> Parametrial invasion → outside cervix/endometrium other than vagina
> **III** pelvic sidewall, lower 1/3 vagina, hydronephrosis, positive nodes
> **IV** bladder or rectal invasion (IVA), mets (IVB)

Tx:

> **Microscopic DZ** (no basement membrane invasion)
>> Conization Bx or loop electrical excision procedure (LEEP) _only_
> **Stages I and IIa**
>> **Total abdominal hysterectomy**(TAH) **+ pelvic LN dissection**
>> **High risk tumors → Chemo-XRT** (cisplatnin based) after surgery
> **Stages IIb to IV**
>> **Chemo-XRT _only_** (cisplatnin based); if that fails or tumor recurs → **pelvic exenteration salvage** (TAH+BSO, vagina, rectum, bladder)
> Can **leave ovaries** w/ cervical CA (unless pelvic exoneration)
> **Hycamtin** – topoisomerase I inhibitor for stage IV cervical CA

Overall 5-YS – 75% (early stage at Dx due to Pap smear)

Vaginal cancer
MC type – squamous cell CA
    SCCA – MC in women > age 50
    Adenocarcinoma – MC in women < age 30
RFs – DES (diethylstilbestrol; can cause clear cell CA of vagina)
Sarcoma Botryoides – rhabdosarcoma that occurs in young girls
Tx: Resection for early stage
    XRT used as primary or adjuvant tx for most vaginal CA
MC vaginal tumor – invasion from surrounding or distant structure

Vulvar cancer
Often in elderly, nulliparous, obese
Usually unilateral
MC type – SCCA
RFs – HPV, HIV, smokers
Goes to inguinal nodes 1st, then pelvic nodes
Want **2 cm margins** w/ excision
Tx:
    Paget's, VIN III or higher (vulvar intra-epithelial neoplasia), or **carcinoma in situ** – all premalignant (Tx: WLE); if **Pagets**→look for other tumors
    Stage I (< 2 cm) →
        WLE + ipsilateral inguinal and femoral node dissection
    Stage II (> 2 cm) or **Stage III** (spread beyond vulva or positive nodes)
        Bilateral vulvectomy + bilateral inguinal/femoral LN dissection
        Postop XRT w/ close margins (< 1 cm)
Overall 5-YS – 75%

Ovarian cysts
Postmenopausal
    If septated, has solid components, papillary projections, increased vascular flow on Duplex U/S → oophrectomy w/ intra-op frozen section; TAH if ovarian CA
    If none of the above:
        Follow w/ Duplex U/S for 1 year, if persists or gets larger → oophrectomy w/ intra-op frozen section; TAH if ovarian CA
Premenopausal
    If septated, has solid components, papillary projections, increased vascular flow Duplex U/S, → oophrectomy w/ intra-op frozen section
        Tx very complicated after this, weighing how aggressive CA is (histology and stage) compared w/ desire for future pregnancy
    If none of the above → can follow w/ Duplex U/S; surgery if suspicious findings appear

Abnormal uterine bleeding
    < age 40 – anovulation (causes infertility)
        Tx: clomifene citrate (Clomid, selective estrogen receptor modulator)
            Inhibits action of estrogen on anterior pituitary gland, causing GnRH release (regular menses and improves fertility)
        Uterine leiomyomas (eg fibroids)
            Sx's: under hormonal influence; bleeding (MC sx), recurrent abortions, infertility, anovulation
            Tx: GnRH analogues (eg leuprolide)
    > age 40 – **CA** or **menopause**;
        Dx – need endometrial biopsy

Other Gynecologic Disorders

Hydatidiform mole (molar pregnancy)

CA risk w/ **partial mole**; complete mole is paternal origin

Tx:

1) **Evacuate uterus** of molar pregnancy (uterine suction or curettage)
2) Follow **Beta HCG** (should fall to 0)

If **invasive molar pregnancy** or **beta-HCG does not fall to 0**
– give **methotrexate** (response nearly 100%)

Wait 1 year before another conception

Toxic shock syndrome

50% due to highly absorbent tampons; other – skin infections

Diagnostic criteria:

1) **Fever** (Temp > 38.9 °C)
2) **Hypotension** (systolic BP < 90 mmHg)
3) **Diffuse rash** (erythema + blanching) w/ **subsequent desquamation** (esp palms and soles)
4) $\geq$ **3 organ system involvement**:

GI – N/V, diarrhea

Mucous membrane hyperemia (vaginal, oral, conjunctival)

Renal failure (Cr 2 x normal)

Hepatic inflammation (AST, ALT > 2x normal)

Thrombocytopenia (plts < 100,000)

CNS (confusion w/ focal findings)

Mechanism

Staph aureus (MC) releases **TSST protein** → causes non-specific binding between MHC class II receptor and T cell receptors

T cell activation causes massive cytokine release (**cytokine storm**) and multisystem DZ

Strep pyogenes can cause toxic-like shock syndrome (usually associated w/ **skin infection**)

Tx: Abx's (vancomycin for staph; high dose PCN if strep) and **ICU care**

Ovarian torsion – Tx: relieve torsion, check for viability, resection if necrotic

Adnexal torsion w/ vascular necrosis – Tx: adnexectomy (ovary resection)

Ovarian vein thrombosis

Sx's: pelvic pain, fever, and a right-sided abdominal mass after pregnancy

Can lead to **thrombosis of hepatic veins** (elevated LFTs w/ ascites), **renal veins** and **IVC**

Can lead to **thrombophlebitis**

Usually presents after **recent child-birth**

Dx: CT scan *(best test)* or U/S

Tx: heparin + abx's (can get infected, esp post partum)

Postpartum pelvic thrombophlebitis

MCC of ovarian vein thrombosis

Tx as above

Post-menopausal vaginal bleeding: Dx – endometrial Bx (suspicious for endometrial CA)

Radical hysterectomy – removes cervix, uterus, parametrium, fallopian tubes, and ovaries

Uterine Prolapse (procidentia)– uterus protrudes through vagina

RFs – multiparity

Tx: weight loss. D/C smoking (↓ cough), pessary, vaginal hysterectomy

Polycystic Ovarian Disease

Sx's – amenorrhea, infertility, hirsutism; Tx: clomiphene citrate (Clomid)

Hormone replacement therapy (menopause) – avoid unopposed estrogen

NEUROSURGERY

Circle of Willis
Circle of arterial circulation in the brain such that it one artery is occluded, the communicating arteries will still allow blood flow

Vertebral arteries – coalesce to form a single **basilar artery**

Basilar artery branches into two **posterior cerebral arteries**

Posterior communicating arteries

These connect **middle cerebral arteries** to **posterior cerebral arteries**

Anterior cerebral arteries – branches of **middle cerebral arteries**

Connected to each other through one **anterior communicating artery**

The **internal carotid artery** becomes the **middle cerebral artery**

Broca's area – <u>speech motor</u>, posterior part of anterior lobe
Wernicke's area – <u>speech comprehension</u>, temporal lobe
Pituitary adenoma, undergoing XRT, pt now in shock

Dx: pituitary apoplexy Tx: steroids

Diaphragm innervation – **phrenic nerve** (cervical nerve roots 3–5)
Microglial cells – brain macrophages

Nerve injury
Neuropraxia – mildest form of injury (MC injury)

No axon or myelin sheath injury but interruption of **conduction impulse**

Temporary loss of function (motor >> sensory)

Generally all recover

Mildest form – foot falls asleep (pressure on sciatic nerve)

Severe – blunt trauma (make take 6-8 weeks to recover)

Axonotmesis

Disruption of **axon w/ preservation of myelin sheath**

Paralysis and loss of sensation

MC w./ crush injury

Wallerian degeneration of nerve occurs (antegrade degeneration towards end plate)

Nerve has to regenerate for recover (1 mm/day) – can take weeks

Neurotmesis

Worst form of injury

Axon and myelin sheath are disrupted

Severe contusion, stretch, complete laceration

May not recover or may need surgery for recovery

Regeneration of **peripheral nerves** occurs at rate of **1 mm/day**

Central nerves do <u>not</u> regenerate

Nodes of Ranvier – bare sections between myelin sheath cells; allow salutatory propagation of action potentials

Sensory – 1st to recover after nerve damage

Hemorrhage
Arteriovenous malformations (AVMs)

50% present with hemorrhage

MC in pts aged < 30; are congenital

Sx's: stiff neck (nuchal rigidity), severe HA, photophobia, neuro defects

The tx of unruptured AVMs is highly controversial

Emergency tx for AVM w/ subarachnoid hemorrhage → see below

Cerebral aneurysms (berry aneurysm)

MC pts aged > 40; most are congenital

Sx's: severe HA, N/V, dizziness, LOC, infarct

Occur at **artery branch points**

85% are in anterior portion of circle of Willis

MC in **anterior cerebral or anterior communicating** artery (35%)

The tx of unruptured intracranial aneurysms is highly controversial

Emergency tx for cerebral aneurysm w/ subarachnoid hemorrhage – see below

Subdural hematoma
>Caused by **torn bridging veins** that cross the subdural space
>Head CT – crescent shape and conforms to brain
>More common the epidural hematomas
>**Higher mortality** than epidural hematoma (associated **brain injury**)
>**Tx:** operate for significant **neuro degeneration** and significant **mass effect**
>>(shift > 10 mm for subdural)

Epidural hematoma
>Caused by injury to **middle meningeal artery** (skull Fx)
>Has lens shape on head CT and pushes brain away
>Pts classically lose consciousness, have a lucid interval, and then lose
>>consciousness again
>**Tx:** operate for significant **neuro degeneration** and significant **mass effect**
>>(shift > 5 mm for epidural)

Subarachnoid hemorrhage (non-traumatic causes)
>**Sx's:** severe HA (thunderclap), vomiting, confusion, LOC, seizures
>>Late neck stiffness, dilation of pupil
>**Etiology** – cerebral aneurysms (85%) and AVMs (10%)
>**Mortality** – 50%
>**Goals:**
>>**ABC's**
>>1) Identify **bleed**
>>>**Get Head CT - If large compressing hematoma found**
>>>>consider early evacuation and clipping
>>2) Prevent **re-bleeding**
>>>Need to **isolate aneurysm** (or AVM) from systemic circulation
>>>Get **transfemoral angiogram** or **cerebral angio CT** to dx
>>>>location
>>>a) **Middle cerebral artery → craniotomy w/ surgical clips**
>>>>likely better (hard to reach w/ angio catheters)
>>>b) **Posterior cerebral artery → endovascular coils** likely
>>>>better (hard to reach area w/ surgery)
>>>↑ed risk of **aneurysm recurrence** w/ coils
>>3) Prevent **vasospasm**
>>>**Maximize cerebral perfusion** to overcome and prevent
>>>>vasospasm
>>>Vasospasm can occur early or as far as 1-2 weeks out
>>>Can be rapidly fatal from **brain ischemia**
>>>**Dx: trans-cranial doppler** can be used to monitor for
>>>>vasospasm (flow < 120 cm/sec)
>>>**Tx and prevention:**
>>>>**Triple H therapy** (hypervolemia, hypertension,
>>>>>hemodilution) – may help prevent
>>>>**Calcium channel blockers** (CCB, eg nimodipine)
>>>>Angio and direct intra-arterial vasodilators or PTA
>>>>**Nimodipine** – cerebro-selective CCB

>Can get subarachnoid hemorrhages with trauma as well

Intracerebral hematomas – temporal lobe MC area
>If very large and causing compression w/ focal deficits should be drained.

Spinal cord injury

Cord injury with neuro deficit → give **high-dose steroids** (decreases swelling)

Complete cord transection
- Areflexia
- Flaccidity
- Anesthesia
- Autonomic paralysis below level of transection

Spinal shock (neurogenic shock) – **hypotension, normal or slow heart rate, and warm extremities** (vasodilated)
- Occurs w/ spinal cord **injuries above T5** (loss of sympathetic tone)
- **Tx:** fluids initially, may need phenylephrine drip (alpha agonist)

Anterior spinal artery syndrome
- **MCC** – acutely ruptured cervical disc
- **Bilateral** loss of **motor, pain, and temp** sensation below level of lesion
- **Preservation** of **position-vibratory sensation** and **light touch**
- About 10% recover to ambulation (worst prognosis of all syndromes)

Brown-Sequard syndrome (incomplete cord transection; hemi-section of cord)
- **MCC** – penetrating injury
- **Loss of** (occurs below level of injury):
    - **Ipsilateral motor**
    - **Contralateral pain and temperature**
- About 90% recover to ambulation

Central cord syndrome
- **MCC** – hyperflexion of the cervical spine
- **Bilateral** loss **motor, pain, and temp** in **upper extremities**
- **Lower extremities spared**

Cauda equina syndrome – pain and weakness in lower extremities
- **Loss of bowel or bladder function**
- Due to compression of lumbar nerve roots

Doral nerve roots (posterior) – generally afferent; carry **sensory neurons**
- **Spinothalamic tract** – pain and temp

Ventral nerve roots (anterior) – generally efferent; carry **motor neurons**
- **Corticospinal tract** – motor
- **Rubrospinal tract** – motor

Brain tumors

- **Sx's:** HA, seizures, progressive neuro deficit, persistent vomiting
- **Adults** – 2/3 supratentorial
- **Children** – 2/3 infratentorial
- **MC primary brain tumor** – gliomas
    - **MC subtype** – glioblastoma multiforme (uniformly fatal)
- **MC mets to brain** – lung
- **MC brain tumor in children** – meduloblastoma
- **MC mets to brain in children** – neuroblastoma

Spine tumors

- **MC benign**
- **MC overall** – neurofibroma
- **Intradural tumors** more likely benign
- **Extradural tumors** are more likely malignant
- **Paraganglioma** – check for metanephrines in urine; MIBG for extramedullary chromatin tissue

Pediatric neurosurgery

Intraventricular hemorrhage (IVH, subependymal hemorrhage)
- **Premature infants** from rupture of fragile vessels in **germinal matrix** (lack of oxygen thought to cause vascular cell death)
- Get **intra-ventricular hemorrhage**
- **RFs** – ECMO, cyanotic congenital heart disease
- **Sx's:** bulging fontanelle, neuro deficits, ↓ BP, ↓ Hct
- **Tx:** place ventricular catheter for drainage and prevention of hydrocephalus

Myelomeningocele

Neural cord defect – herniation of spinal cord and nerve roots through defect in vertebra; looks like big sac off vertebral column

If sac ruptured – surgery needed to prevent infection of spinal cord

MC in lumbar region

Thoracic sympathectomy

Palmar and axillary hyperhidrosis –take T2-T4 sympathetic nerves

MC indication by far

MC cx – compensatory sweating in the lower extremities or abdomen

Avoid taking T1 – can result in Horner's Syndrome (ptosis, miosis-small pupil, and anhydrosis)

Nerve of Knutz

Accessory nerve pathway between T1 and T2 that can result in refractory palmar sweating after sympathectomy

Need to coagulate on bottom of the 2nd rib to divide the nerve of Knutz and avoid this complication

Other indications (rarely done for below)

Complex regional pain syndrome

(Reflex sympathetic dystrophy, causalgia)

Neuron derived pain – usually after trauma or amputation

Continuous pain out of proportion to degree of injury

Medical Tx: gabapentin and amitriptyline; TENS unit

Only use sympathectomy when pain is dramatically relieved by nerve blocks

Location of sympathectomy depends on location of pain

Unresectable pancreatic CA causing pain (lumbar sympathectomy)

Non-revascularizable lower extremity ischemic rest pain (lumbar sympathectomy)

Cranial nerves

Nerve	Name	Motor/ Sensory / Both	Function
I	Olfactory	sensory	Smell
II	Optic	sensory	Sight
III	Oculomotor	motor	Eye
IV	Trochlear	motor	Eye (Superior oblique)
V	Trigeminal (ophthalmic, maxillary, mandibular)	both	1) Muscles of mastication 2) Sensory to face
VI	Abducens	motor	Eye (Lateral rectus)
VII	Facial	both	1) Motor to face 2) Taste anterior 2/3 of tongue
VIII	Vestibulocochlear	sensory	Hearing, balance
IX	Glossopharyngeal	both	1) Swallowing (only stylopharyngeus) 2) Taste to posterior 1/3 of tongue
X	Vagus	both	1) Swallowing 2) Voice, viscera
XI	Accessory	motor	Trapezius (shrug) Sternocleidomastoid (head turn)
XII	Hypoglossal	motor	Tongue movement

GABA (Gamma-Amino-Butyric Acid) – chief neuro-inhibitory neurotransmitter in brain; GABA analogues have anti-convulsing, anti-anxiety, relaxing effects

Anatomy
Osteoblasts
1) **Synthesize osteoid** (non-mineralized bone cortex; mainly **Type I collagen**)
2) **Mineralize osteoid**

Osteoclasts
Cause **bone resorption**
Hormonal regulation of osteoclasts
PTH – ↑s bone resorption (Ca and PO_4 release)
Calcitonin – ↓s bones resorption

Bone healing
1) **Inflammation**
2) **Granulation tissue**
3) **Callus formation**
Hyaline cartilage from chondroblasts
Woven bone from osteoblasts
4) **Lamellar bone deposition** (replaces hyaline cartilage and woven bone)
5) **Remodeling** – compact bone placement
Healing process mainly determined by **periosteum**
Periosteum primary source of precursor cells (eg chondroblasts and osteoblasts)

Cartilage receives nutrients from synovial fluid

Brachial Plexus
Ulnar nerve
Motor
Intrinsic musculature of hand (palmar interossei, palmaris brevis, adductor pollicis, hypothenar eminence); finger abduction (spread fingers)
Wrist flexion
Sensory
5th and ½ 4th fingers
Back of hand
Injury – claw hand; involved in **cubital tunnel syndrome** at elbow

Median nerve
Motor
Thumb apposition (anterior interosseous muscle, the OK sign)
Thumb abduction
Finger flexors
Sensory
Most of palm
1st 3½ fingers on palmar side
Nerve involved in **carpal tunnel syndrome** at wrist
Injury – decreased thumb movement, fingers will be extended

Radial nerve
Motor
Wrist extension
Finger extension
Thumb extension
Triceps
No hand muscles
Sensory – 1st 3½ fingers on dorsal side

Musculocutaneous nerve – motor to biceps, brachialis, and coracobrachialis
Axillary nerve – motor and sensory to deltoid (abduction)

Radial nerve	C5–C8 (superior portion of brachial plexus)
Axillary nerve	C5–C6
Musculocutaneous nerve	C5–C7
Median nerve	C6–T1
Ulnar nerve	C8-T1 (inferior portion of brachial plexus)

Lower extremity nerves

Obturator nerve	hip adduction
Superior gluteal nerve	hip abduction
Inferior gluteal nerve	hip extension
Femoral nerve	knee extension

Bone Sections

Diaphysis – midsection, shaft
Metaphysis - area of epiphyseal growth plate (between diaphysis and epiphysis)
Epiphysis – rounded end of long bone

Herniated Cervical Disc

C1, C2, C3, and C4 (C1–2, C2–3, C3–4)	Neck and scalp pain
C5 (C4–5 disc)	Weak deltoid and biceps
	Weak biceps reflex
C6 (C5–6 disc)	Weak deltoid and biceps
	Weak wrist extensors
	Weak biceps reflex
	Wk brachioradialis reflex
***C7 (MC type, C6–7 disc)	Weak triceps
	Weak triceps reflex
C8 (C7–T1 disc)	Weak triceps
	Wk intrinsic hand muscle
	Weak wrist flexion
	Weak triceps reflex

Dx: MRI (usually only if planning on surgery)
Tx:
>NSAID's, physical therapy, soft collar
>**Surgery If evidence of nerve root compression w/ motor weakness**
>>Tx – discectomy w/ spinal fusion
>
>Surgery also considered for failure of medical Tx to relieve pain / numbness
>**Emergency decompression indications:**
>>1) **Anterior spinal syndrome**
>>2) **Acute loss of motor function**
>>Need to get **emergent MRI**

Radiculopathy – nerve root pain or numbness, poor motor function
Various etiologies (eg herniated disc (MC), spurs, spinal stenosis)
There is no C8 vertebral body although there is a C8 nerve root

Herniated Lumbar Disc

Sx's
>**Back pain** aggravated by activity, can **radiate down leg**
>Relived w/ rest on unaffected side w/ affected leg flexed
>15 x more common than cervical disc herniation
>Herniated disc is **nucleus pulposus**
>Certain movements ↑ inter-vertebral pressure at disc (eg attempting to rise out of a chair and bending over at waist)
>Often have a history of chronic back pain.

L1 to L3 nerves	Weak hip flexion
***L4 nerve** (MC type L4–5 disc)	Weak knee extension (quadriceps)
	Weak patellar reflex
L5 nerve (L5–S1 disc)	Weak dorsiflexion (foot drop)
	↓ sensation in big toe web space
S1 nerve (S1–S2 disc)	Weak plantarflexion
	Weak Achilles reflex
	↓ sensation in lateral foot

Dx: MRI *(best test)*

Tx:

> 90% treated w/ NSAID's and pain meds
>
> With time, disc will usually shrink on its own, decompressing spine
>
> **Failure of conservative tx** (6 weeks) warrants consideration for surgery
>
> Surgical decompression involves removal of part of offending disc
> **(discectomy)**
>
> **Sx's that warrant consideration for emergent decompression due to cord compression include** (ie cauda equina syndrome):
>> Loss of bowel or bladder function
>>
>> Saddle anesthesia
>>
>> Loss of movement
>>
>> Progressive muscle weakness
>>
>> Progressively increasing pain
>>
>> Disc fragments in the cord
>>
>> **Tx:**
>>> **Empiric dexamethasone**-10 mg IV, drip 5.4 mg/kg/hr for 23 hr
>>>
>>> **Possible decompression**

Fractures

Salter Harris Fracture Types in children

> **Type I and I** – closed reduction
>
> **Type III, IV, and V** – crosses epiphyseal plate
>> Can affect growth plate of bone;
>>
>> Need open reduction and internal fixation (ORIF)

Fx's associated w/ **avascular necrosis** – scaphoid, femoral neck, talus (ankle)

Fx's associated w/ **non-union** – clavicle, 5th metatarsal (Jones' fx)

Fx's associated w/ **compartment syndrome** – supracondylar humerus, tibia

RF for non-union – smoking (#1)

Spine fx's (see Trauma Chp)

Upper Extremity

Prolonged hand ischemia (eg laceration of radial and ulnar arteries) - Motor function can remain in digits after prolonged ischemia because motor groups are in proximal forearm.

Clavicle Fx - Tx: usually just sling
> Risk of non-union, vascular impingement, and skin compromise (all indications for surgery)

Shoulder dislocation
> **Anterior** (MC, 90%) Tx: closed reduction
>> Risk of **axillary nerve injury**
>
> **Posterior** (seizures, electrocution). Tx: closed reduction
>> Risk of **axillary artery injury**
>
> Surgery for either of above if **displaced humeral fx** also present

Rotator cuff tears
> **Muscles** (SITS) - supraspinatus, infraspinatus, teres minor, subscapularis
>
> **Acutely** → sling and conservative treatment
>
> **Tx:**
>> **Generally conservative Tx 1st** (NSAIDS, physical therapy, occasional steroid injections)
>>
>> Profound loss of rotator cuff mediated **motion and strength, failure of medical Tx,** or **normal activities affected** Tx - surgery
>>
>> **Surgery** – tendon re-attached to bone

Acromioclavicular separation
> **Non- or minor displacement** (majority, Types I – III) Tx - sling
>
> **Severely displaced** (types IV – VI) Tx - ORIF
>> **Type IV** - Concomitant **coracoclavicular ligament** injury
>>> Clavicle into or through **trapezius**
>>
>> **Type V** – severe **vertical displacement** of clavicle from scapula
>>
>> **Type VI** - severe **inferior displacement** of clavicle below coracoid
>
> Risk of **brachial plexus** and **subclavian vessel injury**

Scapula Fx
>Tx: sling unless **glenoid fossa** involved, then need ORIF

Proximal humeral Fx
>**Non-displaced** Tx: sling
>**Displaced or comminuted** Tx: ORIF
>Risk of **axillary nerve damage**

Midshaft humeral Fx – Tx: sling (almost all)
>Surgery only for failed reduction or neurovascular events
>Risk of **radial nerve damage**

Supracondylar humerus Fx
>**Adults** → ORIF
>**Children**
>>**Type I** (non-displaced) – closed reduction
>>**Type II and III** (partially and totally displaced) – closed reduction and internal fixation w/ Kirschner wire
>
>Risk of **brachial artery damage**
>Risk of **Volkmann's Contracture** (ie compartment syndrome, see below)

Elbow (Ulnar) **dislocations and fx's**
>**Simple** (no fracture) – closed reduction, cast, early mobilization
>**Complex** (associated w/ fx) – ORIF
>**Posterior dislocations** - MC
>**Anterior dislocations** at risk for **brachial artery injury**

Nursemaid's elbow – subluxation of radius at elbow from pulling on an extended, pronated arm; Tx - closed reduction

Monteggia Fx
>Proximal ulnar fracture and proximal radial head dislocation
>Fall w/ hyperpronation
>**Tx: ORIF (adults and children** – need to pin ulnar shaft)

Galeazzi Fx – distal radius fx and dislocation of distal radio-ulnar joint
>**Adults – ORIF**
>**Children** – **closed reduction** preferred, cast
>>ORIF for failed reduction, articular incongruity, or neurovascular involvement

Colles' Fx – fall on outstretched hand, distal radius fx ± distal ulnar dislocation
>**MC fx in children**
>**Tx: closed reduction** for vast majority (adults and children)
>>ORIF for failed reduction, articular incongruity, or neurovascular involvement

Combined radial and ulnar Fx
>**Adults – ORIF**
>**Children** – **closed reduction** preferred
>>ORIF for failed reduction, articular incongruity, or neurovascular involvement
>
>Risk of **ulnar and radial nerve damage** w/ forearm fx's

Scaphoid Fx (eg wrist fx; perilunate wrist fx)
>**MC carpal bone fx** – scaphoid (MC bone involved in wrist fx), 2nd – lunate
>Snuffbox tenderness *(classic);* can have **negative x-ray**
>**Tx:**
>>**Negative X-ray** – *all pts get spica cast to elbow*, follow-up X –rays in 2 weeks to look for fx healing (occult fx)
>>**Non-displaced Fx** (scaphoid or lunate) - spica cast to elbow, 6-8 wks
>>**Displaced Fx** (scaphoid or lunate) – ORIF
>>Risk of **avascular necrosis** w/ scaphoid (Tx: hip bone graft repair)

Scaphoid Dislocation (eg wrist dislocation; perilunate wrist dislocation)
>**MC carpal bone dislocation** – scaphoid (MC bone involved in wrist dislocation); 2nd - lunate
>**Tx:**
>>**Non-displaced** – closed reduction (scaphoid or lunate)
>>**Displaced** (> 1 mm or > 15 degrees, scaphoid or lunate) – ORIF
>>Risk of **avascular necrosis** w/ scaphoid (Tx: hip bone graft repair)

Boxer's fx – 5th metacarpal bone

> **Tx: closed reduction** for most
>
> \> 30 degrees of angulation needs internal fixation (lateral view)

Finger fx – most treated w/ **closed reduction** and splinting; may need pins and internal fixation if severe dislocation or angulation

Volkmann's contracture

> Supracondylar humerus Fx → occludes **anterior interosseous artery** → closed reduction of Fx → artery opens → reperfusion injury, edema, and **forearm compartment syndrome** (flexor compartment)
>
> **Sx's**: pain in forearm w/ passive extension; weakness; tense forearm, hypoesthesia; loss of pulse is late finding
>
> **Median nerve** affected by swelling
>
> Tx: **fasciotomy** (both volar and dorsal compartments)
>
> **Forearm fasciotomy**
>
> > **Volar incision** – curvilinear (lazy S shape) so that all of the major nerves and arteries are decompressed
> >
> > **Dorsal incision**
> >
> > > Longitudinal incision (linear)
> > >
> > > Need to open both the mobile extensor wad and extensor digitorum communus muscle group compartments

Dupuytren's contracture

> **RFs** – diabetes, ETOH, liver DZ, epilepsy
>
> Progressive proliferation of **palmar fascia of hand** results in contractures that MC affect **4th and 5th digits** (can't extend fingers).
>
> **Tx**: NSAIDs, steroid injections; excision of involved fascia for significant contraction

Carpal tunnel syndrome

> **Median nerve** compression by **transverse carpal ligament**
>
> **Tx**: splint, NSAIDs, steroid injections; transverse carpal ligament release if refractory

Trigger finger

> Tenosynovitis of flexor tendon that catches at MCP joint when trying to extend finger
>
> **Tx**: splint, tendon sheath steroid injections (not tendon itself - necrosis)
>
> > If refractory → release pulley system at MCP joint

Suppurative tenosynovitis

> Infection that spreads along flexor tendon sheath (can **destroy tendon**)
>
> Can occur after minor trauma (eg cat or dog bite)
>
> **Sx's** *(4 classic signs)*
>
> > 1) **tendon sheath tenderness**
> >
> > 2) **pain w/ passive motion**
> >
> > 3) **swelling along sheath**
> >
> > 4) **semi-flexed posture of involved digit**
>
> **Tx**: elevation, splinting, and abx's
>
> > If **immunocompromised** (eg DM, HIV, chemo) or **improvement not prompt** → **midaxial longitudinal incision** and **drainage**

Forearm fasciotomies – open both volar and dorsal compartments

Paronychia – bacterial infection where the nail and skin meet on digit; painful

> Infection can proceed underneath nail-bed (**erythema, swollen**)
>
> **Tx**: abx's; warm soaks; **remove nail** if purulent underneath

Felon – infection in finger tip pad (**swollen, erythema**)

> **Tx**: incision over tip of finger and along medial and lateral aspects to prevent necrosis of tip of finger (avoid pad of finger tip – nerve preservation)

Herpetic Whitlow – HSV infection; MC on distal phalynx **vesicles and ulcers** w/ surrounding erythema; Tx: acyclovir for severe cases; self limiting

Biceps tendon rupture – ± repair

Hypothenar Hand Syndrome – ↓ blood flow to hand when used repeatedly as a hammering device at work; MC damages the **ulnar artery**

> Tx: stop activity producing the problem, may need bypass for ulnar artery

Lower extremity
  Pelvic fractures
    MC associated injury – closed head injury
    Need to tx **life threatening hemorrhage** from pelvic fx 1st
    Need to assess whether or not the **pelvic ring is stable**
    Generally, **isolated pubic rami fx's** do not require ORIF
    Generally need **≥ 2 significant Fx's or dislocations** for ring to be
      unstable requiring **ORIF**
        Exceptions
          Isolated pubic symphysis dislocations **> 2.5 cm** (likely
            occult sacro-iliac displacement
          Isolated sacro-iliac joint dislocations **≥ 5 mm** (likely occult
            pubic symphysis dislocation)
    1) **Anterior Pelvis**
        Pubic rami fx's (bilateral rami Fx's also included) w/ minimal
          displacement do not require surgery
            Example - Isolated anterior ring fx (eg pubic rami) w/ minimal
              ischial displacement – Tx: weight bearing as tolerated
            ORIF for associated **SI joint dislocation / fx** *or* **iliac wing fx**
        Pubic symphysis dislocation (open book pelvic fx):
            Tx: weight bearing as tolerated for most
            If **> 2.5 cm** dislocation (diasthesis) - ORIF
            Associated **SI joint dislocation / fx** or **iliac wing fx** – ORIF
            Also consider ORIF w/ concomitant **genitourinary injuries**
    2) **Posterior Pelvis**
        Sacral fx
            Isolated and **impacted or buckle fx**
                Tx: Weight bearing as tolerated, even if displaced
            Severe **sacral impact injuries** w/ displacement can cause
              cauda equine syndrome and need decompression w/
              ORIF (50% w/ severe fx's have nerve injuries)
            Vertical fx w/ associated **rami fx, pubic symphysis
              dislocation, iliac wing fx, or neuro compromise**
                Tx: ORIF
        Sacro-iliac dislocation Tx – ORIF for most
            Most associated w/ **iliac wing, pubic rami, or pubic
              symphysis dislocation / fx**
            If **< 5 mm** dislocation and no **significant associated fx** –
              weight bearing as tolerated
        Iliac Fx
            Isolated anterior iliac spine, iliac crest, *or* iliac wing fx's
                Tx: weight bearing as tolerated (usually from direct blow)
            Associated **rami, pubic symphysis,** or **SI joint** fx (dislocation)
              – ORIF
        Ischial tuberosity fx (isolated) – weight bearing as tolerated
        Coccygeal fx (isolated) – weight bearing as tolerated
        Sacro-coccygeal dislocation (isolated) – weight bearing as
          tolerated
  Hip dislocation (risk of **avascular necrosis**, avoid delayed reduction)
      Posterior (MC 90%) – internal rotation, adduction, shortened leg
          Tx: closed reduction; risk of **sciatic nerve injury**
      Anterior – external rotation, abduction, shortened leg
          Tx: closed reduction; risk of injury to **femoral artery or nerve**
  Hip fx (ie femoral head and acetabulum)
      Almost all treated **surgically**, options:
          Internal fixation – usual if alignment good (young pts)
          Hemiarthroplasty – femoral head and neck replaced w/ metal
            prosthesis (elderly)
          Total hip replacement – like hemiarthroplasty plus replacement of
            socket in pelvis (acetabulum of pelvis; elderly)
      High mortality in **pts aged > 65** (20% mortality in 6 months)

Femoral neck fx – external rotation, abduction, shortened
    ORIF or partial arthroplasty (hemiarthroplasty)
    Risk of **avascular necrosis** if open reduction delayed
Femoral shaft fx – ORIF w/ intramedullary rod (adults and children > age 6)
    Children aged < 6 - spica cast
Lateral knee trauma – can injure the following:
    Anterior cruciate ligament
    Posterior cruciate ligament
    Medial meniscus
    Medial collateral ligament
Anterior cruciate ligament (ACL) **injury** – positive anterior drawer test
    Sx's: swollen knee and **pain w/ pivoting action** (athletes)
    Dx: MRI
    Tx: surgery w/ knee instability (reconstruction w/ patellar tendon or
        hamstring tendon)
    Otherwise physical therapy w/ leg-strengthening exercise
Posterior cruciate ligament injury – positive posterior drawer test
    less common than ACL injury
    Sx's: knee pain and joint effusion
    Dx MRI
    Tx: conservative therapy initially; surgery if that fails
Medial collateral ligament injury – lateral blow to knee
    Tx: small tear – brace; **large tear** – surgery
    At risk for corresponding **medial meniscus** injury
Lateral collateral ligament injury – medial blow to knee
    Tx: small tear – brace; **large tear** – surgery
    At risk for corresponding **lateral meniscus** injury
Meniscus tears – joint line tenderness
    Tx: can treat w/ arthroscopic repair or debridement
Posterior knee dislocation – closed reduction
    All pts need angiogram to R/O popliteal artery injury
Patellar Fx
    Tx: long leg cast for most
    ORIF if comminuted
Tibial plateau, tibial shaft, and **tibia-fibula fx's**
    Tx: ORIF unless open fx, then need **external fixator**
    Risk of **compartment syndrome** w/ tibial plateau fx
Plantaris muscle rupture – pain and mass below popliteal fossa (contracted
    plantaris) and ankle ecchymosis. Unnecessary for normal function so not
    repaired (eg tennis players, still be able to walk on it unlike Achilles' tear)
Achilles tendon tear – re-attachment in OR usual
    non-operative - tendon attaches itself from scar; ↑ risk of **re-rupture**
Ankle Fx
    Tx: most treated w/ **cast immobilization,** non-weight bearing
    Bimalleolar (bony prominence on each side of ankle) **or trimalleolar**
        (bilateral malleolar plus distal tibia) **fractures** need ORIF
Talus Fx (above heel)
    Tx: closed reduction
    ORIF for severe displacement
    Risk of **avascular necrosis**
Calcaneus Fx (heel)
    Tx: cast immobilization if non-displaced
    ORIF for any displacement
    Risk of **compartment syndrome** of foot
    10% have **lumbar spine fx's,** 5% **distal forearm fx's** (from fall)
Metatarsal Fx
    Tx: cast immobilization or brace for 6 weeks
    ORIF for failed conservative tx
    Often **non-union after Jones' fx** (5th metatarsal) – Tx: ORIF
MC injured nerve w/ lower extremity fasciotomy – *superficial peroneal*
    nerve (foot eversion)

Foot-drop after:
> **Lithotomy position** (compression of side of leg while in stirrups) *or;*
> **Fibula head Fx** *or;*
> **Crossing legs for long period** (temporary dysfunction)
> → *common peroneal nerve for all* (Tx: foot brace)
> Common peroneal nerve wraps around the neck of the fibula and divides
> into the deep and superficial peroneal nerves

Swollen erythematous knee, sexually active – aspirate to R/O infection
(gonorrhea)

Lower leg compartments
Anterior
> **Arteries/Nerves** – anterior tibial artery, deep peroneal nerve
> **Muscles** – anterior tibialis, extensor hallucis longus, extensor digitorum
> longus, communis

Lateral
> **Nerves** – superficial peroneal nerve
> **Muscles** – peroneal muscles

Deep posterior
> **Arteries/Nerves** – posterior tibial artery, peroneal artery, tibial nerve
> **Muscles** – flexor hallucis longus, flexor digitorum longus, posterior tibialis

Superficial posterior
> **Nerves** – sural nerve
> **Muscles** – gastrocnemius, soleus, plantaris

Compartment syndrome
> MC in **anterior compartment of leg** (get foot-drop) after **restoration of
> vascular compromise**
>
> **High risk fx's** – supracondylar fracture (Volkmann's contracture), tibial plateau
> fx, calcaneus fx, elbow dislocations
> Any injury that results in **interruption** and then **restoration** of blood flow
> Can also occur from **crush injuries**
> Is a **reperfusion injury** mediated by **PMNs**
> Can occur in any muscle compartment (pressure in compartment exceeds
> capillary filling pressure)
>
> **Sx's:**
>> **Classic scenario** – fx w/ loss of blood flow → repair (> 4-6 hours later) →
>> **pain** and **swelling** soon post-op
>> **1st finding** – **pain** w/ passive motion
>>> **Others** – swelling; paresthesias → anesthesia → paralysis →
>>> poikiothermia → pulseless (late finding)
>>> **Distal pulses** can be present w/ compartment syndrome → last thing
>>> to go
>
> **Dx:**
>> **Based on clinical suspicion** (if suspected → fasciotomy)
>> Pressure **> 30 mmHg** abnormal
>> Undiagnosed compartment syndrome can present as **renal failure**
>> (**myoglobin** release) or hyperkalemia
>
> **Tx:**
>> Fasciotomy, after 5-10 days skin grafts
>> With fasciotomy, you are through the fascia when the **muscle bulges**
>> Incise the **total length of compartment** (eg the length of the leg)
>> **Remove all dead tissue** (myoglobinuria if you don't resect)
>> May just need **amputation** if everything is dead (eg delayed presentation
>> after trauma)
>> Alkalinize urine for **myoglobinuria**
>> Watch for **hyperkalemia**

Pediatric orthopaedics

Osteomyelitis
MC in metaphysis of long bones in children
MC organism – staph
Sx's: pain, ↓ used of extremity
Dx: MRI, bone biopsy
Tx: abx's, incision and drainage

Idiopathic adolescent scoliosis
Prepubertal females, MC right thoracic curve, usually asymptomatic
Tx:

Curves < 20° → observation
Curves 20°–40° → **bracing** to slow progression (can occur w/ growth spurt)
Curves > 40-50° or those likely to progress → **spinal fusion**

Osgood-Schlatter disease
Tibial tubercle apophysitis (tibial tubercle breaks)
Traction injury from quadriceps flexion
Adolescents aged 13–15
Sx's: pain in front of knee
X-ray – irregular or fragmented tibial tubercle
Tx: NSAID's and activity limitation (rare cast to limit activity)

Legg-Calvé-Perthes disease
Idiopathic avascular necrosis of femoral head
Children ≥ age 2
RFs – hypercoaguable state
bilateral in 10%
Sx's: painful limping gait
X-ray – flattening of femoral head
Tx:

Observation –crutches, maintain range of motion w/ limited exercise
Femoral head remodels without sequelae
Surgery if femoral head not covered by acetabulum

Slipped capital femoral epiphysis
Obese male children aged 10-13
The capital (head of femur) slips off femur neck
Risk of **avascular necrosis** of femoral head
Sx's: thigh pain and **painful gait**
X-ray – widening and irregularity of the epiphyseal plate
Tx: surgical pinning

Congenital dislocation of hip
MC in females
Tx (age based):

< 6 months – Pavlik harness (keeps legs abducted and femoral head reduced in acetabulum)
6 months to 2 years – closed reduction
> 2 years – open reduction
↑risk of avascular necrosis w/ closed reduction, need

Clubfoot – Tx: serial casting or splints in orthodox position (makes the foot grow into normal position)

Greenstick fx – due to flexibility in bones of children, bone only partially breaks
Tx: closed reduction and cast

Bone tumors

MC bone tumor – mets (**MC - breast**, #2 prostate)
>   **Tx**: ORIF w/ impending fx (> 50% cortical involvement); followed by XRT
>   **Colon CA rarely goes to bone**
>   XRT for painful bony mets
>   **Pathologic fractures** – Tx: ORIF

MC primary malignant bone tumor – multiple myeloma
>   Tx: chemo for systemic disease; internal fixation for impending fx

MC bony tumor overall – osteoid osteomas
MC bony malignant tumor – osteosarcoma
Presence of **pain** w/ any bone lesion (other than a fx) is highly suggestive of
malignancy (exception – osteoid osteomas)
Most impt prognostic indicator for sarcomas – tumor grade
Malignant Bony tumors

>   **Osteosarcoma** (osteogenic sarcoma)
>>   ****MC primary malignant bony tumor** (35%), MC at **knee (50%)**
>>   **Young pts** (80% aged < 20 years)
>>   **90%** can have **limb sparing resection**
>>   **Dx:**
>>>   **X-ray** – Codman's triangle (periosteal reaction)
>>>   **MRI** – before any biopsy
>>>   **CT chest/abd/pelvis**
>>>   **Bone scan** – look for multifocal DZ
>>>   **Bone biopsy**
>>>>   Only after above diagnostic studies
>>>>   In line of future resection incision
>>   **Path** – osteoid formation in tumor (bone formation)
>>   **Biggest prognostic factor** – tumor grade
>>   **Lung mets**
>>>   Can resect multiple tumors if you leave enough lung behind for
>>>   survival (use wedge resections)
>>>   **Better prognosis** – long **disease free interval** ($\geq$ 2 years) and
>>>   **low number of mets**
>>   Tx: **limb-sparing resection**; consider **pre-op chemo-XRT**
>>   (doxorubicin-based; see Skin and Soft Tissue chp)
>>   **Overall 5-YS** – 65%
>>>   **5-YS w/ lung mets resection** – 35%
>>   **Chemo**
>>>   **Doxorubicin based** (usually w/ cisplatnin and methotrexate)
>>>   Usually given as **neoadjuvant** for limb preserving procedure
>>>   Direct **intra-arterial chemo** may be of benefit

>   **Chondrosarcoma**
>>   **MC in pts aged > 40**
>>   MC in pelvic and shoulder regions
>>   Can arise out of pre-existing **endochondroma** or **osteochondroma**
>>   **X-ray** – cortical scalloping, ill-defined borders, adjacent soft tissue
>>   mass; Usually radiolucent mass
>>   W/U and basic tx as above
>>   Have poor chemo response

>   **Ewing's Sarcoma**
>>   MC in adolescents; **painful swelling**
>>   MC location proximal **diaphysis of femur** (long bones)
>>   30% have distant mets at presentation
>>   **X-ray** – 'onion skin' periosteal reaction
>>   W/U and basic tx as above
>>   **Chemo** – Doxorubicin based (usually w/ ifosfamide and etoposide)
>>>   Almost **all pts get chemo** due to high rate of micrometastases

Benign bone tumors
    Osteochondroma
        MC bony tumor overall
        MC benign bony tumor
        Young pts (80% aged < 20 years)
        Bony stalk-like outgrowth at epiphyseal plate covered by
            cartilagenous cap
        Almost always **grows away from associated joint** and is
            continuous w/ host bone w/o cleavage plane *(characteristic*
            findings)
        Resection only if cosmetic defect or causing sx's
    Osteoid osteomas
        < 1.5 cm, **severe pain at night** improved greatly w/ **ASA**
        Dense sclerotic lesion w/ radiolucent nidus that **lights up w/ IV**
            contrast on CT scan *(characteristic finding)*
        Tx: resection or RF ablation if symptomatic
    Endochondroma
        Tubular bones of **hands** (90%), radiolucent
        Observe unless pathologic fx, then resection and stabilize fx
  Giant cell tumor of bone
    Metaphyseal location, grow to articular surface of involved bone
    Dx: X-ray – Soap bubble appearance
    Surgery w/ **curettage** usual, XRT if inaccessible area
    Post-op XRT if felt malignant (most benign but 30% risk of recurrence; 10%
        malignant degeneration)

Other orthopaedic conditions
  Spondylolisthesis
    Subluxation or slip if one vertebral body over another
    MC in lumbar region
    MCC of lumbar pain in adolescents (eg gymnasts)
    Tx Lumbar Spondylolisthesis:
        Low grade (< 50% offset) **–** NSAIDs, PT, conservative tx for 6-12
            mos; spinal fusion if that fails
        High grade (> 50% offset) – spinal fusion
  Torus fracture – buckling of metaphyseal cortex in children (eg distal radius)
    Tx: cast (3 weeks)
  Open fractures – washout, abx's, external fixation of fx, soft tissue coverage

Epidural Abscess
  Hematogenous or direct spread (spinal or epidural anesthesia)
  RFs – DM, renal failure, ETOH, IVDA, immunosuppression
  MC organism – staph aureus
  Sx's: back pain, fever, possible neuro compromise
  Dx: emergent MRI *(best test)* or CT scan
  Tx:
    Surgery for majority (decompressive laminectomy, debridement) + **abx's**
    Surgical indications:
        Neurologic deficit (signs of cord compression)
        Failure to improve on medical Tx (eg pain, fever, WBCs, ↑ing size)

Malignant Spinal cord compression
  Mets in vertebral canal cause cord compression
  MCC – prostate, breast, lung
  MC level – thoracic
  Sx's: pain, weakness, autonomic dysfunction (urinary retention, ↓ sphincter
    tone), sensory loss
  Dx: whole spine MRI (don't wait for neuro sx's to develop)
  Tx: **Dexamethasone** (10 mg IV then 4 mg IV Q 6 hr)
    Emergent XRT or surgical decompression if compression + neuro deficit
    Surgery <u>superior</u> to XRT in regaining neuro function for solid tumors
        causing cord compression

Spinal stenosis
Occurs in lumbar or cervical areas

Sx's

> **Cervical** – upper extremity weakness/numbness; similar sx's to herniated cervical disc
>
> **Lumbar** – pain w/ walking or prolonged standing relieved by bending forward or sitting

Dx: MRI *(best test)*

Tx:

> **Conservative tx 1st** (NSAID's, etc)
>
> > Temporary soft collar for cervical stenosis
> >
> > Avoid bending and lifting w/ lumbar, weight loss
>
> **Surgery**
>
> > **Cervical stenosis** – laminectomy if nerve compression w/ **motor deficit** or **severe sx's** refractory to medical tx (3-6 mos)
> >
> > **Lumbar stenosis** – laminectomy if nerve compression w/ **motor deficit** or **severe sx's** refractory to medical tx (3-6 mos)

Infectious Arthritis
RFs – immunocompromised, damaged joints, bacterial seeding (IVDA, endocarditis, skin infection)

Sx's: acute onset of monoarticular arthritis;, MC site - **Knee**

pain, swelling, warmth; fevers, chills, sweats

Dx:

> **Arthrocentesis** – WBCs usually > 100,000; PMN's > 90%; gram stain positive in 70%, culture positive in 90%
>
> **> 50,000 WBCs highly suspicious for infectious arthritis**
>
> **Labs** – ↑ WBC, blood cultures positive in 50%
>
> **CT and MRI** useful for suspected hip infection or epidural abscess

Tx:

> **Abx's** (vancomycin usual unless worried about gonorrhea)
>
> **Surgical drainage** indicated in most cases, esp w/ larger joints

Traumatic Amputation
Tx:

> Place limb wrapped in plastic bag in ice-water container for transport to the facility (allows 18 hours of preservation)
>
> **Abx's, wash off limb, tetanus shot**
>
> **Re-implantation technique:**
>
> > **Tendon repair**
> >
> > > 4-0 Tevdek core suture 1 cm back on both ends of tendon
> > >
> > > 5-0 Tevdek interrupted sutures ½ cm back
> >
> > **Nerve repair (**eg median, radial and ulnar nerves w/ wrist amputation)**:** 10-0 prolenes just through epineurium
> >
> > **Vascular repair** (eg radial and ulnar arteries w/ wrist amputation): 8-0 prolene
> >
> > Place in cast for bones to heal

Child w/ tip of finger amputated – re-implant so nail bed can grow properly

Thumb amputation and can't re-implant – consider index finger (or 2nd toe) to thumb area transfer

Most impt finger to re-implant – thumb (best rehab potential of all fingers)

PEDIATRIC SURGERY

Embryology and Development
Foregut – includes lungs, esophagus, stomach, pancreas, liver, gallbladder, bile duct, duodenum proximal to ampulla

Midgut – includes duodenum distal to ampulla, small bowel, large bowel to distal ⅓ of transverse colon

Hindgut – includes distal ⅓ of transverse colon to anal canal

Midgut rotates 270 degrees counterclockwise during normal development

Umbilical vessels – 2 arteries (from iliac arteries) and **1 vein** (drains to portal system and IVC)

↑ed **alk phos** in children vs. adults from **bone growth**

Prematurity
Premature infants – 24 to 37 weeks

Low birth weight – < 2500 g (30% due to pre-term labor)

Premature labor Tx (eg pre-term bleed or pre-term ruptured membranes):

    Tocolysis (see Gynecology chp) – usually can delay delivery 2-7 days

    Dexamethasone (if birth felt imminent and < 34 weeks)

        Stimulates **lung maturation** (Prevents **Respiratory Distress Syndrome**)

        Also reduces chance of **intra-ventricular hemorrhage, patent ductus arteriosus,** and **necrotizing colitis**

    Abx's to group B strep (to mother, if birth felt imminent and < 34 weeks) – amoxicillin and erythromycin (decreases risk of **sepsis**)

Respiratory Distress Syndrome (eg hyaline membrane DZ): **Tx –** surfactant

Immunity at birth
IgA – from mothers milk

IgG – only immunoglobulin to crosses placenta

PMNs have **impaired chemotaxis** (children at risk for **cutaneous** infections)

Maintenance intravenous fluid rate
4 cc/kg/hr for 1st 10 kg

2 cc/kg/hr for 2nd 10 kg

1 cc/kg/hr after above

Maintenance Fluid Type
Neonates – D10 1/4 normal saline (no potassium)

Infants – D10 1/4 normal saline (no potassium until making urine)

Toddlers and school age – D5 1/2 normal saline w/ 20 mEq K

Effective fluid resuscitation
Neonates and infants – urine output of 2-3 cc/kg/hr

Toddlers and school age – urine output of 1 cc/kg/hr

Children (<6 months) have **25% GFR capacity of adults** – poor concentrating ability, need to be careful w/ potassium containing fluids

MCC childhood death – trauma

    Trauma bolus – 20 cc/kg x 2, then blood 10 cc/kg

    Tachycardia – best indicator of shock in children

        Neonate   >150

        Age 0-1 year >120

        Rest   >100

Initial fluid resuscitation for dehydration (eg pyloric stenosis) – normal saline 20 cc/kg

Caloric need

Age (years)	Calories (kcal / d)
0-1	750 (avg)
1-15	1000 + 100 for each year
15-18	2500

Most commons (in childhood unless o/w stated)
- MC malignancy – leukemia (ALL)
- MC tumor – hemangioma
   - MC tumor in newborn – sacrococcygeal teratoma
- MC solid tumor class – CNS tumors
- MC intra-abdominal tumor – neuroblastoma
   - MC in child <2 years – neuroblastoma
   - MC in child >2 years – Wilms tumor
- MC kidney tumor – Wilm's Tumor
- MC liver tumor – hepatoblastoma; (70% of liver tumors in children are malignant)
- MC lung tumor – carcinoid
- MCC duodenal obstruction – malrotation
   - MC in newborns (<1 week) – duodenal atresia
   - MC after newborn period (>1 week) – malrotation
- MCC colon obstruction – Hirschsprung's disease
- MCC painful lower GI bleeding – benign anorectal lesions (fissures, etc)
- MCC painless lower GI bleeding – Meckel's diverticulum
- MCC Upper GI bleeding in years 0–1 – gastritis, esophagitis
- MCC Upper GI bleeding 1 year to adult – esophageal varices, esophagitis
- Double bubble sign (gastric + duodenal dilatation on AXR) – malrotation, duodenal atresia, or annular pancreas

Branchial cleft cyst – can lead to sinus tracts, fistulas, and infection
- 1st Branchial Cleft Cyst – angle of mandible
   - Can connect with external auditory canal
   - Very often associated w/ facial nerve
- 2nd Branchial Cleft Cyst (MC location) – anterior border of SCM muscle
   - Goes through carotid bifurcation and into tonsillar pillar
- 3rd Branchial cleft cyst – deep in SCM, emerges in pyriform sinus
- Tx for all cysts: resection

Thyroglossal duct cyst
- From descent of thyroid from foramen cecum
- May be only thyroid tissue pt has; risk of infection or malignancy
- Presents as a midline cervical mass
- Classically moves up w/ tongue protrusion and swallowing
- Tx: excision of cyst, tract, and central portion of hyoid bone (lateral neck incision) – sistrunk procedure

Hemangioma
- MC tumor of childhood and infancy
- Appears at birth or shortly after
- Usually rapid growth w/ first 12 months of life but then involutes
- Head and neck MC sites
- Tx:
   - Observation – most resolve by age 5-6 (85%)
   - Treatment if lesion:
      - 1) Has uncontrollable growth or:
      - 2) Impairs function (airway, eyelid or ear canal) or:
      - 3) Persistent after age 8
   - Tx
      - Oral steroids (possible intra-lesion steroids as adjunct)
      - Laser or resection if steroids not successful
- Rare cx's of hemangioendothelioma (infants; usually liver hemangiomas)
   - Kasabach-Merritt syndrome – consumptive coagulopathy and thrombocytopenia associated w/ large hemangiomas in newborns (DIC clinical picture)
      - Tx: best option embolization and steroids
      - Resection ± pre-op embolization if completely resectable (unusual)
   - CHF (A-V shunting) – Tx: embolization and steroids
      - Resection ± pre-op embolization if completely resectable (unusual)

Pyogenic granuloma (misnomer, actually a lobular capillary hemangioma)
  Benign, although can **bleed** spontaneously and undergo **necrosis**
  MC location – head and neck (70%)
  Tx: resection

Congenital anomalies of the lung
  Congenital lobar emphysema (hyperinflation)
      Sx's: resp distress or hypotension (same mechanism as tension PTX)
      Cartilage fails to develop in bronchus, leading to air trapping w/
            expiration
      MC location – LUL
      Dx: CXR
            Hyperinflation of lobe
            Compression and **displacement** of other structures
      Tx: lobectomy
  Bronchogenic Cysts
      Sx's: can compress adjacent structures w/ **resp distress** or become
            infected; Newborns can become very ill
      Formed from **abnormal lung tissue** (parenchyma, cartilage) <u>outside</u> lung
      MC cyst of mediastinum
      MC location – right side near carina, slightly posterior
      Are **extra-pulmonary** cysts (rarely intra-pulmonary)
      <u>Not</u> connected to airway
      Often contain milky liquid
      Malignant degeneration reported
      Tx: resection
  Congenital cystic adenomatoid malformations (CCAM)
      Sx's: newborns - resp distress, **older children** - infection
            Rapid decompensation can occur w/ ventilator – need mediastinal
                  decompression by removing cyst
      From **overgrowth of bronchiole tissue** (<u>no</u> cartilage; columnar
            epithelium)
      MC location – lower lobes
      Usually **intra-pulmonary**; can get air-trapping
      Connected to airway bronchus
      Malignant degeneration reported
      Dx: CT scan or water soluble UGI (to R/O diaphragmatic hernia)
      Tx: lobectomy
  Pulmonary sequestration
      Sx's: FTT, DOE, resp distress (tachypnea), pulm infection
            Heart failure, hemorrhage w/ rupture (hemoptysis), aneurysm
            Characteristic **continuous murmur** (DDx- AVM, sequestration, PDA)
      Dx:
            1) **CXR –** consolidated lung mass (non-aerated density)
            2) **CT scan –** lung mass w/ anomalous blood supply
            3) **angio –** can confirm anomalous blood supply
      Path
            Lung tissue but <u>not</u> connected to airway and has **systemic arterial
                  blood supply** (lung tissue can be intra-lobar or extra-lobar)
            MC location – LLL, but <u>no</u> connection to airway
            **Anomalous Arterial supply
                  MC off thoracic aorta
                  Can also come off **abdominal aorta** (celiac) **through inferior
                        pulmonary ligament**
            Intra-lobar – MC pulm venous connection
            Extra-lobar – MC systemic venous drainage (eg azygous vein)
            May have malignant change
      Tx: *need to ligate systemic arterial supply*; lobectomy (or rsxn of mass if
            extra-lobar)

Pulmonary arterio-venous malformation (AVM) – continuous murmur
  Tx: embolization 1st line now

Patent Urachus (see Urology chp)

Patent Omphalomesenteric Duct (Vitelline duct)
Connects ileum and umbilicus
Can have drainage out umbilicus
Tx: resection of the persistent duct

Persistent Omphalomesenteric Vessels (Vitelline vessels)
Artery passes from yolk sac to aorta
Vein from yolk sac to portal vein
MC presents w/ torsion of bowel w/ possible strangulation, necrosis
Tx: de-torse bowel w/ resection if necrotic, ligation of persistent vasculature

Omphalitis
Infection of **umbilical stump** after birth
Can lead to portal vein thrombosis (↑LFTs, can lead to variceal bleeding)
Tx: anticoagulation for portal vein thrombosis if acute; abx's for infection

Hydrocoele in children
Formed from **persistent tunica vaginalis**
May have a connection to peritoneum (**processus vaginalis**, communicating
hydrocele) or this may have been obliterated (non-communicating)
Most disappear by 1 year
Can be in **inguinal canal** or **scrotum**
U/S – will transluminate if in scrotum
Surgical indications:
1) At **age 1 year** if not resolved *or;*
2) **Felt to be communicating** (has persistent processus vaginalis; waxes
and wanes in size)
Tx: resect hydrocele + ligate persistent processus vaginalis (inguinal
approach)

Inguinal hernia in children
Due to persistent **processus vaginalis**
MC in **males,** MC on **right**
Can cause **SBO** or **bowel strangulation** w/ incarceration
RF's – prematurity
Varying degrees – can go all the way to the scrotum or stop short
**Lump in inguinal canal (eg intestine, cecum) at internal ring **differentiates
hernia from hydrocoele**
Get U/S to make sure it's not a **hydrocele** (hydrocoele in scrotum will trans-
illuminate)
Tx:
Incarceration (highest risk age **< 1 year**) – tender, firm swelling
Manual Reduction (firm steady pressure)
Sedation will help reduce inguinal hernias
Trendelenburg position (head down) w/ **knees bent**
Emergent operation if not able to reduce incarceration
If reduced → admit, repair within next 24-48 hours
Non-incarcerated - elective repair within 1 week
Repair – **high ligation** (to age 16 or so)
Make sure testicle in scrotum at end of procedure
Explore contralateral side if **left sided**, **female**, or **child <1 year** (use 3
mm scope though hernia sac, into peritoneum, and look at other side)

Umbilical hernia
Failure of closure of linea alba
Most close by age 3
↑ed in African Americans, prematurity, males
Rarely cause incarceration
Tx: surgery if not closed by **age 5**, if **incarceration,** or if pt has a **VP shunt**

Undescended testicles (cryptorchidism)
- **Path**
  - **RFs** – prematurity, low birth weight
  - Associated w/ many genetic syndromes
  - **Location – 90% in inguinal canal**
    - Can be anywhere from high posterior retroperitoneum to inguinal canal; ectopic or vanished also possible
  - 30% bilateral
  - Can be **underdeveloped or dysplastic** when found
  - **Inguinal hernias** common
  - Need to DDx true **undescended testis** vs. **retractile testis** (ie the testis is descended but occasionally retracts back into inguinal canal)
    - Retractile testis do <u>not</u> need operated on
- **Risks of undescended testicle:**
  - ↑ **Testicular CA** risk (5 x if unilateral, 10 x if bilateral undescended testis)
    - *CA risk stays the same even if testicles brought into scrotum*
    - Get **seminoma**
  - ↓ **Fertility** (likely related to higher temp in abdomen)
  - ↑ **Torsion risk**
- **Tx:**
  - **If bilateral →**
    1) **Early U/S and MRI** to locate (unless you can feel them in canal)
    2) **Chromosomal studies** (eg Klinefelter's, gonadal dysgenesis)
    3) **Hormonal studies** - to make sure there is actually testicular tissue present (HCG can be used to stimulate testosterone production)
    - Screen for **intersex issues** (eg uterus) if genetalia ambiguous
  - **Medical Tx:**
    - **hCG injections** can be performed (variable success)
  - **Wait 4-6 months after birth before surgery**
    - If you cannot feel testis in inguinal canal, you need to get an **MRI** to confirm presence of testis
    - **Tx:**
      - **Orchiopexy** through **inguinal incision** (if testicle in canal)
        - **Attach testis to scrotum** (eg subdartos pouch)
        - **High ligation** of inguinal canal
        - If not able to get testicles down →
          - Close and wait 6 months and try again
          - If won't come down again, perform division of spermatic vessels
      - Need **multiple procedures** if testis in abdomen to get to scrotum
      - Educate parents on need for future testicular exams to screen for testicular CA
      - **Adults w/ crypto-orchidism** – resect testicle (almost certainly non-functional)
  - **Fowler-Stephens principle** – division of testicular vessels and allowing blood supply to vas deferens to keep undescended testis viable; the testicular vessels should be divided away from testis to preserve collaterals
  - **Prune belly syndrome** (rare) – hypoplasia of abdominal wall, urinary tract abnormalities w/ dilated urinary system, and bilateral cryptorchidism

Testicular torsion
- Involved testis almost never viable
- Torsion usually toward midline (twist testis outward when trying to de-torse – 'open the book')
- **Tx: bilateral orchiopexy**
  - If not viable, resection and orchiopexy of contralateral testis
  - Can also get **torsion of testicular appendages** (requires bilateral scrotal exploration – testicle itself *not* tender, <u>no</u> scrotal edema)

Neuroblastoma

MC extra-cranial solid malignancy in children
MC malignancy in infancy period
MC age ≤ **2** (50%)

Sx's

- **MC presentation** – asymptomatic mass
- **Other sx's** – diarrhea, **raccoon eyes** (orbital mets), **HTN**, **unsteady gait** (opsomyoclonus syndrome)

Path

- From **neural crest cells**
- **MC location** – adrenal gland
  - Can occur anywhere on **sympathetic chain**
- **Majority secrete catecholamines** (90%, check urine for VMA, HVA, metanephrines)
- **50% have mets** at Dx (lung and bone)
- Small round blue cells in **Rosette pattern**
- **Spectrum of DZ** – ganglioneuroma (benign) → ganglioneuroblastoma (malignant) → neuroblastoma (most malignant)
- **Worse prognosis:**
  - **Age > 18 months**
  - **Tumor grade** (unfavorable histology, high mitosis-karyorrhexis index, diploid tumors)
  - **Mets**
  - **N-myc oncogene** amplification (regulates **microRNAs**)
- Tumors categorized into **low risk, moderate risk, and high risk** and tx **stratified** based on this assessment
- Initially unresectable tumors may be resectable after chemotherapy

Dx:

- **CT chest/abd/pelvis**
  - ± **stippled calcifications**
  - **Compresses** renal parenchyma rather than invades (DDx vs. Wilm's tumor)
- **MIBG –** can locate tumors

Stage

I	**Localized** area or origin, complete resection
II	**Incomplete resection**, does <u>not</u> cross midline
III	1) **Crosses midline**, ± regional nodal involvement *or;*
	2) **Unilateral** w/ contra-lateral nodes *or;*
	3) **Midline tumor** w/ bilateral nodes *or;*
IV	**Distant mets** (nodes, bone, liver, other organ)
IV-S	1) **Age < 1** *and;*
	2) **Localized tumor** (stage I or II) *and;*
	3) **Distant mets** (liver, skin, bone)

Tx:

- **Low risk** - resection only
- **Moderate Risk**
  1) **Neoadjuvant chemo** (DECC) – doxorubicin, etoposide, cisplatnin, and cyclophosphamide
  2) **Resection**
  3) **XRT** for <u>residual DZ</u>
- **High Risk**
  1) **Neoadjuvant chemo** (DECC-R) – doxorubicin, etoposide, cisplatnin + cyclophosphamide *followed by* **retinoic acid** (Vit A)
  2) **Resection**
  3) **XRT** to <u>primary area</u>
  - Possible **stem cell TXP**

Overall 5-YS – 40%

<u>Wilms tumor</u> (nephroblastoma, kidney tumor)

MC kidney tumor in children

Sx's

> **MC sx** – asymptomatic mass
>
> **Other sx's** – <u>hemi-hypertrophy</u> (highly assoc. w/ Wilm's), hematuria, HTN

Path

> **MC age > 2** (mean 3 years)
>
> 10% bilateral
>
> **Most impt prognostic indicator** – tumor grade (favorable vs. anaplastic)

Dx:

> **Abd CT** – **replacement** of renal parenchyma - <u>not</u> displacement and <u>no</u> calcifications (DDx vs. neuroblastoma)

Stage and Tx:

I	Tumor **limited to kidney** w/ **complete excision** (<u>intact capsule</u>)
	Tx: nephrectomy^, then chemo* (*exclude* doxorubicin)
II	**Beyond kidney but complete excision**
	(through capsule, into blood vessels, or leak after Bx)
	Tx: nephrectomy^, then chemo-XRT*
III	**Unresectable primary**, nodal mets, positive margins, tumor spillage on peritoneal surfaces, or transected thrombus
	Tx: chemo + XRT + nephrectomy
	Pre-op Stage III → neoadjuvant chemo-XRT to downstage tumor, then resect
	If originally stage II, then upstaged after surgery → post-op chemo-XRT
IV	**Hematogenous mets** (eg lung)
	Tx: nephrectomy^, then chemo-XRT* + whole lung XRT
	Add etoposide + cyclophosphamide to chemo
	XRT to other mets areas as well
V	**Bilateral renal involvement**
	Tx: neoadjuvant chemo *then* nephro-sparing surgery

^Nephrectomy includes **lymph node sampling** (hilar, peri-aortic, iliac, celiac *<u>mandatory</u>*)

***Chemo** (VAD) – vincristine, actinomycin, and doxorubicin (see above)
> *All stages get chemo*

Venous extension – occurs through renal vein, tumor can be extracted from IVC

Examine **contralateral kidney** and look for peritoneal implants

Avoid rupture of tumor w/ resection – will ↑ stage

PCP prophylaxis w/ bactrim w/ whole lung XRT

Resection of **resectable lung mets** if still present *<u>after</u>* whole lung XRT

Overall 5-YS – 90%

Genetic Syndromes:

> **Beckwith-Wiedemann syndrome** – macroglossia, macrosomia (birth weight > 90%), abdominal wall defects, ear creases, hypoglycemia (neonatal) – at risk for Wilm's and hepatoblastoma
>
> **WAGR** – Wilm's tumor, Aniridia (absence of iris), Genitourinary anomalies, and mental Retardation
>
> **Denys-Drash** – Wilm's tumor, nephropathy, gonadal dysgenesis

Hepatoblastoma

MC malignant liver tumor in children (80%)

Sx's

MC Sx – asymptomatic mass

Other sx's- Fractures (severe osteopenia), precocious puberty (beta-HCG)

Better prognosis than hepatocellular CA

RFs – low birth weight

Path

↑ **AFP** (90% of pts)

Can be **pedunculated**

Vascular invasion common

Extramedullary hematopoiesis may develop in tumor

Tx:

Very responsive to cisplatnin-based chemo (+ 5-FU and vincristine usual) → Can completely **eradicate lung mets**

Downstage tumors and make them resectable

Neoadjuvant chemo for majority (80%) unless very low stage tumor thought to be completely resectable at time of Dx

Formal resection w/ **lobectomy**

Residual lung mets after chemo – resection if resectable

XRT for positive margins after resection

TXP is an option for residual, unresectable tumor

AFP levels used to follow response to tx

2nd look laparotomy if elevated AFP levels

Meckel's diverticulum

MCC of painless lower GI bleeding in children aged ≤ 2 years

MC presentation in adults – Obstruction

Obstruction from **intussusception** or **volvulus**

Can also get diverticulitis

2's

2 feet from iliocecal valve

2 inches in length

2% of population

Usually present in 1st 2 years of life with **bleeding**

2% symptomatic

2 **tissue types** (pancreatic and gastric)

MC – **pancreatic**

Most likely to be symptomatic – **gastric** (causes bleeding)

Is a **true diverticula** (involves all layers of bowel wall)

Persistent vestigial remnant of **omphalomesenteric duct** (ie **persistent vitelline duct**)

Found on anti-mesenteric border of small bowel

Dx: get **Meckel scan** (99-Tc-pertechnate) if trouble localizing (mucosa lights up)

Tx:

Incidental → usually not removed unless **gastric mucosa** suspected (diverticulum feels **thick**) or has a very **narrow neck**

Diverticulectomy – for uncomplicated diverticulitis (base not involved)

Segmental resection for:

1) **Complicated diverticulitis** (eg perforation)

2) **Neck of diverticulum is > 1/3 diameter of normal bowel lumen** (don't want to narrow lumen)

3) **Base** involved

Gastroschisis

Congenital **abdominal wall defect**

Etiology – intrauterine rupture of **umbilical vein** (omphalomesenteric vessels)

RFs – high risk pregnancies, low birth weight

Path

> **No** peritoneal sac
>
> Usually **right of midline**
>
> **Stiff bowel** from exposure to amniotic fluid
>
> Can have other **congenital anomalies** (10%, less than omphalocele)

Tx:

> **Saline soaked gauzes** (prevent <u>fluid loss</u> from exposed bowel)
>
> **Fluid resuscitation**
>
> **Prophylactic abx's**
>
> Repair when stable
>
> **At operation:**
>
> > Try place bowel back in abdomen and close primarily as long as bowel not compromised
> >
> > Often can't get primary repair and have to attach a **silastic silo** to abdominal wall:
> >
> > > Contains abdominal contents outside body
> > >
> > > Progressively tightened over days-weeks to stretch abd cavity wall and make room for intestines
> >
> > Primary closure at a later date
>
> Check for other abnormalities (eg **malrotation**)

MC serious complication – sepsis

Mortality – 10%

Omphalocele

Congenital **abdominal wall defect**

Etiology – failure of **embryonal development**

Path

> **Midline defect**
>
> **Has peritoneal sac w/ umbilical cord attached**
>
> Associated w/ **multiple congenital anomalies** (50% → causes **worse prognosis then gastroschisis,** eg Down's, cardiac, GI, neuro)
>
> Can contain bowel, liver, spleen, etc

Tx:

> **Saline soaked gauzes** (prevent <u>fluid loss</u> from exposed bowel)
>
> **Fluid resuscitation**
>
> **Prophylactic abx's**
>
> Repair when stable
>
> **At operation:**
>
> > Try place bowel back in abdomen and close primarily as long as bowel not compromised
> >
> > Often can't get primary repair and have to attach a **silastic silo** to abdominal wall:
> >
> > > Contains abdominal contents outside body
> > >
> > > Progressively tightened over days to stretch abd cavity wall and make room for intestines
> >
> > Primary closure at a later date
>
> Check for other abnormalities (eg **malrotation**)

MC serious complication – sepsis

Mortality – 20% (mainly increased due to associated congenital anomalies)

Cantrell pentalogy:

> 1) **Cardiac** defects
> 2) **Pericardium** defects (usually at diaphragmatic pericardium)
> 3) **Sternal** cleft or absence of lower sternum
> 4) **Diaphragmatic** septum transversum absence
> 5) **Omphalocele**

Necrotizing enterocolitis (NEC)
Sx's:
>> **Bloody stools** after **1st feeding in premature neonate** (*classic*)
>> **Others** – feeding intolerance, abd distension, vomiting, lethargy, resp decompensation,
> **RFs:** prematurity, hypoxia, hypotension, anemia, polycythemia, sepsis
> **Dx:**
>> **Serial AXR's** (Q 6 hours)
>>> Check for free air, **pneumotosis** (pathognomonic), portal vein air
>>> **Persistent fixed loop** of bowel gas (ie nothing moving)
>> **Lateral decubitus** best to look for free air
> **Initial Tx:**
>> **Fluid resuscitation**
>> NPO, prophylactic Abx's, NGT, correct coagulation abnormalities (can get bleeding), TPN (medical tx usually for 2 weeks)
>> Serial exams and AXRs (Q 6 hours)
> **Indications for operation:** free air, peritonitis or clinical deterioration
>> → resect dead bowel and bring up ostomies
>> If extremely ill and cannot tolerate laparotomy – consider placing drain in NICU
>> Pneumotosis and/or portal venous air by themselves are <u>not</u> indications for drain or laparotomy
> Mortality 10%
> Need **barium contrast enema** and upper GI w/ SBFT before taking down ostomies to R/O distal obstruction from stenosis
> At risk for **short bowel syndrome** later in life

Intussusception
> **MC age** – 3 months to 3 years
> **Sx's:**
>> **RUQ pain, sausage mass** and **abd distention**
>> **Currant jelly stools** (from vascular congestion, <u>not</u> an indication for resection)
> **Path**
>> Invagination of one loop of intestine into another (**MC – ileocolic**)
>> **Lead points in children:**
>>> **MC** – enlarged Peyer's Patches
>>> Others – Meckel's diverticulum, lymphoma
>> **Recurrence after reduction** – 15%
>>> Surgery if occurs <u>after 2nd time of reduction</u>
> **Tx:**
>> **Reduce w/ air-contrast enema**
>>> **90% successful** (<u>no</u> surgery required if reduced)
>>> Max pressure with **air-contrast enema – 120 mmHg**
>>> Max column height with **barium enema – 1 meter** (3 feet)
>>> ↑**perforation risk beyond these values** → need laparotomy w/ manual reduction if you have reached these values
>>> Incompletely relieved intussusception despite above – laparotomy for manual reduction
>> Need to go to OR with **peritonitis, free air, or if unable to reduce**
>>> **When reducing in OR**, do <u>not</u> place traction on proximal limb of bowel; apply pressure to distal limb and squeeze out proximal bowel
>>> Usually don't require resection unless associated with lead point (eg Meckel's) or perforation
>> **If it occurs a 3rd time** → go to OR to look for lead point
> **Adult w/ intussusception** –most likely has **malignant lead point** (eg colon CA, metastatic melanoma) → OR

Hirschsprung's disease

MCC colonic obstruction in infants
Males (4:1)
Sx's

Infants fail to pass meconium in 1st 24 hours (MC Sx)
Others sx's - distension, constipation, vomiting
Can get **explosive release of watery stool** w/ anorectal exam

Dx:

Barium enema
Often shows **spastic distal colon** and **dilated proximal colon**
Can also be normal
**Rectal biopsy *(best test)* - diagnostic
Absence of ganglion cells in myenteric plexus

Path

Failure of neural crest cells to migrate in caudal direction
In 5%, the entire colon is affected

Tx:

Resect colon proximal to where ganglion cells appear
May need to bring up a **colostomy initially** (eg Hirschsprung's colitis)
Pull-through procedure (connect good residual colon to anus, eg Soave
or Duhamel procedure)
Hirschsprung's colitis
Can be rapidly progressive
Sx's - abd distension, foul smelling diarrhea, lethargy, sepsis
Tx: fluid resuscitation, abx's, rectal irrigation and washout; may need
emergency colectomy w/ colostomy (later hook-up)

Meconium ileus

Thick meconium (ie **1st stool**) causes **distal ileal obstruction**
Sx's: abd distension, bilious vomiting
High association w/ **Cystic Fibrosis**

Dx:

AXR

Dilated loops of small bowel *without* air-fluid levels (meconium is
too thick to separate from bowel wall); colon is decompressed
Ground glass or **soap suds** appearance
Gastrograffin enema (see below)
Sweat chloride test or **PCR for Cl channel defect** (cystic fibrosis
transmembrane conductance regulator, CFTR)

Path

Can cause **ischemia** or perforation w/ **meconium pseudocyst** or free
perforation
Can cause **late strictures** (from ischemia)

Tx:

Initial Tx:

Fluid resuscitation impt (osmotic load w/ gastrograffin enema will
draw fluid, can cause hypotension)
Empiric abx's and **NGT**
Gastrograffin enema *(best test and best Tx)*
Effective in 80%, done under fluoro
Can make Dx and potentially Tx (N-acetylcysteine can be used)
Surgical indications:
Failure of gastrograffin enema
Peritonitis (eg perforation or necrosis)
Clinical deterioration
If surgery required, manual decompression (milk meconium out) and create
tube enterostomy vent for **N-acetylcysteine** antegrade enemas
Pancreatic enzymes for w/ future feeds w/ CF
Cystic Fibrosis
Cx's: progressive lung destruction, pancreatitis, biliary cirrhosis,
coagulopathy (trouble absorbing fat soluble vitamins), infertility,
failure to thrive, late distal intestinal obstruction syndrome

Cornerstone of tx – IV, oral, and inhaled Abx's to ↓ pulmonary infections
Only lung disease requiring **mandatory** *double lung transplantation* (as opposed to single lung – pseudomonas in contralateral lung would infect new lung)
Burkholderia cepacia – particularly virulent organism that ↓s survival after lung TXP; resistant to majority of abx's
Mean survival of CF pts – 36 years

Malrotation

MCC duodenal obstruction in children (90% occur at age ≤ 1 year)
Sx's: sudden onset of **bilious vomiting**
    ****Bilious vomiting** in any child in the first 2 years of life requires an upper GI series to R/O malrotation; this needs to be done emergently

Path
    Failure of normal counter clockwise rotation (270°)
    Ladd's bands cause **duodenal obstruction**, coming out from right retroperitoneum
    Volvulus is associated w/ compromise of SMA, leading to **infarction of entire small bowel**
    Any child w/ bilious vomiting needs an UGI to R/O malrotation

Dx:
    UGI *(best test)* – duodenum does not cross midline, may see obstruction
    Equivocal UGI – barium enema shows cecum in abnormal position

Tx: (Ladd's procedure)
    Resuscitation
    Resect Ladd's bands
    Counterclockwise rotation of bowel (assess viability)
    Place cecum in LLQ (cecopexy)
    Place duodenum in RUQ
    Appendectomy
    Duodenal webs may be present w/ malrotation and can cause persistent bowel obstruction after Ladd's procedure

Pyloric stenosis

Usually presents at **3–12 weeks;** first born **males**
Sx's: projectile vomiting (*classic*, <u>non-bilious</u>)
    Can feel **olive mass** in stomach
U/S – pylorus **≥ 4mm thick, ≥ 14 mm long**
Get <u>hypochloremic, hypokalemic metabolic alkalosis</u>
Tx:
    Fluid Resuscitate before OR
        Normal saline bolus (20 cc/kg)
        D5 1/2 normal saline at 1.5 x maintenance then used
        Potassium replaced as needed <u>after</u> UOP is established
    Pyloromyotomy – RUQ incision; divide vein of Mayo, proximal extent should be circular muscles of stomach

Duodenal atresia

MCC duodenal obstruction in newborns (< 1 week)
MC intestinal atresia
MC type – distal to ampulla of Vater
Etiology – failure of recanalization of the duodenum (<u>not</u> vascular accident)
Sx's: causes **bilious vomiting,** feeding intolerance
    80% distal to ampulla – bilious vomiting
    20% proximal to ampulla – non-bilious vomiting
Associated anomalies
    Duodenal webs (look for these intra-op)
    Down's syndrome (20% have Down's)
    Cardiac, renal, and GI anomalies (eg malrotation)
RFs – Polyhydramnios
Dx: AXR – shows **double-bubble sign** (*classic*, duodenum and stomach)
Tx:

> **Resuscitation**
> Duodeno-duodenostomy or duodeno-jejunostomy
> **Check for chromosomal abnormalities**
> **Duodenal webs** can cause persistent obstruction after repair (Tx: resection of web via longitudinal duodenostomy)

Intestinal atresia (jejunal and ileal)

Etiology – result of **intrauterine vascular accident** (→ ischemia and atresia)
Pre-natal U/S – polyhydramnios
Sx's: bilious emesis, distention; most do not pass meconium
Dx:
> AXR – bowel distension w/ distal decompression
> Get barium enema to look for Hirschsprung's before surgery
> Can be **multiple**

Tx: resection w/ **primary anastomosis** or bring up **ostomies** if too damaged (look for **multiple lesions**)

Cystic duplication

MC in **ileum**; MC on **mesenteric border**; Tx: **resect cyst**

Diaphragmatic hernias

Overall survival 50%
MC on **left side** (80%)
Can have severe **pulmonary hypertension**
80% have **associated anomalies:**
> **Cardiac** and **neural tube** defects; can have **malrotation**
Both lungs are dysfunctional (one from compression by bowel and contralateral lung dysfunction not completely understood)
Sx's: resp distress
Dx:
> **Prenatal –** U/S
> **CXR** - bowel in chest (may see NGT in chest)
Tx:
> **High frequency ventilation**
> **Prostacyclin** (pulmonary vasodilator), **inhaled NO,** May need **ECMO**
> **Stabilize before operating**
> Surgery through **abdominal approach**:
>> Need to reduce bowel and repair diaphragmatic defect ± mesh
>> Look for malrotation
> **Bochdalek's hernia** (MC) – located posterior
> **Morgagni's hernia** (rare) – located anterior (retrosternal)
>> **MC in adults** (pressure creates hernia)– if asymptomatic, leave alone
> **Eventration** – failure of diaphragm to fuse

Tracheoesophageal fistulas

Sx's:
> Newborn **spits up feeds**
> Excessive **drooling**
> **Respiratory symptoms** w/ feeding (aspiration, choking)
> **Can't place NG tube in stomach** (*classic*)
RFs – males, diabetic mothers, polyhydramnios, < 2500 g
Dx
> **CXR/AXR** (almost always give Dx) – contrast studies rarely needed
>> **Distal atresia –** gasless abdomen
>> **Proximal atresia –** distended stomach
> ECHO, renal U/S, spinal and limb X-rays to R/O VACTERL
Path
> **Type C**
>> **MC type** (85%)
>> **Proximal esophageal atresia** (blind pouch)
>> **Distal TEF**
>> **AXR** – distended stomach

Type A
　　2nd MC type (10%)
　　Esophageal atresia and <u>no</u> fistula
　　AXR – gasless abdomen
Type E
　　MC in adulthood
　　H configuration of esophagus and trachea
　　<u>Not</u> associated with atresia
Anomalies → VACTERL = **V**ertebral, **A**norectal (MC - imperforate anus),
　　Cardiac anomalies, **TE** fistula, **R**enal Disorders, and **L**imb anomalies
Tx:
　　Initial tx
　　　　Replogle tube (just goes into proximal segment)
　　　　Semi-upright position (never prone)
　　　　If intubation required, place gastrostomy tube (G-tube)
　　Right thoracotomy for most repairs:
　　　　Perform **primary repair of esophagus** (resect atretic segment) *and*
　　　　　　close hole in trachea
　　　　Bronch to locate fistula and find undiagnosed fistulas or
　　　　　　tracheomalacia
　　　　Circular myotomies – can be made in esophagus to get more length
　　　　　　(1-3, each gives 1 cm) – **submucosa left intact** (blood supply)
　　　　End to end anastomosis, absorbable suture; feeding tube through
　　　　　　anastomosis
　　　　Can close up to **6 cm defects**
　　If primary repair not possible:
　　　　Distal esophagus is oversewn and sutured to pre-vertebral fascia
　　　　Delayed primary repair after **daily proximal esophageal dilatations**
　　　　　　for 1-2 months
　　　　If that fails, esophageal **replacement w/ colon** may be necessary
　　Infants that are **premature, < 2500 gm, or sick →** replogle tube, treat
　　　　respiratory sx's, delayed repair
　　MC Cx of repair – <u>GERD</u>; others - leak, empyema, stricture, fistula
　　Survival related to **birth weight** and **associated anomalies**

Imperforate anus
　　Associated w/ **VACTERL** (see TE Fistula above)
　　High (fistulizes above levators)
　　　　Meconium in **urine or vagina** (fistula to bladder/vagina/prostatic urethra)
　　　　Tx: colostomy, later anal reconstruction w/ **posterior sagittal anoplasty**
　　Low (fistulizes below levators, perineal skin)
　　　　Tx: Perform **posterior sagittal anoplasty** (pull anus down into sphincter
　　　　　　mechanism), **no colostomy needed**
　　Need post-op **anal dilatation** to avoid **stricture**
　　These pts prone to **constipation**
　　Persistent cloaca – rectum, vagina and colon are joined in single channel

Congenital Vascular Malformations
　　Types:
　　　　Arterio-venous (by far **MC type to cause sx's** and **MC requiring tx**)
　　　　Venous only
　　　　Arterial only
　　Surgical indications:
　　　　Hemorrhage
　　　　Ischemia to affected limb
　　　　CHF
　　　　Ulcers
　　　　Functional impairment
　　　　Limb-length discrepancy (AVM limb longer and bigger)
　　Tx: embolization (may be sufficient on its own) and/or **resection**

Choledochal cysts

Young females of Asian descent

Sx's: episodic **abd pain**, **jaundice**, and **RUQ mass** (*classic*, triad found in 50%)
Other sx's – **pancreatitis**, **cholangitis**

Path

From abnormal **reflux of pancreatic enzymes** during uterine development
90% extrahepatic
5-10% CA risk (cholangiocarcinoma)
Can also get **pancreatitis and cholangitis**

Types

Type I: (MC – 85%) saccular or **fusiform dilatation** of common bile
duct (CBD) w/ normal intrahepatic duct.
Type II: isolated **diverticulum** off CBD
Type III or Choledochocele: arise from dilatation of **duodenal
portion of CBD** or where pancreatic duct joins
Type IV: dilatation of both **intrahepatic and extrahepatic** biliary
systems
Type V or Caroli's disease: dilatation of **intra hepatic** ducts *only*

Tx:

Type I – **cyst excision, hepaticojejunostomy** (roux-en-Y) and
cholecystectomy
Type II – **cyst excised completely** and choledochotomy closed **primarily**
Type III – trans-duodenal approach w/ **marsupialization or cyst excision**
Careful identification of ampulla → may need sphincterotomy for
adequate drainage
Type IV (partially intrahepatic) and **type V** (Caroli's disease, totally
intrahepatic) → individualized; will need **partial liver resection,
hepatico-jejunostomy,** or **liver TXP**

Biliary atresia

MCC neonatal jaundice requiring surgery
Jaundice > 2 weeks after birth suggests atresia (**refractory to phototherapy**)

Path

Can involve either extrahepatic or intrahepatic biliary tree or both
Get cholangitis, continued cirrhosis, eventual hepatic failure
↑ed **conjugated bilirubin**
Does <u>not</u> cause kernicterus (conjugated bilirubin does <u>not</u> cross blood-brain
barrier)

Dx

Liver Bx *(best test)* – periportal fibrosis, bile plugging, eventual cirrhosis
U/S and **ERCP** – may reveal atretic biliary tree
Labs – ↑ LFTs

Tx:

Extra-hepatic ducts *only* → **Kasai procedure** (hepaticoporto-jejunostomy)
1/3 get better, 1/3 go on to liver transplant, 1/3 die
Need Kasai procedure **before age 2 months**, o/w get irreversible
liver damage
Steroids after Kasai improves post-op bile flow (no affect on long
term survival)
If intra-hepatic ducts involved → liver TXP

Teratoma (dermoid cyst)
Path
Likely congenital but can present later in life
Germ cell or embryonal tumor
 Germ cell teratomas – occur is testes and ovaries
 Embryonal – MC along midline
  MC location – sacrococcygeal teratoma
MC tumor overall in newborns – sacrococcygeal teratoma
MC presentation in adolescents – ovarian
At risk for **malignancy**
 ↑ **AFP or beta-HCG** indicates malignancy
Can be cystic, solid, or mixed
Tumor Grade
0 – benign
1 – immature, probably benign
2 – immature, possibly malignant
3 – malignant
Cystic teratomas MC grade 0
Tx: excision

Sacrococcygeal teratomas
Females
90% benign at birth (almost all have exophytic component)
Great potential for malignancy (**adenocarcinoma**)
AFP – good marker to follow for recurrence
2-month mark is a huge transition
 < 2 months → 10% malignant
 > 2 months → 60% malignant
Tx:
 Coccygectomy (possible sacral resection) and long-term follow-up
 Re-attachment of coccygeal muscles and ligaments to prevent late
  perineal hernia

Lymphadenopathy
Usually acute suppurative adenitis associated w/ URI or pharyngitis
 If fluctuant → FNA, culture and sensitivity, abx's
 May need incision and drainage if it fails to resolve
Chronic causes – cat scratch fever, atypical mycoplasma
Asymptomatic
 Abx's for 10 days → excisional biopsy if no improvement
 ***This is lymphoma until proved otherwise**
Cystic hygroma
 Classically found in **lateral posterior neck triangle** (usually posterior to
  sternocleidomastoid muscle (SCM)
 MC on left; swollen bulges under skin; can form sinuses and get infected
 Tx: resection
 Branchial cleft cysts are either anterior or through the SCM
 Thyroglossal duct cysts – midline

Other Disorders
Pectus excavatum (sinks in)
 Sternal osteotomy, strut placed
 Repair if causing respiratory symptoms or emotional stress
 Possible improvement of pulmonary dynamics
Pectus carinatum (sticks out, pigeon chest)
 Strut <u>not</u> necessary
 Repair for emotional stress (<u>not</u> shown to improve pulmonary dynamics)

Congenital laryngomalacia
- **MCC airway obstruction in infants**
- **Sx's**
    - Intermittent respiratory distress and stridor
    - Exacerbation w/ supine position
- **Path**
    - **Immature epiglottis cartilage** w/ intermittent collapse of epiglottis over airway
    - Vast majority of children outgrow this by 12 months
- **Tx:**
    - PPI for associated **GERD** (may resolve sx's)
    - Surgery involves **cutting aryepiglottic folds** to let supraglottic airway spring open (rarely need surgery)
    - **Surgical tracheostomy** rarely necessary after surgery

Congenital tracheomalacia
- Elliptical fragmented rings (rather than C shaped)
- Usually w/ associated **TEF or esophageal atresia**
- **Sx's**
    - Expiratory wheeze; can have dying spells w/ feeding
    - Sx's get better within **1-2 years** but surgery not be delayed w/ dying spell
- **Dx:**
    - **CXR** – narrowing on lateral
    - **Awake bronch –** A-P dimension collapses (last test to be performed)
- **Indications for surgery** (<u>rarely</u> need surgery):
    - **Dying spell** (MC indication for surgery)
    - **Resp sx's** (eg recurrent infections)
    - **Unable to wean from vent**
- **Tx:**
    - **Aortopexy** (*best*, aorta sutured to back of sternum, opens up trachea)
    - Tracheostomy also option
    - **Pts w/ both GERD and tracheomalacia –** fix GERD 1st unless dying spell was sx

Choanal atresia
- Obstruction of choanal opening in nose by bone or mucus membrane, usually unilateral
- **Sx's:** intermittent respiratory distress, poor suckling
- **Tx:** surgical excision of obstruction

Laryngeal papillomatosis
- MC tumor of pediatric larynx
- Frequently **involutes after puberty**
- **Tx:** endoscopic removal or laser but frequently come back
- **Etiology** – HPV in the mother

Cerebral palsy – many have GERD

Indications for fundal wrap for GERD in <u>children:</u>
1) **Near-miss SIDS** associated w/ GERD
2) **Barrett's** (<u>not</u> an indication for adults)
3) **Neurologically impaired** w/ severe GERD (eg cerebral palsy) – for aspiration risk

Mediastinal tumors – see Thoracic chp

Branchial Cleft Cysts – see Head and Neck chp

Congenital hyperinsulinema (ie nesidioblastosis) – causes hypoglycemia
- **Tx:** ↑ feedings, steroids, diazoxide, octreotide, calcium channel blocker
- If above fail to relieve sx's → 90% pancreatectomy (w/ intra-op portal vein sampling of insulin levels)

Klinefelter's Syndrome (XXY)
- Hypogonadism, cryptorchidism, sterile, gynecomastia
- **Tx: testosterone** for hypogonadism
- ↑ed **risk of** – breast CA, lymphoma, DM,

SKIN and SOFT TISSUE

Skin Components

Epidermis (top layer) – consists of stratified squamous epithelium
Avascular w/ 4 cell types:

1) **Keratinocytes** – main cell type (95%); originate from basal cells on bottom; provides a mechanical barrier

2) **Melanocytes**
- Neuroectodermal origin (neural crest cells); in basal layer
- **Dendritic processes** transfer **melanin** to the neighboring keratinocytes via **melanosomes**
- Density of melanocytes is same among races, difference in production of melanin

3) **Langerhan's cells**
- Dendritic cells, take up and process antigens and become antigen-presenting cells (MHC class II) in secondary lymphoid tissue
- They lose antigen processing properties after antigen exposure while gaining capacity to interact w/ T-cells
- Derived from **monocytes** (requires stimulation by **colony stimulating factor 1**)
- Have a role in **contact hypersensitivity reactions** (type IV)

4) **Merkel cells** – likely involved w/ touch

Dermis – collagen, elastic fibers, extrafibrillar matrix, scaffold for the epidermis
Mechano-receptors

Pacinian corpuscles – deep pressure and high frequency vibration
Ruffini's Corpuscles – warmth, skin stretch (slippage of objects)
Krause's end-bulbs – cold, low frequency vibration
Meissner's corpuscles – light pressure and tactile sense

Eccrine sweat glands – aqueous sweat (for thermal regulation, is hypotonic)
Apocrine sweat glands – milky type sweat

Highest concentration in palms and soles
Most sweat released is a result of the sympathetic nervous system via acetylcholine

Lipid-soluble drugs – have increased skin absorption
Type I collagen – predominant type; 70% of dermis; provides tensile strength
Tension – the resistance to stretching (collagen)
Elasticity – the ability to regain shape (branching proteins can stretch out to twice normal length)
Cushing's Syndrome Striae – due to loss of tensile strength (**↓ed collagen**) and elasticity

Tissue expanders work by local recruitment, thinning of dermis and epidermis, and mitosis (more cells)
MCC of pedicled or anastomosed free flap necrosis – venous thrombosis
Blood supply to skin for myocutaneous flap – underlying muscle perforators
Trans-rectus abdominal myoplasty (TRAM Flap)

Blood supply – superior epigastric vessels (can't use if previous CABG w/ IMA use)
Cx's – necrosis, ventral hernia, bleeding, infection, abdominal wall weakness
Most important determinant of TRAM flap viability – peri-umbilical muscle perforators to skin

UV radiation

Damages DNA indirectly (90%, free radical formation mainly) and directly (10%, breaks up DNA)
Acts as a **promoter and initiator**
Melanin - single best factor for protecting skin from UV radiation
Absorbs UV radiation and dissipates energy as heat
UVA – can only damage indirectly
UVB – most damaging type
UVC – filtered by the atmosphere

Skin Lesion
DDx: melanoma, BCCA (teleangiectasias), SCCA, seborrheic keratosis, actinic keratosis, pigmented wart, neurofibroma, benign nevus

Dx

1) **Punch biopsy** (5 mm, need to get down to subcutaneous fat)
   No shave biopsy, need to get depth
   Face, hands or feet (cosmetic regions or hard to close) – always want punch Bx
   Can consider punch Bx for lesions in any location (easy office procedure)
   Biopsy at **thickest spot** or **most abnormal looking**
2) **Can perform excisional Bx** w/ 1 mm margin for other areas (as long as it is small)
   Make sure you are into **subcutaneous fat** (need full thickness) w/ Bx (no stitch placed w/ punch)
   Fix in **Formalin**, paraffin embedded permanent section, H and E stain, (**not** frozen section)

Melanoma
Lung MC metastatic location
5% of all skin CA, 70% of deaths from skin CA
Melanoma MC metastasis to **small bowel**
MC site for melanoma – back (men), **legs** (women)
Blue worst color in terms of malignant potential
Worse survival - ↑number of nodes; location on back or posterior arms/neck/scalp (BANS), ocular, mucosal, ulcerated, men, ↑ mitotic rate
Originates from **melanocytes** (neural crest cells) in epidermis basal layer
10% of all melanomas felt to be **familial** in nature
Axillary lymph node melanoma w/ no primary → Tx: complete ALND
Resection of metastases has provided some w/ long disease-free survival
Resectable isolated metastases: Tx: resection
RFs – Fair complexioned people, easy sunburning, previous skin CA or XRT
Markers – **S-100** protein and **HMB-45**
Melanin – single best protector from UV-B damage
No MOHS surgery for melanoma
Signs of melanoma transformation (ABCD rule)
   Asymmetrical
   Border irregularity (angulations, indentation, notching, ulceration, bleeding)
   Color change (blue most ominous, red, darkening)
   Diameter (> 6 mm or enlargement)
Syndromes
   Dysplastic nevus syndrome (**100% risk of melanoma**; have following criteria – > 100 moles, one mole > 8 cm, 1 mole w/ atypical histology)
   Xeroderma pigmentosa – defect in **nucleoside repair enzyme;** get melanoma at young age; may need to avoid sunlight completely
   Giant congenital nevus (± hair; **5-10% risk of melanoma**)
      Do not prophylactically remove these unless small (< 2 cm)
      The larger the nevi, the greater the risk of melanoma
      Tx: frequent F/U to look for change in nevus
      If melanoma found, need to resect whole nevus (may need rotational flap or STSG)
   Familial BK mole syndrome – atypical nevi > 5 mm considered to be precursors to melanoma
Types of Melanoma
   Lentigo maligna (eg Hutchinson's freckle) – **melanoma in situ;** least aggressive, radial growth 1st usual; usually an elevated nodule
   Superficial spreading melanoma (MC type) intermediate malignancy
   Nodular – most aggressive; increased metastasis and deep growth at Dx: Blue-black w/ smooth borders; occurs anywhere
   Acral lentigo – very aggressive; presentation is palms, soles or subungal (pigment can spread to lateral nail folds); African-Americans

Dx:

Primary Diagnosis

1) **Punch biopsy** often used to make initial diagnosis

2) **< 2 cm and non-cosmetic location** – excisional Bx

When you discover melanoma, need w/u for **mets** and **nodal DZ**

Mets w/u:

All **intermediate** and **thick melanomas** (> 1 mm) require:

1) **Chest/Abd/Pelvic CT**

2) **LFT's**

3) **LDH** (marker for metastasis)

Thin melanoma w/ clinically positive nodes need same as above

Risk of mets or nodal DZ:

Thin melanoma (< 1 mm)	< 5%
Intermediate melanoma (1-4 mm)	25%
Thick melanoma (> 4 mm)	50%

Clinically positive nodes or **mets** on CT→ need **PET scan**

Nodal DZ w/u:

All **intermediate** and **thick melanomas** (> 1 mm) get **SLNBx**

Exception - **clinically positive nodes**, then perform formal lymphadenectomy

Thin melanoma (< 1 mm) that need **SLNBx:**

Ulceration

Regression on path (was deeper at one point but regressed)

If into **reticular dermis**

↑**mitotic rate**

**Nodal DZ but can't find primary → formal lymphadenectomy

Either regression of primary or is non-pigmented melanoma

Can consider palliative lymphadenectomy in pt's w/ extensive DZ for positive nodes

Staging (based on depth)

I – < 1 mm or 1-2 mm *without* ulceration

II – > 1 mm (w/ exception of above)

III – positive regional nodes, in-transit metastasis, satellite lesion

IV – distant mets (skin, node, lung, subcutaneous tissue, small bowel)

Tx:

Primary excision (or re-excision) **for melanoma:**

Melanoma in situ (Hutchinson Freckle if on face)- 0.5 cm margin OK	
Thin melanoma (< 1 mm)	1 cm margin
Intermediate melanoma (1-4 mm)	2 cm margin
Thick melanoma (> 4 mm)	2-3 cm margin

Need to get down to underlying **muscle fascia** (not through it; elliptical incision w/ 3:1 ratio length to width)

If going across a **joint,** make an **S-shaped incision**

If you can't primarily close defect:

Non-cosmetic region → STSG

Cosmetic region → FTSG (can take skin from just above the clavicle or behind the ear – lot's of redundant skin)

Foot → pedicled, myofascial, cutaneous skin graft

In-transit mets - resection

SLNBx

Technique

Technetium labeled sulfur colloid 1-4 hours before OR adjacent to the tumor

Lymphazurin injection when in OR and rub in

Gamma probe to find area for incision before prepping (identifies nodes outside traditional basin)

Situation in which gamma is hot in an unexpected area – **sample unexpected area**

W/ dissection, use gamma probe and blue stain to remove:

1) **All blue nodes** *and*

2) **All nodes within 10% of the highest gamma count**

If you find **clinically positive nodes** (bulky nodes) while
dissecting → convert to **formal lymph node dissection**

Path from SLNBx – <u>no</u> frozen sections

Need sequential thin **step sectioning** through each node w/
routine **H and E stains** (all of this for permanent)

Then stain for **S-100** and **HMB-45**

If nodes are positive, need formal lymphadenectomy later (see
below, 2nd procedure)

Formal lymphadenectomy of nodal drainage areas

Indicated for **positive SLNBx** or **clinically positive nodes**

You are trying to clear tumor from these areas (not sample)

4 general nodal basins - Ilio-inguinal, axillary, cervical, and parotid

Lymph node staging based on primary site:

1) **Truncal and extremity melanoma** (below neck):

Line of Sappey – (2 cm above umbilicus to L2/L3)

Above this line → melanoma goes to axillary nodes (in
general)

Below this line → melanoma goes to ilio-inguinal nodes (in
general)

a) **Axillary** – need to take **level I, II, and III nodes** (unlike breast CA
in which you take just level I and II nodes)

May need to divide **pectoralis minor muscle**

Watch for lateral pectoral nerve - innervates pectoralis major

If **supra-clavicular** nodes involved as well, no dsxn → not
going to be able to clear all these nodes (no cure)

b) **Ilioinguinal area has 2 levels** (superficial and deep):

Superficial nodes in femoral triangle

Need **S shaped incision** starting 1 cm medial to **anterior
superior iliac spine**

Goes down to intersection of **sartorius muscle and
femoral adductor muscles**

Take greater saphenous vein and all accompanying
nodes up to inguinal ligament (superficial
nodes)

Open femoral sheath and sample **Cloquet's node**

This is the highest inguinal node

This is the node between the superficial and
deep areas (obturator and iliac area)

Deep nodes (obturator and iliacs)

Indications:

Clinically positive superficial nodes

Obturator or iliac adenopathy on CT scan

Positive Cloquet's node

Obturator or iliacs nodes light up w/ SLNBx

Make separate incision through external abdominal
oblique fascia superior and parallel to inguinal
ligament

Cut through abdominal wall muscles

Retro-peritoneal dissection (pull back the peritoneum)

Can also just **split inguinal ligament** or go through
abdomen

2) **Head and Neck melanoma**

Close to vital structures

May need **special tailoring** (eg carotid) → may only get 1 cm margin

Lymph node spread →

1) Scalp and face **anterior** to pinna <u>(including ear)</u> and superior
to lip → **parotid gland**

2) Lesions **inferior** to lip commissure→ **anterior cervical chain**

3) Lesions **posterior** to pinna → **posterior cervical chain**

a) **Anterior lesions** (including ear):
    SLNBx
        If parotid lights up → superficial parotidectomy
        Clinically positive nodes → **MRND** (level I-V nodes) +
            superficial parotidectomy
        Positive nodes on SLNBx (requires re-operation) → **MRND**
            (level I-V nodes) + **superficial parotidectomy**
        If superficial parotid has tumor → need <u>**total parotidectomy**</u>
b) **Posterior lesions:**
    SLNBx
        Take all blue nodes and any nodes ≥ 10% of the node w/ the
            highest gamma count
        Clinically positive adenopathy → posterior node dissection
        Positive nodes on SLNBx (requires re-operation) → posterior
            node dissection
c) **Inferior lesions:**
    SLNBx
        Clinically positive adenopathy → MRND
        Positive nodes on SLNBx (requires re-operation) → MRND
    Full thickness skin graft (free graft) from behind ear or above
        clavicle for big facial lesions
        Undermine the area some; rotational flap also a possibility

Special situations
Subungal melanoma
    Remove the nail and get a punch Bx
    Thumb melanoma– amputate at the DIP joint
    Any other finger melanoma → amputate at the PIP
    Toe melanoma→ amputate at the MTP joint
Foot melanoma – pedicled, myofascial cutaneous flap for sole of foot
Ear melanoma (pinna = ear) – wedge resection w/ previous outlined
    margins
Eye melanoma – enucleation
Anal canal
    Make sure you have **mets w/u** before contemplating APR
    Thin melanoma → excise to appropriate margins
    Thick melanoma → APR
    Intermediate melanoma → case by case basis, thicker lesions lean
        towards APR; Discuss w/ pt

Systemic tx
Dacarbazine *(first line)* for positive nodes (stage IIIb) or mets (stage IV)
Interferon, IL-2, and **tumor vaccines** can be used for **positive nodes** or
    mets (all have marginal results)
XRT – considered for multiple node DZ (> 4 nodes); palliation (eg bone pain)
Delayed clinically positive nodes after previous melanoma resection
    → mets W/U as above, **formal lymphadenectomy** if no systemic mets

Basal cell

**MC malignancy in US (4x MC than squamous)

MC location - head and neck, upper lip

From epidermis – basal epithelial cells and hair follicles

Pearly, rolled appearance, slow growth, ulcerative deep invasion

Rare mets or nodal spread

MC type – nodular form

Morpheaform most aggressive; **collagenase** production

Path – peripheral palisading of nuclei, stromal retraction

Tx:

> Need 0.3-0.5 cm margins
>
> Regional lymph node dissection for clinically positive nodes
>
> Chemo-XRT – limited benefit for inoperable DZ or mets
>
> > Also for neuro, lymphatic or vessel invasion
>
> **Lip CA** – needs to involve the mucosa or not lip CA
>
> > 0.75 cm margins, If **> 1/3 of lip** resected, need **skin flap**

Squamous cell CA

Erythema, papulonodular with crust, ulceration, red-brown color

Possible surrounding induration satellite nodules

Mets - Melanoma > Squamous cell CA > Basal cell CA

RFs - post-XRT, old burn scars, actinic keratoses, xeroderma pigmentosum, Bowen's DZ, atrophic epidermis, arsenics, hydrocarbons (coal tar), chlorophenols, nitrates, HPV, immunosuppression, UV radiation, fair skin people, previous skin CA, chronic draining fistulas

RFs for mets – poorly differentiated, ↑ depth, recurrent CA, immunosuppressed

Tx:

> ****Need 1 cm margins for most**
>
> > **Cosmetic location or high risk** - Mohs surgery (margin mapping w/ conservative slices; <u>NOT</u> used w/ melanoma); minimizes resection area (eg on face)
> >
> > **Need 2 cm margins for:**
> >
> > > 1) **Marjolin's ulcer** – need 2 cm margin
> > >
> > > 2) **Penile CA** (penectomy, possibly partial if distal lesion)
> > >
> > > 3) **Vulvar CA**
> >
> > ****Special areas**
> >
> > > **Lip CA** – needs to involve mucosa or its not lip CA (considered anterior oral cavity tumor, see Head and Neck chp)
> > >
> > > **Anal canal CA** and **anal margin CA** (see Rectum + Anus chp)
>
> **Nodes**
>
> > **Indications for prophylactic nodal dissection:**
> >
> > > 1) **> 2 cm** in circumference *or:*
> > >
> > > 2) **> 4 mm** deep *or:*
> > >
> > > 3) **All Parotid Basin Lesions (**ear**, temple, forehead, anterior scalp) – 20% risk of parotid nodal involvement (all need **prophylactic superficial parotidectomy**)
> > >
> > > For above, follow technique for formal lymph node dissection described in melanoma section (eg, MRND, ALND, ilioinguinal LND) – *except* parotid basin lesion
> > >
> > > **Parotid basin lesions →** superficial parotidectomy, if positive for tumor → total parotidectomy + MRND
> > >
> > > *No role* for sentinel lymph node biopsy proven yet
> >
> > **Clinically positive nodes →** regional lymph node dissection
> >
> > > **Parotid basin lesion w/ clinically positive nodes –** total parotidectomy + MRND
>
> **Chemo-XRT** - used if neuro, nodal, or vessel invasion; positive margins

Soft tissue sarcoma

MC sarcoma – malignant fibrous histiosarcoma (#2 liposarcoma)
MC site – extremities (50%, **MC area** - thigh)
50% in **children** (embryonic mesoderm)
RFs – **Asbestos** (mesothelioma), **PVC and arsenic** (angiosarcoma), **Chronic lymphedema** (lymphangiosarcoma); **XRT**
Desmin – marker for rhabdomyosarcoma
Hematogenous spread, <u>not</u> to lymphatics (nodal mets rare)
    Do <u>not</u> need lymph node dissection
MC mets – lung
Most impt prognostic indicator – tumor grade (undifferentiated worse)
    Part of staging sarcomas

Sx's
    Asymptomatic mass (MC), bowel obstruction, neuro or vascular deficit
    For **retroperitoneal sarcomas**, need to think about **lymphoma (sx's** - fevers, chills, night sweats)
    Full neuro, muscular, and **vascular exam** of affected area (document these for later)

Dx:
    MRI of primary area for all <u>before Bx</u> to r/o **neuro, bone**, or **vascular invasion**
    Chest/abd/pelvic CT
    LFT's
    Biopsy:
        1) **Core needle biopsy** (along long axis plane of future incision for en bloc resection)
        2) If core needle <u>not</u> feasible or insufficient tissue:
            Longitudinal Excisional biopsy if < 4 cm → then go back for margins if sarcoma
            Longitudinal Incisional biopsy if > 4 cm (resect biopsy skin site if biopsy shows sarcoma)
            Both of above along **long axis plane of future incision** for en bloc resection (eg incision along **long axis** of extremity)

Tx:
    Need elliptical incision around the previous Bx site
    Want at least **2 cm margin** for tumor
    Try to get at least **1 un-involved fascial plane** medially and laterally
    90% do <u>NOT</u> need amputation → try to perform limb-sparing operation
    Complete resection best chance for survival
    Pre-op chemo-XRT (doxorubicin based) - may allow **limb sparing** surgery
        MAID – mesna, doxorubicin [Adriamycin], ifosfamide, dacarbazine
    Post-op chemo-XRT indications (doxorubicin based) - **high-grade, close margins**, or tumors **>5 cm**
    5-YS with complete resection – 40%

Special Issues:
    Close margins → **place clips** to mark site will XRT these later
    Close involvement of vascular supply → will pick this up on pre-op MRI
        Plan ahead for arterial or venous reconstruction if invasion of vessels
        Otherwise try to leave vessels intact (tumor is close but not invading) and place clips for post-op XRT
    Close involvement of nerve
        1) **Take nerve** if its already **non-functional** (possible amputation, depends on function of limb)
        2) **If nerve is functional** → shave tumor off, place clips, XRT later
    Close involvement of bone → will pick this up on MRI
        Counsel pt ahead of time that may require amputation
        Do your best to try and get tumor off bone if at all possible
        Place clips, XRT that area later
    Isolated mets w/o evidence of systemic DZ (eg lung or liver) → resect as long as you leave enough liver or lung to live
    Local recurrence → re-stage the pt
        Chest/Abd/Pelvic CT and **LFT's**

MRI of primary area – looking for bone, neuro, or vascular involvement

Resection if resectable

Distant recurrence (eg lung) → re-stage pt

Chest/abd/pelvic CT and **LFT's**

MRI of the primary area – looking for bone, neuro, or vascular involvement

Make sure you have local control

Resection if resectable

Presentation w/ primary sarcoma and lung met

(synchronous met, general recommendations)

Make sure both the lesions are potentially resectable

Resect the primary 1st

Then go after the met in **6 weeks** (allow for recovery)

In general, metastatic lesions do not metastasize

Situation in which you feel the **mets is going to be difficult to resect** → go after met 1st

Saves potentially disabling surgery (ie amputation) in pt w/ unresectable DZ

Best prognosis mets:

Disease free interval > 12 months

< 4 mets

Doubling time > 20 days

Complete resection

Primary control

Head and neck sarcomas

MC in **pediatric population** (**MC type** - rhabdomyosarcoma)

Difficulty getting margins due to proximity to vital structures (eg carotid, spinal cord)

Retroperitoneal sarcoma

MC type – liposarcoma

Need to make sure this is not lymphoma (night sweats, fever or chills; adenopathy)

Want en bloc resection

Take everything you have to – eg kidney, spleen, colon, portion of liver

<25% resectable w/ negative margins due to proximity to vital organ structures

Best chance for survival is a **negative margin resection**

Midline incision for pelvic and retroperitoneal sarcomas

Poor prognosis due to:

Delay in diagnosis

Difficulty w/ total resection and getting negative margins

Difficulty getting XRT to retroperitoneal and pelvic tumors

Local recurrence 40%

Often have a pseudocapsule but cannot shell out → leaves residual tumor

Visceral and retroperitoneal sarcomas

MC type – leiomyosarcomas; others - liposarcomas

Kaposi's sarcoma (KS; highly vascular sarcoma)

ALL* are caused by *human herpes virus 8 (HHV 8)

From **lymphatic endothelium** that forms vascular channels

Epidemiology

Endemic (sub-Saharan Africans; NOT HIV related)

Classic – old men, Mediterranean

Transplant related – ↑ since calcineurin inhibitors

Epidemic – AIDS (300 x more likely than after TXP)

MC neoplasm in AIDS pt

Sx's

MC sites - **oral** and **pharyngeal** mucosa (odynophagia, dysphagia; bleeding); others skin, respiratory or GI tract

Slow growing - rarely causes death w/ AIDS

Tx:

Surgery generally not tx of choice – primary goal is **palliation**
Exceptions - intestinal hemorrhage
HAART Tx (see Infection chp) will often shrink AIDS related KS
Systemic Tx: interferon-alpha, liposomal anthracyclines (eg Doxil) or paclitaxel
Local Tx: XRT, intra-lesional vinblastine, cryosurgery, XRT

Childhood rhabdomyosarcoma
MC soft tissue sarcoma in children – rhabdomyosarcoma
Can manifest in head, ear, neck, vagina, extremities and trunk (poorest prognosis)
MC malignant aural tumor of childhood
MC subtype – embryonal
Worst prognosis subtype – alveolar
Tx: as above
Botryoides tumor – vaginal rhabdomyosarcoma (sx's – bleeding)

Bone sarcomas (see Orthopaedics chp)
MC metastatic at time of dx
Osteosarcoma
MC location – knee
MC population – children
From **metaphyseal cells**

Genetic syndromes

Neurofibromatosis (von Recklinghausen's DZ; autosomal dominant)
Affects all **neural crest cells** (schwann cells, melanocytes, endoneurial fibroblasts)
Disordered **skin pigmentation** (café au lait spots, axillary freckling)
< 10% actually get CA
1) **Type I NF** (**neurofibromin** gene mutation, normally inhibits GTPase)
    a) **CNS** (optic nerve, acoustic neuroma)
    b) **Peripheral nerve sheath** (neurofibroma, neurolemma)
    c) **Pheochromocytoma**
2) **Type II NF** (**merlin** gene mutation, cytoskeletal protein)
    → *only get acoustic neuromas*
Schwannomatosis – multiple schwannomas

Li-Fraumeni syndrome (autosomal dominant)
Wide range of CA - breast, brain, acute leukemia, soft tissue sarcomas, bone sarcomas, adrenal cortical carcinoma
Often present in **childhood** (eg rhabdomyosarcoma)
Mutation in **p53 tumor suppressor**

Hereditary retinoblastoma
RB-1 gene defect (retinoblastoma)
55% sporadic, 45% inherited
MC in childhood
Best 5-YS of all childhood CA – 98%
Also at risk for pineal tumors and other sarcomas
Tx options include: chemo, cryotherapy, radioactive plaques, laser therapy, XRT and surgery

Tuberous sclerosis (tuberous sclerosis complex, autosomal dominant)
Get hamartomas (angiomyolipoma)
Affects brain kidneys, heart, eyes, lungs, and skin
70% sporadic, 30% inherited
Sx's: seizures, developmental delay, skin abnormalities, lung and kidney tumors
Skin – hypomelanotic macules, subependymal nodules
Mutations of **TSC1** (Hamartin) or **TSC2** (Tuberin) – tumor suppressor genes (GTPase which suppresses mTOR signaling pathway)

Gardner's syndrome (autosomal dominant)

FAP + extra-colonic tumors (abd desmoid tumors, osteomas of skull, thyroid CA, epidermoid cysts, fibromas sebaceous cysts)

Sx's: multiple impacted and supernumerary teeth, multiple jaw osteomas (cotton-wool appearance), odontomas, congenital hypertrophy of retinal pigment epithelium

APC gene (APC gene binds glycogensynthasekinase [GSK] and is involved in cell cycle regulation and movement)

Other Skin Lesions

Merkel cell carcinoma

Neuroendocrine tumor

Highly aggressive w/ early regional and systemic spread

Path

Can spread through skin and lymph nodes

Commonly have mets (MC bone) and lymph node spread

Red to purple papulo-nodules

80% have Merkel Cell Polyomavirus

Have neuron-specific enolase (NSE), cytokeratin, and neurofilament protein staining

Keratin antibodies show peri-nuclear pattern

Tx:

All pts need SLNBx or formal lymph node dissection

Resection w/ 2-3 cm margin

Post-op Chemo-XRT

5-YS for all patients – 60%

Dermatofibrosarcoma Protuberans (RFs – arsenic)

Low grade sarcoma (3% malignancy potential → fibrosarcoma)

Usually presents as a protuberance on the back

Forms in dermis from fibroblasts

95% have chromosome 17,22 translocation (PDGF expressed instead of collagen)

Tx: wide local excision only (very low grade, 3 cm margin)

Lipomas – rarely malignant liposarcomas

Often on back, neck, between shoulders

MC mesenchymal neoplasm

Neuromas – nerve sheath tumors (neurofibromas, neurolemma)

Genetic predisposition w/ neurofibromatosis (von Recklinghausen's disease, see above)

Angiomyolipoma – benign vascular leiomyoma

Can arise in kidney or extremities; painful

Tx: excision

Keratoses

Actinic keratosis

Premalignant; dark or light; tan, pink, or red

Sun damaged areas

Tx:

Diclofenac sodium, liquid nitrogen, 5-fluorouracil cream, photodynamic therapy, laser, surgery

Excisional biopsy if suspicious

Seborrheic keratosis

NOT premalignant (keratinocytes)

Trunk on elderly pts

Can be dark looking or look like warts (can be mistaken for melanoma)

Arsenical keratosis – association w/ squamous cell carcinoma

Glomus Tumor of Skin (from glomus body, not glomus cells)

Painful tumor comprised of blood vessels and nerves

Benign

MC location –terminal aspect of digit near fingernail

Tx: tumor excision

Not a paraganglioma

Paraganglioma (chemodectoma) – rarely malignant (3%); neural crest cell

> Part of **autonomic nervous system**
>> From **glomus cells** (chemo-receptors that regulate blood pressure and blood flow to various area of body)
>
>> **MC location overall** – abdomen
>> **MC ENT location** – carotid body (can also occur in ear)
>> **MC thoracic location** – aortic arch body
>> Can secrete **norepinephrine**
>> highly **vascular**
>> **Tx:** tumor excision

Hutchinson's freckle

> MC in elderly and on face; premalignant, not very aggressive (see melanoma above for tx)

Desmoid tumors

> Low grade fibrosarcomas that tend to recur
>
> **Occur in fascial planes**
>
> **RFs** – trauma, estrogen, previous surgery, pregnancy, women
>
> **Sx's:** painless mass, obstruction
>
> **MC location – <u>anterior abdominal wall</u>**
>> **Intra-abdominal desmoids** are associated with Gardner's syndrome and retroperitoneal fibrosis
>
> High risk of local recurrence; no distant spread
>
> **Tx:**
>> **Surgery w/ WLE** if possible
>> **Chemo-XRT** if vital structure involved or would end up taking entire bowel
>> NSAID's, anti-estrogens, Imatinab (Gleevac)

Bowen's disease (non-perineal region)

> **Squamous cell carcinoma in situ**
>
> Dysplastic cells that are confined to **epidermis**, not invading dermis
>
> **RFs**
>> **HPV infection** (perineal Bowen's)
>> **UV radiation**
>> **Chronic skin injury or dermatosis**
>
> Gradually enlarging, well demarcated **erythematous plaque** w/ irregular border and surface crusting or scaling
>
> 10% turn into invasive CA
>
> 80% women, 80% in lower legs
>
> **Tx:**
>> Excision with 4 mm margins *(best option)* – non-perineal
>>> MOHS surgery also an option
>>> Others - cautery, cryo-ablation, CO2 laser options
>>
>> **For perineal Bowen's** (ie due to HPV infection, surgery is not the first option (see Rectum and Anus chp)
>
> **Perineal region MC location for Bowen's**

Keratoacanthoma

> From **pilo-sebaceous glands**
>
> Have rolled edges and crater filled with **keratin**
>
> Rapid growth over a few weeks to months, followed by spontaneous resolution over 4-6 months
>
> Rarely turns into squamous cell CA and can be confused w/ squamous cell CA
>
> **Tx:**
>> Resection to prevent CA (even though rare)
>> If not going to resect, always biopsy to be sure.

Hyperhydrosis

> Perfuse sweating, especially noticeable in palms.
>
> **Tx:**
>> Try a variety of anti-perspirants over 3 months
>> **Sympathectomy** if affecting lifestyle
>>> Ligate T2-T4 sympathetic chain (hook cautery)
>>> Not above T2 ganglion – will get Horner's Syndrome

Need to get **crossing nerve of Kuntz on the 2nd rib**

MC Cx – compensatory sweating in face, trunks, and legs
(15%)

Hidradenitis

Apocrine sweat gland infection, more common in women

MC sites – axilla and groin

MC organisms – Staph/strep

Tx: abx's and improved hygiene initially; may need resection

Chronic axillary hidradenitis – need excision extending from fascia
to skin (removing apocrine glands)

Benign cysts

Epidermal inclusion cyst (MC) – completely mature epidermis w/
creamy keratin material; **Tx:** resection

Trichilemmal cyst – scalp, keratin filled cyst from hair follicle; no
epidermis; **Tx:** resection

Ganglion cyst – over joints in hand or foot (MC – wrist, 80%)
Filled with collagenous synovial type material

Tx: aspiration cures 50%, recurrence after resection 5%
(remove check valve at joint capsule to ↓recurrence)

Dermoid cyst

Cystic Teratoma (skin, hair, sweat glands, bone, cartilage)

Rare CA (squamous cell CA)

Often midline abdominal and sacral areas, occiput and nose

Found along body fusion planes

Tx: resection

Pilonidal cyst – congenital coccygeal sinus w/ ingrown hair
Can get infected; males, **Tx:** excision

Xanthoma – yellow cholesterol-rich; tendons and other areas, contain
histiocytes, can be associated w/ familial hypercholesterolemia;
benign. Tx: excision

Warts (verruca vulgaris) – HPV origin, contagious, self- inoculable, may
cause pain; often on hands and feet

Tx: salicylic acid *(best therapy),* liquid nitrogen, podophyllum resin
paint, surgery, laser

HPV 1, 2, and 3 – common warts

HPV 6 and 11 – 90% of genital warts

HPV 16 and 18 – 70% cervical CA

Gardasil – vaccine to prevent infection for HPV 6, 11, 16, and 18

Keloids

Autosomal dominant; dark skinned people higher risk

Can be dark looking

Collagen (Type I and III) **goes** <u>beyond</u> **original scar**
(main differentiation w/ hypertrophic scar)

From **failure of collagen breakdown**

Tx: Intra-lesional steroid injection after keloid excision *(best Tx)*
others – silicone gel sheet or injection (preferably before
development of keloids), pressure garments

Hypertrophic scar tissue

Higher risk in dark skinned people

Often on **flexor surfaces** of upper torso

Collagen stays within confines of scar

Often w/ burns or wounds taking a long time to heal

Tx: **steroids, silicone,** and/or **pressure garments**

Lip lacerations – most important issue is to line up vermillion border

Imiquimod (cream)

Activates immune cells by ligating the membrane bound toll-like
receptor (TLR-7) which is involved in pathogen recognition

Immune cells activated include Langerhan's cells, natural killer cells,
macrophages, and B lymphocytes

Used for some basal cell CA, Bowen's, superficial squamous CA,
actinic keratoses, genital warts

Sacral Decubitus Ulcer (pressure sores)
Look to see how deep the wound is on exam

Ulcer Stage	Exam	Tx
I	Erythema, pain, no skin loss	Keep pressure off
II	Partial skin loss w/ yellow debris	Local treatment below, keep pressure off
III	Full-thickness skin loss, has subcutaneous tissue exposure	Sharp debridement necessary, likely need myocutaneous flap
IV	Bony cortex	Need myocutaneous flaps

Tx:

Keep pressure off the area → place pt on **kin-air bed**
Assess and optimize nutrition w/ protein shakes or feeding tube
Consider diverting stool w/ **colostomy** (stage III and IV)
Debride wound in OR (consider additional short course of enzyme debridement w/ Accuzyme or Panifil)
Bx and send cultures
Abx's

No flap if the pt has an **active infection**
When wound looking good, place **gluteal myocutaneous flap**
Scrape off bony cortex if lesion extends to bone when placing myocutaneous flap (send for cultures)
Place gluteal myocutaneous flap
Keep on abx's for 6 weeks if the **bony cortex** was involved
Get **bone scan** at 6 weeks to see if there is still **active infection** in bone, keep on abx's if so

Retroperitoneal fibrosis
RFs – autoimmune DZ, CA, drugs (eg methysergide, beta-blockers, hydralazine), previous XRT, infections (TB)
Sx's: usually related to **trapped ureters** and **obstruction** (hydronephrosis) **lymphatic obstruction**.
Dx: intravenous pyelogram *(best test)* – see trapped ureters (compression)
Tx:
Steroids + immunosuppression (eg Tamoxifen, Imuran, Infliximab)
Surgery if renal function becomes compromised *(**free up ureters and wrap in omentum)** – R/O CA
Percutaneous nephrostomy tube if pyelonephritis develops, abx's, then free up ureters at later procedure

Mesenteric tumors
Of primary tumors, most are **cystic**
Malignant tumors – closer to **root** of mesentery
Benign tumors – peripheral
MC Malignant – liposarcoma; others – leiomyosarcomas, GIST
MC benign – lipomas; others – lymphangiomas, benign GIST tumors
Dx: abd CT
Tx: resection

Omental tumors
MC omental solid tumor - metastatic disease
Omentectomy for mets has role for some cancers (eg ovarian CA)
Primary solid omental tumors rare; 30% malignant
Same types as mesenteric tumors (MC liposarcoma)
No biopsy → can bleed
Tx: resection

Retroperitoneal tumors
15% in children, others in 5–6th decade
Malignant > benign
Sx's: vague abd and back pain
MC malignant retroperitoneal tumor – lymphoma
MC malignant retroperitoneal solid tumor – liposarcoma

Peritoneal membrane
Saline absorbed at 35 cc/hr
Blood absorbed through fenestrated lymphatic channels
Most drugs <u>not</u> removed w/ peritoneal dialysis
NH_3, Ca, Fe, and **lead** are removed w/ peritoneal dialysis
Movement into peritoneal cavity w/ hypertonic intraperitoneal saline load → 300–
500 cc/hr; can cause **hypotension**

Lymphangiomas
Cystic, fluid filled, benign proliferation of lymphatic vessels
Types
Cutaneous lesions (microcystic) – 2 components
1) clear to purple colored, small clustered **vesicles**
2) underlying **cystic mass**
No real tx necessary unless for cosmetic reasons
Tx: definitive Tx is **excision** (including underlying mass); but often
just **cauterized**
Cystic hygroma (macrocystic)
Classically found in **lateral posterior neck triangle**
MC on left; swollen bulges under skin; form sinuses; get infected
Tx: resection
Lymphangioma Cavernosum
Deep under skin; bulging mass, filled w/ lymph
Usually affects tongue and lips
Can form sinuses and get infected
Tx: resection

STATISTICS

Basic Rules

Type I error

Rejects null hypothesis incorrectly (rejecting the null hypothesis when it is true)

Assumed there was a difference when no difference actually exists

Type II error

Accepts null hypothesis incorrectly

Falsely assumed there was no difference when an actual difference exists

MC due to a **small sample size** (ie a larger sample size would have picked up the difference)

Null hypothesis

The hypothesis that no difference exists between groups

A $p < 0.05$ rejects the null hypothesis

$p < 0.05$ =

>95% likelihood that the difference between populations is true

<5% likelihood that the difference is not true and occurred by chance alone

Variance – the spread of data around a mean value

Parameter – a population

Numeric terms – eg 2, 7, 7, 8, 9, 12, 14

Mode – the most frequently occurring value = 7

Mean – the average = 9

This is the best measure of **central tendency** when **values are distributed normally** (ie you do not have outliers)

There are no outliers in the above set of numbers, so the mean value is a good measure of central tendency

Median – the middle value of a set of data (eg 50th percentile) = 8

This is the best measure of **central tendency** when **values are not distributed equally** (ie you have outliers)

Take example above, but add 85 and 86 (eg 2, 7, 7, 8, 9, 12, 14, 85, 86)

The **mean** would now be = 26

This is not a good representation of **central tendency** due to the outliers 85 and 86

The **median** would now be = 9

This is a better representation of central tendency

Any set of numbers (eg INR values, weight loss, WBC counts, Hct's, temp's) can be used for the above

95% confidence interval

Instead of estimating the parameter by a single value (eg mean), this also includes an interval likely to include the parameter

Confidence intervals are used to indicate reliability of an estimate

Example:

Following **lap banding**, mean weight loss for your pts is 125 lb

95% of your pts have a weight loss between 100 and 150 lb

The 95% confidence interval for amount of weight loss in your population is (100,150)

or there is a 95% probability that following gastric bypass, your pt will lose somewhere between 100 and 150 lb

Written as: mean weight loss 125 lb [100,150]

The more narrow the confidence interval, the more accurate the estimate

Example – for **gastric bypass**, mean weight loss was 130 lb [120,140]; 130 would be a more accurate estimate of weight loss in this population than 125 in the above lap banding population)

Prevalence

Number of people w/ disease in a population

(eg number of patients in US w/ lung CA)

Longstanding diseases will ↑ prevalence

Incidence

Number of new cases diagnosed over a certain time frame (MC annually)

(eg number of pt in US newly diagnosed with lung CA in 2009)

Relative risk

= incidence in exposed population / incidence in unexposed population

Odds ratio – odds of an event occurring in one group (group 1) compared to odds of that event occurring in a separate group (group 2). The higher the odds ratio, the more likely the condition or event is going to occur in the first group.

Power of test (probability of making correct conclusion)

= 1 – probability of type II error

Likelihood that the conclusion of test is true

Larger sample size increases power (by ↓ing the likelihood of a type II error)

Clinical Trials and studies

Randomized controlled trial (prospective study)

Prospective study w/ random assignment to treatment and non-treatment groups

Avoids treatment bias

Double-blind controlled trial (prospective study)

A prospective study in which both pt and doctor are blind to treatment

Avoids observational bias

Thought to be the best form of trials

Cohort study (prospective study)

Cohort – a group of people who share a common characteristic

Cohort study – a prospective study comparing the cohort to either the general population of another group that lacks the characteristic

Example: prospectively following teenagers who smoke and comparing them to other teenagers who do not smoke in terms of developing lung CA

Case–control study (retrospective study)

Retrospective study in which those w/ the disease are compared to a similar population w/o the disease

The frequency of the suspected risk factor is then compared between the two groups

Meta-analysis – combining the data from **different studies**

Quantitative variables (numbers)

Student's t test

Two independent groups and variable is **quantitative**

Compares means (eg mean weight between group A and B)

Eg – a new preservation solution is used a the time of lung transplant harvest and pO2 values are measured after transplantation. The average pO2 in the experimental group is 350 mmHg. The average pO2 in the control group is 250 mmHg. A student's T test is used here to figure out if the 2 groups are significantly different

Paired t tests

Variable is **quantitative** w/ **before and after studies**

(eg mean weight before and after treatment, comparing drug vs. placebo)

ANOVA (analysis of variance)

Compares **quantitative** variables (eg means) for more than 2 groups

(eg mean weight between groups A, B, C, and D)

Qualitative variables

Nonparametric statistics
Compare categorical (qualitative) variables (eg race, sex, diseases, meds)
Non-numerical categories

Chi-squared test
Compares two groups based on **categorical** (eg qualitative) **variables** (eg number of obese pts w/ and w/o development of hyperlipidemia vs. number of non-obese pts w/ and w/o development hyperlipidemia)

Kaplan-Meier estimator –estimates survival

	Positive Test	**Negative Test**
Pts w/ disease	True-positive (TP)	False-negative (FN)
Pts w/o disease	False-positive (FP)	True-negative (TN)

Sensitivity
Ability to detect disease = true-positives/(true-positives + false-negatives)
Indicates number of people who have the disease who test positive
With high sensitivity, a **negative test** result means pt is very unlikely to have disease

Specificity
Ability to state no DZ present = true-negatives/(true-negatives + false-positives)
Indicates number of people who do not have the disease who test negative
With high specificity, a **positive test** result means patient is very likely to have disease

Positive predictive value
= true-positives/(true-positives + false-positives)
Proportion of pts w/ a positive result who actually have the disease.
This value does depend on prevalence of disease within a population.
Tests with a very high positive predictive value have a low false positive rate and a positive result suggests the patient is very likely to have the disease

Negative predictive value
= true-negatives/(true-negatives + false-negatives)
Determines the likelihood of not having the disease given a negative result.
A test with a high negative predictive value will have a low false negative rate

Accuracy
= true-positives + true-negatives / true-positives + true-negatives + false-positives + false-negatives

Predictive value – dependent on disease prevalence
Sensitivity and specificity – independent of prevalence

Prevention

Primary Prevention – avoiding disease altogether (ie vaccinations for HPV)

Secondary Prevention – focuses on early detection of the disease to prevent progression (ie pap smears, stress test, screening colonoscopy, screening mammograms, blood pressure checks)

Tertiary Prevention – decreasing the morbidity related to an established disease (i.e. controlling blood pressure in patients w/ HTN, screening and treatment of diabetics w/ eye, foot, and renal problems; HMG-CoA reductase inhibitors in pts w/hyperlipidemia)

Appendix

↑	increase, increased *or* high	cGMP	cyclic guanosine 3,5'-mono-phosphate
↓	decrease, decreased *or* low		
2,3-DPG	2,3-diphosphoglycerate	chemo	chemotherapy
5-FU	5-fluorouracil	CHF	chronic heart failure
AAA	abdominal aortic aneurysm	CI	cardiac index
Ab	antibody	CMV	cytomegalovirus
Abd	abdominal	CN	cranial nerve
Abx	antibiotic(s)	CNS	central nervous system
ACE	angiotensin converting enzyme	CO	cardiac output
ACh	acetylcholine	COPD	chronic obstructive pulmonary disease
ACT	activated clotting time	CPAP	continuous positive airway pressure
ACTH	adrenocorticotropic hormone	CPP	cerebral perfusion pressure
AD	autosomal dominant	CPR	cardiopulmonary resuscitation
ADH	antidiuretic hormone	Cr	creatinine
AFP	alpha-fetoprotein	CRBSI	catheter related blood stream infection
Ag	antigen		
AIDS	acquired immunodeficiency syndrome	CRH	corticotropin (ACTH)-releasing hormone
AKA	above knee amputation	Cryo	cryoprecipitate
ALND	axillary lymph node dissection	CSA	cyclosporin A
ALT	alanine aminotransferase	CSF	cerebrospinal fluid
angio	angiography	CT	computed tomography
ANOVA	analysis of variance	CVA	cerebrovascular accident (stroke)
APACHE	acute physiology and chronic health evaluation	CVVH	continuous veno-venous hemodialysis
APC	antigen presenting cell	CvO_2	venous oxygen content
APR	abdominoperineal resection	CVP	central venous pressure
APUD	amine precursor uptake and decarboxylation	Cx	complication
		CXR	chest x-ray
ARB	angiotensin II receptor blocker	D/C	discontinue
ARDS	acute/adult respiratory distress syndrome	DAG	diacylglycerol
		DCIS	ductal carcinoma in situ
ASA	acetylsalicylic acid	DDAVP	desmopressin acetate, 1-desamino-8-d-arginine-vasopressin
ASD	atrial septal defect		
AST	aspartate aminotransferase	DES	diethylstilbestrol
ATGAM	antithymocyte gamma globulin	DIC	disseminated intravascular coagulation
AT-III	antithrombin III	DIT	diiodotyrosine
ATN	acute tubular necrosis	DKA	diabetic ketoacidosis
ATP	adenosine triphosphate	DLCO	lung diffusing capacity for carbon monoxide
ATPase	adenosine triphosphatase		
A-V	arteriovenous	DM	diabetes mellitus
AV	atrioventricular	DPL	diagnostic peritoneal lavage
AVM	arteriovenous malformation	DTRs	deep tendon reflexes
AVN	avascular necrosis	DVT	deep venous thrombosis
AXR	abdominal x-ray	Dx	diagnosis
BCG	bacille Calmette-Guérin	DZ	disease
BKA	below-knee amputation	EBV	Epstein-Barr virus
BM	bowel movement	ECA	external carotid artery
CNBx	core needle biopsy	ECHO	echocardiogram
BPH	benign prostatic hyperplasia	ECMO	extracorporeal membrane oxygenation
BSA	body surface area		
BT shunt	Blalock-Taussig shunt	EDRF	endothelium-derived relaxing factor
BUN	blood urea nitrogen	EDV	end diastolic volume
Bx	biopsy	EEG	electroencephalogram
Ca	calcium	EF	ejection fraction
CA	cancer, carcinoma	EGD	esophagogastroduodenoscopy
CABG	coronary artery bypass graft	EGJ	esophago-gastric junction
cAMP	cyclic adenosine monophosphate	EGF	epidermal growth factor
		EKG	electrocardiogram
CaO_2	arterial oxygen content	ELAM	endothelial leukocyte adhesion molecule
CBD	common bile duct		
CCK	cholecystokinin	Epi	epinephrine
cCMP	3',5'-cyclic monophosphate (cytidine)	ER	emergency room *or* endoplasmic reticulum
CD	cluster of differentiation (eg CD4, CD8)	ERCP	endoscopic retrograde cholangiopancreatography
CEA	carcinoembryonic antigen	ERV	expiratory reserve volume
CEA	carotid endarterectomy	ESR	erythrocyte sedimentation rate

ESWL	extracorporeal shock wave lithotripsy	HSV	herpes simplex virus
ET	endotracheal	HTLV-1	human T-cell leukemia virus 1
ETCO$_2$	end tidal CO$_2$	HTN	hypertension
ETOH	ethanol, alcohol	HUS	hemolytic uremic syndrome
ETT	endotracheal tube	HVA	homovanillic acid
EUS	endoscopic ultrasound	IABP	intra-aortic balloon pump
F/U	follow-up	IBW	ideal body weight
FAP	familial adenomatous polyposis	ICA	internal corotid artery
		ICAM	intracellular adhesion molecule
FAST	focused abdominal sonography for trauma	ICP	intracranial pressure
		ICU	intensive care unit
Fc	antibody fragment, crystallizable	Ig	immunoglobulin
		IJ	internal jugular vein
FEV$_1$	forced expiratory volume in 1 second	IL	interleukin
		IMA	inferior mesenteric artery or internal mammary artery
FFP	fresh frozen plasma		
FGF	fibroblastic growth factor	IMF	intermaxillary fixation
FiO$_2$	fraction of inspired oxygen	IMV	inferior mesenteric vein
FNA	fine needle aspiration	INF	interferon
FRC	functional residual capacity	INH	isoniazid
FS	frozen section	INR	International Normalized Ratio
FSH	follicle stimulating hormone	ITP	Immune (idiopathic) thrombocytopenic purpura
FTSG	full-thickness skin graft		
FTT	failure to thrive	IV	intravenous
Fx	fracture	IVC	inferior vena cava
G6PD	glucose-6-phosphate dehydrogenase	IVF	intravenous fluid
		IVP	intravenous pyelogram
GCS	Glasgow Coma Scale	L	liter
GCSF	granulocyte colony– stimulating factor	LA	left atrium
		LAD	left anterior descending (coronary artery)
GDA	gastroduodenal artery		
GERD	gastroesophageal reflux disease	LAK	lymphokine-activated killer
		LATS	long acting thyroid stimulator
GFR	glomerular filtration rate	LAR	low anterior resection
GH	growth hormone	LCIS	lobular carcinoma in situ
GHRH	growth hormone-releasing hormone	LD$_{50}$	dose that will kill 50% of test subjects
		LDH	lactate dehydrogenase
GI	gastrointestinal	LES	lower esophageal sphincter
GIP	gastric inhibitory peptide	LFT	liver function test
GIST	gastrointestinal stromal tumors	LGIB	lower gastrointestinal bleed
		LH	luteotropic hormone
GNR	gram-negative rods	LHRH	luteinizing hormone–releasing hormone
GnRH	gonadotropin-releasing hormone		
		LLQ	left lower quadrant
GPC	gram-positive cocci	LMWH	low molecular weight heparin
GPR	gram-positive rod	LN	lymph nodes
GRP	gastrin-releasing peptide	LR	lactated ringers
GSH	glutathione	LS ratio	lecithin:sphingomyelin ratio
GU	genitourinary	LV	left ventricle or left ventricular
H and P	history and physical	LVEDV	left ventricular end-diastolic volume
HA	headache		
HBIG	hepatitis B immunoglobulin	LVEF	left ventricular ejection fraction
HBV	hepatitis B virus	LVESV	left ventricular end-systolic volume
HCG	human chorionic gonadotropin	LVOT	left ventricular outflow tract
HCl	hydrochloric acid	MAC	minimum alveolar concentration
Hct	hematocrit	MALT	mucosal-associated lympho- proliferative tissue
HCV	hepatitis C virus		
Hgb	hemoglobin	MAO	monoamine oxidase
HIDA	hepatic iminodiacetic acid	MAOI	monoamine oxidase inhibitor
HIT	heparin-induced thrombocytopenia	MAP	mean arterial pressure
		MDR	multi-drug resistant
HIV	human immunodeficiency virus	MEN	multiple endocrine neoplasia
		MF	mucus fistula
HLA	human leukocyte antigen	MHC	major histocompatibility complex
HMG-CoA	β-hydroxy-β-methylglutaryl- CoA	MI	myocardial infarction
		MIBG	radioactive iodine meta- idobenzoguanidine
HMW	high molecular weight		
HP	Hartman's pouch	MIT	monoiodotyrosine
HPF	high-power field	MMC	migrating motor complexes
HPV	human papillomavirus	MRA	magnetic resonance angiogram
HR	heart rate	MRCP	magnetic resonance cholangiopancreatography

MRM	modified radical mastectomy	PTA	percutaneous transluminal angioplasty
MRND	modified radical neck dissection	PTC	percutaneous transhepatic cholangiography
MRSA	methicillin-resistant *S. aureus*	PTCA	percutaneous transluminal coronary angioplasty
MS	mental status		
MSH	melanocyte-stimulating hormone	PTFE	polytetrafluoroethylene
		PTH	parathyroid hormone
MTP	metatarsophalangeal	PTHrP	parathyroid hormone-related peptide
MTX	methotrexate	PTT	partial thromboplastin time
N/V	nausea and vomiting	PTU	propylthiouracil
NADH	nicotinamide adenine dinucleotide	PTX	pneumothorax
		PUD	peptic ulcer disease
NADPH	nicotinamide adenine dinucleotide phosphate	PVC	premature ventricular contraction
		PVR	pulmonary vascular resistance
NE	norepinephrine		
NEC	necrotizing enterocolitis	Px	prevention preventative therapy
NGT	nasogastric tube		
NHL	non-Hodgkin's lymphoma	Qp/Qs	pulmonary-to-systemic flow ratio
NIF	negative inspiratory force	R/O	rule out
NO	nitric oxide	RA	right atrium
NPO	nil per os (nothing by mouth)	RBC	red blood cell
NS	normal saline (solution)	RLL	right lower lobe
NSAID	nonsteroidal anti-inflammatory drug	RLN	recurrent laryngeal nerve
		ROM	range of motion
NSE	neuron-specific enolase	RPR	rapid plasma reagin
NTG	nitroglycerine	RQ	respiratory quotient
OCP	oral contraceptive pills	RR	respiratory rate or relative risk
OKT3	murine monoclonal anti-CD3 antibody therapy	RUG	retrograde urethrogram
		RUL	right upper lobe
Op-DDD	2,4'-dichlorodiphenyl-dichloroethane (mitotane)	RUQ	right upper quadrant
		RV	residual volume
OPSI	overwhelming post-splenectomy sepsis syndrome	RV	right ventricle
		S/E	side effect
		SBFT	small bowel follow-through
OR	operating room	SBO	small bowel obstruction
ORIF	open reduction and internal fixation	SBP	spontaneous bacterial peritonitis
		SBP	systolic blood pressure
O/W	otherwise	SC	subcutaneous
PA	pulmonary artery	SCCA	squamous cell carcinoma
PABA	*p*-aminobenzoic acid	SCD	sequential compression device
PADP	pulmonary artery diastolic pressure	SCM	sternocleidomastoid
		SFA	superficial femoral artery
PAF	platelet activating factor	SIRS	systemic inflammatory response syndrome
PAS	periodic acid–Schiff stain		
PCN	penicillin	SLE	systemic lupus erythematosus
PCR	polymerase chain	SMA	superior mesenteric artery
PDA	patent ductus arteriosus	SMV	superior mesenteric vein
PDGF	platelet-derived growth factor	SOB	shortness of breath
PE	pulmonary embolism	SSI	surgical site infection
PECAM	platelet/endothelial cell adhesion molecule	SSRI	selective serotonin reuptake inhibitor
		STSG	split-thickness skin graft
PEEP	positive end-expiratory pressure	SVC	superior vena cava
		SvO$_2$	mixed venous oxygen saturation
PEG	percutaneous endoscopic gastrostomy	SVR	systemic vascular resistance
		SVT	supraventricular tachycardia
Plts	platelets	Sx's	signs and/or symptoms
PMHx	past medical history	SZ	seizure
PMN	polymorphonuclear leukocytes		
		T bili	total bilirubin
PNMT	phenylethanolamine-N-methyl-transferase	TAG	triacylglyceride
		TAH	total abdominal hysterectomy
POD	postoperative day	TB	tuberculosis
PNA	pneumonia	TBG	thyroid-binding globulin
PPI	proton pump inhibitor	TCA	tricyclic anti-depressant
PPN	peripheral line parenteral nutrition	TCOM	transcutaneous oxygen measurement
PRBC	packed red blood cells	TCR	T-cell receptor
PSA	prostate-specific antigen	TE	tracheoesophageal
PSSS	postsplenectomy sepsis syndrome (see OPSI)	TEN	toxic epidermal necrolysis
		TFT	thyroid function test
PT	prothrombin time	TGF-beta	transforming growth factor-beta
Pt	patient	TIA	transient ischemic attack

TIPS	transjugular intrahepatic portosystemic shunt		UES	upper esophageal sphincter
			UGI	upper gastrointestinal
TLC	total lung capacity		UGIB	upper gastrointestinal bleed
TMJ	temporomandibular joint		URI	upper respiratory tract infection
TNF	tumor necrosis factor		UTI	urinary tract infection
TOS	thoracic outlet syndrome		UV	ultraviolet
tPA	tissue plasminogen activator		V/Q	ventilation/perfusion
TPN	total parenteral nutrition		VC	vital capacity
TRALI	transfusion-related acute lung injury		VCAM	vascular cell adhesion molecule
			V-fib	ventricular fibrillation
TRAM	transverse rectus abdominis myocutaneous flap		VIP	vasoactive intestinal peptide
			VIPoma	vasoactive intestinal peptide–producing tumor
TRH	thyrotropin-releasing hormone			
TRUS	trans-rectal ultrasound		VLDL	very-low-density lipids
TSH	thyroid-stimulating hormone		VMA	vanillylmandelic acid
TSI	thyroid-stimulating immunoglobulin		VO_2	oxygen consumption
			VP-16	etoposide
TTP	thrombotic thrombocytopenic purpura		VRE	vancomycin-resistant *Enterococcus*
			VSD	ventricular septal defect
TURP	transurethral resection of prostate; transurethral prostatectomy		vWD	von Willebrand's disease
			vWF	von Willebrand factor
			W/U	work-up
TV	tidal volume		WBC	white blood cell
Tx	treatment		WDHA	watery diarrhea, hypokalemia, achlorhydria
TXA_2	thromboxane A_2			
TXP	transplant		WLE	wide local excision
U/S	ultrasound		XRT	radiation therapy
UC	ulcerative colitis		Z-E/ZES	Zollinger-Ellison syndrome
UDCA	ursodeoxycholic acid			

INDEX

Choanal atresia, 423
Cholangiocarcinoma, 307
Cholangiohepatitis, Oriental, 302
Cholangiosarcoma, 294
Cholangitis, 302
Cholecystitis, 298
Cholecystokinin (CCK), 242
Choledochal cyst, 421
Cholesteatoma, 154
Cholesterol, synthesis, 281
Cholesterolosis, 301
Cholestyramine, 63
Chromium deficiency, 88t
Chronic granulomatous disease, 22
Chronic renal failure, 65
Chylomicrons, 82
Chylothorax, 212
Circle of Willis, 391
Cirrhosis, 283
Cis-atracurium, 70
Claudication, 225
Clavicle fracture, 397
Cleft lip, 157
Cleft palate, 157
Clindamycin, 59
Clopidogrel 14
Clostridium difficile colitis, 49
Clostridium perfringens infection, 48
Clubfoot, 40
Coagulation factors, cascade 7
Coarctation of aorta, 214
Cobalamin deficiency, 88t
Coccidioidomycosis, 50
Cohort study, 439
Coin lesion, lung, 206
Collagen, 25
Collateral circulation, lower extremity, 225
Collateral ligaments, injury, 401
Colles fracture, 398
Colon
    anatomy + physiology, 343
    obstruction, 349
    polyps, 359
    venous drainage, 343
Colon cancer, 352-357
Colonic inertia, 344
Colonoscopy, screening 357
Colon trauma, 111
Colorectal cancer, 352-357
Common bile duct
    injury, 113, 302
    strictures, 312
Compartment syndrome, 117, 402
    abdominal, 140
Complement system, 22
Compliance, lung 136
Condylomata acuminata, 370
Congenital adrenal hyperplasia, 159
Congenital anomalies of lung, 409
Congenital cystic adenoid
    malformation, 409

Congenital heart disease
    atrial septal defect, 213
    coarctation of aorta, 214
    hypoplastic left heart, 214
    patent ductus arteriosus, 214
    tetralogy of Fallot, 214
    transposition of great vessels, 214
    truncus arteriosus, 214
    vascular rings, 214
    ventricular septal defect, 213
Congenital incontinence, 382
Congenital lobar hyperinflation, 409
Congenital vascular malformation, 420
Conn's syndrome, 163
Contrast dyes, renal toxicity, 134
Controlled trial, 439
Cooper's ligaments, 182
COPD (chronic obstructive pulmonary
    disease), 65, 137
CO_2 pneumoperitoneum, 142
Copper deficiency, 88t
Cori cycle, 85, 280
Coronary artery bypass grafting, 215
Coronary artery disease, 215
Coumadin, 15
Cranial nerves, 394t
    injury in carotid endarterectomy, 223
Craniopharyngioma, 166
Critical illness polyneuropathy, 70, 141
Crohn's disease, 329-333, 347t
Cronkite-Canada syndrome, 359
Cruciate ligaments, injury, 401
Cryoprecipitate, 16
Cryptococcus, 50
Cryptorchidism, 411
Crypts of Lieberkühn, 327
Cullen's sign, 310
Curling's ulcer, burn injury, 147
Cushing's disease, 161
Cushing's striae, 424
Cushing's syndrome, 161
Cysteine stones, 377
Cystic artery, 296
Cystic duplication, 419
Cystic hygroma, 155, 422, 437
Cystic medial necrosis syndromes, 236
Cystosarcoma phyllodes, 195
Cytokines, 20
Cytomegalovirus, 36, 54

Dacron graft, 142
D cells, 242
Dead space ventilation, 136
DeBakey classification, aortic dissection, 219
Deep venous thrombosis, 10
Delta bilirubin, 301
Demerol, 69
Denonvillier's fascia, 344
Dentate line, 367
DeQuervain's thyroiditis, 175
Dermis, 424

THE COMPREHENSIVE ABSITE REV